CLINICAL MANAGEMENT OF PITUITARY DISORDERS

Seminars in Neurological Surgery

SEMINARS IN NEUROLOGICAL SURGERY SERIES

Pediatric Neurological Surgery
Edited by Mark S. O'Brien

Spinal Deformities and Neurological Dysfunction
Edited by Shelley N. Chou and Edward L. Seljeskog

Surgery of the Posterior Fossa
Edited by William Buchheit and Raymond Truex, Jr.

Neural Trauma
Edited by A. John Popp, Robert S. Bourke, Louis R. Nelson, and Harold K. Kimelberg

Clinical Management of Pituitary Disorders
Edited by George T. Tindall and William F. Collins

SEMINARS IN NEUROLOGICAL SURGERY

Clinical Management of Pituitary Disorders

Sponsored by the Subcommittee on Continuing Education II (Expanded Program), American Association of Neurological Surgeons, and Congress of Neurological Surgeons

Edited by

George T. Tindall, M.D.
Professor of Surgery
Chief of Neurosurgery
Emory University School of Medicine
Atlanta, Georgia

William F. Collins, M.D.
Harvey and Kate Cushing Professor of Surgery
Professor and Chief
Section of Neurosurgery
Yale University School of Medicine
New Haven, Connecticut

Raven Press ■ New York

Raven Press, 1140 Avenue of the Americas, New York, New York 10036

Made in the United States of America

Library of Congress in Publication Data
Main entry under title:

Clinical management of pituitary disorders.

(Seminars in neurological surgery)
Includes bibliographies and index
1. Pituitary body – Surgery 2. Pituitary body – Tumors. 3. Pituitary body – Diseases. I. Tindall, George T. II. Collins, William Francis, 1924–
III. Committee on Continuing Education II (Expanded Program)
IV. Series: Seminars in neurological surgery series.
RD599.5.P58C54 616.4′ 7 77-90599
ISBN 0–89004–362–0

Preface

. . . There is every reason to believe that cases of clinically recognizable pituitary disease are at least as common as our cases of clinically recognizable thyroid disease.

Harvey Cushing, 1912
The Pituitary Body and Its Disorders

Perhaps Dr. Cushing used the comparison of pituitary and thyroid disease to stress to his readers their need to learn more about the pituitary and its dysfunction, or perhaps he just used the comparison as an improbably finite frequency to generate interest in the pituitary body among physicians. No matter his intent, recent advances in endocrinology, neuroradiology, and neurosurgery have made his statement prophetic, for the diagnosis of pituitary dysfunction and particularly the diagnosis of pituitary adenoma is in many medical centers as frequent as the diagnosis of adenoma in any endocrine gland. These advances include the measurement of circulating pituitary hormones, the identification of many of the hypothalamic factors controlling pituitary function, the accurate definition of sella and parasella structures with polytomography and computerized axial tomography, and the refinement and reintroduction of the transsphenoidal surgical approach to the sella by Guiot in Paris and Hardy in Montreal. These advances, along with generating widespread interest in the management of pituitary disorders, especially pituitary tumors, have allowed earlier and more precise diagnosis of pituitary tumors and more effective and safer therapy. The reduction in operative mortality and morbidity with transsphenoidal microsurgery and the ability to selectively excise pituitary tumors while sparing the residual normal pituitary gland represents a major contribution in pituitary surgery. These advances have also uncovered many unanswered questions concerning pituitary tumors that before their advent were irrelevant to the clinical problem of the pituitary gland being treated by physicians.

The primary purpose of this volume is to present the current state of the art on the clinical aspects of the pituitary gland as viewed through a variety of disciplines including, among others, neurosurgery, endocrinology, radiation therapy, and neuropathology. Problems in diagnosis, therapy, and evaluation as they are reflected in the current state of the art are also examined. We hope the reader feels as we do that this goal has been accomplished and that this volume will be a valuable reference source for neurosurgeons, endocrinologists, and other physicians with an interest in the pituitary gland.

George T. Tindall, M.D.
(Atlanta, Georgia)

William F. Collins, M.D.
(New Haven, Connecticut)

Acknowledgments

The editors would like to express their appreciation to the Committee on Continuing Education of the Joint Education Committee of the American Association of Neurological Surgeons and the Congress of Neurological Surgeons for their support and guidance.

Editing the proceedings has not only been a labor of love but an educational experience and the editors are thankful for the cooperation from each contributor, both to the book and to the symposium on which this book is based. Dr. Soman of Yale University School of Medicine did not participate in the symposium but prepared a manuscript on the medical management of acromegaly. His cooperation is gratefully acknowledged.

The editors also wish to acknowledge the advice and assistance of Larry Meyer and the rest of the staff at Raven Press, and Grace Groover, Daphne Eitel, and David Adams for valuable help in typing, bibliographic searches, and proofing—those tedious, time-consuming aspects so necessary in publication.

Contents

Contributors

H. Dwight Cavanagh, *Department of Ophthalmology, Emory University School of Medicine, Atlanta, Georgia 30322*

James H. Christy, *Department of Medicine (Endocrinology), Emory University School of Medicine, Atlanta, Georgia 30322*

William F. Collins, *Department of Surgery, Section of Neurosurgery, Yale University School of Medicine, New Haven, Connecticut 06510*

Paul A. Fitzgerald, *Metabolic Research Unit and Department of Medicine, University of California at San Francisco, San Francisco, California 94143*

Alan S. Fleischer, *Department of Surgery, Division of Neurosurgery, Emory University School of Medicine, Atlanta, Georgia 30322*

David G. Hardy, *Department of Neurosurgery, University of Florida Health Center, Gainesville, Florida 32610*

Jules Hardy, *Department of Surgery, Service of Neurosurgery, Notre-Dame Hospital and University of Montreal, Montreal, Canada H2L 4K8*

James C. Hoffman, Jr., *Department of Radiology, Section of Neurovascular Radiology, Emory University School of Medicine, Atlanta, Georgia 30322*

O. Wayne Houser, *Department of Diagnostic Radiology (Neuroradiology), Mayo Clinic, Mayo Medical School, Rochester, Minnesota 55901*

Eugene B. Kern, *Department of Otorhinolaryngology, Mayo Clinic, Mayo Medical School, Rochester, Minnesota 55901*

Raymond N. Kjellberg, *Department of Surgery, Harvard Medical School, Boston, Massachusetts 02114*

Bernard Kliman, *Department of Medicine, Harvard Medical School, Boston, Massachusetts 02114*

Edward R. Laws, Jr., *Department of Neurologic Surgery, Mayo Clinic, Mayo Medical School, Rochester, Minnesota 55901*

C. Scott McLanahan, *Department of Surgery, Division of Neurosurgery, Emory University School of Medicine, Atlanta, Georgia 30322*

Jimmy D. Neill, *Department of Physiology, Emory University School of Medicine, Atlanta, Georgia 30322*

Lawrence H. Pitts, *Department of Neurological Surgery, University of California at San Francisco, San Francisco, California 94143*

Albert L. Rhoton, Jr., *Department of Neurosurgery, University of Florida Health Center, Gainesville, Florida 32610*

Francoisẽ Robert, *Department of Pathology, Notre-Dame Hospital and University of Montreal, Montreal, Canada H2L 4K8*

Glenn E. Sheline, *Department of Radiation Oncology, University of California, San Francisco, California 94143*

Vijay R. Soman, *Department of Medicine, Yale University School of Medicine, New Haven, Connecticut 06510*

Maurice Somma, *Department of Medicine, Service of Endocrinology, Notre-Dame Hospital and University of Montreal, Montreal, Canada H2L 4K8*

George Stefanis, *Department of Surgery, Division of Neurosurgery, Emory University School of Medicine, Atlanta, Georgia 30322*

Yung-Fong Sung, *Department of Anesthesiology, Division of Neurosurgical Anesthesia, Emory University Hospital, Atlanta, Georgia 30322*

Yoshio Takei, *Department of Pathology and Laboratory Medicine, Emory University School of Medicine, Atlanta, Georgia 30322*

George T. Tindall, *Department of Surgery, Division of Neurosurgery, Emory University School of Medicine, Atlanta, Georgia 30322*

Suzie C. Tindall, *Department of Surgery, Division of Neurosurgery, Emory University School of Medicine, Atlanta, Georgia 30322*

J. Blake Tyrrell, *Metabolic Research Unit and Department of Medicine, University of California at San Francisco, San Francisco, California 94143*

Charles B. Wilson, *Department of Neurological Surgery, University of California, San Francisco at San Francisco, California 94143*

Earl A. Zimmerman, *Department of Neurology, College of Physicians and Surgeons, Columbia University, New York, New York 10032*

Clinical Management of Pituitary Disorders,
edited by G. T. Tindall and W. F. Collins.
Raven Press, New York © 1979.

1

Microsurgical Anatomy of the Sphenoid Bone, Cavernous Sinus, and Sellar Region

Albert L. Rhoton Jr. and David G. Hardy

Department of Neurological Surgery, University of Florida Health Center, Gainesville, Florida 32610

Microsurgery has played a significant role in improving the operative approaches to the sellar region. The purpose of this chapter, based on previously reported studies by the authors (4,10,16,17), is to review the microsurgical anatomy important when performing the various transcranial and subcranial approaches to the sphenoid bone and sellar region, and to provide a step-by-step guide to the transsphenoidal approach in the laboratory.

The sphenoid bone is located in the center of the cranial base. Some part of it is exposed in transcranial operations through the anterior, middle, and posterior cranial fossae and in the subcranial approaches through the nose and orbit. The sphenoid ridge is an important landmark in the frontotemporal approach to many aneurysms and sellar lesions. The intimate contact of the body of the sphenoid bone with the nasal cavity below and the pituitary gland above has led to the transsphenoidal route being the operative approach of choice for selected sellar tumors.

The sphenoid bone has many important arterial and venous relationships: the carotid arteries groove each side of the sphenoid bone and may bulge into the sphenoid sinus; the basilar artery rests against its posterior surface; the circle of Willis is located above its central portion; and the middle cerebral artery courses parallel to the sphenoid ridge of the lesser wing. The cavernous sinuses rest against the sphenoid bone, and intercavernous venous connections line the walls of the sella turcica and dorsum sella.

The neural relationships of the sphenoid bone are among the most complex of any structure: the olfactory tracts, gyrus rectus, and posterior part of the frontal lobe rest against the smooth upper surface of the lesser wing; the temporal lobe rests against the inner surface of the greater wing; the pons and mesencephalon lie posterior to the clival portion; the optic chiasm lies posterior to the chiasmatic sulcus; and the second through sixth cranial nerves are intimately related to the sphenoid bone. All exit the skull through either the optic canal, superior orbital fissure, foramen rotundum, or the foramen ovale, all foramina located in the sphenoid bone.

Dissections of the cranial base in the laboratory, especially those involving the temporal bone, have become a standard part of the training of the otologic surgeon. The experience with the microneurosurgery training program at the University of Florida has revealed that the performance of transsphenoidal dissections of the sphenoid bone and sellar region using surgical magnification can play an important role in increasing the neurosurgeon's knowledge and skill (12,17).

OSSEUS RELATIONSHIPS

The whole skull with the calvarium and mandible removed is used for this review of osseus relationships.

Anterior View

Look directly at the anterior part of the skull (Fig. 1A) and trace the articulations of the sphenoid bone with the frontal, ethmoid, and zygomatic bones and the maxillae. In the anterior view the sphenoid bone forms part of the posterior wall and roof of the orbit.

Superior View

In the superior view (Fig. 1B) locate the articulations with the frontal, ethmoid, temporal, and occipital bones.

Lateral View

In the lateral view (Fig. 1C) locate the junctions of the sphenoid bone with the maxilla and the zygomatic, frontal, and temporal bones. The greater wing of the sphenoid bone projects above the zygoma, and the pterygoid plates project below in the lateral view.

The pterion and the "keyhole" are two important anatomic landmarks in the region of the greater wing in the lateral view. The pterion is located over the upper part of the greater wing. The "keyhole" is located just behind the junction of the temporal line and the zygomatic process of the frontal bone several centimeters anterior to the pterion. A burr hole placed over the pterion will be located at the lateral end of the sphenoid ridge. Bone in the region of the pterion is often removed to improve the operative exposure along the sylvian fissure. A burr hole placed at the keyhole will expose the orbit at its lower margin and dura over the frontal lobe at its upper margin.

Inferior View

In the inferior view (Fig. 1D) locate the junctions of the sphenoid bone with the maxillae and the occipital, temporal, and zygomatic bones. The vomer is outlined in the inferior view even though it is a separate bone because in disarticulated skulls it usually remains attached to the sphenoid bone.

TOPOGRAPHIC ANATOMY

A disarticulated dry sphenoid bone should be used for this exercise. The bones can be obtained from an anatomic supply dealer.

Anterior View

Hold the dry sphenoid bone in your hand so you are looking at the anterior surface (Fig. 2A–D). The sphenoid bone resembles a bat with wings outstretched. Locate the central portion (called the body); the lesser wings, which spread outward from the superolateral part of the body; the two greater wings, which spread upward from the lower part of the body; and the superior orbital fissure between the greater and lesser wings. Identify the vomer, the pterygoid processes, and the medial and lateral pterygoid plates, which are directed downward.

The body of the sphenoid bone is more or less cubical and contains the sphenoid sinus. From the anterior aspect the body is divided into two halves by the midline or sphenoidal crest, which articulates anteriorly and superiorly with the ethmoid bone. Locate the sphenoid ostia, the paired entrances into the sphenoid sinus, on each side of the midline crest.

The superior orbital fissure, through which the oculomotor, trochlear, and abducens nerves and the ophthalmic division of the trigeminal nerve pass, is formed on its inferior and lateral margins by the greater wing and on its superior margin by the lesser wing. The inferior surface of the lesser wing forms the posterior part of the roof of each orbit and the exposed surface of the greater wing forms the posterior wall of the orbit. Identify the optic canals at the superomedial margin of the superior orbital fissure. Note that the optic canal passes inferolaterally from its intracranial end. Locate the pterygoid canal and foramen rotundum, which transmits the pterygoid nerve and the maxillary division of the trigeminal nerve, respectively. Look through the sphenoid ostia into the sinus. Try to determine which of the three types of sphenoid sinus is present. The 6× or 10× magnification provided by the surgical microscope will prove helpful in this determination. Hamberger et al. (7) classified the sphenoid sinus into three types: conchal, presellar, and sellar types, depending on the extent to which the sphenoid bone is pneumatized. In the conchal type the area below the sella is a solid block of bone without an air cavity (Fig. 2A). In the presellar type of sphenoid sinus, the air cavity does not penetrate beyond a vertical plane parallel to the sellar wall (Fig. 2B). The sellar type of sphenoid sinus is the

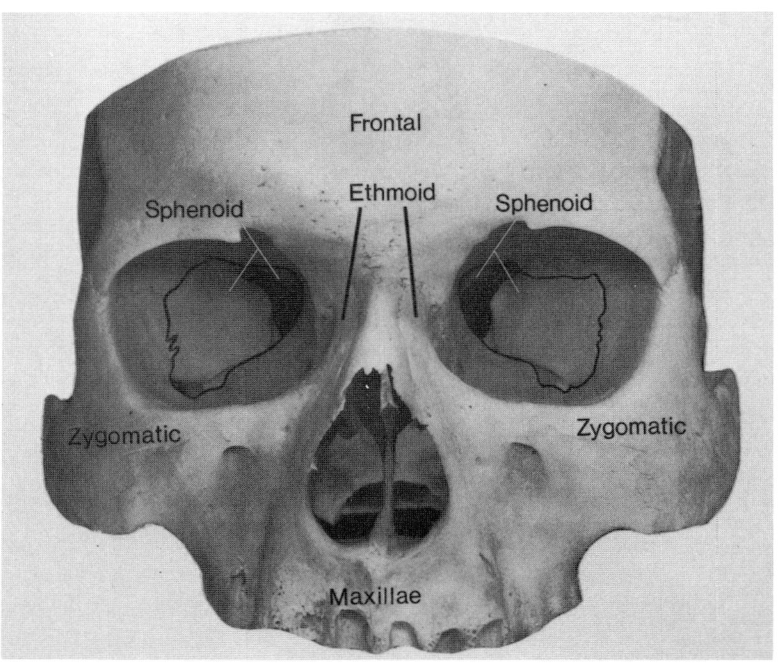

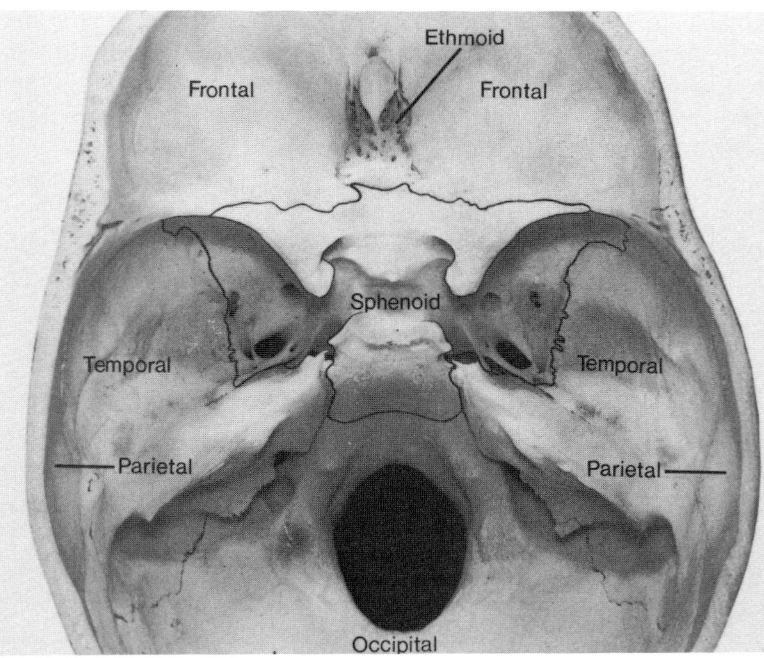

FIG. 1A and B. Osseus relationships of the sphenoid bone. Sphenoid bone is outlined in each view. **A** *(top):* Anterior view. **B** *(bottom):* Superior view. (From ref. 17.)

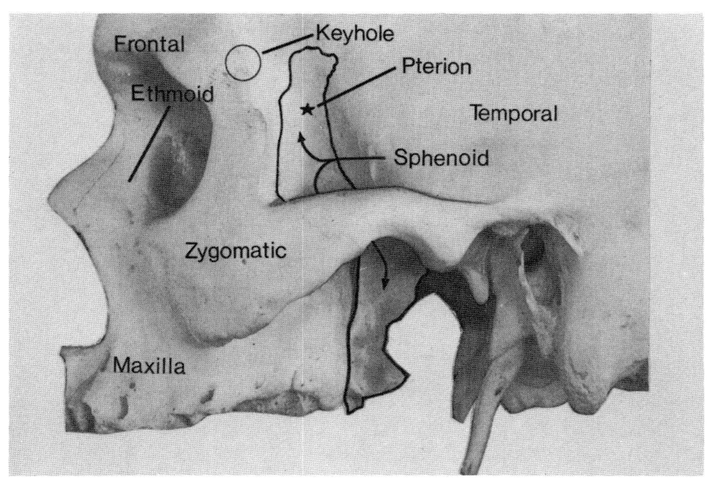

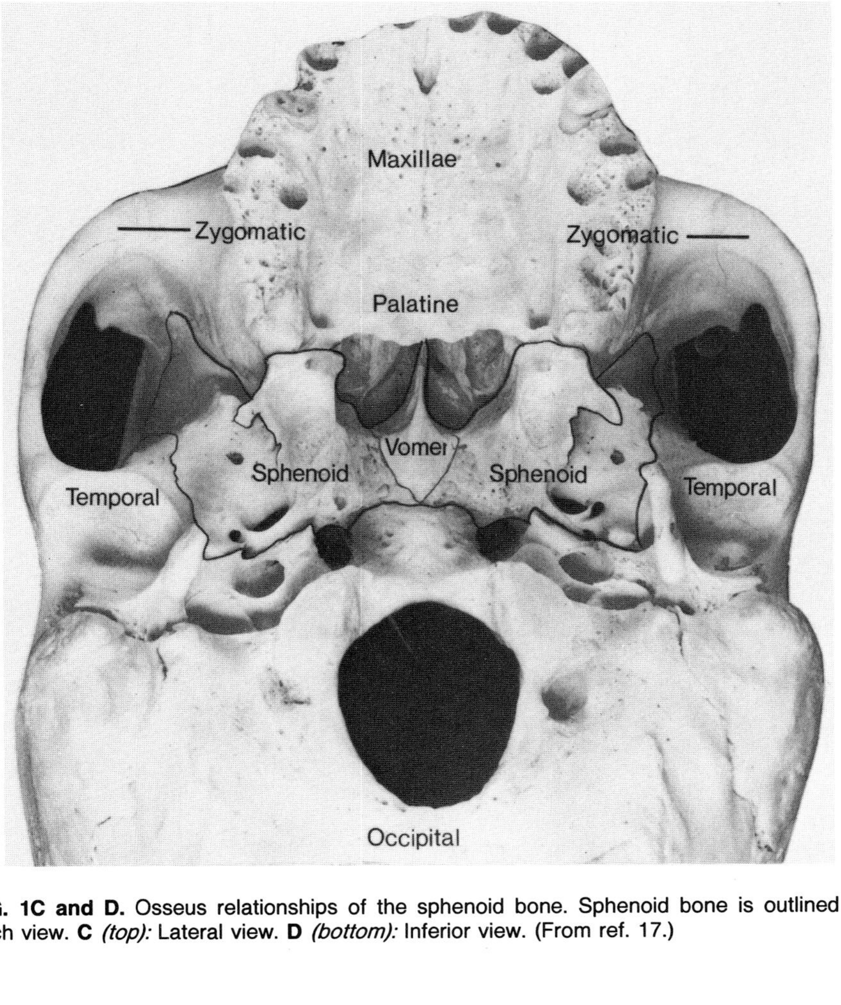

FIG. 1C and D. Osseus relationships of the sphenoid bone. Sphenoid bone is outlined in each view. **C** *(top):* Lateral view. **D** *(bottom):* Inferior view. (From ref. 17.)

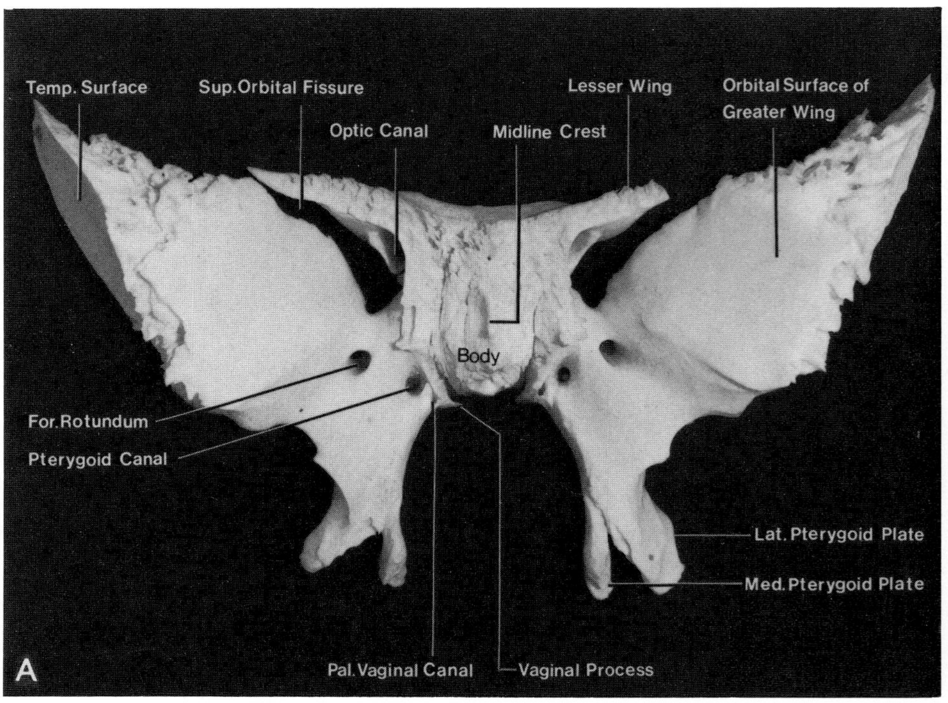

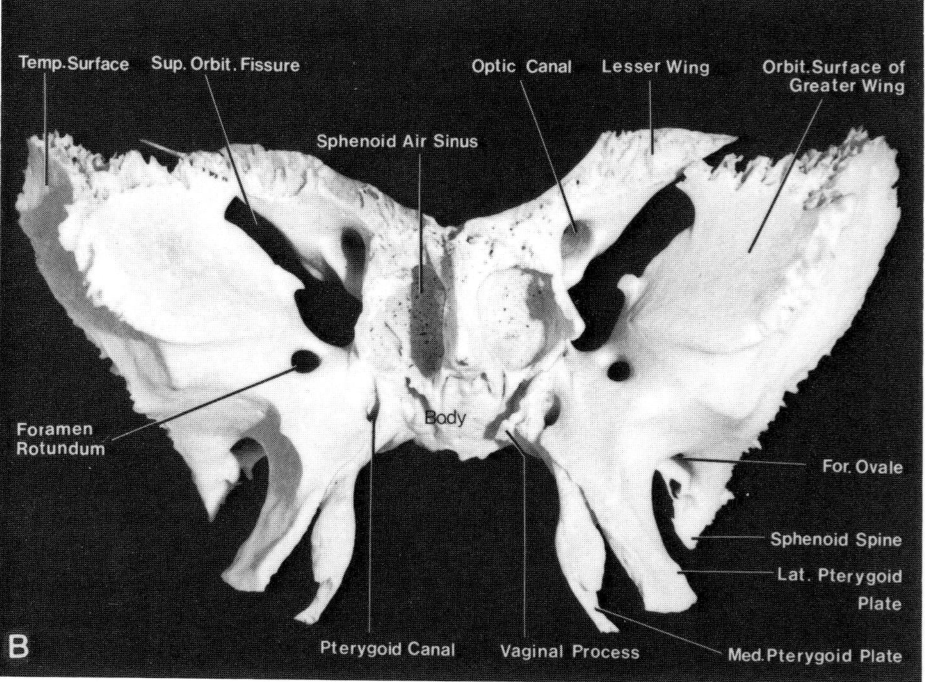

FIG. 2A and B. Anterior view of the sphenoid bone. **A:** Conchal type sphenoid bone. **B:** Bone with presellar-type sphenoid sinus. (From ref. 17.)

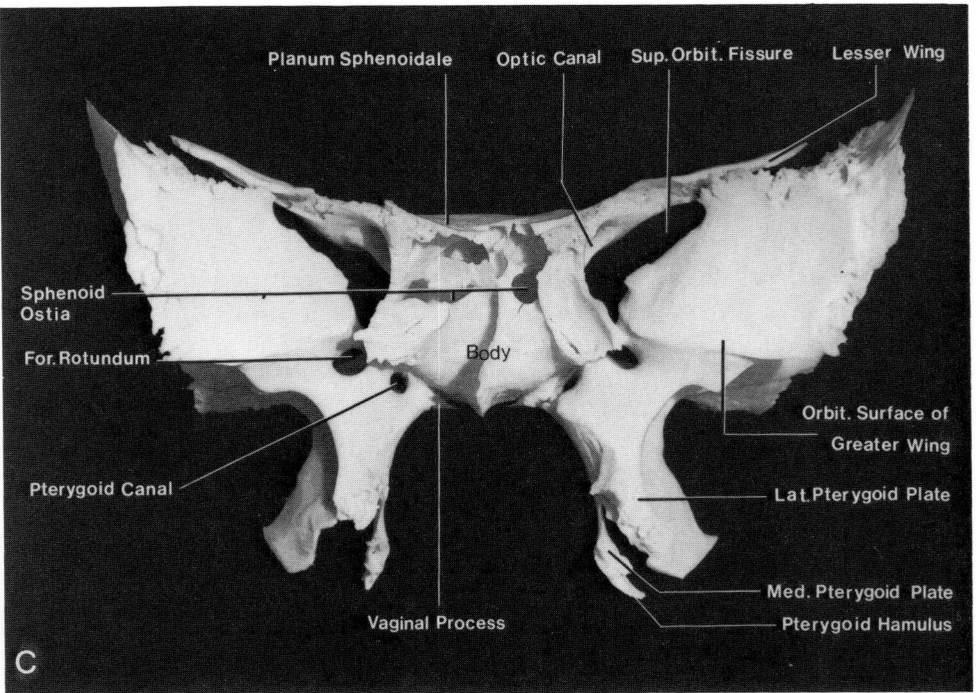

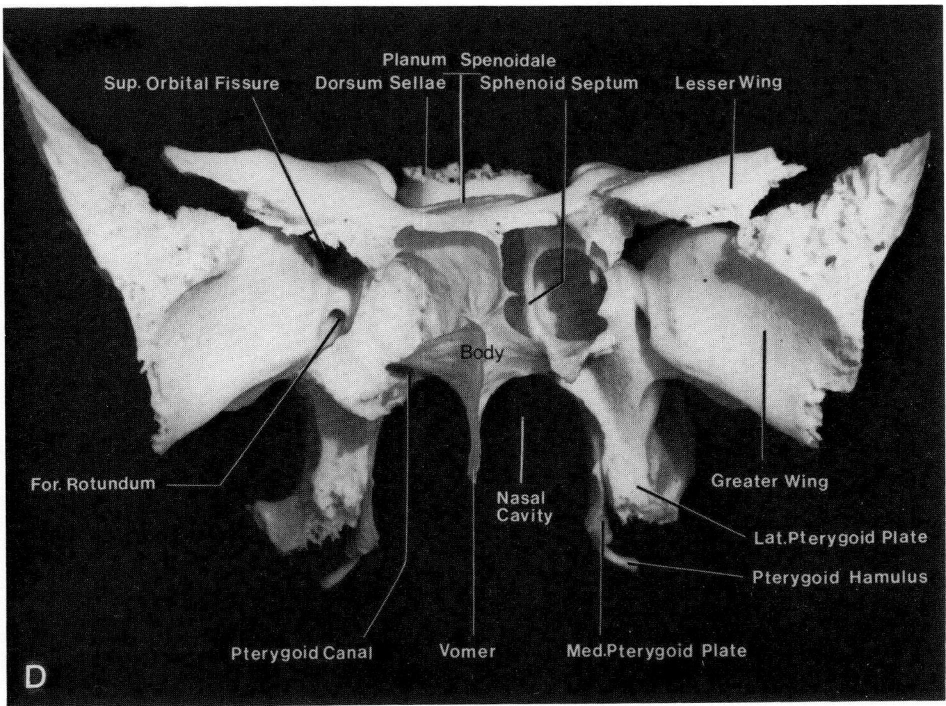

FIG. 2C and D. Anterior view of the sphenoid bone. **C:** Bone with sellar-type sphenoid sinus and well-defined sphenoid ostia. **D:** Bone with sellar-type sphenoid sinus with poorly defined sphenoid ostia and obliquely oriented sphenoidal septae. (From ref. 17.)

most common, and here the air cavity extends into the body of the sphenoid below the sella and as far posteriorly as the clivus (Fig. 2C,D).

Superior View

Identify the body of the sphenoid bone medially and the greater and lesser wings laterally in the superior view (Fig. 3). The pituitary fossa occupies the central part of the body and is bounded anteriorly by the tuberculum sellae and posteriorly by the dorsum sellae. Locate the chiasmatic groove, a shallow depression between the optic foramina which is bounded posteriorly by the tuberculum sellae and anteriorly by the planum sphenoidale. The frontal lobes and the olfactory tracts rest against the smooth upper surface of the lesser wing and the planum sphenoidale. The posterior margin of the lesser wing forms a free edge called the sphenoid ridge, which projects into the lateral cerebral fissure to separate the frontal and temporal lobes.

Locate the anterior clinoid process at the medial end of the lesser wing, the middle clinoid process lateral to the tuberculum sellae, and the posterior clinoid process at the superolateral margin of the dorsum sellae. The dorsum sellae is continuous with the clivus. The upper part of the clivus is formed by the sphenoid

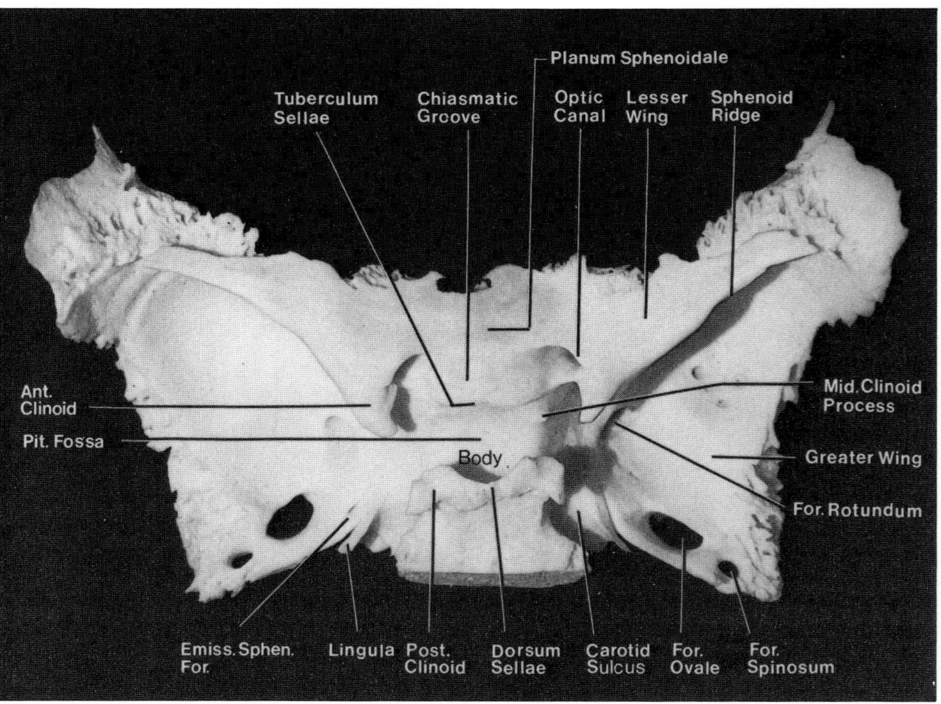

FIG. 3. Superior view of the sphenoid bone. (From ref. 17.)

bone and the lower part by the occipital bone. Identify the carotid sulcus lateral to the body of the sphenoid bone and the lingula, which forms the lateral wall of the posterior part of the sulcus.

The superior aspect of each greater wing is concave upward and is filled by the tip of each temporal lobe. The foramen rotundum, through which the maxillary division of the trigeminal nerve passes, is located at the junction of the body and greater wing. Locate the foramen ovale and foramen spinosum along the posterior margin of the greater wing: The former transmits the mandibular division of the trigeminal nerve and the latter the middle meningeal artery.

Inferior View

Hold the sphenoid bone so you are looking at the inferior surface (Fig. 4). The vomer, a separate bone, frequently remains attached to the anterior half of the body of the sphenoid, and its most anterior portion separates the sphenoid ostia. The lesser wings arise from the anterior portion of the body, and the greater wings from the middle and posterior parts. The pterygoid processes project inferiorly from the posterolateral part of the body. Locate the foramen rotundum behind the superior orbital fissure, and the foramina ovale and spino-

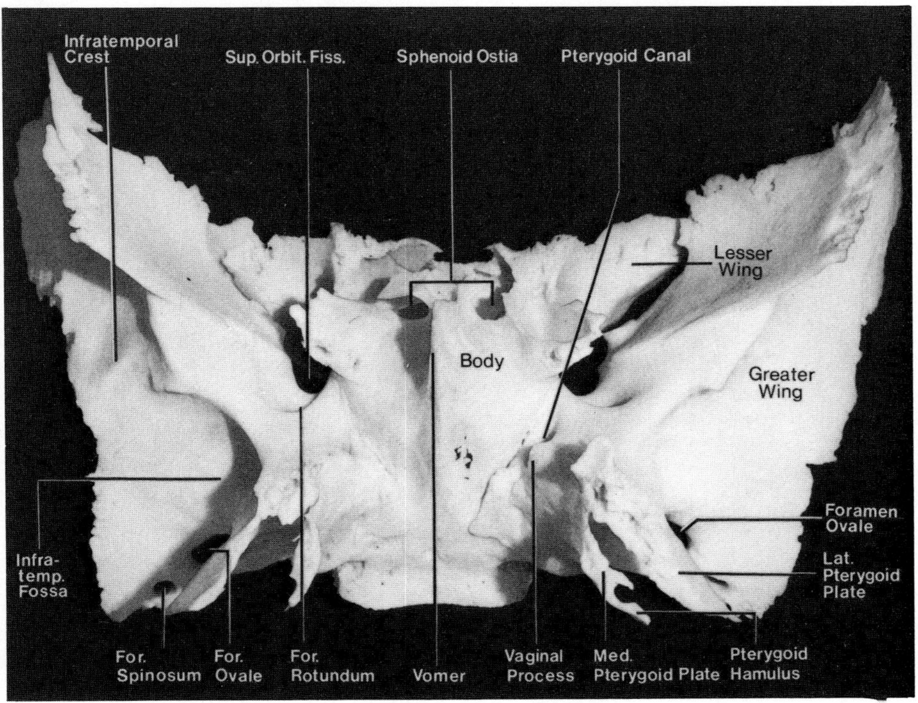

FIG. 4. Inferior view of the sphenoid bone. (From ref. 17.)

sum along the posterior margin of the greater wing. The infratemporal crest divides the inferior from the lateral parts of the greater wing. The lateral pterygoid muscles arise between the infratemporal crest and the lateral pterygoid plate. The area lateral to the infratemporal line gives origin to the temporalis muscle. The pterygoid canal is located at the base of the medial pterygoid lamina and is bounded medially by the vaginal process.

Posterior View

The batlike shape of the sphenoid bone may best be appreciated from the posterior aspect (Fig. 5). In the midline, from posteriorly to anteriorly, locate

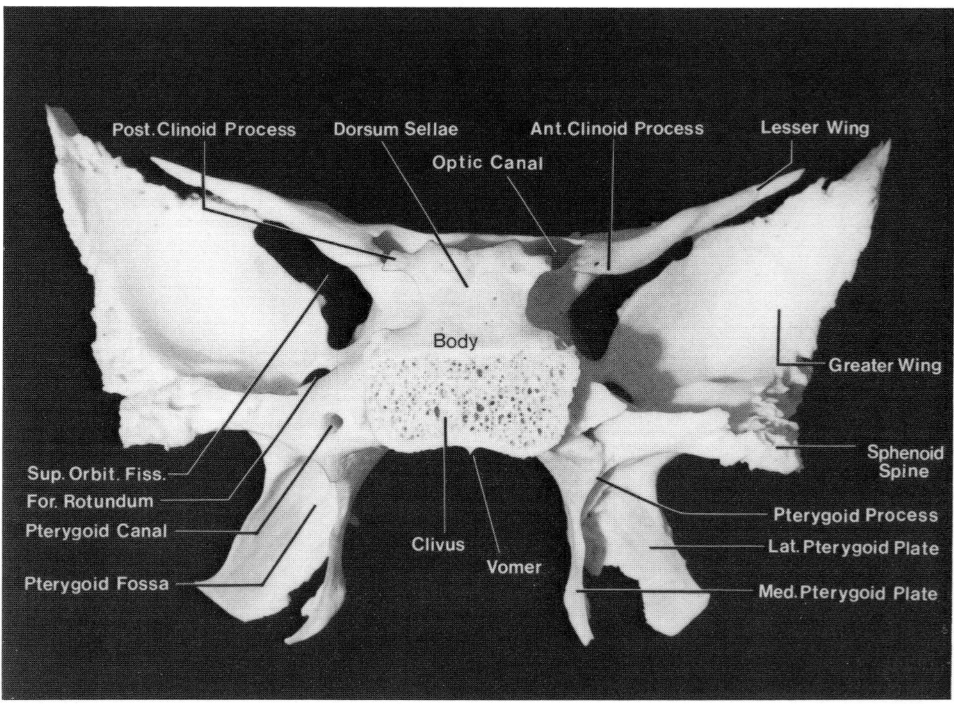

FIG. 5. Posterior view of the sphenoid bone. (From ref. 17.)

the clivus, dorsum sellae, and anterior clinoid process. The greater and lesser wings extend laterally from the body and are separated by the obliquely lying superior orbital fissure. The foramen rotundum is below the superior orbital fissure. The spine of the sphenoid bone projects from the inferolateral margin of the greater wing. Inferiorly, in the midline, the vomer projects into the nasal cavity. Locate the pterygoid canal near the base of the pterygoid processes.

Lateral View

Hold the bone so you are looking directly at the lateral surface (Fig. 6). Identify the body of the sphenoid bone, and on its upper surface locate the anterior clinoid process anteriorly, the dorsum sellae and posterior clinoid process posteriorly, and the pituitary fossa in its midportion. The course of the carotid artery along the body is marked by a shallow groove, the carotid sulcus. The lingula projects upward to form the lateral border of the posterior part of the carotid sulcus. In the carotid sulcus the carotid artery is surrounded by the cavernous sinus.

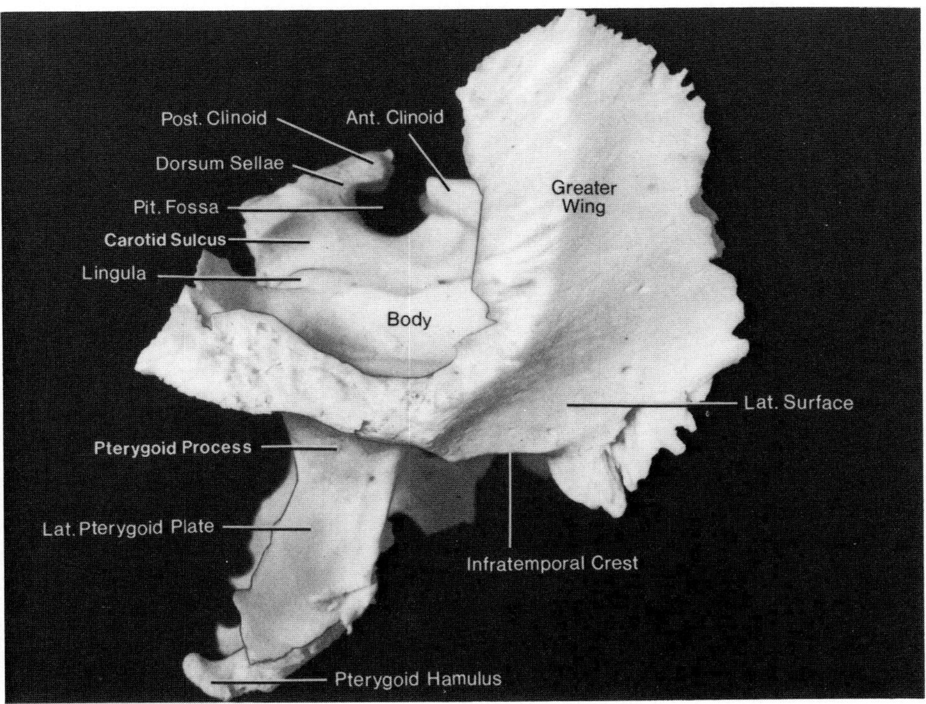

FIG. 6. Lateral view of the temporal bone. (From ref. 17.)

Locate the upward projections of the greater wing and the downward projecting pterygoid process. The infratemporal crest divides the lateral from the infratemporal surface of the bone. The lateral surface of the greater wing gives origin to the temporalis muscle. The lateral pterygoid muscles arise from the infratemporal surface.

SELLAR REGION FROM ABOVE

Transcranial Approach

Although the transsphenoidal surgical approach is the one most frequently used for tumors of the pituitary gland, there are still specific occasions when some transcranial approach may be appropriate. For example, some surgeons prefer the transfrontal approach for all tumors with large suprasellar extensions, especially those in which the sella is small or a suprasellar extension is asymmetrically located (19). The most common variations of the transfrontal intracranial approach are the subchiasmatic approach between the optic nerves and below the chiasm (Fig. 7); the opticocarotid approach between the carotid artery and the optic nerve; the transfrontal-transsphenoidal approach, achieved by drilling off the planum sphenoidale to approach the sella by a combined route; and the lamina terminalis approach posterior to the chiasm, medial to the optic tracts and below the anterior cerebral artery (15,19).

The description which follows is aimed at acquainting the reader with the anatomy of the sellar region as seen by the transfrontal approach.

Chiasmatic Configuration and Tuberculum Sellae

The relationship of the chiasm to the sella (Figs. 8 and 9) is an important determinant of the ease with which the pituitary fossa may be exposed by the transfrontal surgical route. The normal chiasm overlies the diaphragma sellae and the pituitary, the prefixed chiasm overlies the tuberculum sellae, and the postfixed chiasm overlies the dorsum sellae. In approximately 70% of cases the chiasm is in the normal position. Of the remaining 30%, about half are "prefixed" and half "postfixed" (1,16).

A prominent tuberculum sellae may restrict access to the sellae even in the presence of a normal chiasm. The tuberculum may vary from being almost flat to protruding upward as much as 3 mm, and it may project posteriorly to the margin of a normal chiasm (16).

The limited transfrontal approach exposure provided by a prefixed chiasm, a normal chiasm with a small area between the tuberculum and the chiasm, and a superior protruding tuberculum sellae may be enlarged by using the transfrontal–transsphenoidal approach advocated by Rand (15). In this approach access is obtained by opening into the sphenoid sinus from above by drilling through the tuberculum and planum sphenoidale, thus converting the approach to a "transfrontal–transsphenoidal" one. If the chiasm is normal or "postfixed," a subchiasmatic approach below the chiasm is possible. If the chiasm is prefixed and the tumor is seen through a thin, stretched anterior wall of the third ventricle, the lamina terminalis approach may be used. If the space between the carotid artery and the optic nerve has been enlarged (e.g., by a lateral or parasellar extension of tumor), the opticocarotid approach may be utilized (19). Whichever approach is adopted, it is important to avoid retraction of the optic nerves. If more space is needed in the opticocarotid approach, the carotid artery, rather than the optic nerve, may be gently retracted.

Carotid Artery, Optic Nerve, Anterior Clinoid Process

An understanding of the relationship of the carotid artery, optic nerve, and anterior clinoid process is fundamental to all surgical approaches to the sellar and parasellar areas (Figs. 10 and 11). The carotid artery and the optic nerve are medial to the anterior clinoid process. The artery exits the cavernous sinus beneath and slightly lateral to the optic nerve. The optic nerve pursues a posteromedial course toward the chiasm and the carotid artery a posterolateral course toward its bifurcation into the anterior and middle cerebral arteries.

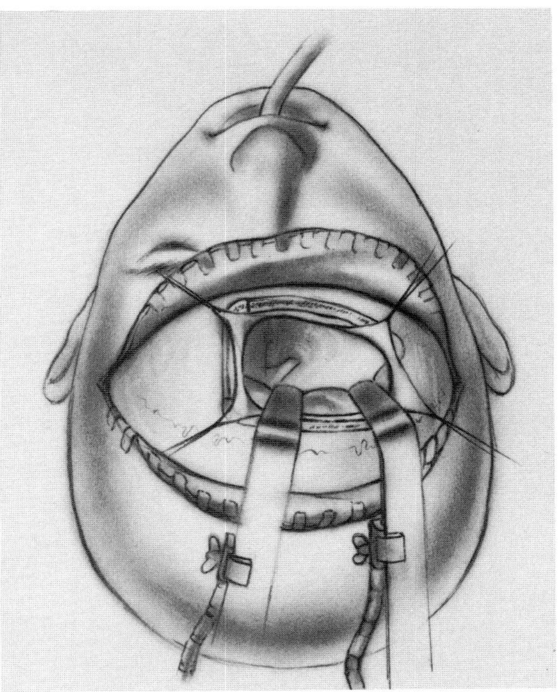

FIG. 7. Above: Transfrontal operative exposure used for **A–F** (see pages 13–15). Transfrontal subchiasmatic approach to a suprasellar craniopharyngioma. **A–F** were retouched from 16-mm movie frames taken at the time of removal of a tumor that was deeply indenting the third ventricle. **A:** Tumor protrudes between optic nerves and a prefixed optic chiasm. **B:** A needle is introduced for attempted aspiration of a cyst in this tumor, which proved to be solid. **C:** Whitish particles of calcified tumor are being removed with a cup forceps. **D:** Scissors amputates some of the tumor. **E:** Tumor capsule is being pushed inferiorly away from chiasm. **F:** Tip of a pointed dissector rests against the upper margin of the dorsum sellae after complete tumor removal. (From ref. 19.)

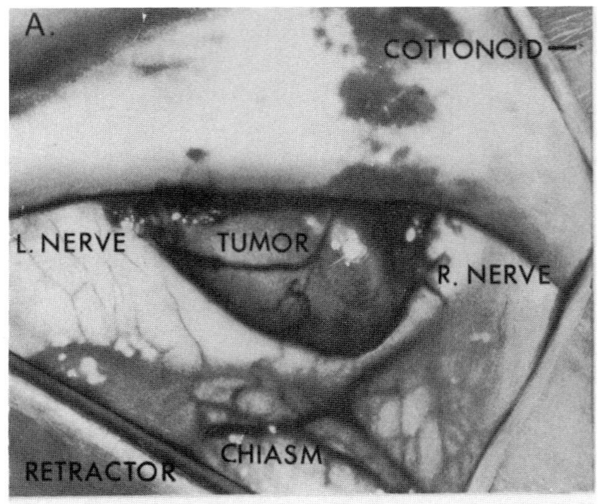
A.
COTTONOID
L. NERVE
TUMOR
R. NERVE
CHIASM
RETRACTOR

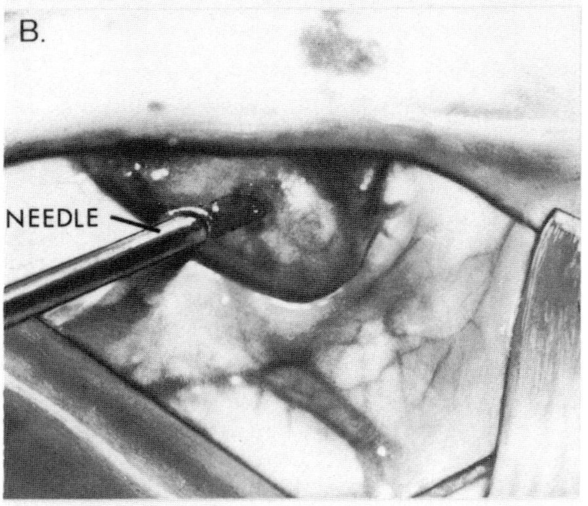
B.
NEEDLE

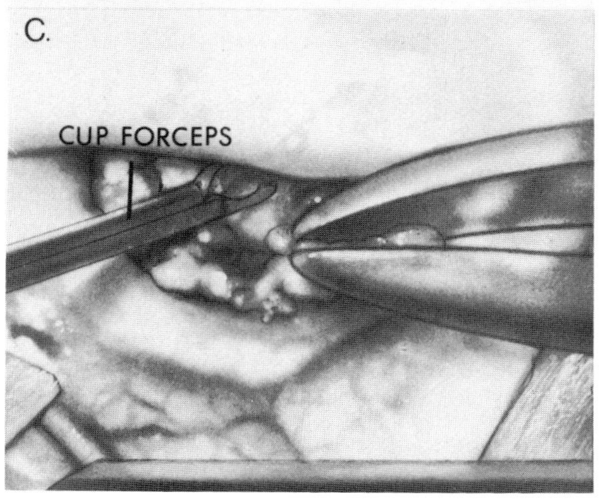
C.
CUP FORCEPS

FIG. 7A–C

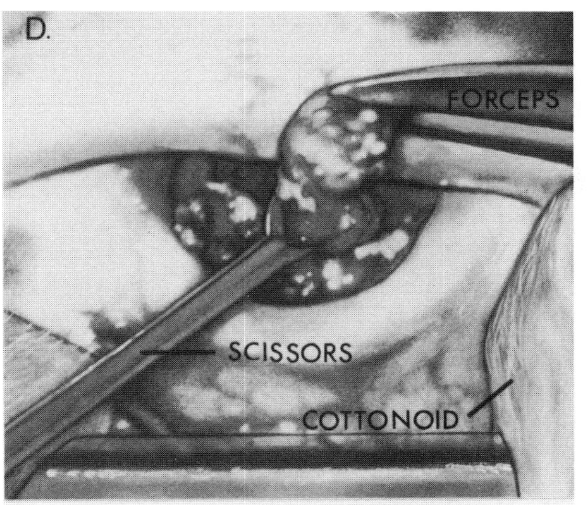
D.
FORCEPS
SCISSORS
COTTONOID

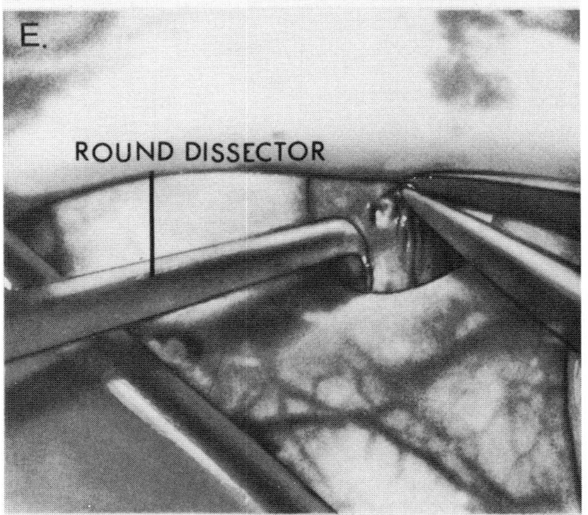
E.
ROUND DISSECTOR

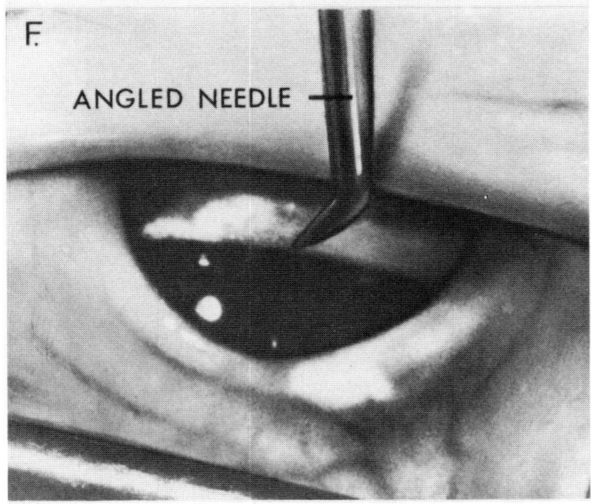
F.
ANGLED NEEDLE

FIG. 7D–F

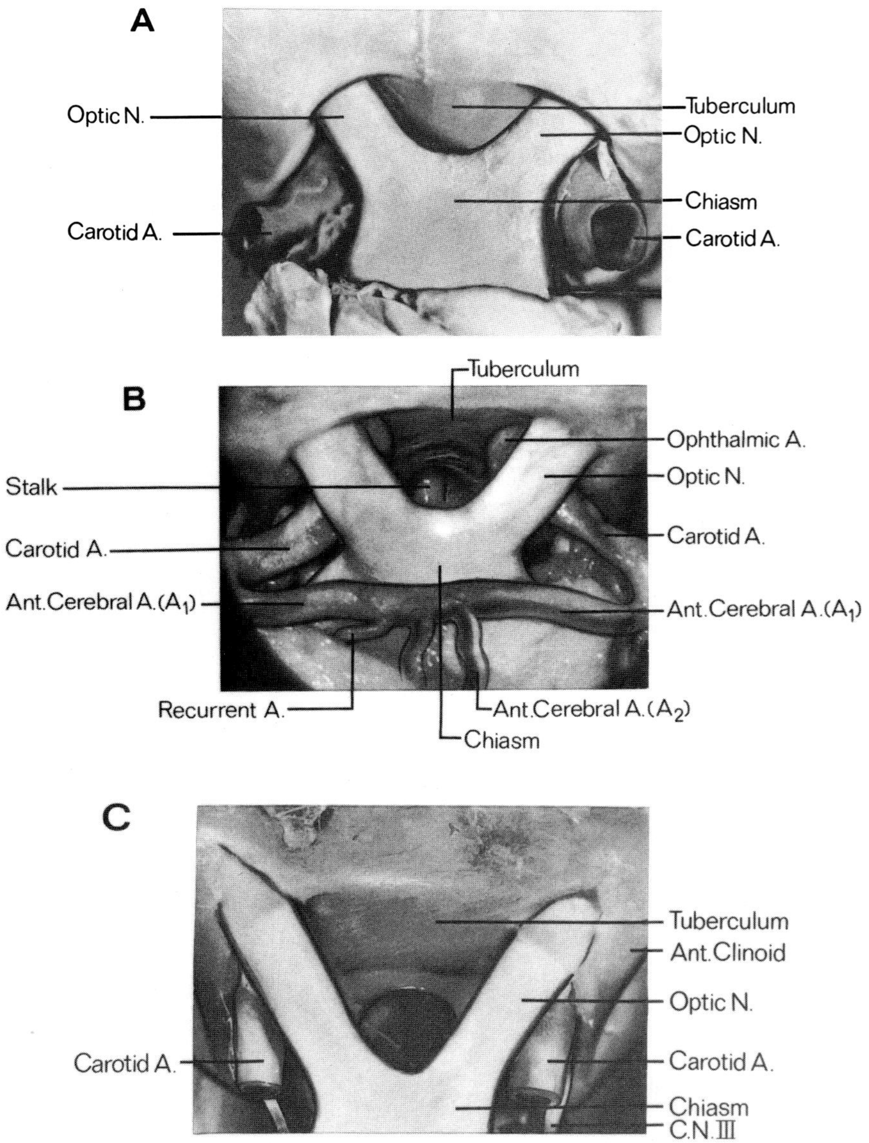

A

Optic N.
Tuberculum
Optic N.
Chiasm
Carotid A.
Carotid A.

B

Tuberculum
Ophthalmic A.
Stalk
Optic N.
Carotid A.
Carotid A.
Ant.Cerebral A.(A_1)
Ant.Cerebral A.(A_1)
Recurrent A.
Ant.Cerebral A.(A_2)
Chiasm

C

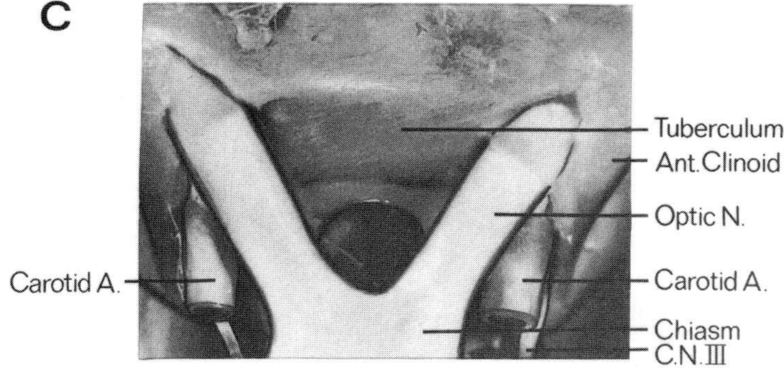

FIG. 8. Superior view of the sellar region. **A:** Prefixed chiasm. **B:** Normal chiasm. The ophthalmic artery protrudes medial to the right optic nerve. The anterior cerebral arteries pass dorsal to the chiasm. The left recurrent artery arises from the A-1 segment of the left anterior cerebral artery. The pituitary stalk lies between the optic nerves. **C:** Postfixed chiasm. Diaphragma sellae and pituitary gland are removed. Cranial nerve III lies ventral to the carotid arteries. (From ref. 16.)

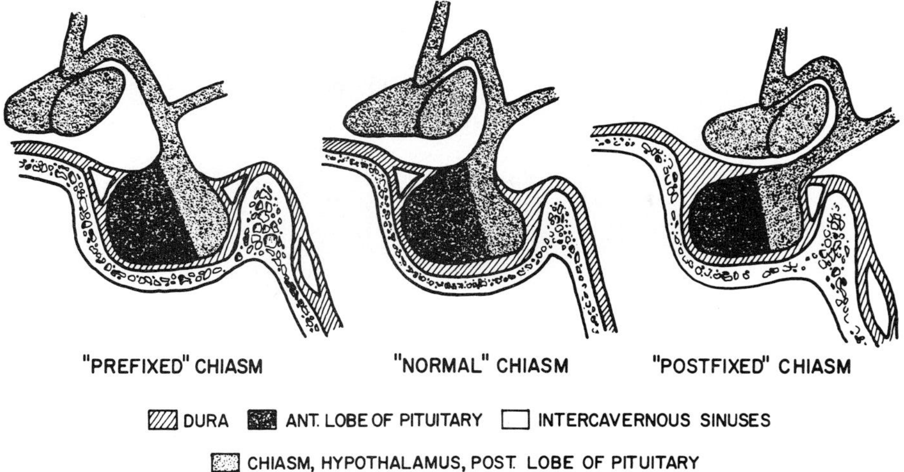

FIG. 9. Three sagittal sections of the sellar region showing neural structures, chiasm, posterior lobe pituitary and hypothalamus, anterior lobe pituitary, dura, and intracavernous venous connections. Prefixed chiasm above tuberculum **(left)**, normal chiasm above diaphragma **(center)**, and postfixed chiasm above dorsum **(right)**. (From ref. 19.)

Optic Canal

The optic nerve proximal to its entrance into the optic canal (Fig. 11) is covered by a reflected leaf of dura, the falciform process, which extends medially from the anterior clinoid process across the top of the optic nerve. The length of nerve covered by dura only at the intracranial end of the optic canal may vary from less than 1 mm to as great as 1 cm. Coagulation of the dura above the optic nerve just proximal to the optic canal on the assumption that bone separates the dura from the nerve could lead to nerve injury. Compression of the optic nerves against the sharp edge of the falciform process may result in a visual field deficit even if the compressing lesion does not damage the nerve enough to cause visual loss. In unroofing the optic canal, the full length must be unroofed before its narrowest point is passed because the narrowest part is closer to the orbital than the intracranial end. The optic canals average 5 mm in length and are of a conical configuration, tapering to a narrow waist near the orbit. The ophthalmic artery is found inferolateral to the optic nerve when the periosteum lining the optic canal is opened. Normally the optic nerve is separated medially from the sphenoid sinus by a thin plate of bone, but in a few cases this bone is absent and the optic nerves may protrude directly into the sphenoid sinus and are separated from the sinus by only mucosa and the dural sheath of the nerve (4,16).

Extraocular Nerves

The extraocular nerves (Figs. 10 and 11) are frequently compressed or injured near their entrance into the dura. The oculomotor nerve enters the dura lateral

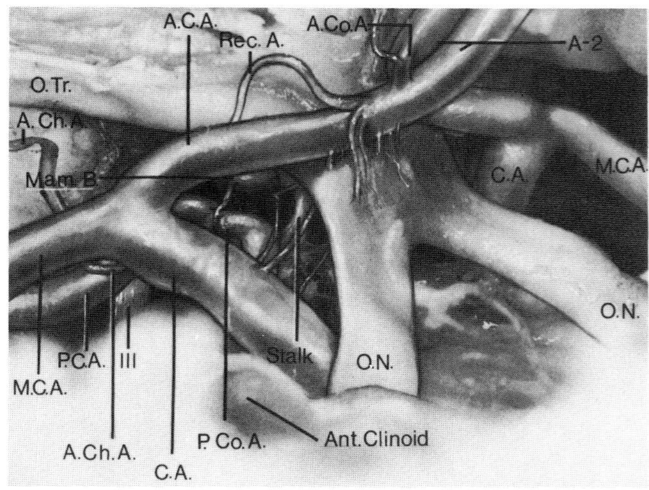

FIG. 10A

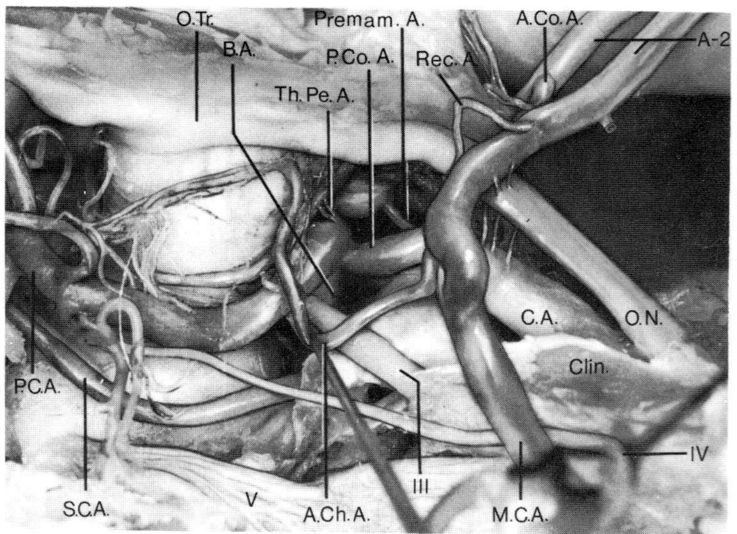

FIG. 10B

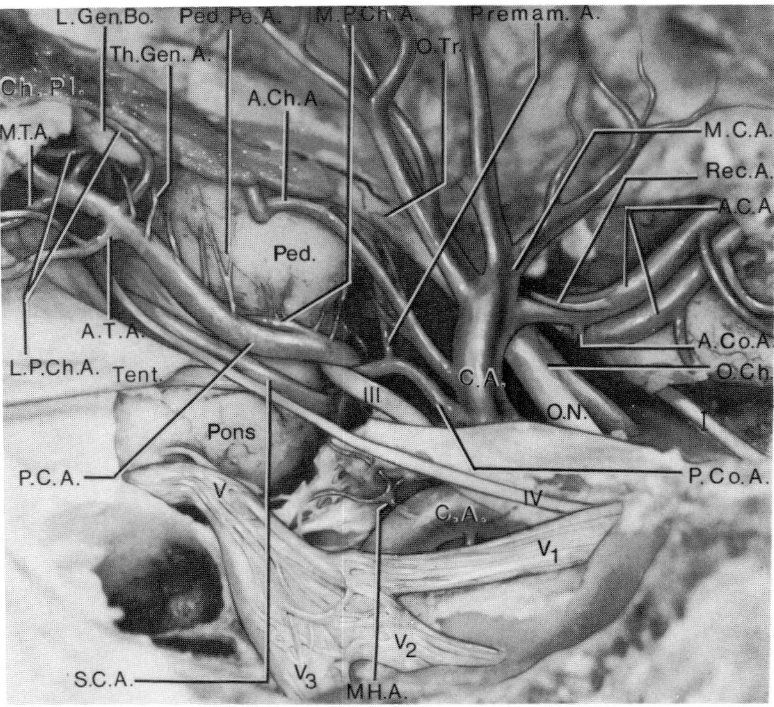

FIG. 10. Right anterior and lateral views of the suprasellar area. **A:** Right anterolateral view. Anterior clinoid process (Ant.Clinoid), lateral to optic nerve (O.N.), and carotid artery (C.A.). Perforating arteries pass from the carotid to terminate in the optic chiasm and tract (O.Tr.) and the hypothalamus anterior to the mamillary body (Mam.B.). Right posterior communicating artery (P.Co.A.) is medial to the carotid artery. Anterior choroidal artery (A.Ch.A.) arises from the carotid and passes above the posterior cerebral artery (P.C.A.). The third nerve (III) lies below the right posterior cerebral artery. The right recurrent artery of Heubner (Rec.A.) arises from the anterior cerebral artery (A.C.A.) proximal to the anterior communicating artery (A.Co.A.). (M.C.A.) middle cerebral artery. (A-2) anterior cerebral artery distal to the anterior communicating artery. (From ref. 20.) **B:** Right lateral view with temporal lobe removed. Anterior clinoid (Clin.) is lateral to the carotid artery. Premamillary (Premam.A.) arises from the posterior communicating artery. Thalamoperforating arteries (Th.Pe.A.) arise from the proximal posterior cerebral artery. The optic tract passes around the peduncle to the lateral geniculate body. Arterioles pass from the carotid artery to the optic nerve. The basilar artery (B.A.) is medial to the third and fourth (IV) cranial nerves. The trigeminal nerve (V) is below the superior cerebellar artery (S.C.A.). (From ref. 20.) **C:** Lateral view. The lateral wall of the cavernous sinus is removed, exposing the third, fourth, and fifth cranial nerves, the three divisions of the trigeminal nerve (V_1, V_2, V_3), and the intracavernous portion of the carotid artery. The anterior choroidal artery arises distal to the posterior communicating artery and gives branches to the optic tract, cerebral peduncle (Ped.), choroid plexus (Ch.Pl.), and lateral geniculate body (L.Gen.Bo.). The meningohypophyseal artery (M.H.A.) arises from the carotid artery. The lateral (L.P.Ch.A.) and medial (M.P.Ch.A.) posterior choroidal arteries, the peduncular perforating artery (Ped.P.C.A.), and the anterior (A.T.A.) and middle temporal (M.T.A.) arteries arise from the posterior cerebral artery. (O.Ch.) optic chiasm. (From ref. 22.)

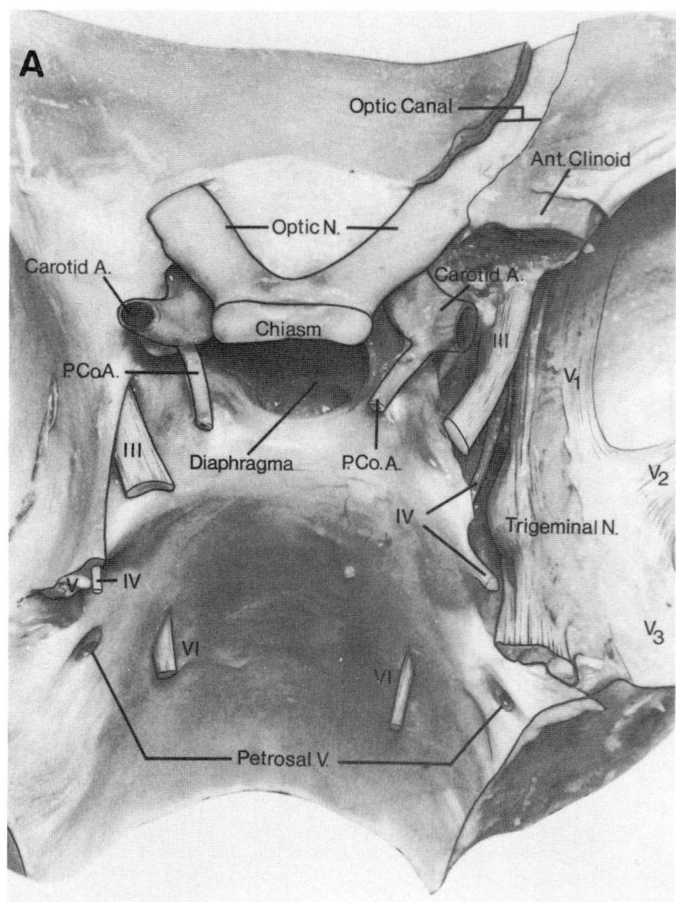

FIG. 11. Sellar region with bone over optic canal removed. **A:** Superior view. The tip of the anterior clinoid (Ant.Clinoid) process and the dura over the right cavernous sinus is removed. The origin of the posterior communicating artery (P.Co.A.) from the carotid artery (Carotid A.) is directed posteromedially. The oculomotor (III) nerves enter the dura lateral to the dorsum sellae, medial to the tentorial attachment to the anterior clinoid process. The trochlear (IV) nerves enter the dura along the anteromedial edge of the tentorium and pass forward in the cavernous sinus. The abducens nerves (VI) enter the dura of the upper clivus. The right trigeminal nerve (Trigeminal N.) and its first (V_1), second (V_2), and third (V_3) divisions are seen below the oculomotor nerve. The diaphragma sellae is concave upward. Petrosal vein (Petrosal V.) enters the superior petrosal sinus. **B:** Optic chiasm is reflected forward to expose the origin of the ophthalmic arteries (Ophth.A.) from the carotid arteries. **C:** Superolateral view of the same dissection shown in **A** showing the relationship of the optic nerve, carotid artery, and ophthalmic artery to extraocular nerves and the cavernous sinus. The trigeminal nerve has been reflected forward to expose the abducens nerve. The intercavernous portion of the carotid artery gives origin to the meningohypophyseal trunk and its branches and the inferior hypophyseal (Inf.Hypophyseal A.), tentorial (Tentorial A.), and dorsal meningeal (Dorsal Meningeal A.) arteries. The artery of the inferior cavernous sinus (Ant.Inf.Cav.Sinus) passes over the abducens nerve. A sympathetic plexus is seen around the carotid artery. (From ref. 17.)

B
Chiasm
Optic Canal
Ant. Clinoid
Optic N.
Ant. Clinoid
Ophth. A.
Carotid. A
III
V1
III
P.Co.A.
Diaphragma
P.Co.A.
Trigeminal N.
IV
IV
VI

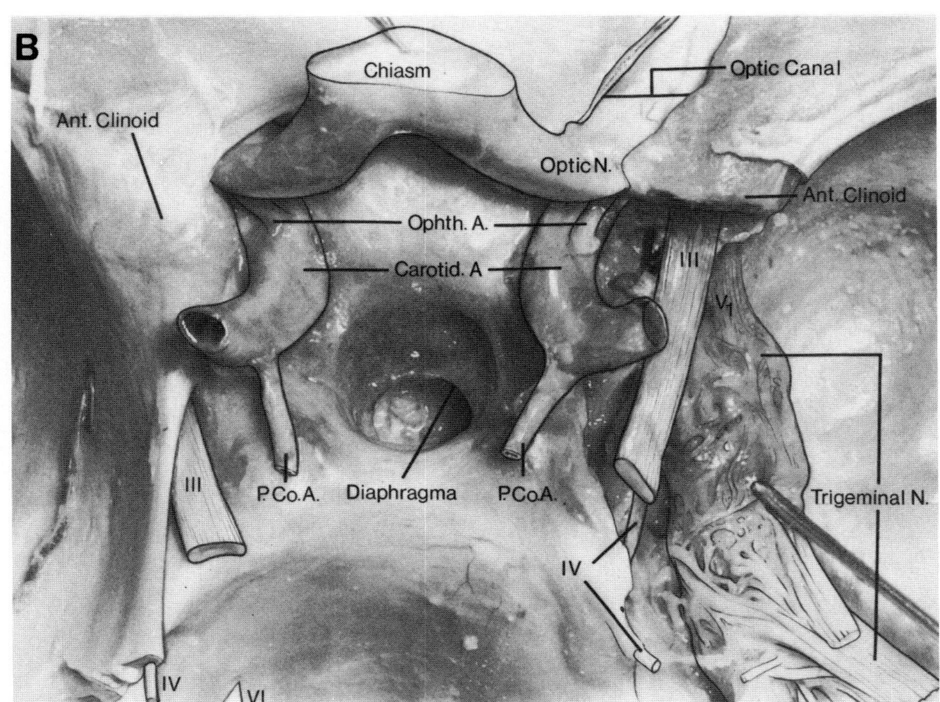

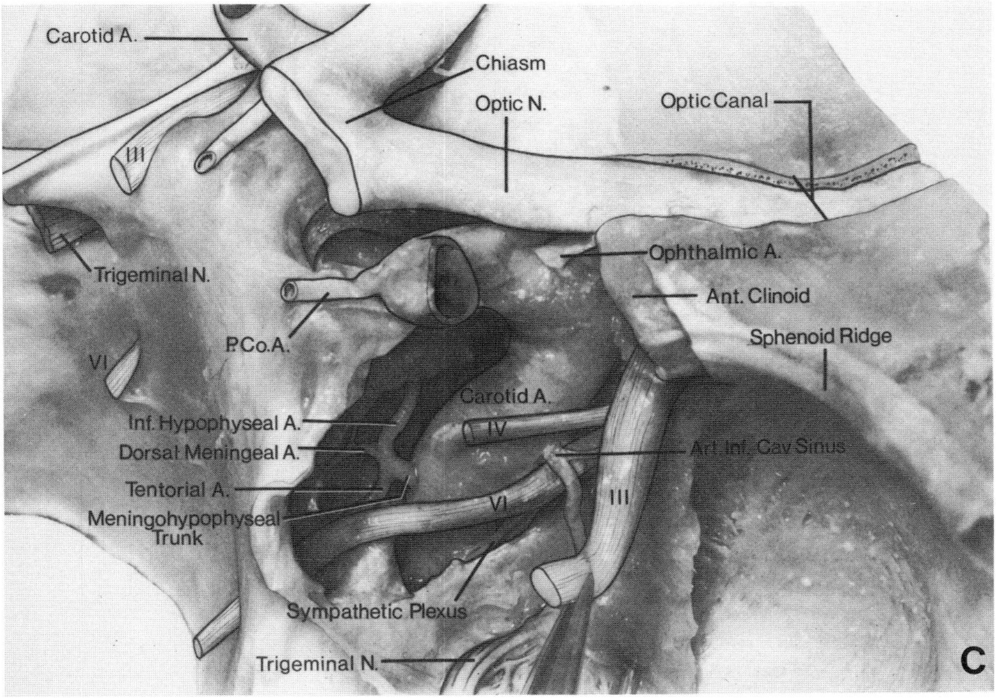

Carotid A.
Chiasm
Optic N.
Optic Canal
III
Trigeminal N.
Ophthalmic A.
P.Co.A.
Ant. Clinoid
Sphenoid Ridge
VI
Carotid A.
Inf. Hypophyseal A.
IV
Dorsal Meningeal A.
Art. Inf. Cav Sinus
Tentorial A.
III
VI
Meningohypophyseal Trunk
Sympathetic Plexus
Trigeminal N.
C

to the posterior clinoid process and medial to a dural band passing from the tentorium cerebelli toward the anterior clinoid process. The trochlear nerve enters the dura of the anteromedial part of the tentorium cerebelli, and the abducens nerve pierces the dura of the upper clivus, which covers the posterior wall of the cavernous sinus.

Suprasellar Arteries

Circle of Willis

All the arterial components of the circle of Willis and the adjacent carotid artery give origin to multiple perforating branches which may become stretched over suprasellar tumors (20,22) (Fig. 12). The supraclinoid portion of the carotid artery, in addition to giving off the posterior communicating and anterior choroidal arteries, also give off perforating branches which include the superior hypophyseal artery and other branches passing to the optic nerve, chiasm, anterior hypothalamus, and anterior perforated substance. The posterior part of the circle of Willis and the upper centimeter of the basilar artery also send a series of perforating arteries through the suprasellar area into the diencephalon and midbrain which may become stretched around suprasellar tumors or aneurysms. The largest perforating branches arising from the posterior part of the circle of Willis are the thalamoperforating and medial posterior choroidal arteries.

Ophthalmic Artery

The ophthalmic artery is the first branch of the internal carotid artery above the cavernous sinus. Its origin and proximal segment may be visible below the optic nerve without retracting the nerve, although elevation of the optic nerve away from the carotid artery is usually required to see the preforaminal segment. The artery arises above the supraclinoid segment at the carotid artery in most cases, but it may also arise within the cavernous sinus or be absent in a few cases (10,16).

The ophthalmic artery origin has a variable relationship to the tip of the anterior clinoid process. Its origin may vary from as far as 5 mm anterior to 7 mm posterior to the clinoid tip and 2 to 10 mm medial to the clinoid (10). Most arise anterior and approximately 5 mm medial to the tip. In our studies, 14% of ophthalmic arteries exited from the carotid artery and immediately entered the optic canal; in the remaining 86% the maximal preforaminal length was 7 mm and the mean 3 mm (10).

Posterior Communicating Artery

The posterior communicating artery arises from the posterior medial wall of the carotid artery. Its posterior course varies depending on whether the artery provides the major supply to the distal posterior cerebral artery. If it is normal, with the main posterior cerebral artery supply arising from the basilar artery, it is directed posteromedially above the oculomotor nerve toward the interpeduncular fossa. If the posterior cerebral artery arises from the carotid artery, it is directed posterolaterally below the optic tract. The oculomotor nerve pierces the dura 2 to 7 mm (average 5 mm) posterior to the initial supraclinoid segment of the carotid artery (10). Aneurysms arising from the internal carotid artery at the origin of the posterior communicating artery frequently point back and down, and compress the oculomotor nerve near its entrance into the dural roof of the cavernous sinus. The posterior communicating artery gives rise to multiple perforating branches which might be stretched over the tip of the suprasellar tumors.

Anterior Choroidal Artery

The origin and initial segment of the anterior choroidal artery may be visible between the posterior communicating artery and the bifurcation of the internal carotid artery. The initial segment of the anterior choroidal artery is directed posterolateral below the optic tract around the side of the brainstem and sends branches into the optic tract and optic radiations as well as into the temporal lobe, internal capsule, diencephalon, and midbrain.

Anterior Cerebral–Anterior Communicating–Recurrent Artery Complex

Each anterior cerebral artery (Fig. 13) courses over the superior surface of the optic chiasm or nerves to join the anterior communicating artery (14). The junction of the anterior communicating artery with the right and left A-1 segments is usually above the chiasm rather than above the optic nerves. In our studies 70% were above the chiasm and 30% were in a prefixed position above the optic nerves. The shorter A-1 segments are stretched tightly over the chiasm, and the longer ones pass anteriorly over the nerves. The arteries with a more forward course are often tortuous and elongated, and some may course forward and rest on the tuberculum sellae or planum sphenoidale. The anterior cerebral and anterior communicating arteries give rise to multiple branches which terminate in the superior surface of the optic chiasm, the anterior hypothalamus, the anterior perforating substance, and the region of the optic tract.

The recurrent artery of Heubner also arises from the anterior cerebral artery and runs above the chiasm adjacent to the anterior cerebral artery. The recurrent artery arose proximal or distal to the anterior communicating artery in 14% and 78%, respectively, and at the level of the anterior communicating artery in 8% (14). The recurrent artery courses anterior to the A-1 segment of the

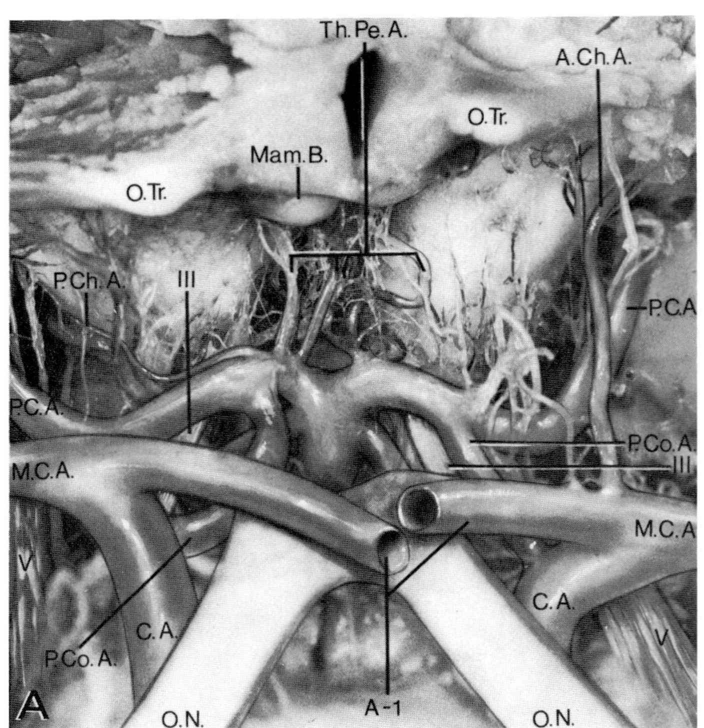
Th. Pe. A.
A.Ch. A.
O.Tr.
Mam. B.
O.Tr.
P.Ch. A.
III
P.C.A.
P.C.A.
P.Co. A.
III
M.C.A.
M.C.A.
V
C.A.
P.Co. A.
C.A.
V
A
O.N.
A-1
O.N.

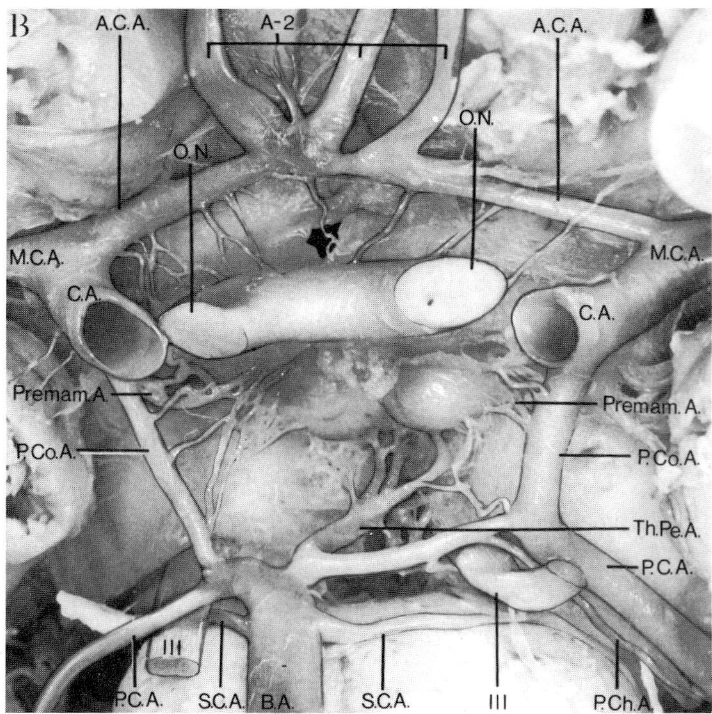
B
A.C.A.
A-2
A.C.A.
O.N.
O.N.
M.C.A.
M.C.A.
C.A.
C.A.
Premam. A.
Premam. A.
P.Co.A.
P.Co.A.
Th.Pe.A.
P.C.A.
III
P.C.A.
S.C.A.
B.A.
S.C.A.
III
P.Ch.A.

FIG. 12A and B. Superior view of the arteries in the suprasellar area. **A:** The posterior part of the optic chiasm is split at junction with optic tracts (O.Tr.) to give this view. The proximal portion of the anterior cerebral arteries (A-1) arise from the carotid arteries (C.A.) and pass above the optic nerves (O.N.) and chiasm; the anterior third ventricle lies above the mammillary bodies (Mam.B.). The thalamoperforating arteries (Th.Pe.A.) terminate in the retromammillary area and the interpeduncular fossa. The right posterior choroidal artery (P.Ch.A.) originates from the posterior cerebral artery (P.C.A.). Small branches arise from the posterior cerebral artery and terminate in the peduncle. The left third nerve (III) courses medial to the posterior communicating artery (P.Co.A.). The right posterior communicating artery joins the posterior cerebral artery medial to the third nerve. The left anterior choroidal artery (A.Ch.A.) passes to the peduncle and optic tract. Trigeminal nerves (V) are lateral to the carotid artery. (M.C.A.) middle cerebral artery. **B:** Inferior view of the circle of Willis. Fetal type of left posterior cerebral artery. The left third nerve courses under the posterior cerebral artery distal to its junction with the posterior communicating artery and the right under the part proximal to the communicating artery. The left thalamoperforating and the posterior choroidal (P.Ch.A.) arteries originate from the proximal part of the posterior cerebral artery. The right premammillary artery (Premam.A.) emerges from the anterior and the left from the middle third of the posterior communicating artery. Small posterior communicating branches course superiorly and medially, terminating in the premammillary area. The left thalamoperforating and right premammillary arteries are well developed in spite of the small trunk of origin. The superior cerebellar artery (S.C.A.) arises below the posterior cerebral artery. No branches arise on the anterior surface of the basilar artery (B.A.) (A-2) distal part of the anterior cerebral artery. (From ref. 20.)

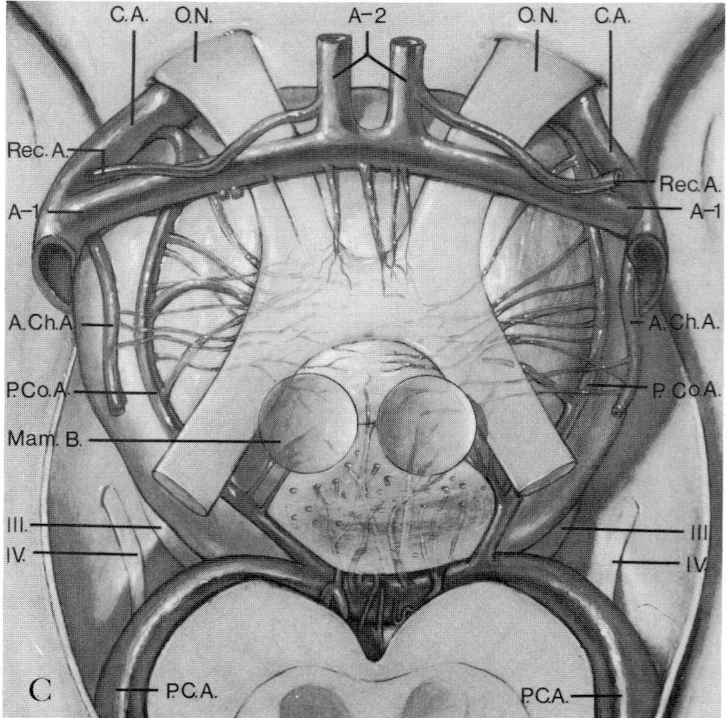

FIG. 12C. Superior view of the suprasellar area. Arterial branches stretch around the superior extension of a pituitary tumor. Anterior cerebral arteries send branches to the superior surface of the optic nerves and chiasm. The posterior communicating, internal carotid, and posterior cerebral arteries send branches into the area below and behind the chiasm. Recurrent arteries (Rec.A.) arise just distal to the anterior communicating artery. (IV) trochlear nerve. (From ref. 20.)

anterior cerebral artery and would have been seen when elevating the frontal lobe prior to visualizing the A-1 segment in about two-thirds of cases. Of the remaining one-third, most coursed superior to A-1 (14).

Diaphragma Sellae

The diaphragma sella (Figs. 11 and 14) forms the roof of the sella turcica. It covers the pituitary gland, except for a small central opening in its center, which transmits the pituitary stalk. The diaphragma is more rectangular than circular, tends to be convex or concave rather than flat, and is thinner around the infundibulum and somewhat thicker at the periphery; the opening in its center is large when compared to the size of the pituitary stalk. It frequently is a thin, tenuous structure which would not be an adequate barrier for protecting

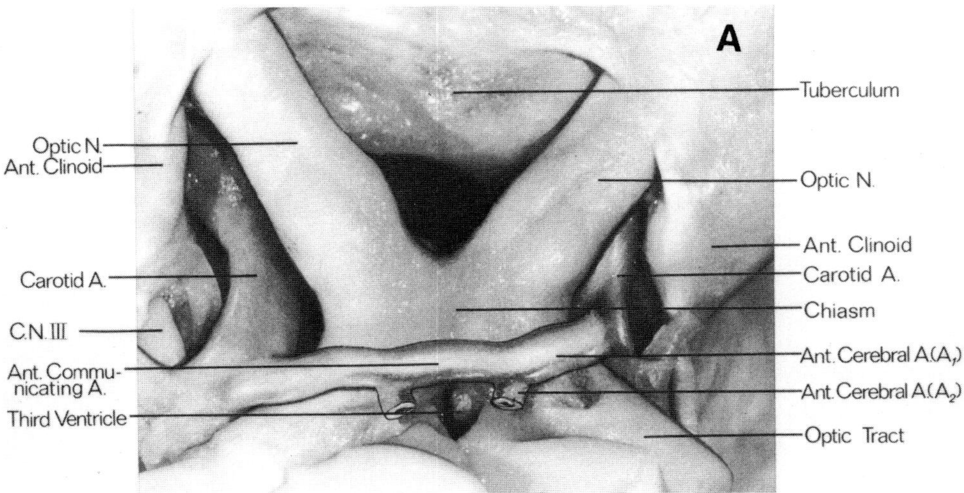

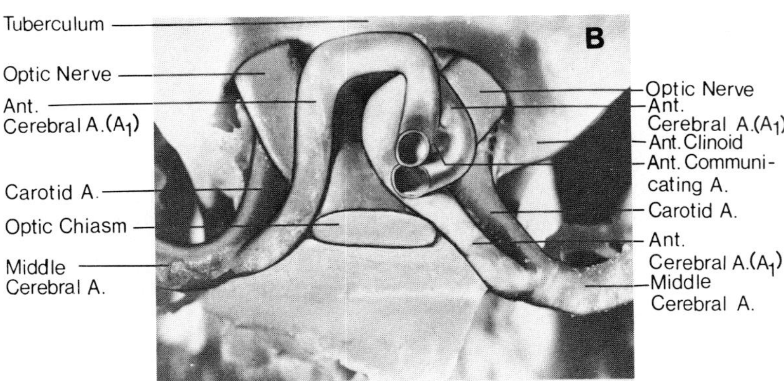

FIG. 13. Superior views of sellar region. **A:** Carotid arteries are lateral to the optic nerves; anterior cerebral arteries are stretched across the superior surface of the optic chiasm; and the right optic nerve is shorter than the left. **B:** Long, tortuous anterior cerebral arteries are above the optic chiasm. The A-1 segment of the right anterior cerebral artery loops in a complete circle between its origin from the carotid artery and its junction with its mate from the opposite side at the anterior communicating artery. A tortuous left anterior cerebral artery rests against the tuberculum sellae covering the prechiasmatic space. (From ref. 16.)

the suprasellar structures during transsphenoidal surgery. An outpouching of the arachnoid protrudes through the central opening in the diaphragma into the sella turcica in about half of the specimens. Although Hardy (9) maintains that this diverticulum can usually be retracted unruptured during transsphenoidal surgery, it does represent a potential source of postoperative cerebrospinal fluid leakage.

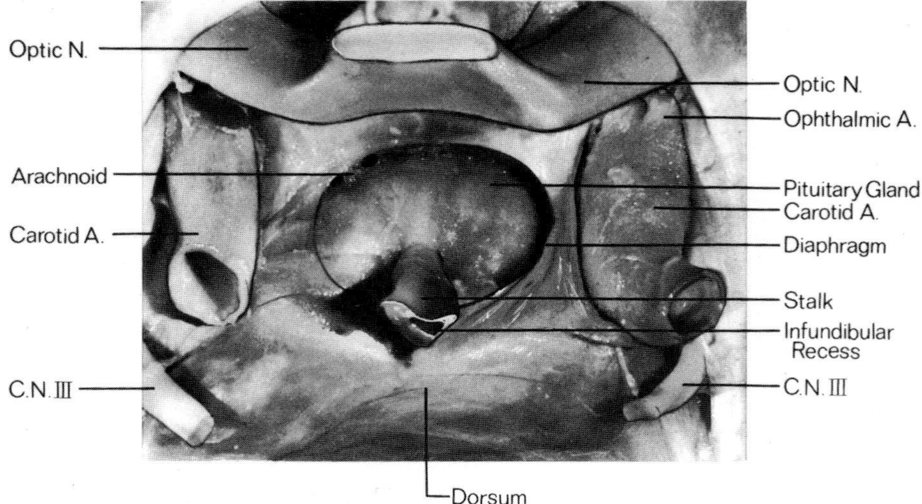

FIG. 14. Superior view of the sellar region. The optic chiasm is reflected forward. A congenitally absent diaphragma exposes the superior surface of the gland. Cranial nerve III is posterior to the carotid arteries. The right ophthalmic artery arises below the optic nerve. (From ref. 16.)

Pituitary Gland

When opening the diaphragma, you will note that the superior surface of the posterior lobe of the pituitary gland is lighter in color than the anterior lobe, and that the anterior lobe wraps around the lower part of the pituitary stalk to form the pars tuberalis.

When removing the gland from the sella, the posterior lobe (Figs. 15 and 16) will be found to be more densely adherent to the sellar wall than the anterior lobe. The gland's width is equal to or greater than either its depth or its length in most specimens. Its inferior surface usually conforms to the shape of the sellar floor, but its lateral and superior margins vary in shape because these walls are composed of soft tissue rather than bone. If there is a large opening in the diaphragma, the gland tends to be concave superiorly in the area around the stalk. The superior surface may become triangular as a result of being compressed laterally and posteriorly by the carotid arteries.

As the anterior lobe is separated from the posterior lobe there is a tendency for the pars tuberalis to be retained with the posterior lobe. Intermediate lobe cysts are frequently encountered during separation of the anterior and posterior lobes.

A determination of the dimensions and volume of the sella turcica as seen on X-ray may prove helpful. The depth of the sella is the greatest distance between the floor and a perpendicular line connecting the tuberculum and dorsum

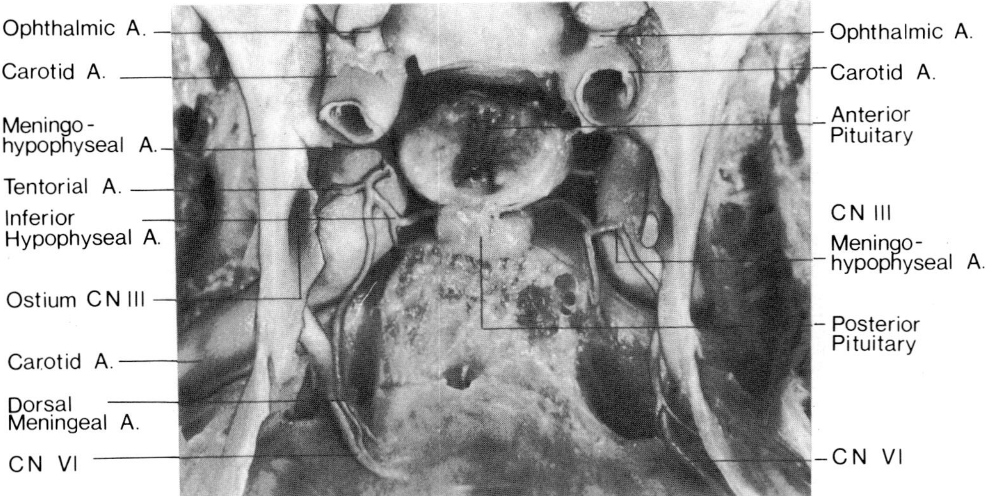

FIG. 15A. Superior view of the cavernous sinus, anterior and posterior lobe of the pituitary, intracavernous portion of the carotid artery, and the meningohypophyseal trunk with its three branches: the inferior hypophyseal, tentorial, and dorsal meningeal arteries. The ophthalmic artery arises from the anterior surface of the carotid artery above the clinoid and enters the optic canal under the optic nerve. The dorsum was removed to expose the posterior lobe of the pituitary. Cranial nerve VI receives a branch from the dorsal meningeal artery and courses laterally around the carotid artery. The dural ostium of cranial nerve III *(left)* is in the roof of the cavernous sinus, and cranial nerve III *(right)* enters its dural ostium. The carotid artery is exposed in the medial part of the foramen lacerum *(left)*. (From ref. 10.)

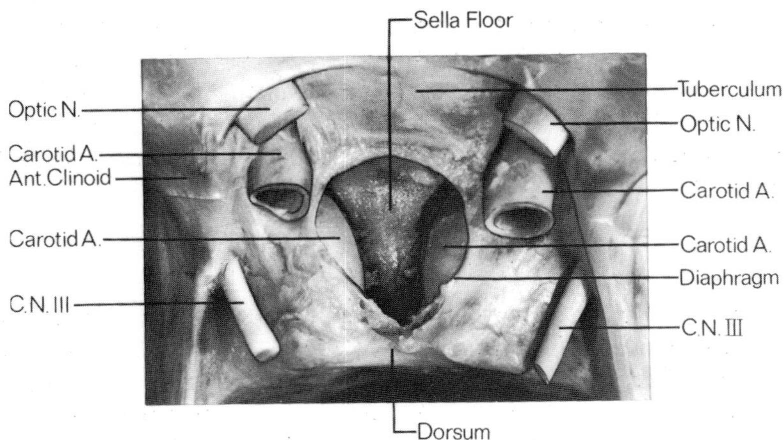

FIG. 15B. Superior view of the sellar region showing optic nerves, carotid arteries, and cranial nerve III. Carotid arteries bulge into the pituitary fossa. (From ref. 16.)

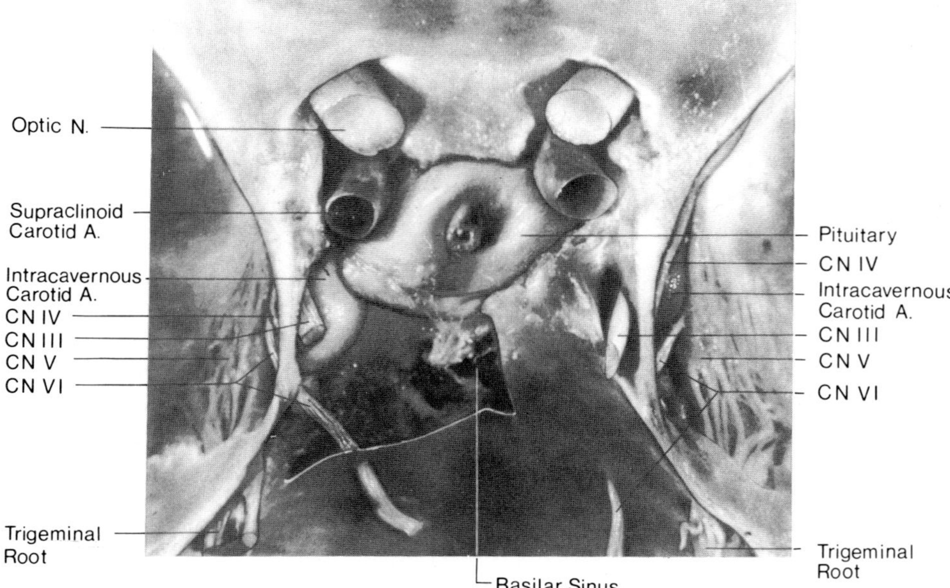

FIG. 15C. Superior view of the sellar region and both cavernous sinuses. The carotid artery indents the lateral margin of the pituitary gland, and a tongue of pituitary extends over the top of the artery. Cranial nerve VI passes through the dura and around the lateral margin of the carotid artery. Cranial nerve III enters the roof of the cavernous sinus lateral to the dorsum sellae. Cranial nerves III through VI are seen in the lateral wall of the cavernous sinus. (From ref. 10.)

sellae. Sellar length—defined as the greatest anteroposterior diameter of the pituitary fossa—may occur at the level of the tuberculum sellae or below. Sellar width is defined as the width of the horizontal plateau of the sellar floor. The volume is calculated by applying the simplified mathematical formula for the volume of an ellipsoid: volume (cm^3) = 0.5 (length × width × depth in mm)/100. The upper limit of normal depth is 13 mm, length 17 mm, and volume 1,100 mm (16).

Pituitary Gland and Carotid Artery

The distance separating the medial margin of the carotid artery and the lateral surface of the pituitary gland usually varies from 1 to 3 mm; however, in some specimens the artery protrudes through the medial wall of the cavernous sinus and indents the gland (Fig. 15). Heavy arterial bleeding during transsphenoidal hypophysectomy has been reported to be caused by carotid artery injury but may also arise from a tear in an arterial branch of the carotid artery (e.g., the inferior hypophyseal artery) or by avulsion of a small capsular branch from the carotid artery (11).

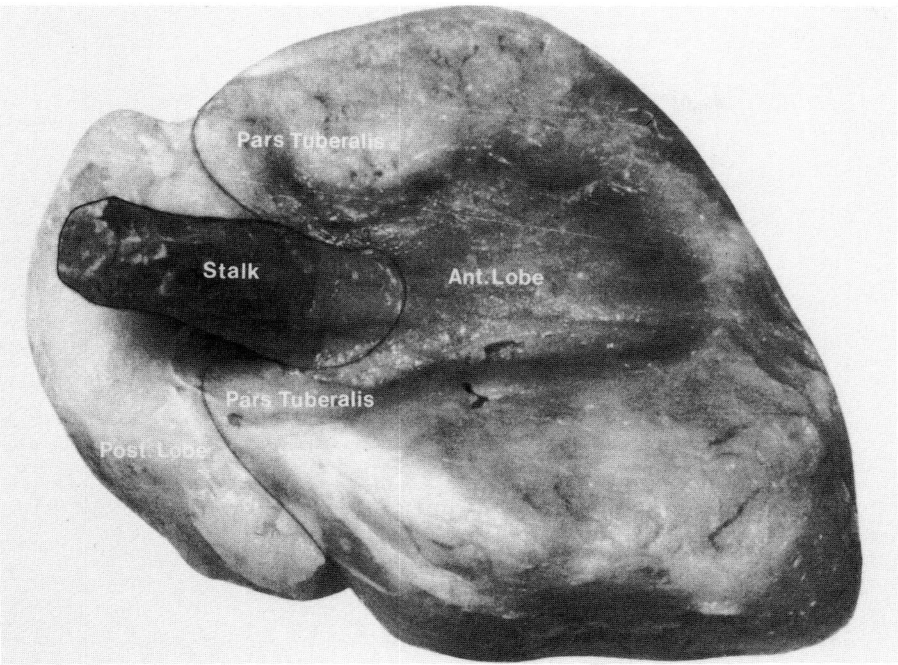

FIG. 16A. Pituitary gland: superolateral view. The posterior lobe is a lighter color and has a different consistency than the anterior lobe. The pars tuberalis partially encircles the stalk. The gland is concave around the stalk. (From ref. 17.)

If the carotid arteries indent the lateral surface of the gland, the gland loses its rounded shape and conforms to the wall of the artery, often developing protrusions above or below the artery. Intrasellar tumors are subjected to the same forces, which prevent them from being spherical, and the increased pressure within the tumor increases the degree to which the tumor insinuates into surrounding crevices and tissue planes. Separation of these extensions from the main mass of gland or tumor may explain cases in which functioning gland remains after hypophysectomy and others in which the tumor and elevated pituitary hormone levels recur long after the hormone levels have fallen to zero immediately following adenoma removal.

Intercavernous Venous Connections

Venous sinuses may be found in the margins of the diaphragma and around the gland. The intercavernous connections (Figs. 17 and 18) within the sella are named on the basis of their relationship to the pituitary gland; the anterior intercavernous sinuses pass anterior to the hypophysis, and the posterior intercav-

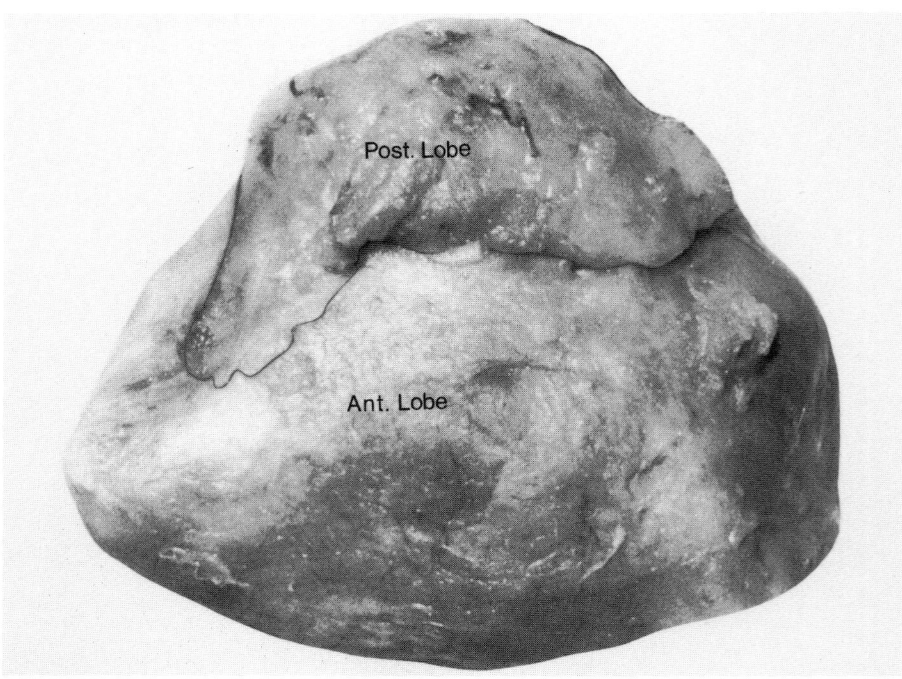

FIG. 16B. Pituitary gland: inferior view. Note the relationship of the anterior and posterior lobes. (From ref. 17.)

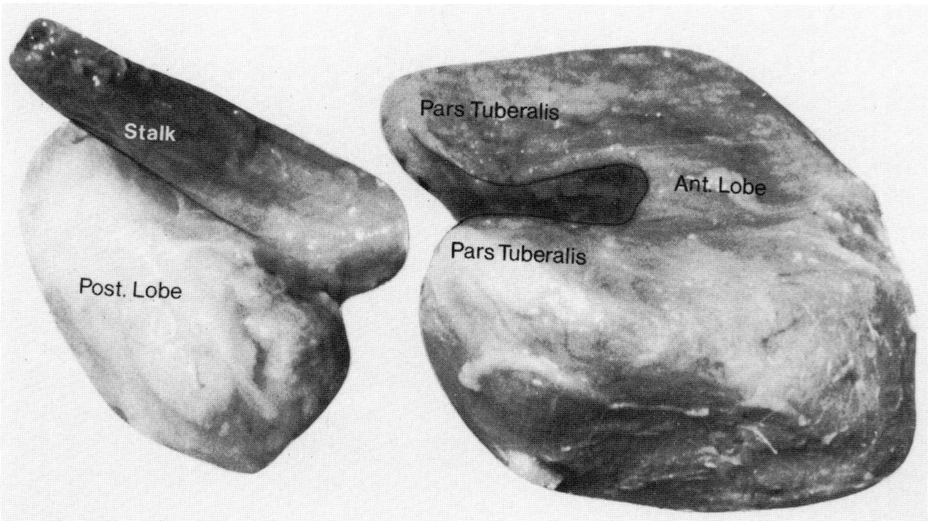

FIG. 16C. Pituitary gland: anterior and posterior lobe separated. The pars tuberalis partially encircles the stalk. (From ref. 17.)

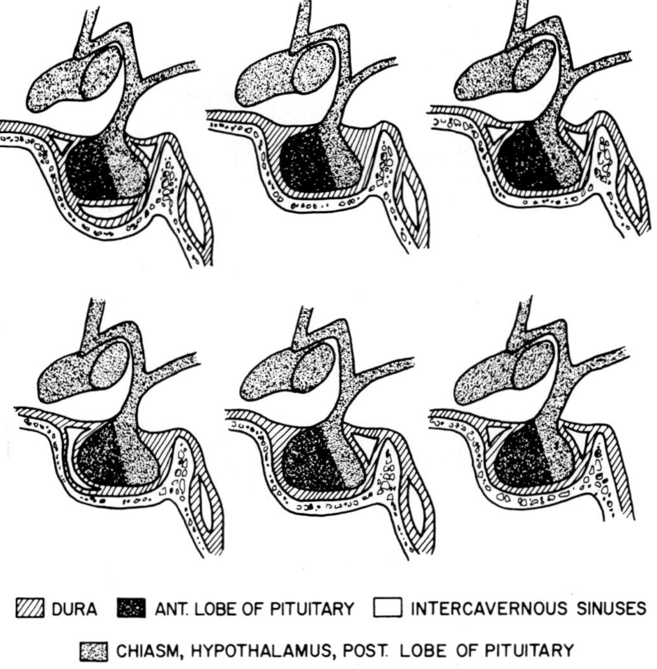

FIG. 17. Six sagittal sections of the sellar region showing variations in the intercavernous venous connections within the dura. The variations shown include combinations of anterior, posterior, and inferior intercavernous connections and the frequent presence of a basilar sinus posterior to the dorsum. Either the anterior **(lower center)** or posterior **(lower left)** intercavernous connection or both **(top center)** may be absent. The anterior intercavernous sinus may extend along the whole anterior margin of the gland **(lower left).** The basilar sinus may be absent **(lower right).** (From ref. 16.)

ernous sinuses pass behind the gland. Actually, these intercavernous connections can occur at any site along the anterior, inferior, or posterior surface of the gland. The anterior sinus is usually larger than the posterior sinus, but either or both may be absent. If the anterior and posterior connections coexist, the whole structure constitutes the "circular sinus." Entering an anterior intercavernous connection which extends downward in front of the gland during transsphenoidal surgery may produce brisk bleeding. However, this usually stops with temporary compression of the channel or with light monopolar diathermy, which serves to glue the walls of the channel together.

A large intercavernous venous connection called the basilar sinus often passes posterior to the dorsum sellae and upper clivus. The basilar sinus connects the posterior aspect of both cavernous sinuses and is usually the largest and most constant intercavernous connection across the midline. The superior and inferior petrosal sinuses join the basilar sinus. The abducens nerve often enters the posterior part of the cavernous sinus by passing through the basilar sinus.

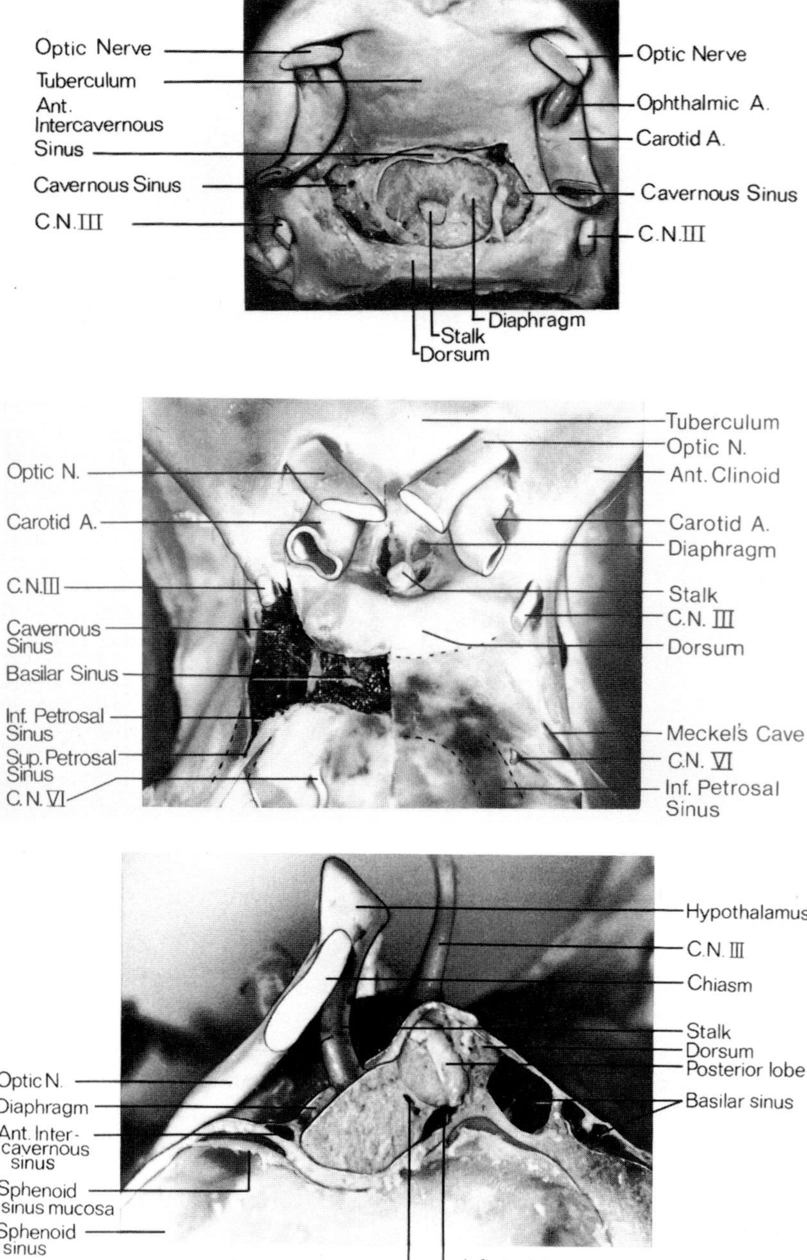

FIG. 18. Superior views of the sellar region. **A** *(top):* Ophthalmic arteries arise from the superior aspect of the carotid artery and course laterally beneath the optic nerves to the optic foramen. The dura over the cavernous and anterior intercavernous sinuses has been removed to show the venous connection across the midline. **B** *(middle):* Superior view of the sellar region showing

Arteriovenous fistulas between the branches of the meningohypophyseal trunk, especially the dorsal meningeal branch and the basilar sinus, may produce all the signs and symptoms associated with a fistula between the internal carotid artery and the cavernous sinus (10).

Cavernous Sinus

Lateral Wall and Roof

The cavernous sinus surrounds the horizontal portion of the carotid artery and a segment of the abducens nerve (Figs. 19 and 20). The oculomotor, troch-

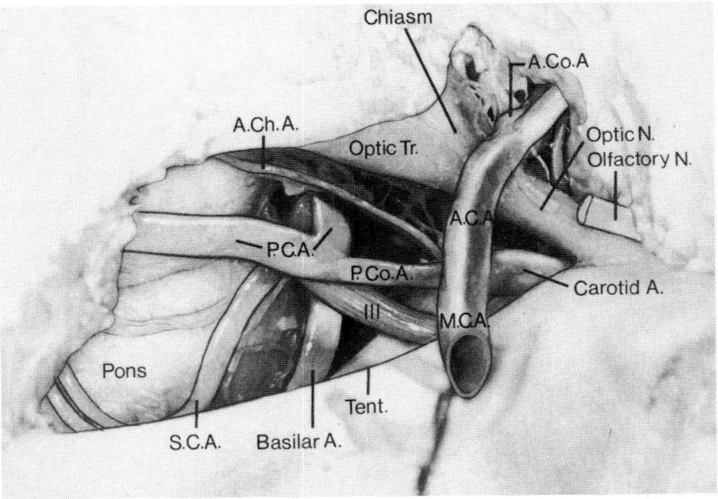

FIG. 19A. Right lateral view of the cavernous sinus and sellar area. Right lateral view, with dura over the cavernous sinus intact. Basilar (Basilar A.) and superior cerebellar (S.C.A.) arteries are seen medial to the tentorial edge (Tent.). Arteries seen in the suprasellar area are the anterior (A.Co.A.) and posterior (P.Co.A.) communicating; posterior (P.C.A.), middle (M.C.A.), and anterior (A.C.A.) cerebral; anterior choroidal (A.Ch.A.); and carotid (Carotid A.). The oculomotor nerve (III) passes forward between the posterior cerebral and superior cerebellar arteries. The optic nerve passes posteriorly to become the optic tract (Optic Tr.). The olfactory nerve is above the optic nerve. (From ref. 17.)

---

optic nerves, carotid arteries, cranial nerves III and VI, and the pituitary stalk. The basilar sinus connects the posterior portion of the two cavernous sinuses. The dura over the posterior aspect of the left cavernous sinus and the left half of the basilar sinus was removed. The course of the basilar, inferior petrosal, and superior petrosal sinus within the dura is shown by the dotted lines. **C** *(bottom):* Midline sagittal section of the sellar region showing the optic nerve and chiasm, cranial nerve III, inferior part of the hypothalamus, and the pituitary stalk and gland. The anterior and inferior intercavernous sinuses are small. The basilar sinus, dorsal to the clivus and joining the posterior aspect of the two cavernous sinuses, is the largest connection across the midline. The anterior sellar wall bulging into the sphenoid sinus is very thin. (From ref. 16.)

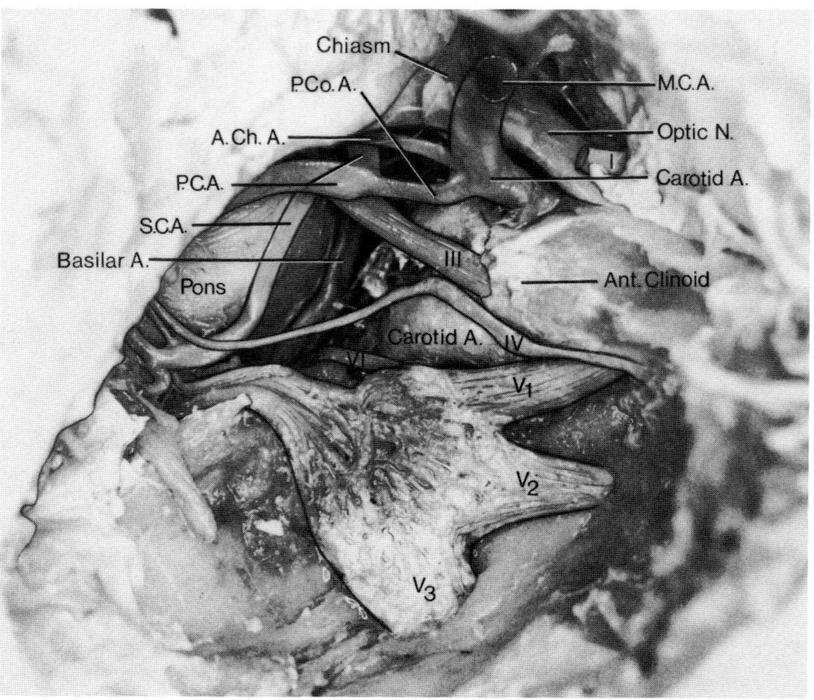

FIG. 19B. Right lateral view of the cavernous sinus and sellar area. The dura over the lateral wall of the cavernous sinus is removed to expose the trigeminal nerve and its ophthalmic (V_1), maxillary (V_2), and mandibular (V_3) divisions, the intracavernous portion of the carotid artery, and the trochlear (IV) and abducens (VI) nerves. The anterior clinoid (Ant.Clinoid) process is below the carotid artery. (From ref. 17.)

lear, and ophthalmic divisions of the trigeminal nerve are found in the roof and lateral wall of the sinus. The lateral wall of the cavernous sinus extends from the superior orbital fissure in front to the apex of the petrous portion of the temporal bone behind. The oculomotor nerve enters the roof of the sinus lateral to the dorsum sellae. The trochlear nerve enters the roof of the sinus posterolateral to the third nerve, and both nerves enter the dura immediately below and medial to the free edge of the tentorium. The ophthalmic division of the trigeminal nerve enters the low part of the lateral wall of the sinus and runs obliquely upward to exit through the superior orbital fissure. The abducens nerve enters the posterior wall of the sinus by passing through the dura lining the upper clivus and courses forward between the intracavernous carotid artery medially and the ophthalmic division laterally. It frequently splits into multiple rootlets in its course lateral to the carotid artery.

Parkinson's Triangle and the Intracavernous Portion of the Carotid Artery

Parkinson described a triangle within the lateral wall of the cavernous sinus through which the intracavernous portion of the carotid artery and its branches

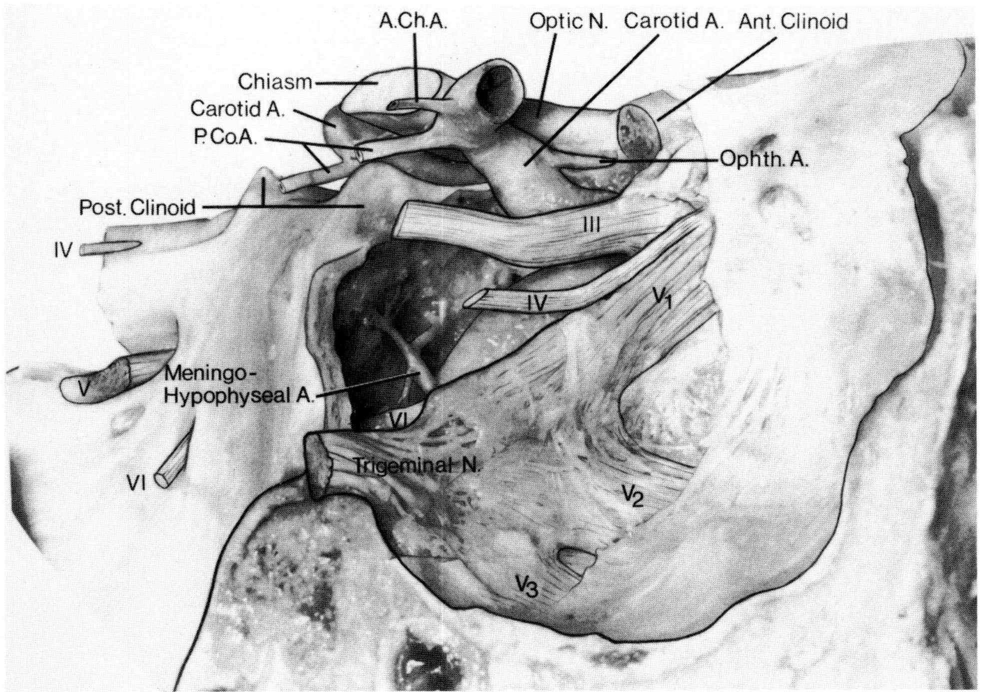

FIG. 19C. Right lateral view of the cavernous sinus and sellar area. Brain is removed to show the relationship of the cavernous sinus to the clivus and suprasellar structures. The meningohypophyseal artery arises from the intracavernous carotid artery. Removal of the anterior clinoid process reveals the origin of the ophthalmic artery (Ophth.A.). (From ref. 17.)

might be exposed for the surgical treatment of carotid cavernous fistulas (13). The boundaries of the triangle are the lower border of the fourth nerve superiorly, the upper margin of the fifth nerve inferiorly, and the slope along the dorsum sellae and clivus posteriorly (Figs. 19 and 20).

Parkinson opened into the cavernous sinus by incising the dura within Parkinson's triangle starting approximately 6 mm below the dural entrance of the third nerve and extending anteriorly for 2 cm parallel to the slope of the third and fourth nerves, and retracting the leaves of the dura. The intracavernous course of the extraocular nerves can be located through this opening. Retracting the ophthalmic division of the trigeminal nerve inferolaterally exposes the abducens nerve between the trigeminal nerve and the carotid artery. We found in previous studies that it may be difficult to expose all branches of the intracavernous portion of the carotid artery through this opening.

Carotid Artery and Trigeminal Nerve

The intracavernous portion of the carotid artery (Figs. 19 and 20) begins lateral to the posterior clinoid process, where it exits the foramen lacerum and

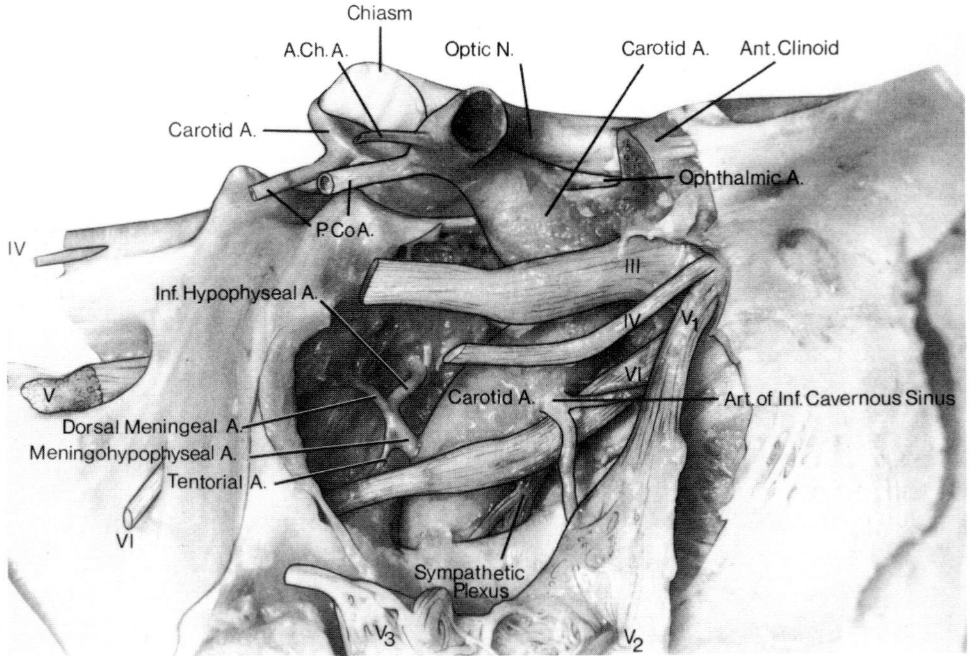

FIG. 19D. Right lateral view of the cavernous sinus and sellar area. The trigeminal nerve is reflected forward to show the abducens nerve; the origin of the meningohypophyseal artery and its tentorial, dorsal meningeal, and inferior hypophyseal branches; and the artery of the inferior cavernous sinus (Art.Inf.Cav.Sinus). The sympathetic plexus is around the carotid artery. (From ref. 17.)

turns abruptly forward to enter the cavernous sinus. It then passes forward in a horizontal direction for approximately 2 cm and terminates by passing upward along the medial side to the anterior clinoid process to perforate the roof of the cavernous sinus. Just proximal to the cavernous sinus in the foramen lacerum, the artery lies beneath the trigeminal nerve and may be separated from it by dura and bone. In a previous study a portion of this bone was found to be deficient in 86% of cases, and only dura separated the artery from the nerve (10). Bundles of sympathetic nerve fibers may be seen on the wall of the carotid artery in the foramen lacerum. The cavernous portion of the artery is relatively fixed by the bony ring formed by the anterior and middle clinoid processes and the carotid sulcus, but despite this large extensions of pituitary tumor may produce lateral displacement of the artery (2).

Branches of the Intracavernous Carotid Artery

The branches of the intracavernous portion of the carotid artery are the meningohypophyseal trunk, the artery of the inferior cavernous sinus, and

McConnell's capsular arteries (Figs. 19 and 20). The ophthalmic artery may also take origin from the carotid within the sinus in a few cases (16). The most proximal branch of the intracavernous carotid artery, the meningohypophyseal trunk, usually arises below the level of the dorsum sellae near the apex of the curve between the petrous and intracavernous segments of the artery. The three branches of the meningohypophyseal artery are the tentorial artery (of Bernasconi-Cassinari), which courses toward the tentorium; the inferior hypophyseal artery, which courses medially to supply the posterior part of the capsule of the pituitary gland; and the dorsal meningeal artery, which perforates the dura of the posterior wall of the sinus to supply the region of the clivus and the sixth nerve.

The artery of the inferior cavernous sinus originates from the lateral side of the horizontal segment of the carotid artery distal to the origin of the meningohypophyseal trunk. It passes above the abducens nerve and downward medially to the first trigeminal division to supply the dura of the lateral wall of the sinus. In a few cases it arises from the meningohypophyseal trunk.

McConnell's capsular arteries, if present, arise from the medial side of the carotid artery and pass to the capsule of the gland, distal to the point of origin of the artery of the inferior cavernous sinus.

Sphenoid Sinus

Pneumatization of the Sphenoid Sinus

The sphenoid sinus is subject to considerable variation in size and shape and to variation in the degree of pneumatization (4,8,17,18) (Figs. 2,21–23). It is present as minute cavities at birth, but its main development takes place after puberty. In early life, it extends backward into the presellar area and subsequently expands into the area below and behind the sella turcica, reaching its full size during adolescence. As the sinus enlarges, it may partially encircle the optic canals. When the sinus is exceptionally large, it extends into the roots of the pterygoid processes or greater wing of the sphenoid bone and may even extend into the basilar part of the occipital bone. As age advances, the sinus frequently undergoes further enlargement associated with absorption of its bony walls. Occasionally there are gaps in its bone with the mucous membrane lying directly against the dura mater. In our previous study in adult cadavers, this sinus was found to be of a presellar type in 24% and of the sellar type in 75% (16). If the infrequent conchal type is present, the thickness of bone separating the sella turcica from the sphenoid sinus is at least 10 mm.

The measurement of the distance from the anterior margin of the sinus to the sellar floor defines the length of the path within the sinus through which instruments must pass to reach the sellar wall. This measurement is important when selecting instruments for transsphenoidal surgery. The speculum most

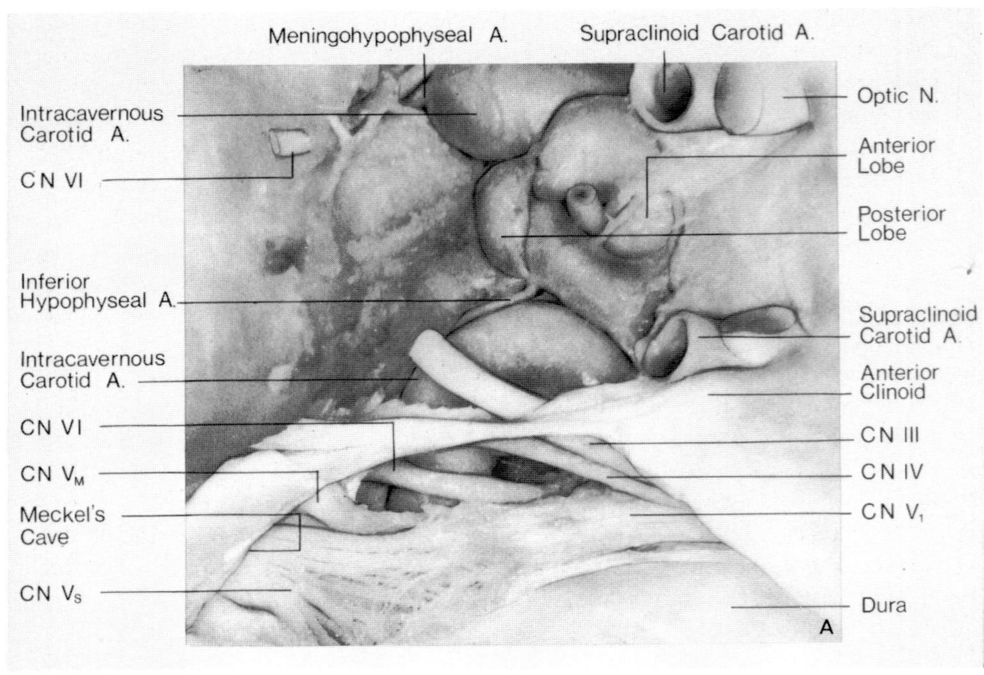
Meningohypophyseal A.
Supraclinoid Carotid A.
Intracavernous Carotid A.
CN VI
Inferior Hypophyseal A.
Intracavernous Carotid A.
CN VI
CN V_M
Meckel's Cave
CN V_S
Optic N.
Anterior Lobe
Posterior Lobe
Supraclinoid Carotid A.
Anterior Clinoid
CN III
CN IV
CN V_1
Dura
A

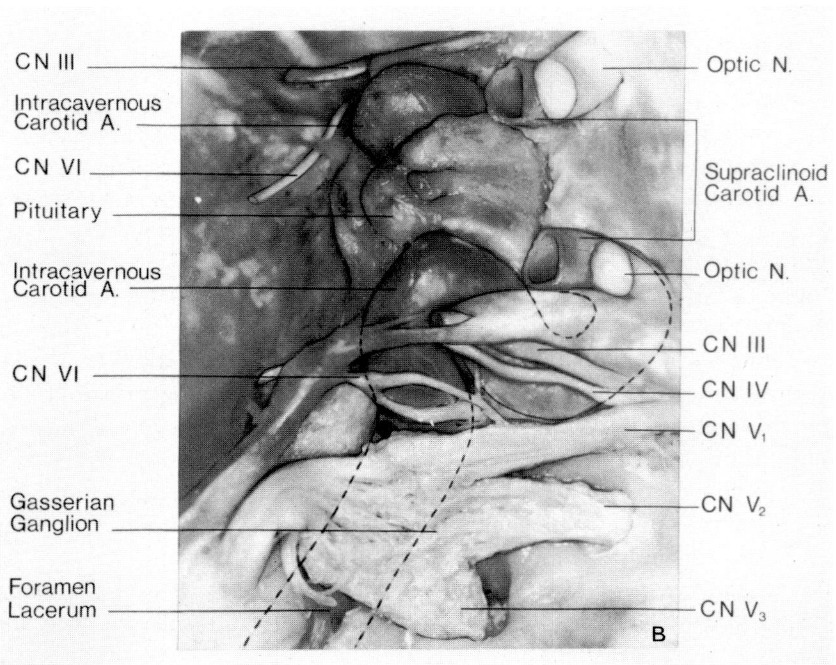
CN III
Intracavernous Carotid A.
CN VI
Pituitary
Intracavernous Carotid A.
CN VI
Gasserian Ganglion
Foramen Lacerum
Optic N.
Supraclinoid Carotid A.
Optic N.
CN III
CN IV
CN V_1
CN V_2
CN V_3
B

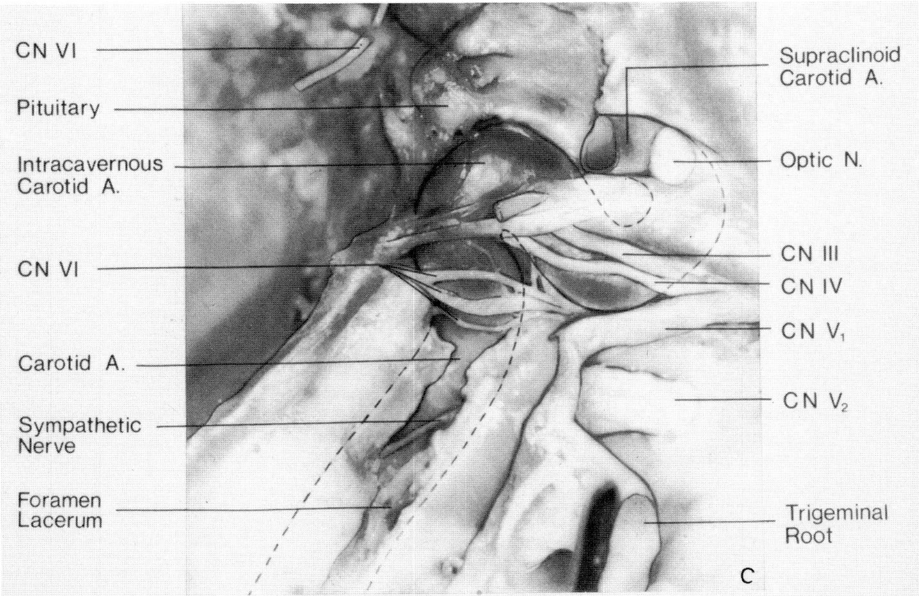

FIG. 20. Superolateral view of the pituitary gland, right cavernous sinus, and intracavernous structures including the carotid artery and cranial nerves III, IV, and VI. **A:** The lateral dural wall of the cavernous sinus is removed. The tortuous carotid artery bulges superiorly, pushing the interclinoid ligament and cavernous sinus roof upward and indenting the lateral margin of the pituitary gland. The inferior hypophyseal artery passes to the pituitary gland. Cranial nerves III and IV enter the roof of the cavernous sinus by passing through the interclinoid ligament. Cranial nerve VI on the left side enters the dura posterior to the dorsum and passes laterally around the left carotid artery. Cranial nerve VI is above the superior margin of the trigeminal sensory (CN V_s) and motor (CN V_m) roots, and only the first division (CN V_1) is exposed distal to the ganglion. **B:** Further dural removal exposes the trigeminal root and its second (CN V_2) and their (CN V_3) divisions. The foramen lacerum is exposed lateral to the gasserian ganglion. The trigeminal root is reflected laterally to show a second branch of cranial nerve, VI, as it passes lateral to the carotid artery. **C:** The trigeminal root is reflected forward, exposing the carotid artery in the foramen lacerum. A sympathetic nerve bundle is on the surface of the carotid artery in the foramen lacerum. Three rootlets of cranial nerve VI are seen passing around the carotid. The outline of the carotid artery is marked with a broken line in the areas where it is out of view in the petrous bone and in the cavernous sinus. (From ref. 10.)

commonly used for transsphenoidal surgery is 9 cm in length, and its tip should be placed anterior to the sphenoid sinus. When reaching the floor of the sellae, the depth of the sphenoid sinus (2 cm or more) is added to the 9 cm length of the speculum (4). Thus after traversing a distance of 11 to 12 cm, the dissecting instruments must then enter the sella and be able to reach above the sella if a suprasellar tumor is present. As the distance may be greater in the presence of acromegaly, it is important that transsphenoidal instruments have shafts at least 12 cm in length.

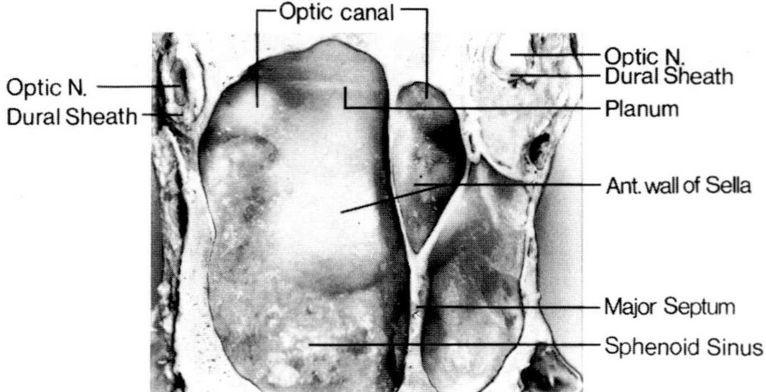

FIG. 21A. Anterior view of the sphenoid sinus. Anterior wall of the sella bulges into the posterior part of the sinus. The optic canals bulge into the superolateral part of the sinus. The major septum is located off the midline and separates the sinus into asymmetrical cavities. (From ref. 16.)

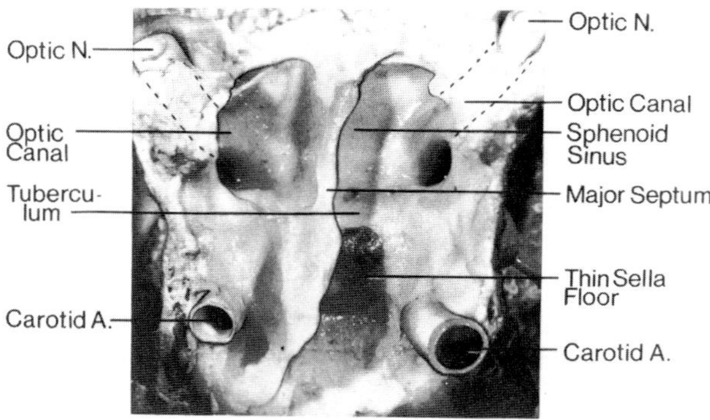

FIG. 21B. Anterior view of the sphenoid sinus. Inferior surface of the sella as seen through the upper half of the sphenoid sinus. Optic canals bulge into superolateral parts of the sinus, and carotid arteries bulge into posterolateral parts of the sinus. The major septum deviates off the midline as it approaches the sellar floor. The sellar floor to the right of the septum is so thin that light transmits through it. (From ref. 16.)

Sphenoid Septae

The septae within the sphenoid sinus (Fig. 24) vary greatly in size, shape, thickness, location, completeness, and relation to the sellar floor. The cavities within the sinus are seldom symmetrical from side to side and are often subdivided by irregular minor septae. The septae are often located off the midline as they cross the floor of the sella. In our previous study a single major septum separated the sinus into two large cavities in only 68% of specimens, and even in these cases the septae were often located off the midline or were deflected to one side (16). The most common type of sphenoid sinus has multiple small

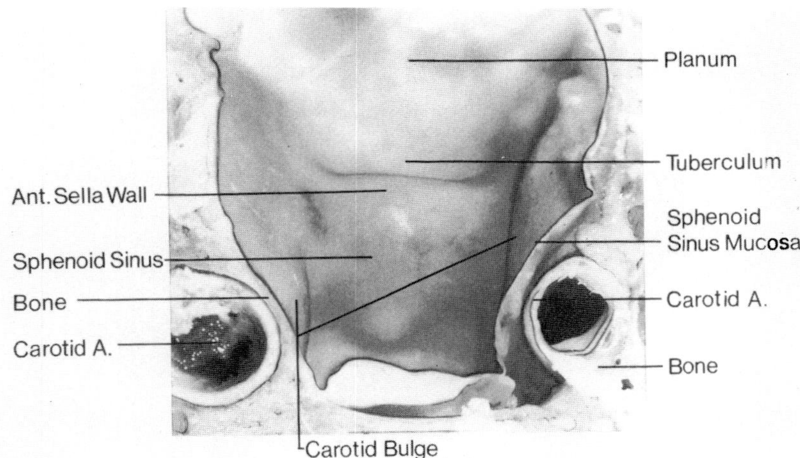

FIG. 21C. Anterior view of the sphenoid sinus. Inferior view of the sella through the sphenoid sinus. The sinus is composed of a single large cavity and is not divided by a septum. The right carotid artery is separated from the sinus by only sinus mucosa. The left carotid artery is covered by bone less than 1 mm thick. (From ref. 16.)

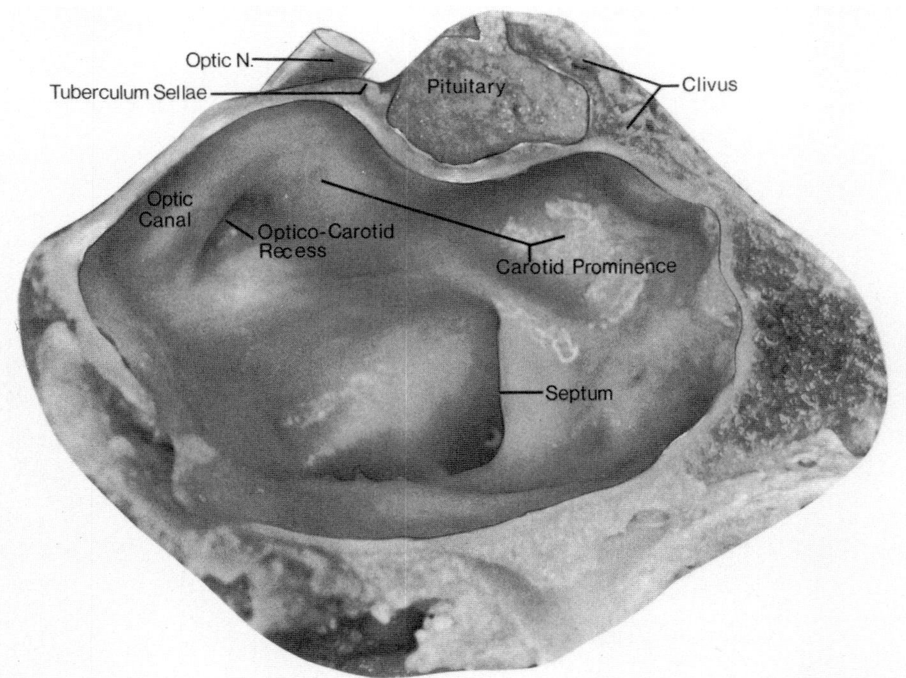

FIG. 22. Stepwise dissection of the lateral wall of the right half of a sellar-type sphenoid sinus and adjacent structures (see pages 43–45). **Step A:** The sphenoid sinus and sellar area are divided in the midsagittal plane. The optic nerve (Optic N.) is seen proximal to the optic canal. The opticocarotid recess separates the carotid prominence and optic canal. The septum in the posterior part of the sinus is incomplete. (From ref. 4.)

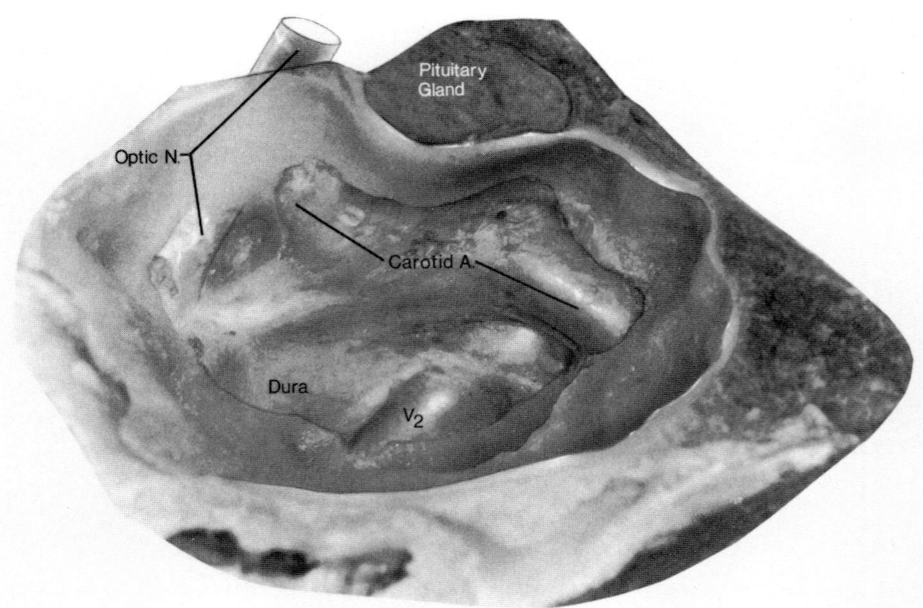

FIG. 22. Step B: The sinus mucosa and thin bone of the lateral sinus wall are removed to expose dura covering the carotid artery (Carotid A.), the second trigeminal division (V_2) just distal to trigeminal ganglion, and the optic nerve. (From ref. 4.)

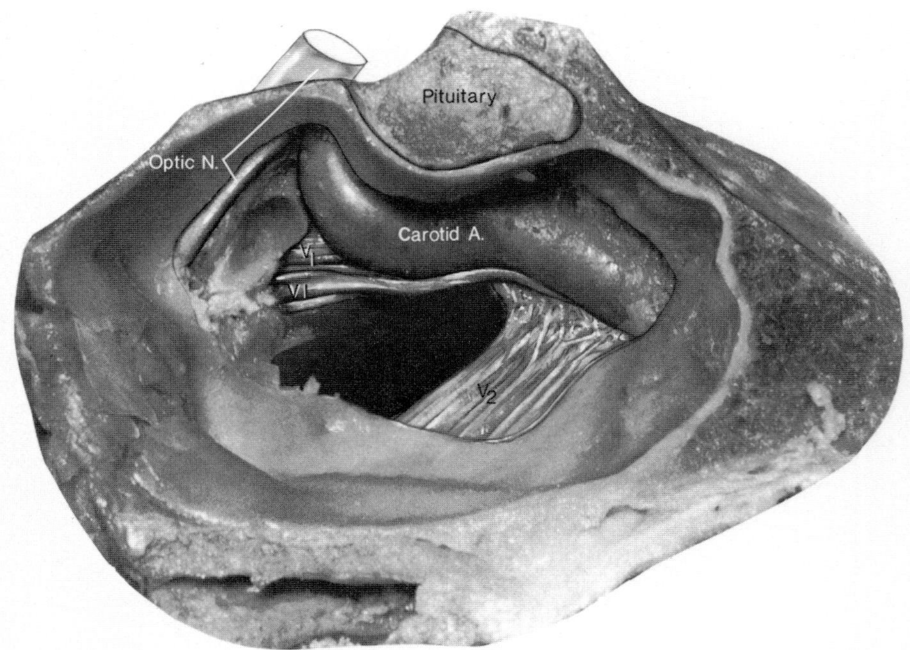

FIG. 22. Step C: The dura is opened to expose the carotid artery, the optic nerve in the optic canal, the second trigeminal division below the carotid artery, the abducens nerve (VI) between the first trigeminal division (V_1), and the carotid artery. (From ref. 4.)

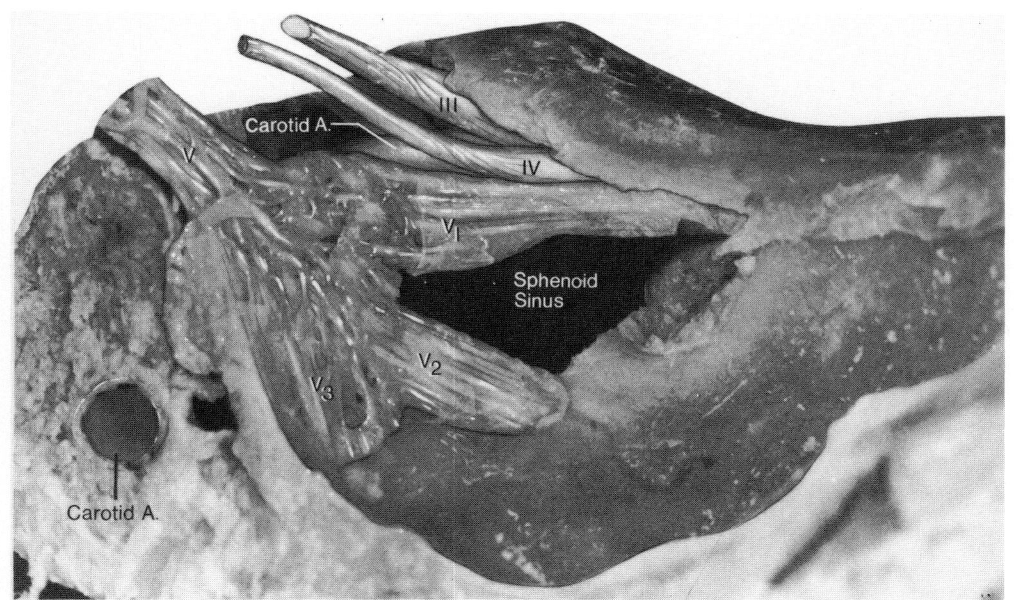

FIG. 22. Step D: Lateral view of the specimen showing area of the cavernous sinus. The oculomotor (III) and trochlear (IV) nerves are seen above. The intracavernous portion of the carotid artery is seen medial to the trigeminal root (V) and the ophthalmic, maxillary, and mandibular divisions (V_3) of the trigeminal nerve. The petrous portion of the carotid artery is seen in cross section below the trigeminal nerve. The opening into the sphenoid sinus is located between the first and second trigeminal divisions. (From ref. 4.)

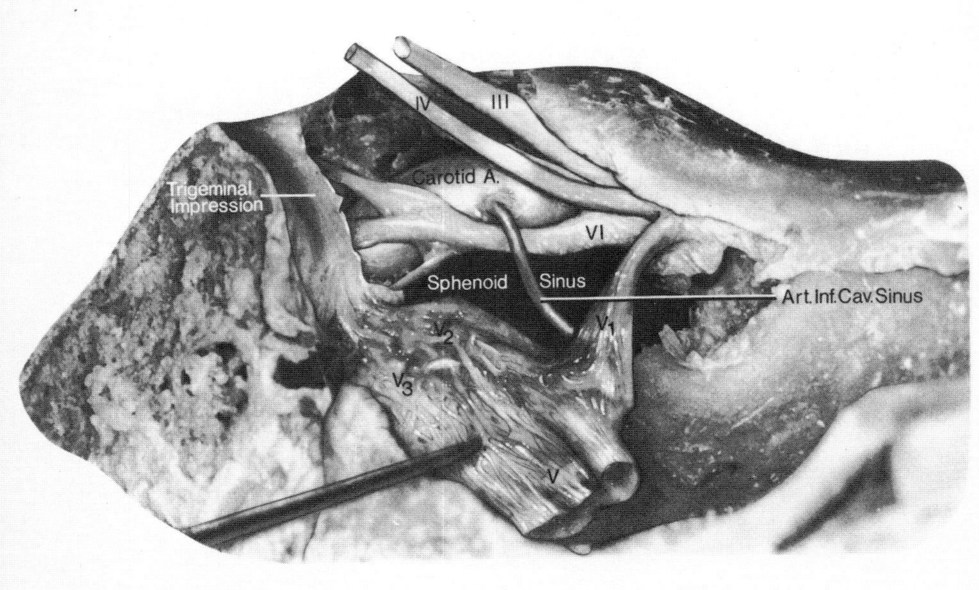

FIG. 22. Step E: Trigeminal nerve is reflected forward to expose the carotid artery, trigeminal impression, the artery of the inferior cavernous sinus (Art.Inf.Cav.Sinus), and the abducens nerve, which splits into three bundles as it passes around the carotid artery. (From ref. 4.)

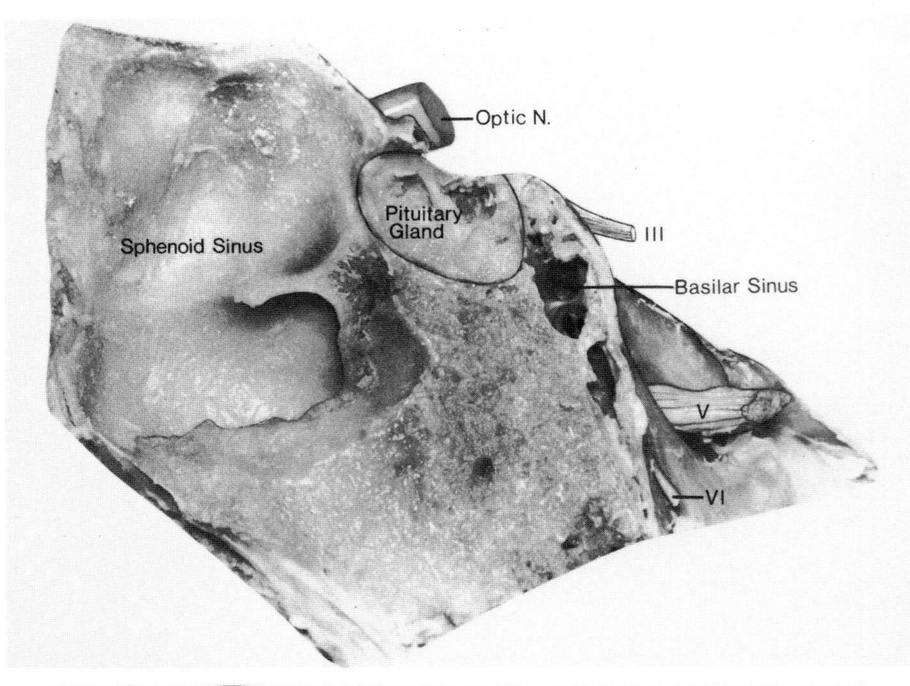

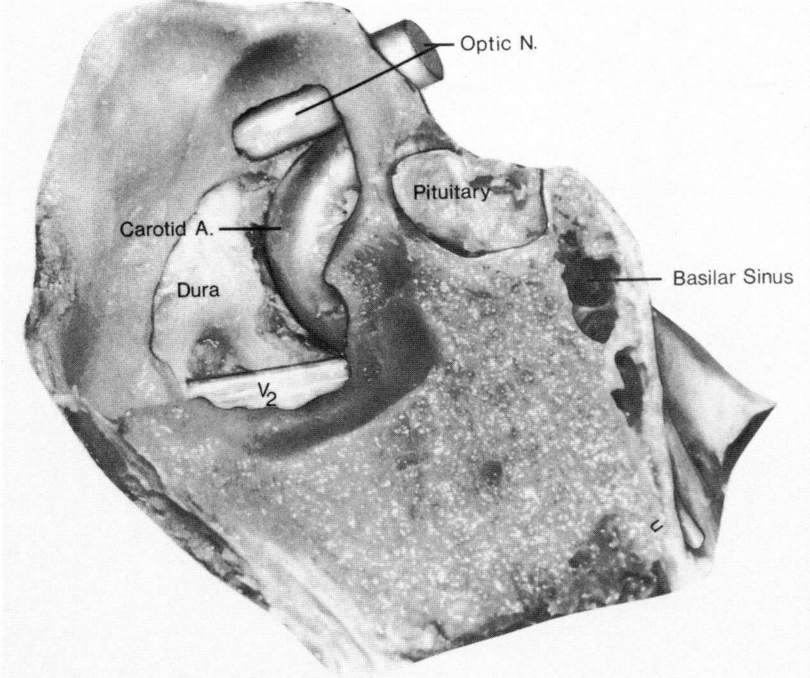

FIG. 23. Stepwise dissection of the lateral wall of the right half of a presellar-type sphenoid sinus and adjacent structures. **A:** The sphenoid sinus and sellar area are divided in the midsagittal plane. The sinus air cavity does not extend posteriorly below the sellar floor. The optic nerve is above the pituitary gland. The oculomotor (III), trigeminal (V), and abducens (VI) nerves are posterior to the clivus. A large dural venous sinus (Basilar Sinus) is posterior to the clivus. **B:** The sinus mucosa and thin bone of the lateral wall are removed to expose the carotid artery, second trigeminal division (V_2), optic nerve in optic canal, and dura. (From. ref. 4.)

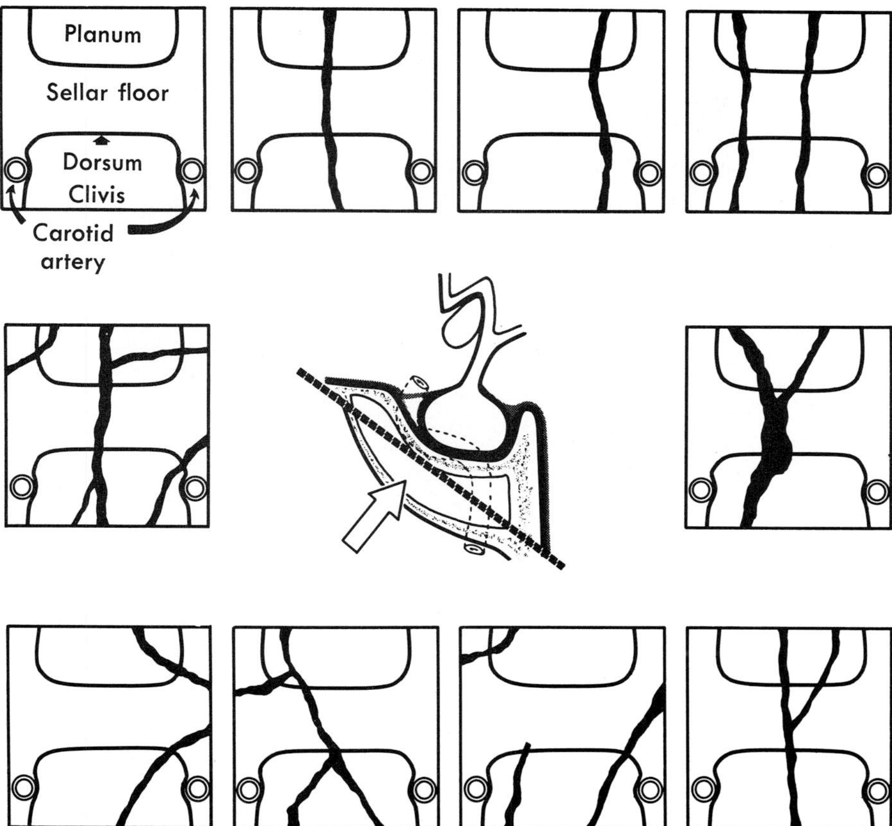

FIG. 24. Septa in sphenoid sinus. The broken line on the central diagram shows the plane of the section of each specimen from which the drawings were taken, and the large arrow shows the direction of view of the specimens. The planum is above, the dorsum and clivus are below, and the sella is in an intermediate position on each diagram. The heavy dark lines on the drawings show the location of the septa in the sphenoid sinus. A wide variety of septae separate the sinus into cavities that vary in size and shape, seldom being symmetrical from side to side. (From ref. 16.)

cavities in the large paired sinuses. The smaller cavities are separated by septae oriented in all directions. Anteroposterior tomograms of the sella are essential to define the relationship of the septae to the floor of the sella for transsphenoidal surgery. Major septae may be found as far as 8 mm off the midline (16).

Lateral Wall of Sphenoid Sinus

The carotid artery frequently produces a serpigenous prominence into the sinus wall below the floor and along the anterior margin of the sella (Figs. 22,23,25). The optic canals usually protrude into the superolateral portion of

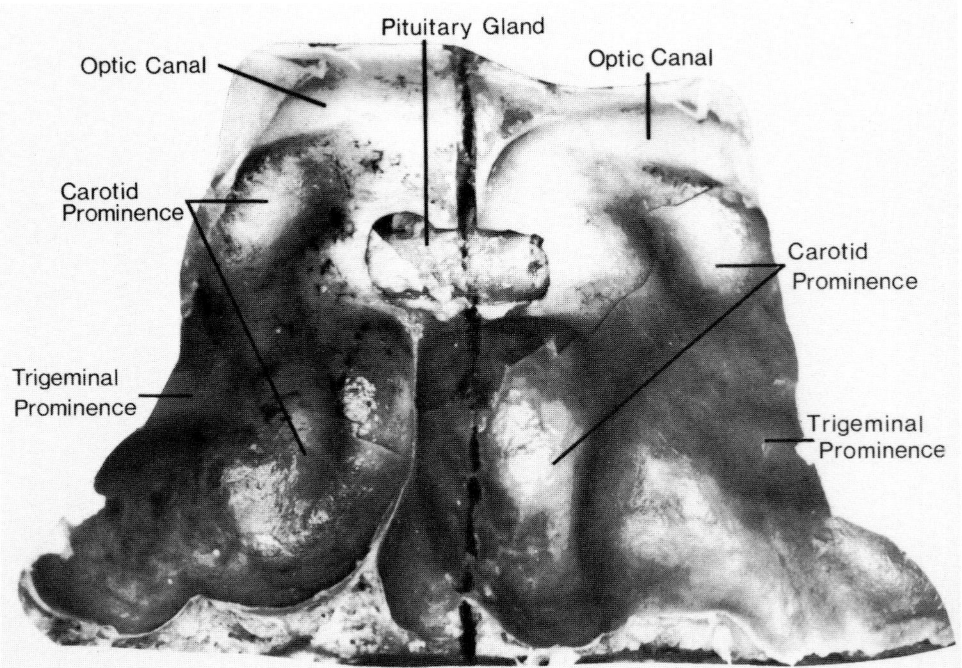

FIG. 25A. Anterior views of a sellar-type sphenoid sinus. The anterior wall of the sella is removed to expose the pituitary gland. The specimen was split in midline. The air cavity is wider below than above, as is typical in a well-pneumatized specimen. The optic canals are above. Carotid prominences are lateral to the sella. The trigeminal prominence is below the carotid prominence. (From ref. 4.)

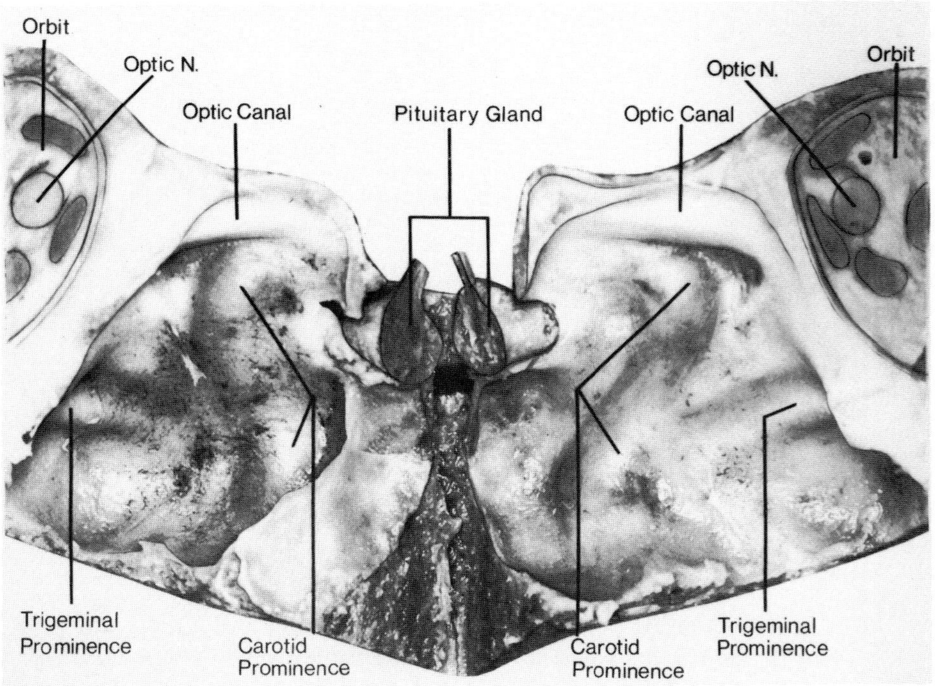

FIG. 25B. Anterior views of a sellar-type sphenoid sinus. The specimen is opened slightly to provide a better view of the lateral wall and the carotid and trigeminal prominences. (From ref. 4.)

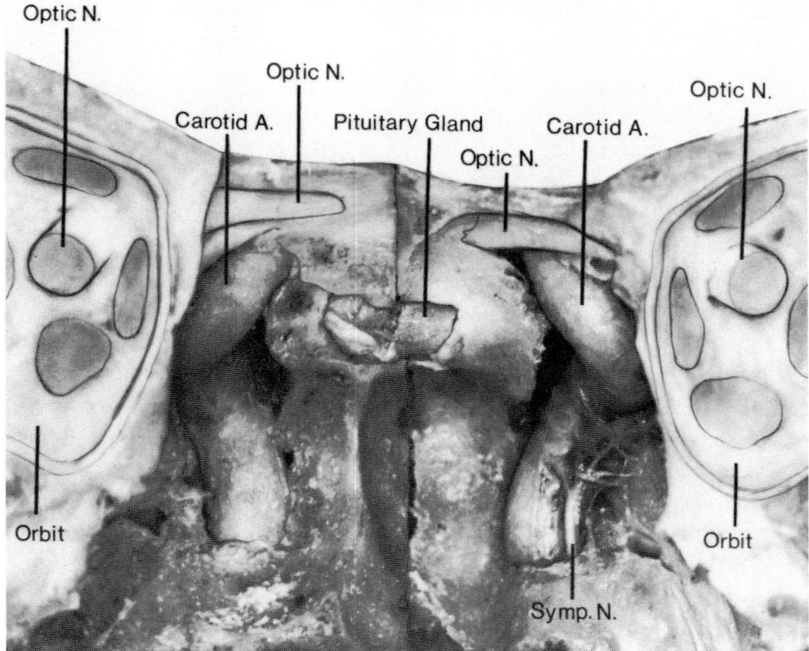

FIG. 25C. Anterior views of a sellar-type sphenoid sinus. Mucosa, dura, and bone of the lateral wall of the sinus are removed to expose parasphenoidal segments of the carotid artery. Sympathetic nerves (Symp.N.) are anterior to the left carotid artery. Orbital contents appear laterally. (From ref. 4.)

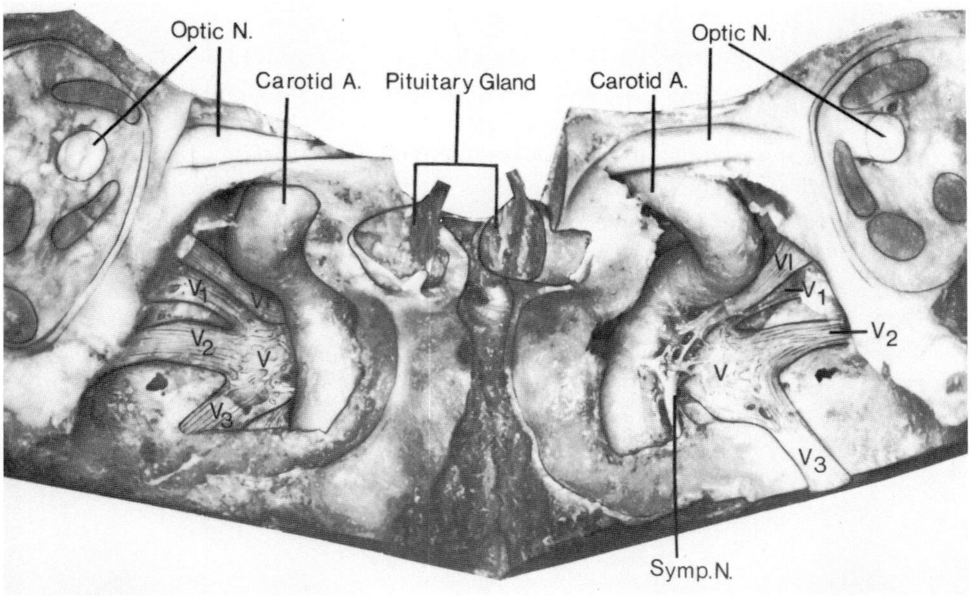

FIG. 25D. Anterior views of a sellar-type sphenoid sinus. Specimen is spread slightly to show abducens (VI) and ophthalmic (V_1), maxillary (V_2), and mandibular (V_3) divisions of the trigeminal nerve (V). (From ref. 4.)

the sinus, and the second division of the trigeminal nerve into the inferolateral part. A diverticulum of the sinus, called the opticocarotid recess, often projects laterally between the optic canal and the carotid prominence.

Removing the mucosa and bone from the lateral wall of the sinus exposes the dura covering the medial surface of the cavernous sinus and optic canals. Opening this dura exposes the carotid arteries and optic and trigeminal nerves within the sinus. The sixth cranial nerve is located between the lateral side of the carotid artery and the medial side of the first trigeminal division. The second and third trigeminal divisions are seen in the lower margin of the opening through the lateral wall of the sphenoid sinus. In half of the cases the optic and trigeminal nerves and the carotid arteries have areas where bone 0.5 mm or less in thickness separate them from the mucosa of the sphenoid sinus, and in a few cases the bone separating these structures from the sinus is absent (4,16). The absence of such bony protection within the walls of the sinus may explain some of the cases of cranial nerve deficits and carotid artery injury reported following transsphenoidal surgery (16). The bone is often thinner over the carotid arteries than over the anterior margin of the pituitary gland.

DISSECTION EXERCISES FOR THE TRANSSPHENOIDAL APPROACH

Although the transsphenoidal approach for sellar tumors was first used by Schloffer in 1907 and Cushing in 1912, the approach subsequently fell into disfavor because of the high incidence of complications and because of the difficulty operating through such a deep, narrow exposure (3,21). However, in 1958 Guiot reintroduced the technique, this time using radiofluoroscopy to visualize, in the lateral view, the depth and position of the surgical instruments (5,6). This, in combination with the intense illumination and magnification provided by the operating microscope, afforded the possibility of a safe operation and more accurate visualization of normal and pathological tissues (Fig. 26). These innovations led to the technique becoming the method of choice for removal of microadenomas of the pituitary gland and selected other sellar tumors. Even those with suprasellar extensions may be approached by this route if they extend above an enlarged sella. Since its reintroduction, the approach has been used extensively by Hardy and others and now forms part of the standard neurosurgical repertoire (8,9). The approach has also been used for clival and upper midline posterior fossa lesions.

Materials and Equipment

Dry sphenoid bones, those in which all soft tissues have been removed chemically and the bone dried, and a number of dry skulls with the calvaria removed to allow inspection of the pituitary fossa are needed. The dry skulls and disarticulated sphenoid bones can be obtained from an anatomic supply dealer.

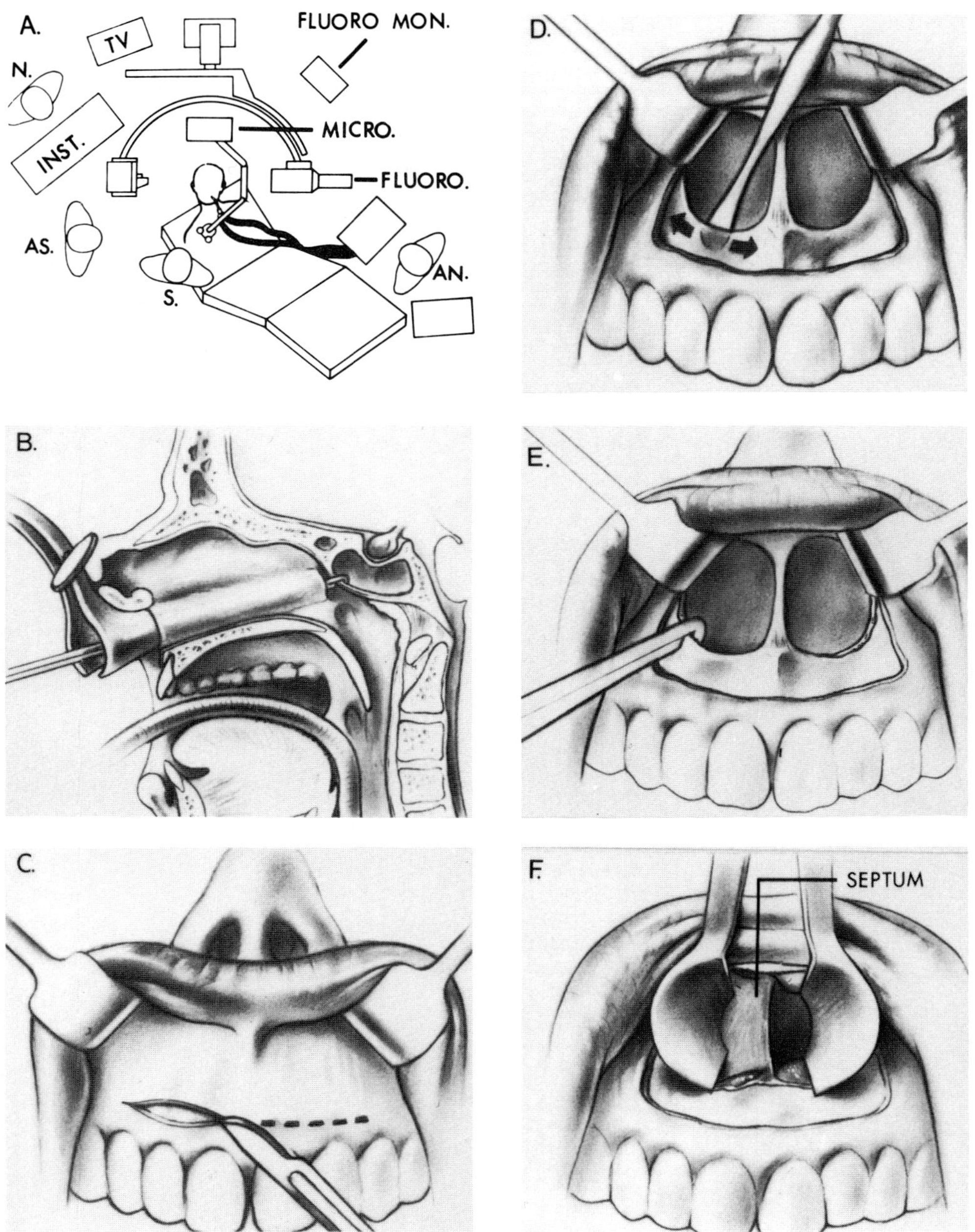

FIG. 26A–F. Transsphenoidal approach to sellar lesions. **A:** Operating room floor plan used for transsphenoidal surgery (AN) anesthesiologist. (AS) surgical assistant. (FLUORO) fluoroscopy unit. (FLUORO MON) fluoroscopy monitor. (INST) instrument tray. (MICRO) ceiling-mounted surgical microscope. (N) nurse. (S) surgeon. (TV) television monitor from surgical microscope. **B:** Hardy oronasal transsphenoidal approach to sella. Hardy speculum lifts upper lip and spreads nasal mucosa away from septum to provide exposure. **C:** Sublabial incision. **D:** Mucosa being elevated from floor of nose. **E:** Bony cavum being enlarged. **F:** Bivalve speculum introduced a short distance prior to incising nasal cartilage in front of vomer. Cartilage is attached to mucosa on right side. (From ref. 19.)

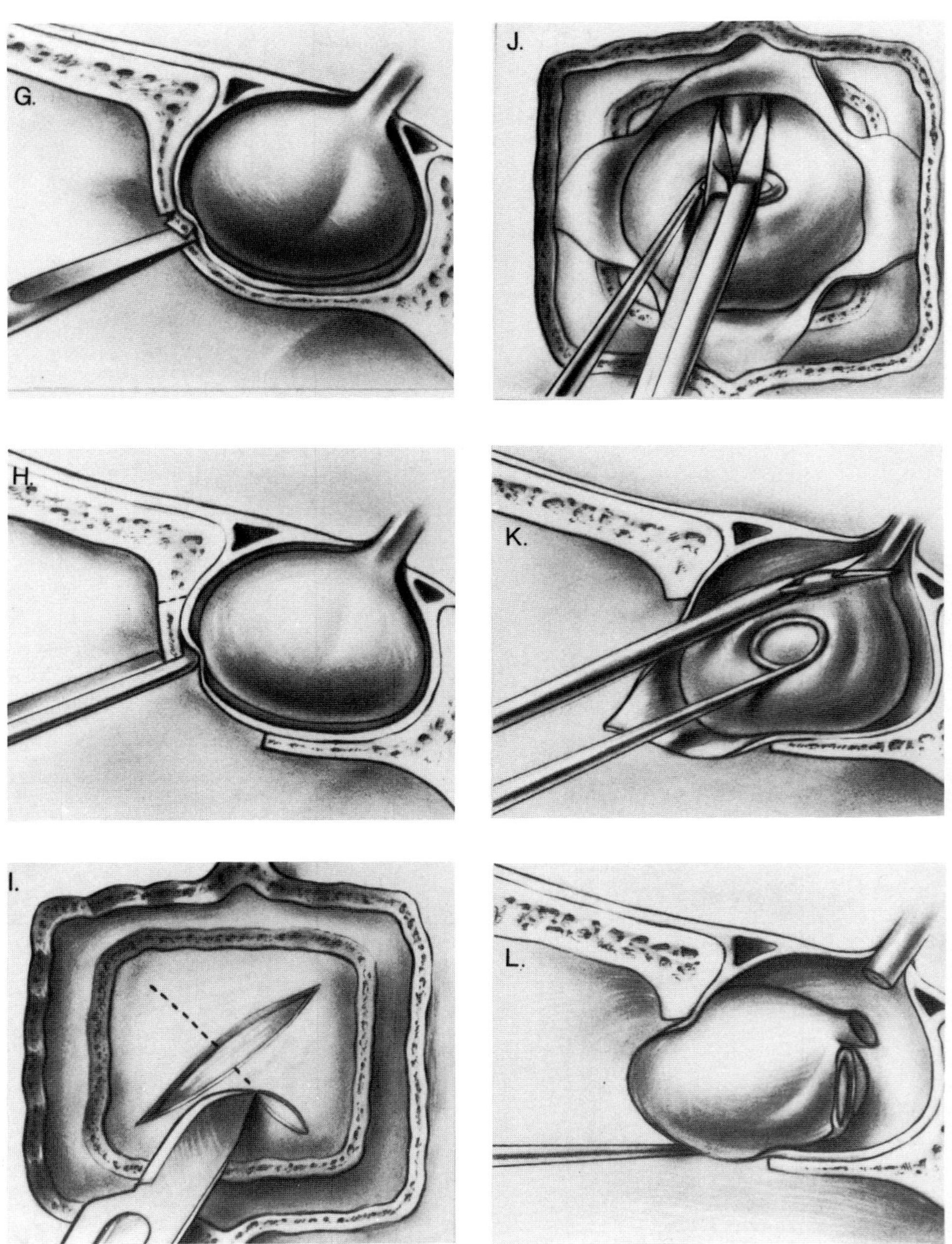

FIG. 26G–L. Transsphenoidal approach to sellar lesions. **G:** Sellar floor opened in midline with a small osteotome. **H:** Kerrison rongeur enlarges sellar opening. **I:** Cruciate incision of dura. **J:** Hardy technique of total hypophysectomy with low stalk section. Anterior view of sella with dura opened and gland depressed for low section of stalk. **K:** Lateral view of stalk section. Blunt ring curette depresses gland. **L:** Removal of gland after separation from sellar dura. (From ref. 19.)

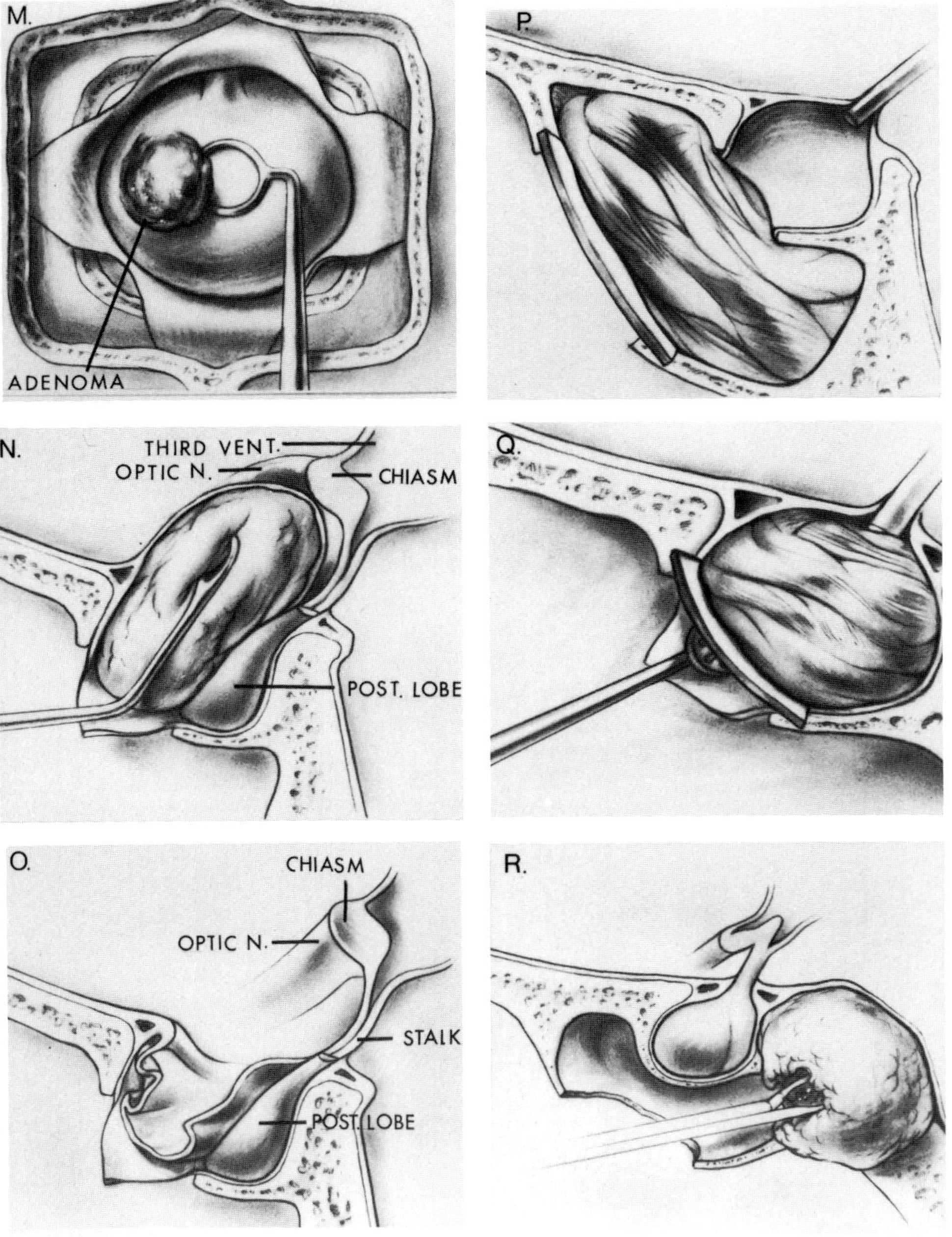

FIG. 26M–R. Transsphenoidal approach to sellar lesions. **M:** Anterior view of removal of microadenoma using blunt ring curette. **N:** Lateral view of intracapsular removal of tumor with suprasellar extension. Pituitary stalk and posterior lobe behind the tumor. **O:** Collapse of tumor capsule into sella following tumor removal. Posterior lobe and stalk are preserved. **P:** Incorrect closure (muscle packed in sphenoid sinus and not sella) associated with a high incidence of rhinorrhea. **Q:** Correct method of closure with sella (not sphenoid sinus) packed with muscle held in place with a cartilage splint. **R:** A clivus chordoma being removed with cup forceps. (From ref. 19.)

Wet sphenoid bone specimens—those with dura mater, nerves, and soft tissue intact—can be prepared at autopsy or from cadavers as described elsewhere (17). Although whole heads from which the brain has been removed are preferred for the transsphenoidal dissections, they may not be readily available, in which case wet sphenoid blocks may be prepared from cadaveric or autopsy material. The wet sphenoid blocks and dry sphenoid bones are mounted in a House-Urban temporal bone holder for completing these dissections (Fig. 27A–C).

The equipment needed for these dissections is as follows (Fig. 27A):

1. Surgical operating microscope: Zeiss Opmi I with 300 mm objective lens, 10× or 12.5× eyepieces, and straight binocular tube
2. Drill, triple arm, reversible, 10,000 to 24,000 rpm (Teledyne-Emesco) with 2- and 3-mm cutting burrs
3. Suction: operating wall suction or portable pump with suction tubes No. 5, 7, and 9 French size
4. House-Urban temporal bone holder (V. Mueller)
5. Bone-holding forceps: Caldwell-Luc or Jansen-Middleton
6. Straight bone rongeurs
7. Kerrison-type rongeurs: 8 inches long, 2 mm tip, 90° down and 90° up
8. Hardy bivalve transsphenoidal speculum: 8 to 9 cm long (Codman)
9. Small periosteal elevators: Adson or Freer
10. Pituitary cup forceps: straight with 3 mm cup

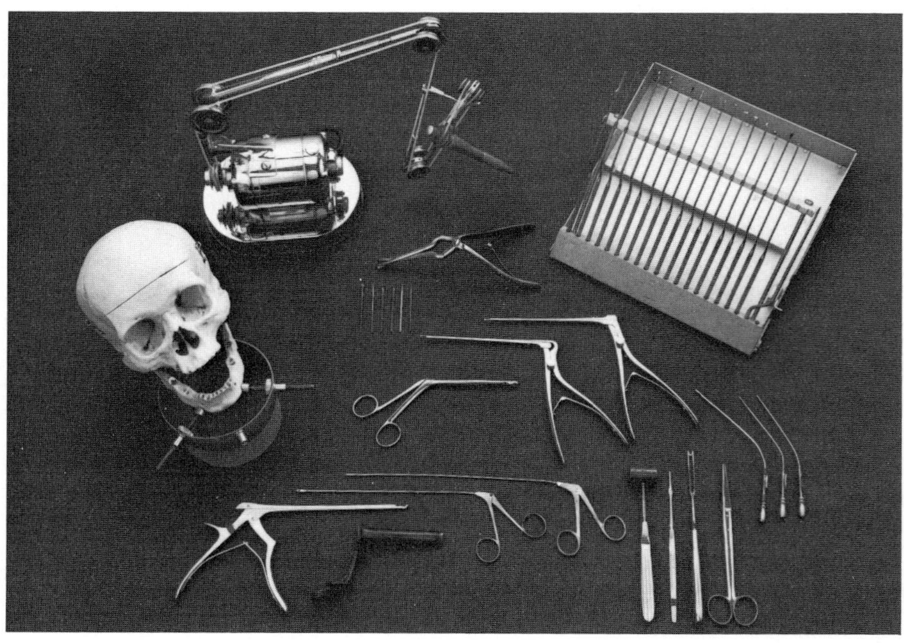

FIG. 27A. Equipment for sphenoid bone and sellar dissections.

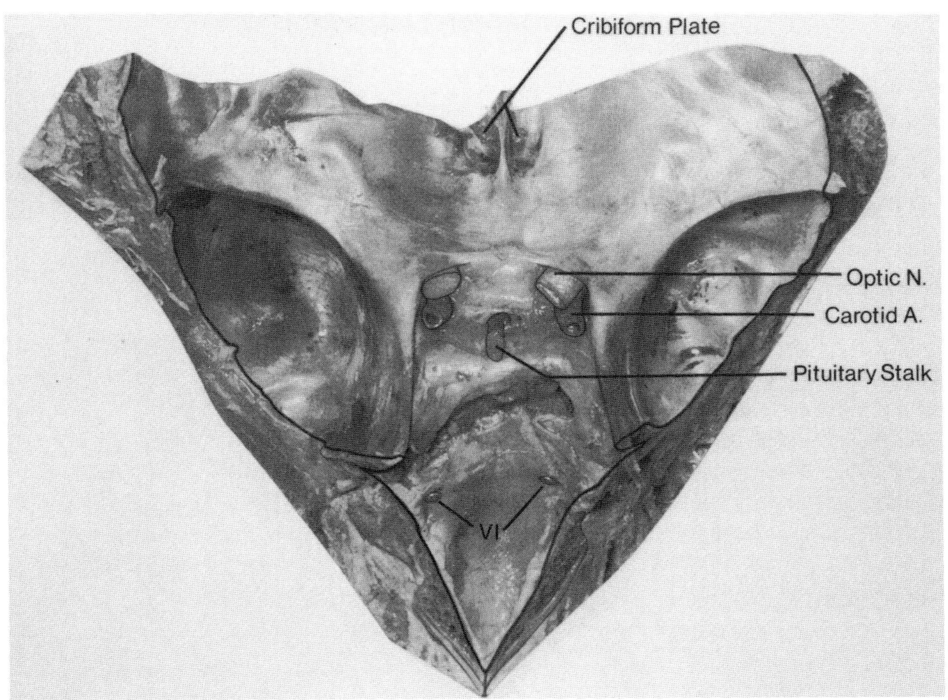

FIG. 27B. Sphenoid tissue block used for study.

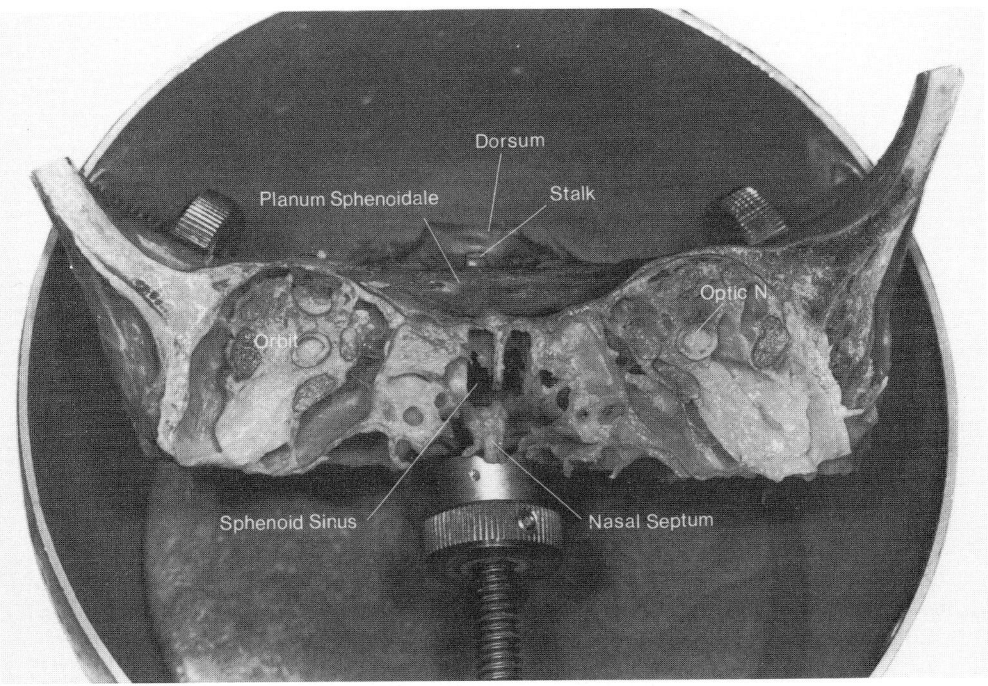

FIG. 27C. Specimen mounted in temporal bone holder for dissection.

11. Bayonet forceps with 10 to 12 cm blades
12. Alligator-type pituitary scissors
13. Rhoton transsphenoidal pituitary dissection set (V. Mueller) (includes enucleators, trident, osteotome, and bayonetted knife
14. Hammer for use with osteotome

A guide to the use of this equipment is recorded elsewhere (12).

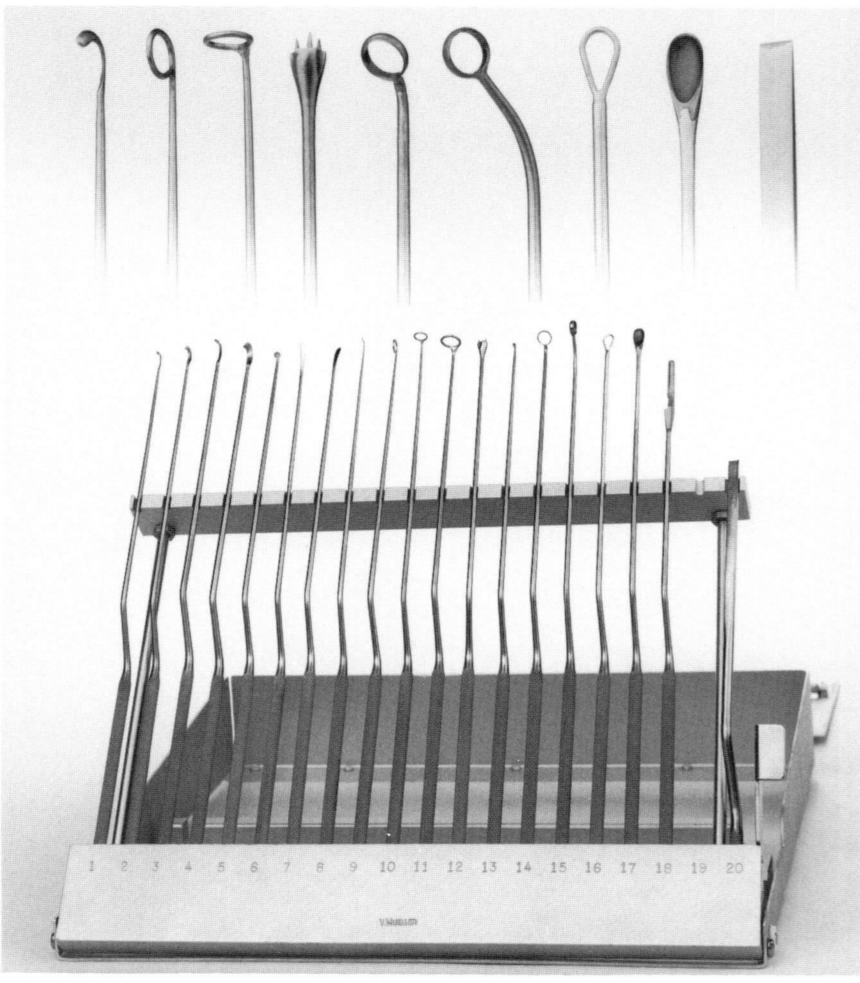

FIG. 27D. Instruments for transsphenoidal surgery. *Below:* Instruments with shafts 12.5 cm in length in rack for easy storage and protection of tips. *Upper:* Inserts show types of tips on instruments. The author (A.L.R.) prefers the blunt ring curettes (second, third, and seventh from left) for dissection in parasellar and suprasellar area. Some of the instruments have malleable tips which can be bent in different directions to follow unusual extensions of tumor. The trident (fourth from left) is used for inserting nasal septal cartilage for closure of sella turcica. Instrument on right is an osteotome used for opening the anterior wall of the sella turcica.

Dry Bone Dissection

Dry bone dissection is preferably conducted using a whole skull (Fig. 28A). The calvarium should be removed to allow inspection of the sella from above after the exercise has been completed. It can also be done on a dry sphenoid bone.

Step 1: Identification of external landmarks and sphenoid ostia (Fig. 28B): Place the skull or dry temporal bone in the bone holder with the anterior aspect facing you. Incline the head holder to give 10° to 15° of extension from the direct face-to-face position. Identify the alveolar process of the maxilla, its lateral rami, and the nasal spine. These form the inferior margin of the nasal orifice.

Step 2: Enlargement of the nasal orifice (Fig. 28C): Using rongeurs, remove the anterior spinous process of the maxilla and the margins of the lateral rami to "square off" the inferior margin of the nasal orifice. The author (A.L.R.)

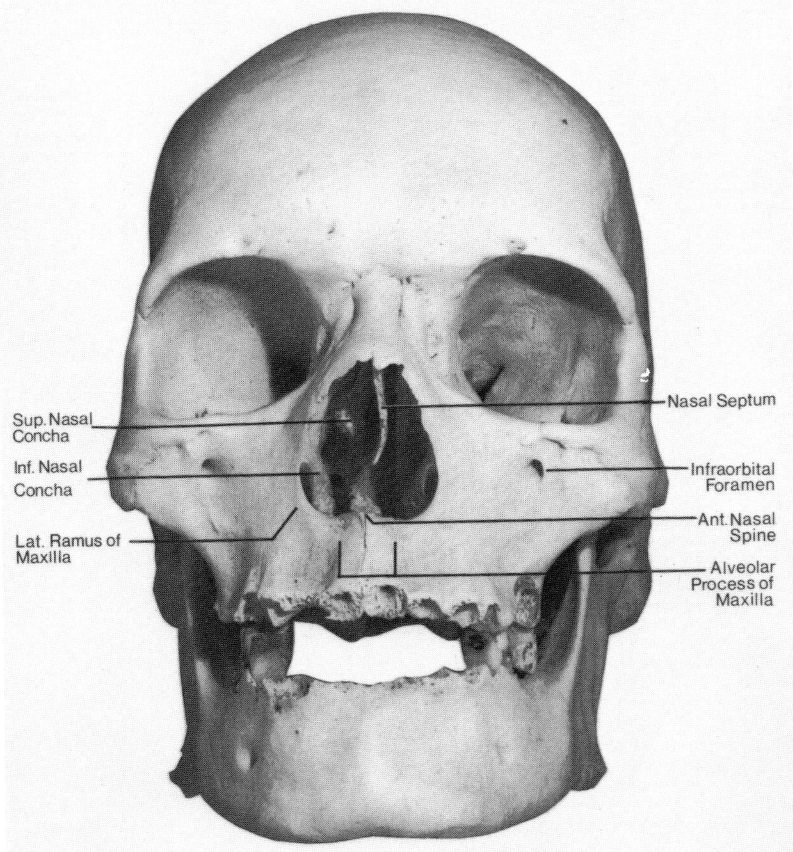

FIG. 28A. Transsphenoidal dry bone dissection. Anterior view of the skull showing osseus structures important in transnasal approaches to the sella turcica. (From ref. 17.)

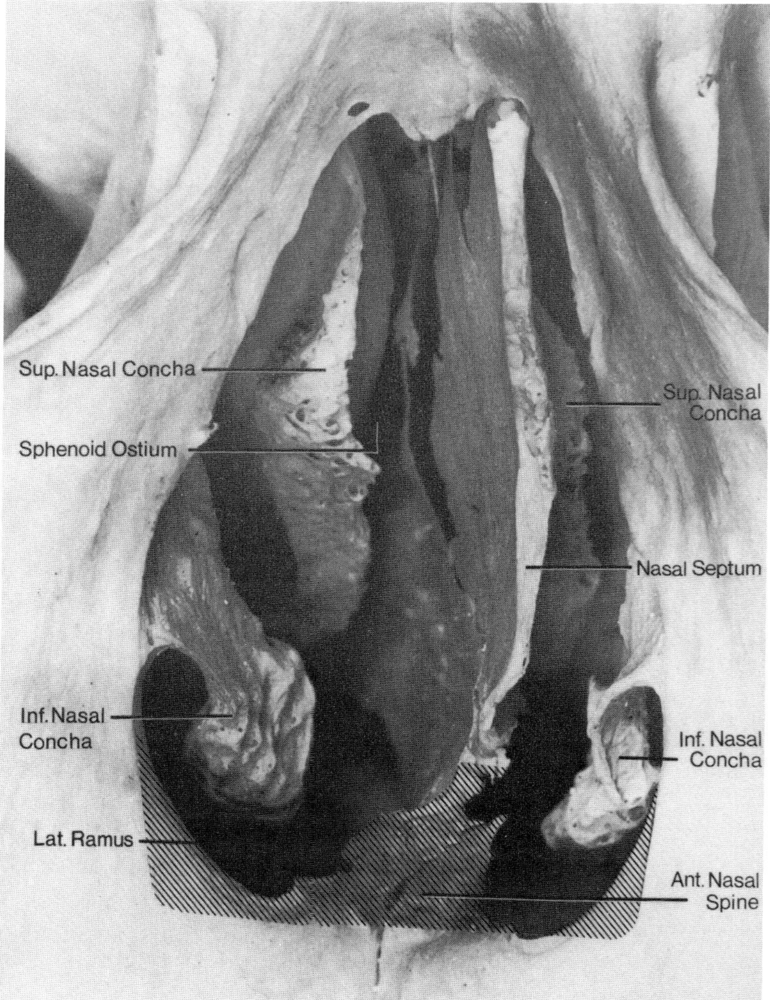

FIG. 28B. Transsphenoidal dry bone dissection. Anterior view of the nasal orifice showing the area of bone (oblique lines), including lateral rami and nasal spine, to be removed to square off the nasal orifice. (From ref. 17.)

avoids removing either the nasal spine or the lateral rami in the live patient. With experience, one can easily work around the nasal spine. Care should be taken to avoid breaking off the thin edge of the lateral rami during the opening of the speculum because healing may produce an annoying callus beside the nose.

Using 10× magnification, look into the nasal cavity and identify the nasal septum, the nasal conchae, the ostia of the sphenoid sinus, and the cribriform plates. The sphenoid ostia may be obscured by the superior and middle nasal conchae. Crush or remove with rongeurs the superior, middle, and inferior

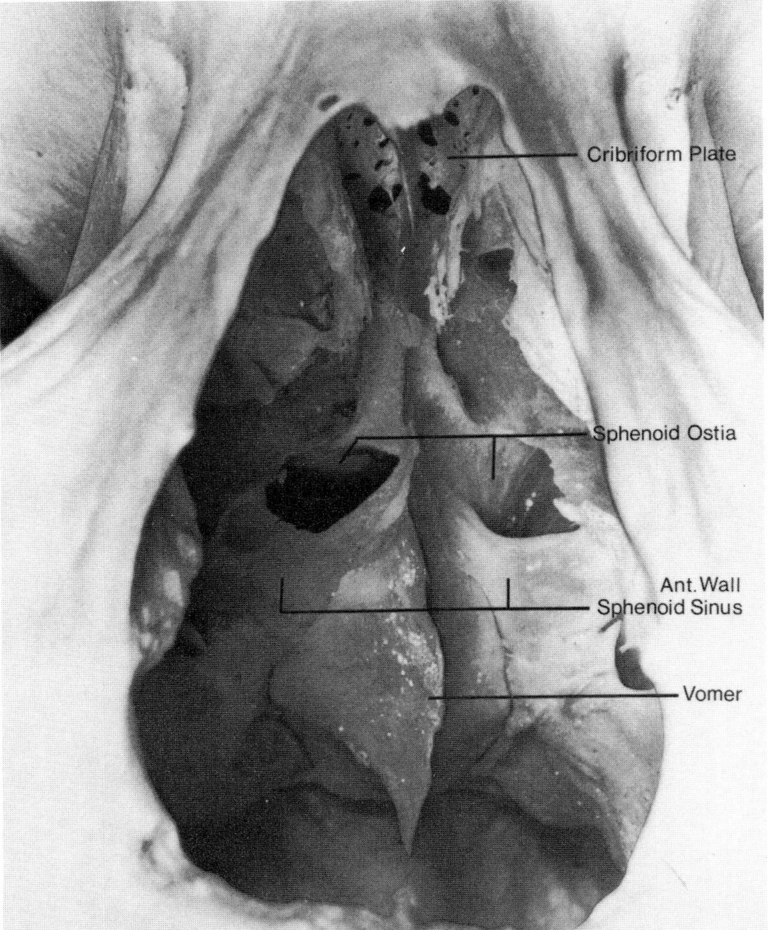

FIG. 28C. Transsphenoidal dry bone dissection. View into nasal cavity, showing sphenoid ostia, cribriform plate, anterior wall of the sphenoid sinus, and the vomer. (From ref. 17.)

nasal conchae until the vomer is clearly visible. Removal of the conchae is not required in transsphenoidal surgery, but it is done here to permit a review of important surgical landmarks. The vomer is invariably midline and is the most reliable guide to locating the midline position essential for this operative approach.

The sphenoid ostia are situated on either side of the perpendicular plate of the ethmoid bone at its junction with the vomer. The ostia should mark the upper margins of the opening into the sphenoid sinus. Identify the cribriform plates, which are located anterior to the sphenoid ostia. Dissection misdirected into the area of the cribriform plate may result in a cerebrospinal fluid (CSF) leak or a loss of the sense of smell.

Place the Hardy bivalve speculum in the nasal cavity so the vomer projects

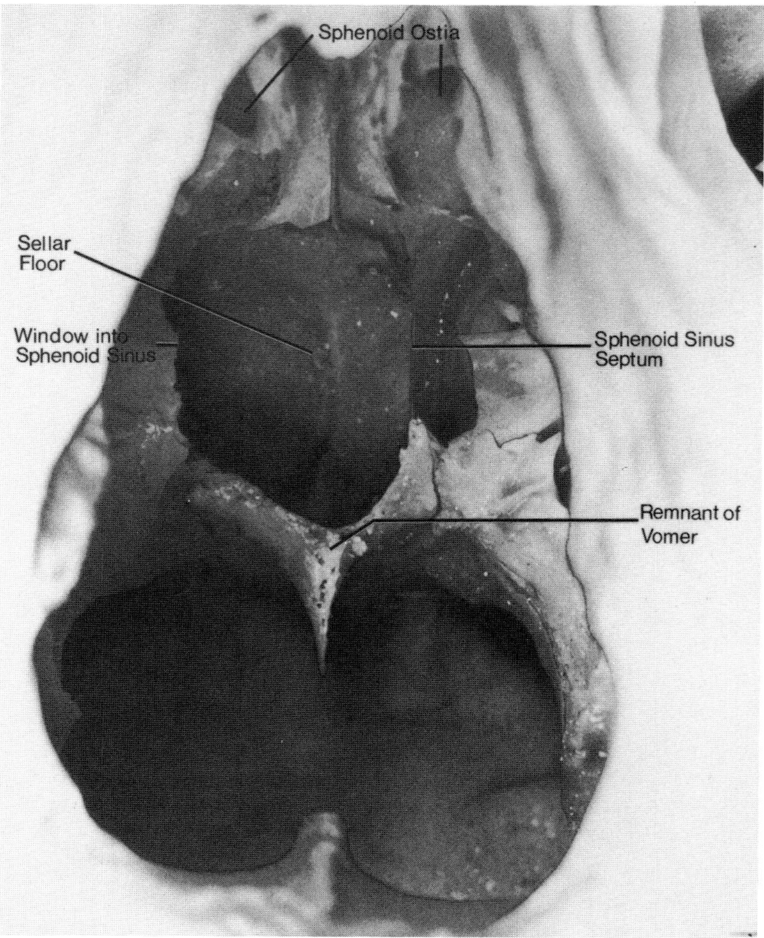

FIG. 28D. Transsphenoidal dry bone dissection. Part of vomer and anterior wall of the sphenoid sinus are removed to expose the sellar floor. Opening does not extend above the sphenoid ostia. Septum in the sphenoid sinus is located to the left of the midline. (From ref. 17.)

inferiorly directly in the midline at the end of the speculum. When the speculum is correctly positioned, the ostia usually lie at the superior end of the exposure. When you are satisfied that the speculum is correctly placed, its position should not be changed because this is the best assurance of the correct incline approach to the sellar floor.

Step 3: Removal of vomer: opening of sphenoid sinus (Fig. 28D): Remove the vomer using the Jansen-Middleton or other suitable forceps. In these specimens it usually comes away in one piece and brings with it the anterior wall of the sphenoid sinus. If the bone is very thick, it may require piecemeal removal with a bone rongeurs or removal using the dental drill.

Enlarge the opening in the anterior wall of the sphenoid sinus to give a

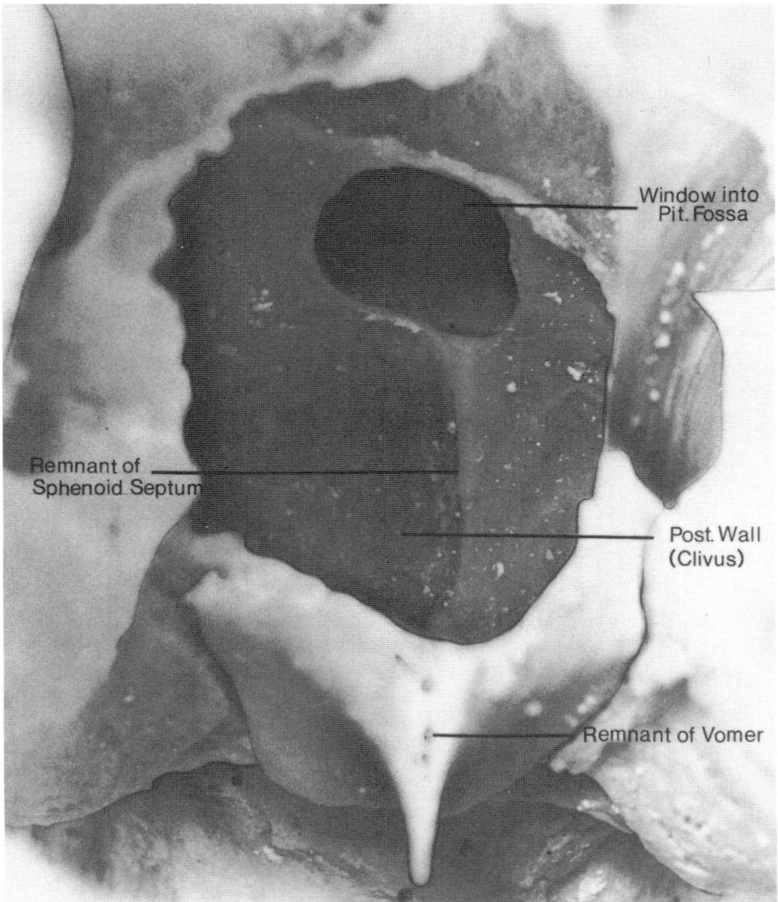

FIG. 28E. Transsphenoidal dry bone dissection. Window opening into sella. Posterior wall of sphenoid sinus forms the anterior wall of the clivus. (From ref. 17.)

1.5-cm square. Note the configuration of the interior of the sinus and the presence of the sphenoid septae. The septae vary in number and position and frequently deviate from the midline. They should therefore not be used as a guide to the midline in this part of the dissection or at operation.

The floor of the sella is usually seen as a smooth bulge in the superior wall of the sinus, and if your positioning has been correct it should lie directly at the end of the speculum. The chiasmatic sulcus may produce a subsidiary bulge into the sinus, which, lying superior to the sellar floor, should not be mistaken for the sella. The nasal speculum should not be advanced into the sinus because this does not increase the exposure and may, in the live patient, cause damage to the poorly protected arteries and nerves within the lateral walls of the sinus (4,16).

Step 4: Opening of sellar floor (Fig. 28E,F): Using the small osteotome or

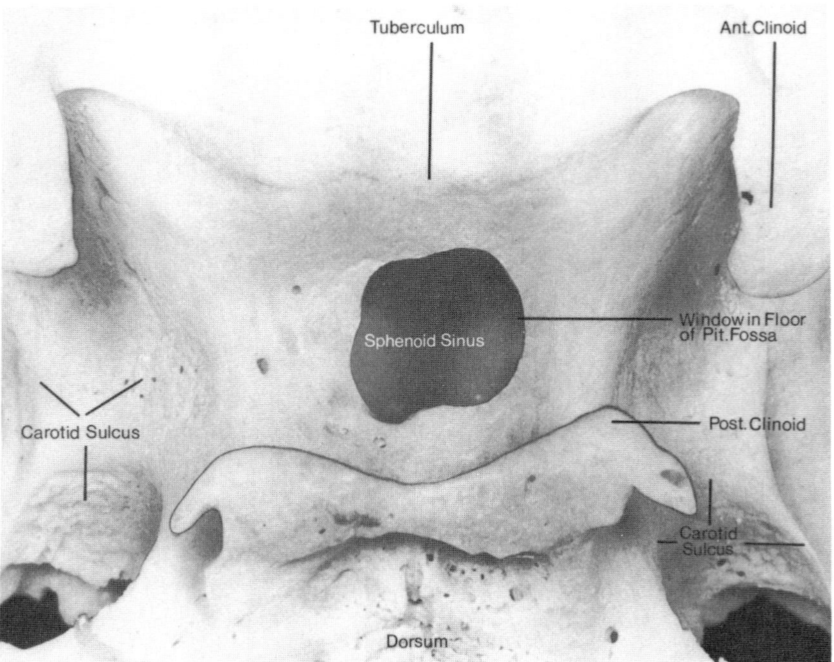

FIG. 28F. Transsphenoidal dry bone dissection. Superior view of opening into floor of the sella turcica. The opening should not include the chiasmatic sulcus or the tuberculum because openings here are very difficult to close. (From ref. 17.)

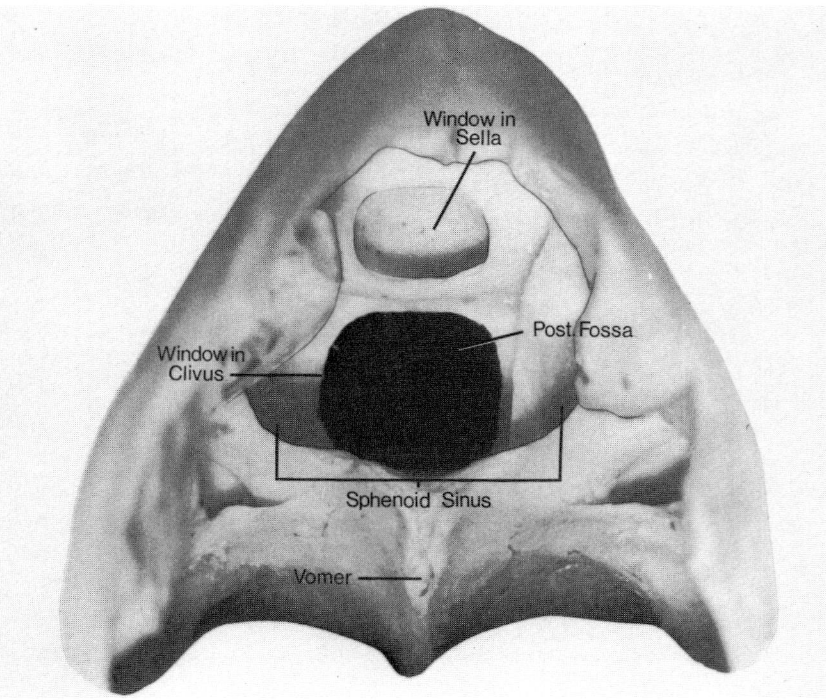

FIG. 28G. Transsphenoidal dry bone dissection. Opening from sphenoid sinus through the clivus is completed. (From ref. 17.)

the drill, make an opening through the sellar floor and enlarge this to a size sufficient to allow passage of a 9.0-mm right-angle enucleator and other pituitary instruments. Check the position of the opening by looking inside the skull. If your approach has been correct, you should now have a centrally placed aperture within the floor of the sella. The opening should not extend along the anterior wall to the chiasmatic sulcus or tuberculum sellae because an opening in this area is difficult to close and may be associated with a high incidence of CSF leakage.

Examine the thickness of the sellar floor. A thin sellar floor facilitates the transsphenoidal approach to the gland. In nearly all adults the floor is less than 1 mm thick, and in two-thirds it is less than 0.5 mm (1,16). In the latter case breaching the floor can usually be accomplished by pressure on the bone with a blunt dissector or a curette, or a gentle tap with an osteotome. If the bone is thicker than 1 mm it may be necessary to use the firm but controlled tap of a hammer against the osteotome or a drill to open the sellar cavity.

Step 5: Transclival exposure (Fig. 28G,H): Direct your attention to the poste-

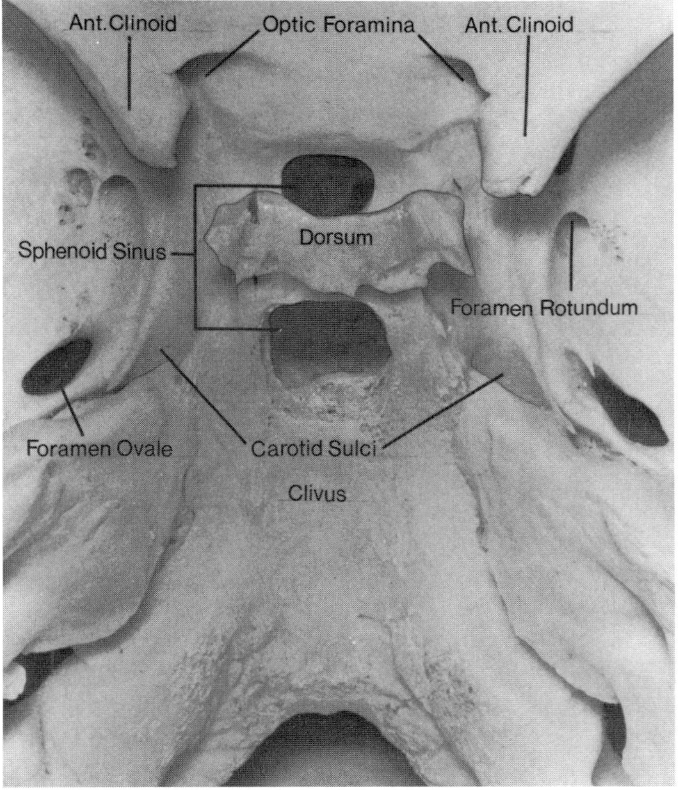

FIG. 28H. Transsphenoidal dry bone dissection. Superior view of opening through the sella floor and clivus. (From ref. 17.)

rior wall of the sphenoid sinus below the sella and using the osteotome or drill make an opening in the midline of the clivus. After completing the initial opening, it can be enlarged using a Kerrison rongeur. The opening should extend to, but not include, the sellar floor and downward to the inferior margin of the sphenoid sinus. If necessary, the opening could be extended upward by removing the floor of the sella and downward by removing the lower wall of the sphenoid sinus. Look inside the skull to check the position of the opening.

Wet Specimen Dissection

Wet specimen dissection may be done on an intact cadaveric head or using a wet sphenoid block. If a sphenoid block is used, steps 1 through 3 are omitted.

Step 1: Enlargement of nasal orifice (Fig. 26C–F, 29A): Place the head directly facing you with 10° to 15° of head extension. Retract the upper lip to expose the gingival margin and, using 6× magnification, incise this transversely, extending your incision from one canine fossa to the other. Using a periosteal elevator, elevate the upper lip until the nasal orifice, the anterior spinous process of the maxilla, and the nasal part of the hard palate are exposed.

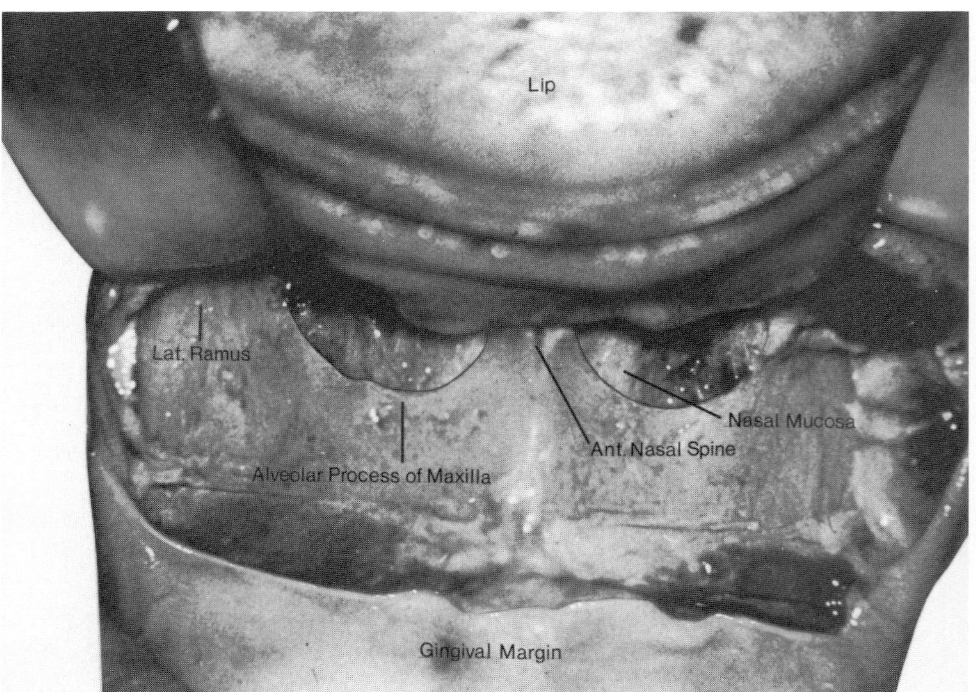

FIG. 29A. Transsphenoidal dissection on wet specimen (see pages 64–71). **A:** Lip is elevated to expose anterior nasal and lateral ramus. (From ref. 17.)

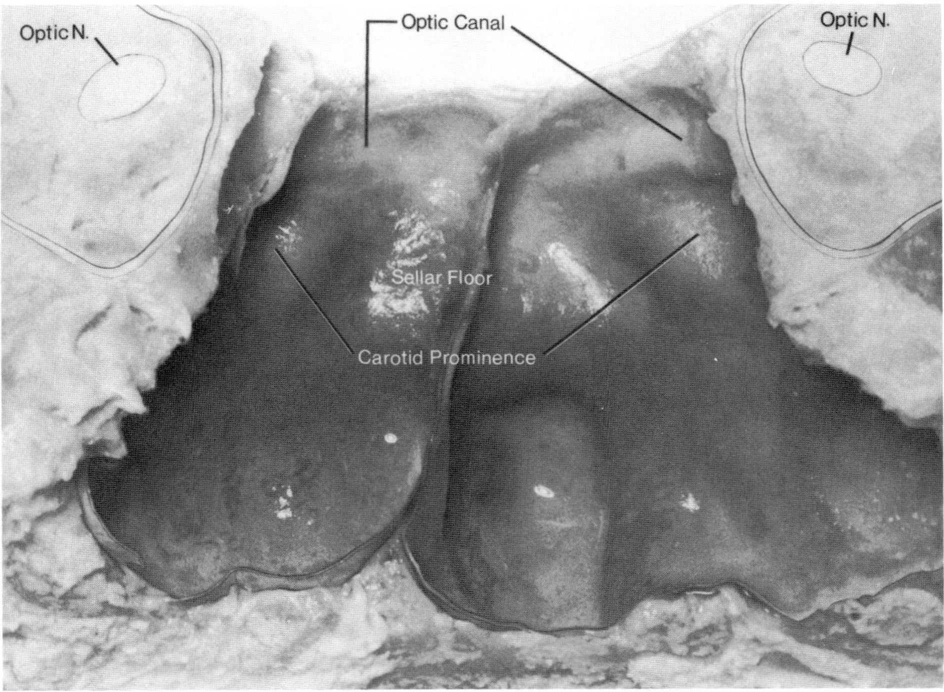

FIG. 29B. Sphenoid sinus and sellar floor is exposed on a wet sphenoid bone section. Sellar type sinus. (From ref. 17.)

Using a Kerrison rongeur remove the margins of the lateral rami and alveolar process of the maxilla, and using the osteotome remove the anterior spinous process of the maxilla. In the live patient, the author (A.L.R.) prefers to preserve and work around the anterior spinous process. If it is removed, it should be repositioned on completion of the procedure to prevent postoperative drooping of the tip of the nose.

Step 2: Removal of nasal septum (Fig. 26F): Use a periosteal elevator to separate the mucosa from the floor of the nasal cavity and from the sides of the nasal septum. Examine the cartilage of the nasal septum; and using a knife, scissors, or a Ballinger swivel knife, remove the posterior half of the lower one-third of the septum and retain it. An anterior strut of cartilage should be preserved to maintain a normal postoperative nasal contour.

Step 3: Insertion of nasal speculum and opening of sphenoid sinus (Figs. 26F, 29B): Insert the nasal speculum between the mucosa on one side and the adjacent side of the nasal septum, with the handle facing superiorly, and open the blades. This retracts the remaining cartilaginous nasal septum and the mucosa of the walls of the nasal cavity. Opening the blades of the speculum is usually enough to crush or displace the turbinates sufficiently for adequate exposure. If the

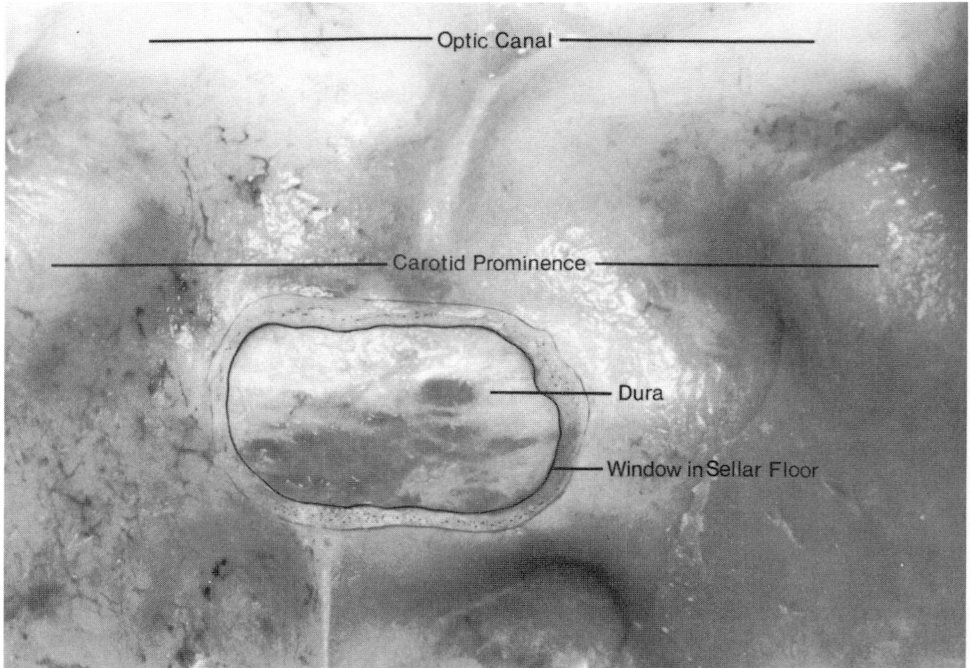

FIG. 29C. Anterior sellar wall was removed using an osteotome and Kerrison-type rongeurs to expose the dura over the pituitary gland. Optic canals and carotid prominences are superolateral to the sellar window. (From ref. 17.)

speculum has been inserted correctly the vomer will be in the midline, and there is no need to reposition it during the remainder of the procedure.

Using a bone rongeurs, bite through the anterior crest of the vomer to open into the anterior wall of the sphenoid sinus. The anterior wall of the sinus may also be opened with the osteotome. Enlarge the opening into the sphenoid sinus until it is a 1.5-cm square using a Kerrison rongeur.

Step 4: Opening of sellar floor (Figs. 26G,H, 29C): Incise the mucosa of the sphenoid sinus and push it laterally. It is not necessary to remove all the mucosa from the walls of the sinus. Remove or displace enough mucosa to obtain a clear view of the cavity of the sinus, its septae, and the anterior sellar wall. The optic canals may be identified in the superolateral part of the presellar portion of the sphenoid sinus, and the carotid arteries may produce a prominence in the lateral walls anterior to the sella. Neither the optic canal nor the carotid prominence is visible at operation, and they should not be searched for in the live patient; however, their presence in the cadaver may be readily determined by inspection and palpation. In a few cases the nerves and arteries are covered by only dura and sinus mucosa, and in others the bone covering the optic nerves is very thin. Therefore the optic nerves could be injured in the transsphenoidal approach if vigorous attempts were made to strip or curette the mucosa from the walls of the sinus or if the nasal speculum is advanced to lie within the sinus and forcefully opened against its lateral walls (4,16).

Septae within the sinus should be removed using the osteotome, Kerrison rongeur, and cup forceps. Identify the bulge of the sellar floor. If the sinus is of a presellar or conchal type, the sellar bulge may not be apparent, but the floor of the sella should be directly ahead if the speculum has been positioned correctly. Using the 6-mm osteotome, make a window in the sellar floor and enlarge the opening to a 1-cm square using the Kerrison-type pituitary rongeur. It may be necessary to use the drill to breach the sellar floor. If so, try to stop drilling while there is still a thin plate of bone over the sella. Remove this thin plate with a bayonetted curette.

Step 5: Removal of pituitary gland (Figs. 26I–L, 29D–H): Using a No. 11 scalpel blade on a bayonet knife handle, incise the dura on the diagonal from corner to corner rather than up and down and side to side. The upper leaf of dura may be further incised in the midline to give adequate exposure over the top of the gland. Examine the dura to see if the incision has entered or crossed an intercavernous sinus. Identify the extracapsular plane of cleavage between the gland and the sellar dura. Using a dissector, depress the superior surface

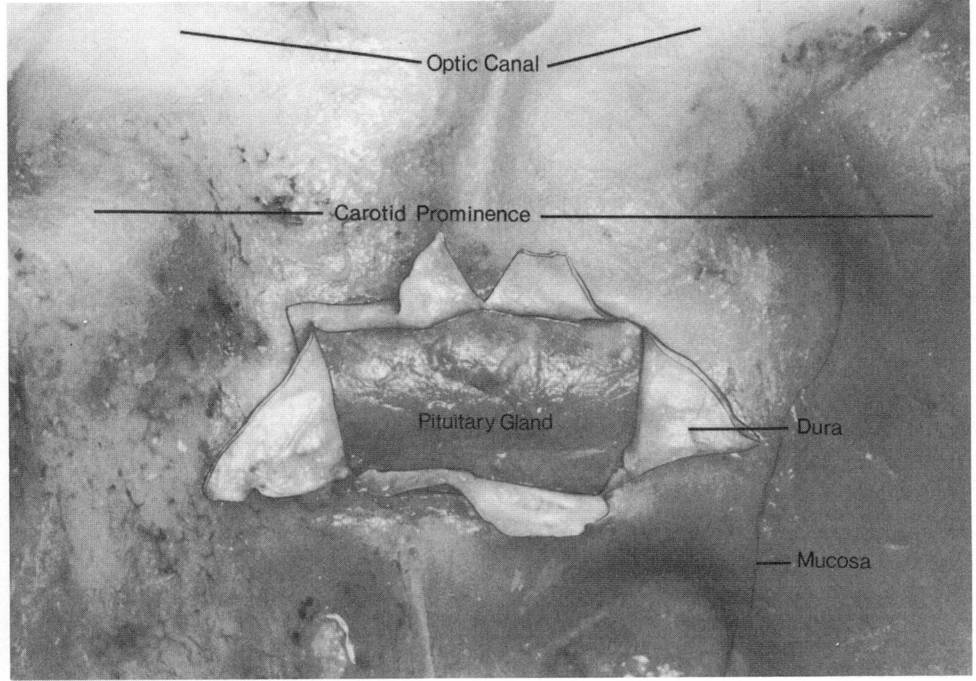

FIG. 29D. Sellar dura is opened from corner to corner. This gives greater exposure than a horizontal and vertical cruciate incision. (From ref. 17.)

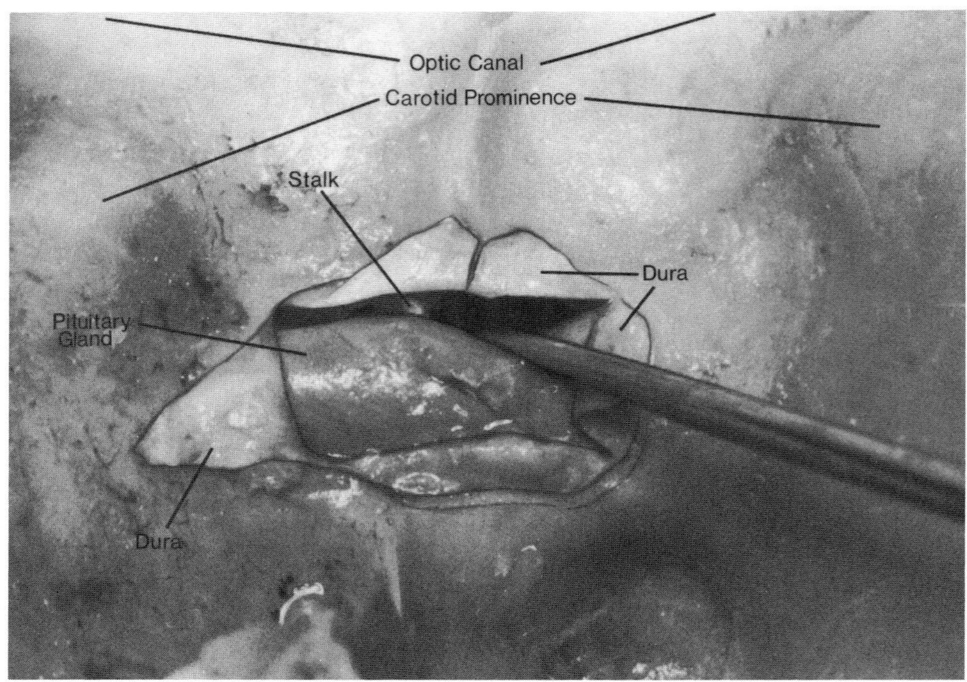

FIG. 29E. The superior surface of the gland is depressed to expose the stalk. (From ref. 17.)

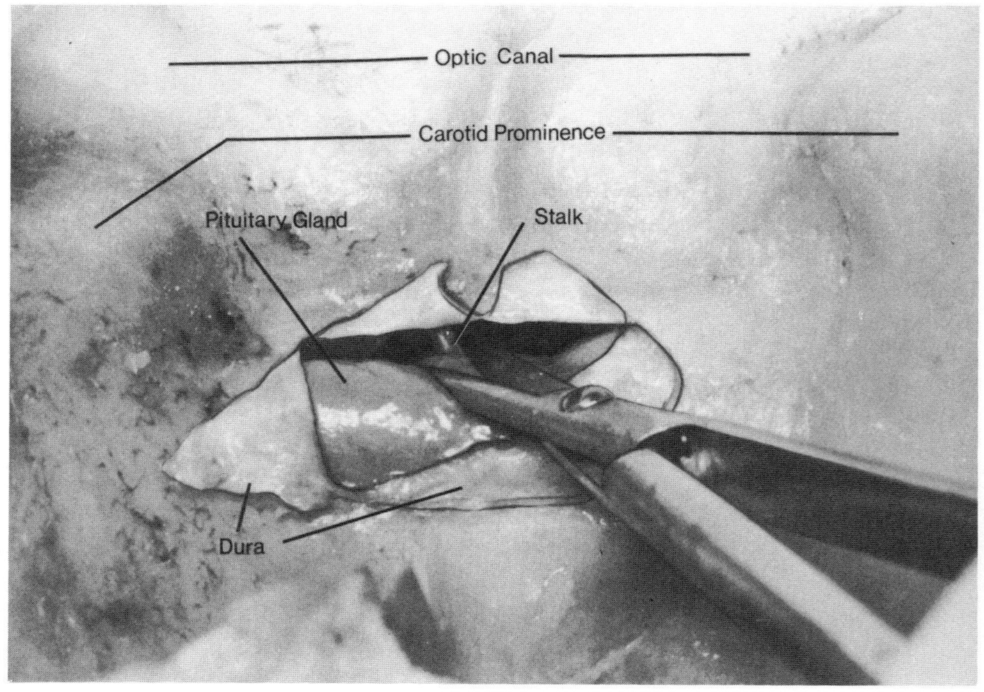

FIG. 29F. Stalk is divided and the gland removed. (From ref. 17.)

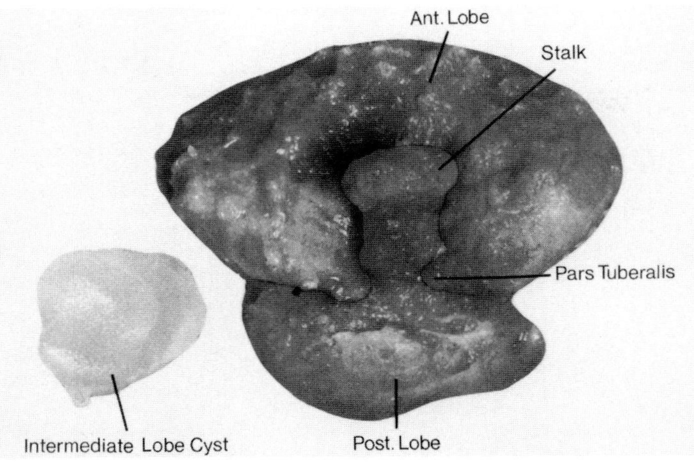

FIG. 29G. Intact gland and stalk after removal. (From ref. 17.)

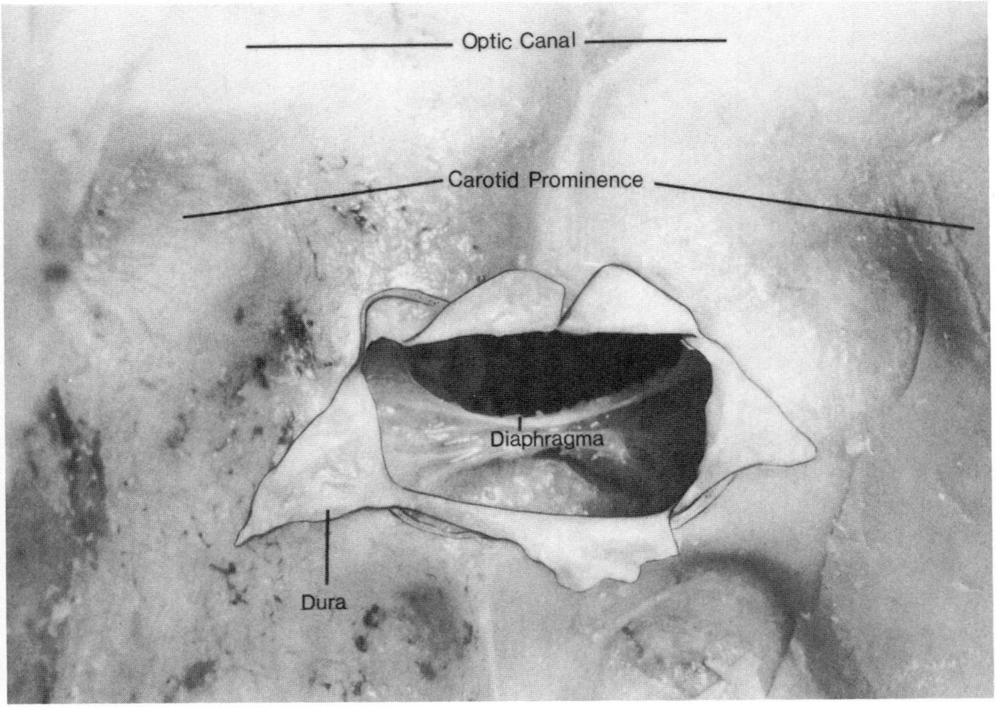

FIG. 29H. Diaphragma is exposed in roof of sella. Diaphragmal opening is large in comparison to the pituitary stalk. (From ref. 17.)

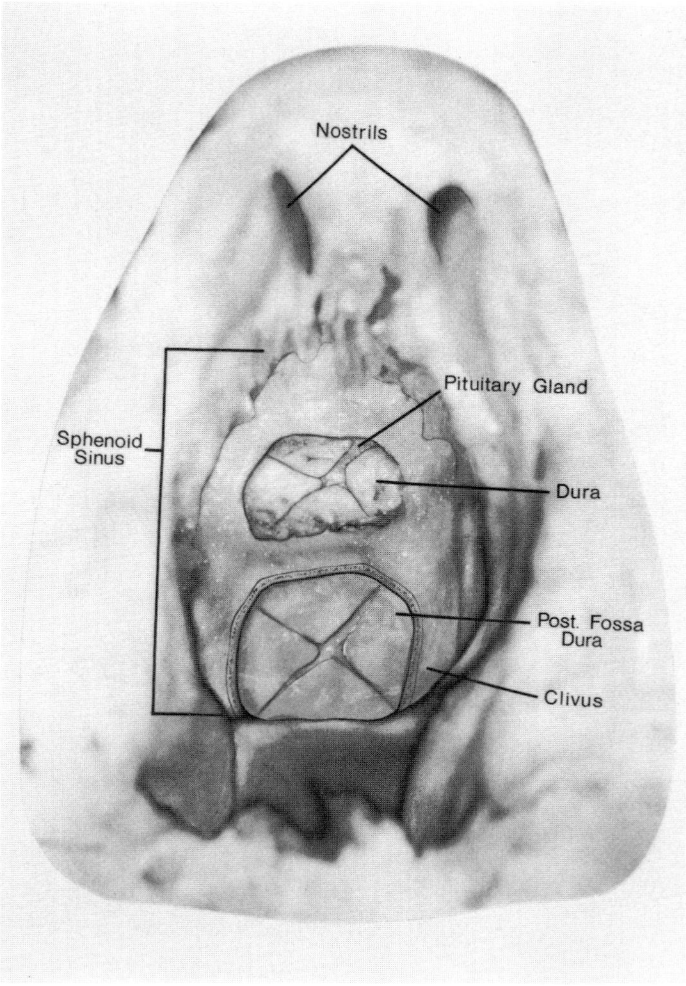

FIG. 29I. The posterior (clival) wall of the sinus is opened to provide transsphenoidal transclival exposure. (From ref. 17.)

of the gland to identify the pituitary stalk; and with alligator pituitary scissors, divide the stalk as close to the gland as possible. Remove the gland in one piece with an enucleator.

Note the thickness of the diaphragma, the size of its opening, and the arrangement of the arachnoid around the pituitary stalk. Variations in gland shape are not uncommon and may cause difficulty in accomplishing complete hypophysectomy. There is usually a space between the gland and the medial margin of the carotid artery, but in some cases the artery may protrude through the medial wall of the cavernous sinus and may indent and displace the gland

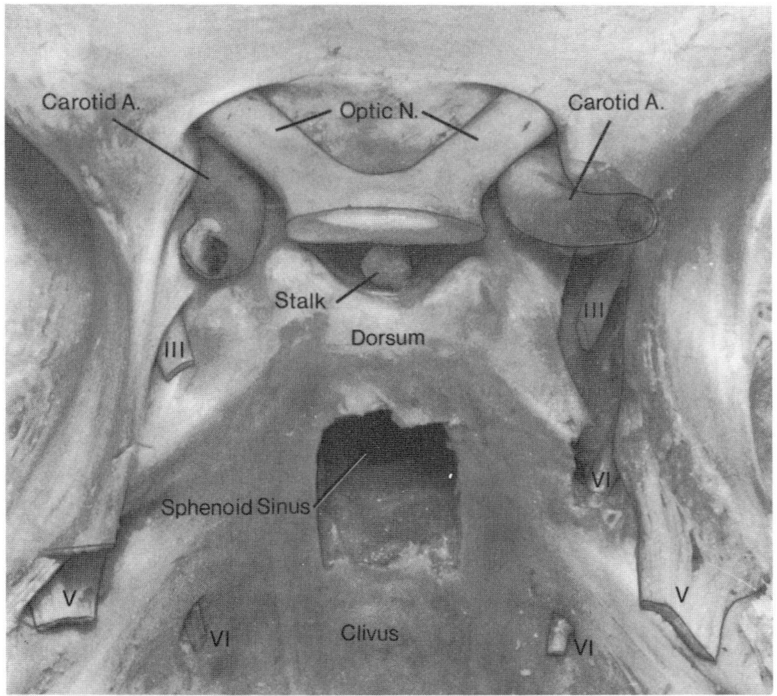

FIG. 29J. Superior view of sellar region showing the opening from the sphenoid sinus through the clivus. (From ref. 17.)

(16). Using 16× magnification, try to identify the carotid arteries through the sellar window.

Step 6: Closing the sella (Fig. 26P,Q): Using cotton or gelfoam as a substitute for muscle or fat, plug the cavity of the sella and, from the cartilage removed from the nasal septum, fashion a stint to plug the defect in the floor of the sella. With forceps and the trident, insert the cartilaginous stint inside the sellar floor so it fits snugly over the defect opening in the sella.

Step 7: Transclival approach (Fig. 26G–R, 29I,J): Direct your attention to the posterior wall of the sphenoid sinus. Remove any mucosa and septae necessary to reach the wall of the sinus surface anterior to the clivus. Using the drill or osteotome, make a small opening in the midline and enlarge it using the Kerrison rongeur, taking care not to open the dura. Using the bayonetted knife handle and a No. 11 blade, open the dura from corner to corner. The opening can be enlarged upward by removing the lower margin of the sella and pushing the pituitary gland upward and downward by removing the floor of the sphenoid sinus. Examine your specimen from above and see if the opening has extended laterally to the abducens nerve or through the basilar sinus within the dura of the clivus. Now remove the speculum and allow the lip to return to its normal position. With a few catgut stitches, approximate the gingival margin.

When you have identified all of these structures in the sellar region and cavernous sinus and have completed the transsphenoidal dissections in the wet and dry specimen, you should have an excellent knowledge of and familiarity with this important region.

ACKNOWLEDGMENTS

Supported in part by the American Heart Association, Broward County Chapter, and the National Institutes of Health, grant NS 10978–03.

REFERENCES

1. Bergland, R. M., Ray, B. S., and Torack, R. M. (1968): Anatomical variations in the pituitary gland and adjacent structures in 225 human autopsy cases. *J. Neurosurg.,* 28:93–99.
2. Bull, J. W. D., and Schunk, H. (1962): The significance of displacement of the cavernous portion of the internal carotid artery. *Br. J. Radiol.,* 35:801–814.
3. Cushing, H. (1912): *The Pituitary Body and Its Disorders.* Lippincott, Philadelphia.
4. Fujii, K., Chambers, S. M., and Rhoton, A. L., Jr. (1978): Neurovascular relationships of the sphenoid sinus: A microsurgical study. *J. Neurosurg.,* 50:31–39.
5. Guiot, G. (1958): *Adenomes Hypophysaires.* Masson & Cie, Paris.
6. Guiot, G. (1973): Transsphenoidal approach in surgical treatment of pituitary adenomas: General principles and indications in non-functioning adenomas. *Excerpta Medica International Congress Series,* No. 303:159–179.
7. Hamberger, C. A., Hammer, G., Norlen, G., and Sjögren, B. (1961): Transsphenoidal hypophysectomy. *Arch. Otolaryngol.,* 74:2–8.
8. Hardy, J. (1969): Microneurosurgery of the hypophysis: A subnasal transsphenoidal approach with television magnification and televised radiofluoroscopy control. In: *Microneurosurgery,* edited by R. W. Rand, pp. 87–103. Mosby, St. Louis.
9. Hardy, J. (1971): Transsphenoidal hypophysectomy. *J. Neurosurg.,* 34:582–594.
10. Harris, F. S., and Rhoton, A. L., Jr. (1976): Anatomy of the cavernous sinus: A microsurgical study. *J. Neurosurg.,* 45:169–180.
11. Laws, E. R., and Kern, E. B. (1976): Complications of transsphenoidal surgery. *Clin. Neurosurg.,* 23:401–416.
12. Pait, T. G., Zeal, A., Harris, F. S., Paullus, W. S., and Rhoton, A. L., Jr. (1977): Microsurgical anatomy and dissection of the temporal bone. *Surg. Neurol.,* 8:363–391.
13. Parkinson, D. (1967): Transcavernous repair of carotid-cavernous fistula: A case report. *J. Neurosurg.,* 26:420–424.
14. Perlmutter, D., and Rhoton, A. L., Jr. (1976): Microsurgical anatomy of the anterior cerebral-anterior communicating-recurrent artery complex. *J. Neurosurg.,* 45:259–271.
15. Rand, R. W. (1969): Transfrontal transsphenoidal craniotomy in pituitary and related tumors using microneurosurgical techniques. In: *Microneurosurgery,* edited by R. W. Rand, pp. 74–86. Mosby, St. Louis.
16. Renn, W. H., and Rhoton, A. L., Jr. (1975): Microsurgical anatomy of the sellar region. *J. Neurosurg.,* 43:288–298.
17. Rhoton, A. L., Jr., Hardy, D. G., and Chambers, S. M. (1979): Microsurgical anatomy and dissection of the sphenoid bone, cavernous sinus and sellar region. *Surg. Neurol.,* 12:63–104.
18. Rhoton, A. L., Jr., Harris, F. S., and Renn, W. H. (1977): Microsurgical anatomy of the sellar region and cavernous sinus. *Clin. Neurosurg.,* 24:54–85.
19. Rhoton, A. L., Jr., and Maniscalco, J. (1977): Microsurgery of the sellar region. *Neuro-ophthalmology,* 9:106–127.

20. Saeki, N., and Rhoton, A. L., Jr. (1977): Microsurgical anatomy of the upper basilar artery and the posterior circle of Willis. *J. Neurosurg.,* 46:563–577.
21. Schloffer, H. (1907): Erfolgreiche operation eines hypophysentumors auf nalalem wege. *Wien. Klin. Wochenschr.,* 20:621.
22. Zeal, A. A., and Rhoton, A. L., Jr. (1978): Microsurgical anatomy of the posterior cerebral artery. *J. Neurosurg.,* 48:534–551.

Clinical Management of Pituitary Disorders,
edited by G. T. Tindall and W. F. Collins.
Raven Press, New York © 1979.

2

Recent Advances in Neuroendocrinology

Jimmy D. Neill

Department of Physiology, School of Medicine, Emory University, Atlanta, Georgia 30322

Neuroendocrinology was established as an identifiable field of study in 1955 by the publication of Harris's (16) classic monograph. This work illustrated the dependence of pituitary hormone secretion on proximity to the brain. Since no neuronal connections exist between the brain and the anterior pituitary, he proposed that regulation occurred via the short vascular pathway that links these organs. According to his neurohumoral hypothesis, hypothalamic substances (hypophysiotropic hormones) were secreted by nerve endings of the hypothalamic median eminence into this specialized vascular communication system (hypophyseal portal vascular system).

During the intervening years his hypothesis was amply confirmed. Moreover, the identity of three hypophysiotropic hormones—thyrotropin-releasing hormone (TRH), luteinizing hormone-releasing hormone (LHRH), and somatostatin—is now established. These three hormones are peptides, and their isolation, structural determination, and synthesis have been well publicized (15,27). In this chapter I present evidence that dopamine is a prolactin-inhibiting factor (PIF) which acts directly on the pituitary gland to inhibit prolactin secretion in physiologic concentrations, and hence it must be considered the fourth hypophysiotropic hormone to be identified. There remains evidence, however, that a separate PIF exists, probably a peptide, and that its secretion is regulated by dopamine acting as a neurotransmitter in the hypothalamus.

Recently a series of new neuropeptides were isolated from hypothalamic tissue that can be shown experimentally to alter pituitary hormone secretion (31). However, they do not appear to be hypophysiotropic factors but instead act at the hypothalamus to influence pituitary hormone secretion, presumably by altering the release of hypophysiotropic factors. These new neuropeptides are substance P, neurotensin, the enkephalins, β-endorphin, vasoactive intestinal polypeptide, and bombesin. Although it is difficult to rationalize their exact regulatory roles in pituitary hormone secretion, simply because of a lack of information, their possible uses as pharmacologic (even therapeutic) agents, are exciting indeed.

ESTABLISHED HYPOPHYSIOTROPIC HORMONES (TRH, LHRH, AND SOMATOSTATIN)

Three peptides are now firmly established as hypophysiotropic hormones: TRH, composed of three amino acids; LHRH, composed of 10 amino acids; and somatostatin or growth hormone-inhibiting hormone, containing 14 amino acids (Table 1). All three have been demonstrated to affect release of pituitary hormones by a direct action on the pituitary gland either *in vitro* or *in vivo* after removal of the influence of the hypothalamus by median eminence lesions or transection of the hypophyseal stalk (31). TRH releases TSH and prolactin, LHRH releases LH and follicle-stimulating hormone (FSH), and somatostatin inhibits growth hormone and TSH release (31). The three hormones have been found in hypophyseal stalk blood in higher concentrations than in the peripheral circulation, demonstrating that they are secreted by the median eminence. LHRH secretion has been shown to correlate with the ovulatory surge of LH secretion (21).

Early studies using radioimmunoassays revealed that the highest concentrations of these hypophysiotropic hormones were found in the median eminence, with lesser concentrations being found in the anterior hypothalamus. More recent applications of immunocytochemical localization techniques (7,17) have confirmed that axonal endings abutting on the primary capillaries of the hypophyseal portal system contain high concentrations of the hypophysiotropic hormones (Fig. 1) (7,17). Location of the cell bodies contributing these axonal endings has been more difficult, but a consensus has developed that some arise from the arcuate nucleus although the majority arise from the suprachiasmatic portion of the anterior hypothalamic area (Fig. 2) (7).

TABLE 1. *Hypophysiotropic hormones of established structure and function*

Name	Structure	Function
TRH[a]	Pyro-Glu-His-Pro-NH_2	Releases TSH and prolactin
LHRH[b]	Pyro-Glu-His-Trp-Ser-Tyr-Gly-Leu-Arg-Pro-Gly-NH_2	Releases LH and FSH
Somatostatin[c]	H-Ala-Gly-Cys-Lys-Asn-Phe-Phe-Trp-Lys-Thr-Phe-Thr-Ser-Cys-OH	Inhibits GH and TSH release
Dopamine[d]	(HO)(OH)C_6H_3—CH$_2$—CH$_2$—NH_2 [structural formula: benzene ring with HO and OH; side chain H H / —C—C—NH_2 / H H]	Inhibits prolactin release

[a] Thyrotropin (TSH)-releasing hormone.
[b] Luteinizing hormone (LH)-releasing hormone.
[c] Growth hormone (GH)-inhibiting hormone.
[d] Prolactin-inhibiting factor (PIF). A putative peptide PIF also is believed to exist.

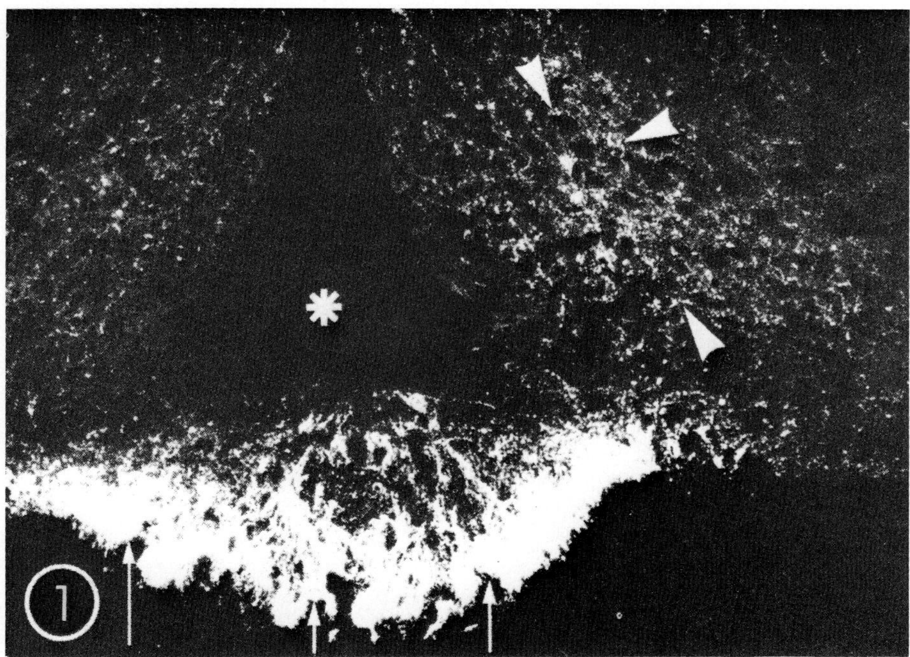

FIG. 1. Immunofluorescence micrograph of a coronal section of a rat hypothalamus showing the localization of somatostatin. The arrows indicate high concentrations of somatostatin adjacent to the primary capillaries of the pituitary portal vascular system in the median eminence. The arrowheads indicate nerve terminals in the arcuate nucleus. The asterisk marks the third ventricle (From ref. 7.)

OTHER HYPOTHALAMIC RELEASING AND INHIBITING FACTORS

Releasing or inhibiting factors have been described for every hormone secreted by the adenophypophysis (Table 2). The releasing factor for ACTH was the first to be described but remains unidentified chemically despite strenuous efforts to isolate it (31). Vasopressin also releases ACTH, but it is much less potent than hypothalamic corticotropin-releasing factor (CRF) preparations. The existence of a growth hormone-releasing factor (GRF) has been reported by numerous groups, but its identity remains unknown (31). Both it and somatostatin are believed to be important for the regulation of ongoing growth hormone secretion. For instance, in rats growth hormone is secreted in a pulsatile pattern and neutralization of somatostatin by injections of an antiserum to somatostatin elevates growth hormone levels. However, the pulsatile pattern of growth hormone secretion continues, presumably due to the secretion of a GRF (10,28).

α-Melanocyte-stimulating hormone (α-MSH) is secreted by the pars intermedia of the rat adenohypophysis. Its secretion is tonically inhibited by the hypothalamus as demonstrated by increased secretion when intermediate lobes are incubated *in vitro* or after hypothalamic lesions (31). The intermediate lobe is

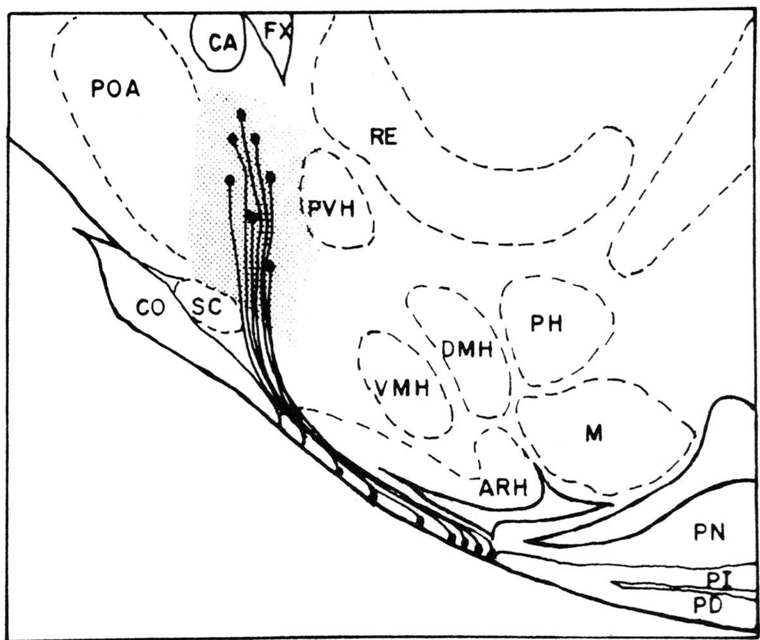

FIG. 2. Parasagittal section of the rat hypothalamus showing the location of neuronal cell bodies for LHRH, TRH, and somatostatin that project to the external layer of the median eminence. They have been localized by immunocytochemical techniques and by lesions and transections. (ARH) arcuate nucleus. (CA) anterior commissure. (CO) optic chiasm. (DMH) dorsomedial nucleus. (FX) fornix. (M) mammillary nucleus. (PD) anterior pituitary gland. (PH) posterior hypothalamic nucleus. (PI) intermediate lobe of the pituitary gland. (PN) posterior lobe of the pituitary. (POA) preoptic area. (PVH) paraventricular nucleus. (RE) reuniens nucleus of the thalamus. (SC) suprachiasmatic nucleus. (VMH) ventromedial nucleus. (From ref. 7.)

densely innervated by dopaminergic neurons, and dopamine has been shown to inhibit MSH secretion. However, in addition, a peptide melanocyte-inhibiting factor (MIF) has been described and is identical to the N-terminal tripeptide sequence of oxytocin. Hypothalamic extracts containing MSH-releasing activity have also been reported. One group reported that MSH-RF was identical to a

TABLE 2. *Hypophysiotropic factors of established function but unknown structure*

Name	Function
Corticotropin-releasing factor (CRF)	Releases ACTH
Growth hormone-releasing factor (GRF)	Releases GH
Prolactin-releasing factor (PRF)	Releases prolactin
Prolactin-inhibiting factor (PIF)	Inhibits prolactin release
Melanocyte-stimulating hormone-releasing factor (MSH-RF)	Releases MSH
Melanocyte-stimulating hormone-inhibiting factor (MSH-IF)	Inhibits MSH release

pentapeptide sequence found in oxytocin, but other groups report that this peptide is inactive in releasing MSH in mammals (31).

At least two inhibiting factors and two releasing factors have been reported to regulate prolactin secretion. These factors are described in detail in the next section.

HYPOTHALAMIC REGULATION OF PROLACTIN SECRETION

Hypophysiotropic Factors

PIFs

At present the hypothalamic regulation of prolactin secretion appears to be the most complex of all the hormones secreted by the adenohypophysis. As noted earlier, at least two inhibiting factors and at least two releasing factors have been described for prolactin (31).

The earliest studies on prolactin secretion indicated that the hypothalamus was inhibitory to prolactin secretion. Everett, in his classic studies (9), demonstrated that transplantation of the pituitary gland under the kidney capsule resulted in maintenance of ovarian corpora lutea, an indication of elevated prolactin secretion. The discovery that tranquilizing drugs—known to deplete the hypothalamus of catecholamine stores—elevated prolactin secretion (19), and Fuxe's (12) discovery that a high concentration of dopamine was present in axonal endings in the median eminence (12) led to the view that dopamine either was a neurotransmitter that regulated PIF release or was PIF itself (19). Although this much-debated question remains incompletely resolved, current evidence suggests that dopamine has both actions.

Recent studies indicate that dopamine is a physiological PIF acting directly on the pituitary to inhibit prolactin secretion. Dopamine inhibits prolactin secretion when added to pituitaries incubated *in vitro* (19). Specific receptors for dopamine have been found in the pituitary, presumably on lactotrophs (5). In addition, Porter's group (3) demonstrated that dopamine is a secretory product of the rat median eminence by showing that plasma collected from the hypophyseal stalk contained more dopamine than did plasma collected from the peripheral circulation (3). We confirmed this finding in the rat but, in addition, showed that the amount of dopamine in stalk plasma was sufficient to account for most of the hypothalamic inhibition of prolactin secretion (22). In these studies we blocked endogenous dopamine secretion with α-methyl-*p*-tyrosine, which results in a 100-fold increase in plasma prolactin levels. We then initiated dopamine infusions into the peripheral circulation at a rate to achieve dopamine concentrations in peripheral plasma that equaled those normally found in portal blood. A 70% inhibition of prolactin secretion occurred, leading us to conclude that dopamine is a physiological PIF. However, because prolactin secretion was not fully inhibited by physiological dopamine infusions, it appears that an additional PIF exists (13).

We performed similar studies in the rhesus monkey (Neill, Plotsky, Frawley, and Tindall, *unpublished*). We collected hypophyseal stalk blood via a transorbital surgical approach for measuring the dopamine concentration using a liquid chromatographic–electrochemical technique. As shown in Table 3, dopamine concentrations in hypophyseal stalk plasma of the monkey ranged from 0.37 to 1.26 ng/ml. The overall mean for all animals was 0.76 ng/ml. Since dopamine was undetectable in serum obtained from the saphenous vein (Table 3), it is apparent that dopamine is a secretory product of the median eminence in rhesus monkeys.

Next we determined the infusion rate of dopamine that would achieve plasma dopamine concentrations similar to those found in stalk plasma. Indwelling cannulas were placed in the two saphenous veins of each of seven monkeys, one for an infusion of dopamine and the other for blood sampling (for measurement of dopamine). We found that a dopamine infusion rate of 0.1 μg/min/kg body weight produced dopamine levels of approximately 0.7 ng/ml (Fig. 3), levels similar to those previously measured in stalk plasma.

Having established a rate of dopamine infusion that might be considered "physiological," we infused that amount of dopamine into the peripheral circulation of hypophyseal stalk-sectioned animals to determine its effect on prolactin secretion. Stalk-transected animals were used to remove the influence of the hypothalamus (including endogenous dopamine secretion), and they were also treated with estradiol in amounts to mimic midfollicular levels of the menstrual cycle since stalk blood had been collected from monkeys in the follicular phase for dopamine measurements (Table 3). The results are shown in Fig. 4. A "physiological" dopamine infusion inhibited plasma prolactin levels by about 70% compared to stalk-sectioned control animals receiving a saline infusion. However, the prolactin was not suppressed to levels normally observed in intact follicular phase monkeys. Thus, as with our results in rats, dopamine appears to be a physiologically significant PIF, but it does not account for the full inhibition normally exerted by the hypothalamus on prolactin secretion.

TABLE 3. *Dopamine concentrations in hypophyseal stalk plasma of rhesus monkeys*

Animal no.	Stalk plasma dopamine (ng/ml)				Peripheral plasma dopamine (ng/ml)
	Hour 1	Hour 2	Hour 3	Mean	
F95	0.40	—	—	0.40	<0.1
F70	0.44	0.37	—	0.41	<0.1
F74	0.99	0.48	0.60	0.69	<0.1
F89	0.84	0.56	—	0.70	<0.1
F78	0.65	0.86	0.76	0.76	<0.1
F5	1.12	1.05	1.26	1.14	<0.1
F4	1.19	1.26	—	1.23	<0.1
Mean				0.76	

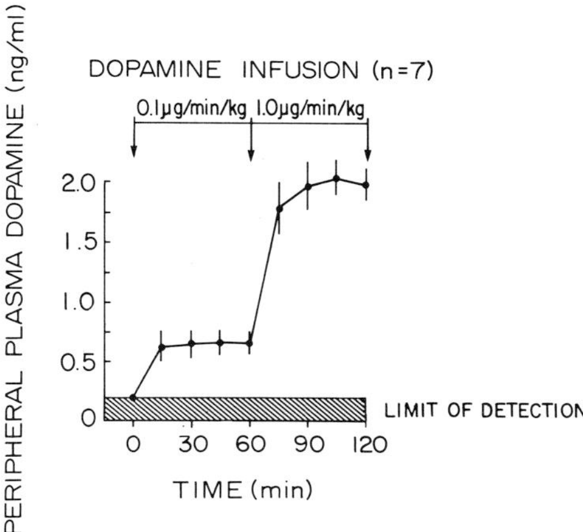

FIG. 3. Dopamine concentrations in peripheral plasma achieved by dopamine infusions into a saphenous vein of rhesus monkeys. A dopamine infusion of 0.1 μg/min/kg achieved plasma dopamine concentrations of approximately 0.7 ng/ml, similar to those found in hypophyseal stalk plasma (0.76 ng/ml; see Table 3).

Our results are consonant with numerous other observations for a non-dopamine PIF. Arimura and Schally (2) reported the isolation of a non-dopamine PIF; structural analysis of the isolated material revealed that it was γ-aminobutyric acid (GABA). The significance of GABA as a PIF is difficult to assess. Its minimal effective dose for inhibition of prolactin secretion from pituitaries incubated *in vitro* is about 100 ng/ml compared to about 10 ng/ml for dopamine (2).

At least two groups reported the existence of a PIF whose activity can be

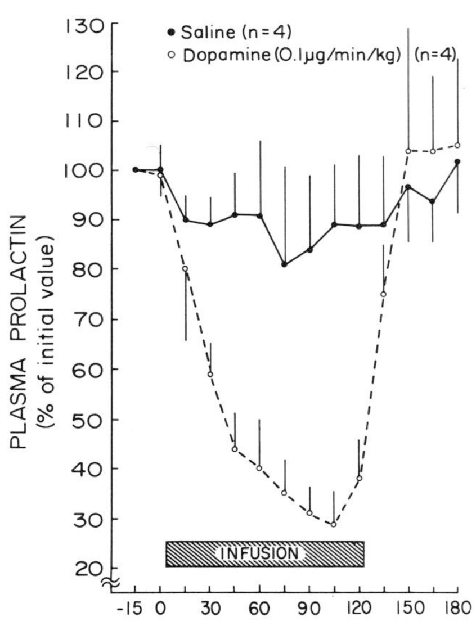

FIG. 4. Effect of physiologic dopamine concentrations on peripheral plasma prolactin levels of stalk-transected monkeys. Dopamine was infused into the saphenous vein at a rate (0.1 μg/min/kg) set to achieve concentrations similar to those found in hypophyseal stalk plasma (see Table 3 and Fig. 3).

destroyed by incubation with proteolytic enzymes, suggesting that their PIF was peptide in nature (14,30). Kordon's group recently reported that a PIF could be extracted from hypothalamic tissue but not from other areas of the brain, and that its action to inhibit prolactin release *in vitro* could not be prevented with dopamine receptor blockers. In the same experiments these blockers were fully effective in preventing dopamine-induced inhibition of prolactin secretion (8).

Thus considerable evidence supports the existence of a PIF, in addition to dopamine, and that it may be a peptide or GABA. An illustration of the complexity of this control system and why it has been so difficult to unravel is provided by experiments suggesting that secretion of a non-dopamine PIF is dopamine-dependent. More PIF activity was released into the medium of incubating median eminence tissues in the presence of dopamine than in its absence (23). The PIF released was assayed by its ability to inhibit prolactin secretion *in vitro* in a system in which nondopamine PIF could be distinguished from dopamine through the use of dopamine-receptor blockers. Thus it is apparent that when a dopaminergic drug is administered to an intact animal and changes in prolactin secretion are observed, the drug may have acted directly on either the pituitary, the hypothalamus, or both to alter prolactin secretion.

PRFs

Just as there appear to be two PIFs, there is evidence for the existence of at least two PRFs. As noted earlier (Table 1), TRH is known to release prolactin by a direct action on the pituitary gland. Some investigators have had difficulty accepting that TRH is a physiologically significant PRF because their expectation has not been met that the patterns of TSH and prolactin secretion would always be coincident in various physiological states. This monolithic view seems less reasonable if we admit that the responsiveness of the pituitary gland might not always be equal; hence the pituitary might be more responsive to TRH in terms of TSH secretion at certain times and less so at others, and *vice versa* with respect to prolactin secretion. Moreover, with the discovery that somatostatin inhibits TSH secretion, but not prolactin secretion, it becomes obvious that the level of somatostatin secretion differentially affects the pituitary's response to TRH (31).

Nevertheless, TRH cannot yet be considered a physiologically important PRF. Studies similar to those we performed with dopamine and prolactin secretion are needed (Table 3; Fig. 3 and 4). That is, the amount of TRH in hypophyseal stalk blood must be established and then those concentrations delivered into animals in which hypothalamic influence is removed to determine if prolactin (and TSH) secretion is stimulated. Only then can we accept or reject TRH as a physiologically significant PRF.

Numerous reports have appeared of PRF activity in hypothalamic extracts that cannot be accounted for by TRH. As an example, Reichlin and his colleagues

(4) recently reported that purified hypothalamic extract, incubated with serum enzymes to destroy TRH and vasopressin, was still effective in stimulating prolactin release *in vitro.* This and numerous other reports of a similar nature lend confidence that a non-TRH PRF exists (31). However, further studies are required before its identity can be established.

Neurotransmitters

Various substances established as neurotransmitters in other neural systems, (e.g., catecholamines, serotonin, GABA, histamine, and acetylcholine) have profound effects on prolactin secretion (31). Except for dopamine, as discussed earlier, these neurotransmitters are thought to act at the hypothalamic level rather than at the pituitary to affect prolactin release. Their roles may be that of classic synaptic transmitters, transmitting incoming information from the periphery via second-order neurons onto the hypophysiotropic neurons (first order), or they may play some role in the tonic stimulation or inhibition of the activity of hypophysiotropic hormones. Whatever their roles, powerful drugs have become available that alter the activity of primarily catecholaminergic neurons. The biochemical or morphological site of action of these drugs is known in many instances (Fig. 5 and 6; Table 4) and are worthy of some consideration in detail.

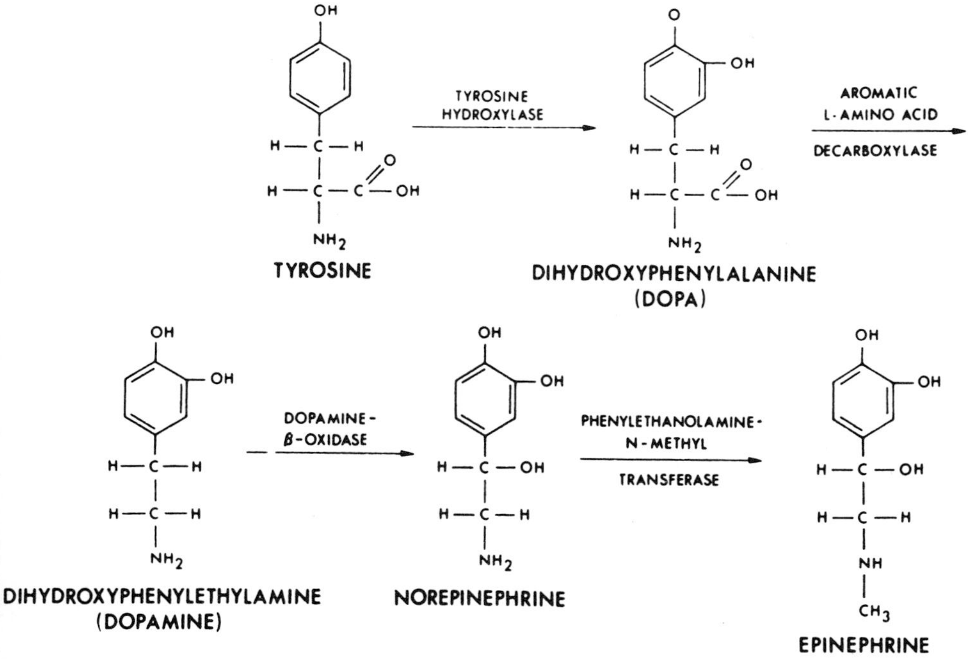

FIG. 5. Metabolic pathways for synthesis of dopamine, norepinephrine, and epinephrine.

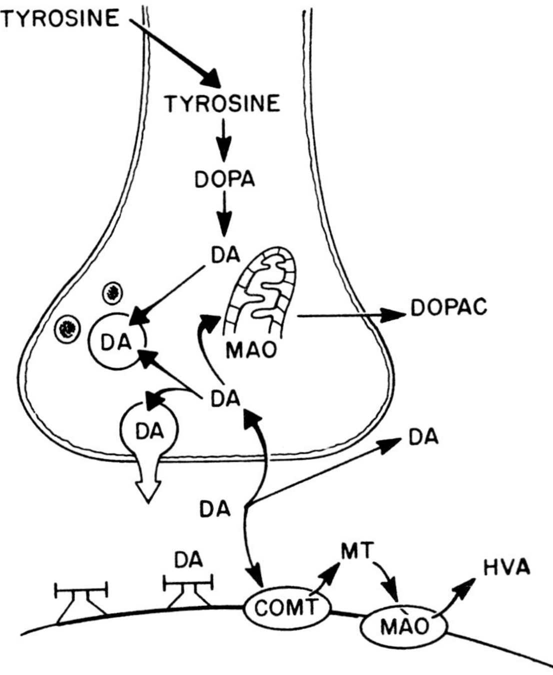

FIG. 6. A central dopaminergic synapse. (DOPA) dihydroxyphenylalanine. (DA) dopamine. (DOPAC) dihydroxyphenylacetic acid. (MAO) monoamine oxidase. (COMT) catechol-O-methyltransferase. (MT) 3-methoxytyramine. (HVA) homovanillic acid. (From ref. 20.)

The precursors, products, and enzymes involved in the synthesis of the catecholamines are shown in Fig. 5 (20). Dopaminergic neurons lack the enzymes necessary for synthesis of norepinephrine and epinephrine, and hence dopamine is stored in and released from granules within the nerve terminals. A generalized central or peripheral dopaminergic synapse is illustrated in Fig. 6. Not all of the details shown are established for hypothalamic dopaminergic neurons, but it seems likely that this is a satisfactory model.

The first step in the synthesis of dopamine is the active transport of amino acid tyrosine into the nerve cell (Fig. 6) (20). After its entry into the neuron, tyrosine is hydroxylated to form L-DOPA by the enzyme tyrosine hydroxylase. L-DOPA is decarboxylated to form dopamine by the enzyme L-aminodecarboxylase. After its synthesis, dopamine is stored in granules within the nerve terminals where it is protected from degradation (Fig. 6). Dopamine is released from the nerve terminal within the granule. This occurs in response to neuronal depolarization; granules are extruded from the axonal endings. Specific receptor sites for dopamine are believed to exist on the postsynaptic cell body of hypophysiotropic neurons. Binding of the dopamine to the receptor site activates the secretion of the hypophysiotropic hormone (PIF?). The fate of free dopamine

TABLE 4. *Catecholaminergic drugs and their effects on prolactin secretion*

Drug	Trade name	Mechanisms of action	Effects on catecholamines	Effect on prolactin secretion[a]
Precursors				
L-DOPA	Larodopa	Increases substrate for DA[b]	Increases DA and NE[b] levels in the brain	–
Receptor stimulators				
Apomorphine	—	Stimulates DA	Mimics DA effects	–
Bromergocriptine	Parlodel	Receptors		
Receptor blockers				
Pimozide	—	Blocks DA receptors	Prevents DA effects	+
Haloperidol	Haldol	Blocks DA receptors	Prevents DA effects	
Chlorpromazine	Largactil Thorazine	Blocks DA receptors	Prevents DA effects	
Enzyme inhibitors				
α-Methyl-p-tyrosine	—	Inhibits tyrosine hydroxylase	Blocks formation of DA and NE	+
Disulfram fusaric acid	Antabuse	Blocks dopamine-β-oxidase	Blocks formation of NE with consequent increase in DA	–
Precursor analog				
α-Methyldopa	Aldomet	Converted into methylated monoamine	Acts as false transmitter	+
Presynaptic storage blockers				
Reserpine	Serpasil	Inhibits storage and reuptake of biogenic amines by granules	Depletion of DA, NE, and serotonin in terminals	+
Tricylic antidepressants	Imipramine Chlorimipramine	Blocks reuptake by nerve terminals	Depletes terminals of catecholamines and serotonin	+
Mixed function				
Amphetamines	—	Releases biogenic amines, blocks reuptake	Increases NE turnover, increases availability of NE	+
Catecholaminergic nerve ending poison				
6-Hydroxydopamine	—	Localizes to catecholamine nerve ending	Destroys dopaminergic and noradrenergic terminals	+

Modified from ref. 20.

[a](+) Stimulation of prolactin secretion. (–) Inhibition of prolactin secretion.

[b](DA) dopamine. (NE) norepinephrine.

in the synaptic cleft not bound to a receptor site is fourfold. It may be (a) taken up into the presynaptic nerve ending and incorporated into a storage granule; (b) taken up by the presynaptic nerve ending and destroyed by monoamine oxidase to form homovanillic acid and dihydroxyphenylacetic acid, both of which are inert; (c) diffused away into the interstitial fluid surrounding the nerve terminals; and (d) destroyed by an enzyme, catechol-0-methyltransferase, to form 3-methoxytyramine (Fig. 6) (20).

Many drugs have been developed that affect dopaminergic activity at one of these numerous sites of action. A partial list of such drugs, their sites of action, and their effect on prolactin secretion are shown in Table 4 (20). Examination of this list reveals that drugs may affect substrate level (L-DOPA), block dopamine synthesis by action on tyrosine hydroxylase, deplete presynaptic granular stores of dopamine, block reuptake, and block or activate dopamine receptors. Experimental use of these drugs has contributed to our understanding of the prolactin control system as well as to ameliorating one of its derangements: the amenorrhea–galactorrhea syndrome.

Neuropeptides

A variety of new peptides have been discovered during the last few years that have profound behavioral and homeostatic effects (7,17,24,31). Among their actions is an effect on pituitary hormone secretion and, in particular, prolactin secretion. Table 5 contains a list of these peptides with their amino acid sequences. These peptides are found in high concentration in the hypothalamus, and all stimulate prolactin secretion when administered systemically or intracranially into experimental animals. However, they are believed not to be hypophysiotropic factors because they are ineffective stimulators of prolactin secretion when applied directly onto pituitary cells cultured *in vitro* (VIP is a possible exception as discussed below) (25,31). Thus they are believed to modulate the release of PIFs and PRFs in stimulating prolactin secretion. Whether these effects are physiological or only pharmacological remains to be determined.

Substance P (Table 5) is a hypotensive agent when administered systemically. It has been localized in the dorsal root of the spinal cord where it is believed to serve as an excitatory synaptic transmitter of primary sensory neurons (24). It is also found in high concentrations in the hypothalamus, particularly in the preoptic region, but little is found in the median eminence (7).

Neurotensin (Table 5) is also hypotensive when administered systemically but, in addition, is hyperglycemic via suppression of insulin and stimulation of glucagon secretion. It stimulates contractions of the ileum but brings about relaxation of the duodenum (31). Neurotensin is found spread throughout the brain but appears in particularly high concentration in the hypothalamus (6).

Bombesin (Table 5) was originally isolated from the skin of the frog *(Bombina bombina)* (1). When administered systemically, it increases blood pressure, stimulates gastric acid secretion, and lowers body temperature. It is the most potent

TABLE 5. *Hypothalamic peptides that affect prolactin secretion indirectly*

Name	Structure
Substance P	Arg-Pro-Lys-Pro-Gln-Gln-Phe-Phe-Gly-Leu-Met-NH_2
Neurotensin	*p*Glu-Leu-Tyr-Glu-Asn-Lys-Pro-Arg-Arg-Pro-Tyr-Ile-Leu-OH
Bombesin	*p*Glu-Gln-Arg-Leu-Gly-Asn-Gln-Trp-Ala-Val-Gly-His-Leu-Met-NH_2
Leu-enkephalin	Tyr-Gly-Gly-Phe-Leu-OH
Met-enkephalin	Tyr-Gly-Gly-Phe-Met-OH
β-Endorphin	Tyr-Gly-Gly-Phe-Met-Thr-Ser-Glu-Lys-Ser-Gln-Thr-Pro-Leu-Val-Thr-Leu-Phe-Lys-Asn-Ala-Ile-Val-Lys-Asn-Ala-His-Lys-Lys-Gly-Gln-OH
Vasoactive intestinal polypeptide (VIP)	His-Ser-Asp-Ala-Val-Phe-Thr-Asp-Asn-Tyr-Thr-Arg-Leu-Arg-Lys-Gln-Met-Ala-Val-Lys-Lys-Tyr-Leu-Asn-Ser-Ile-Leu-Asn-NH_2

of all the neuropeptides discovered thus far that stimulate prolactin secretion (25). Like the other neuropeptides, it is found throughout the brain but with particularly high concentrations in the hypothalamus (32).

The enkephalins and β-endorphin (Table 5) are called opioid peptides because they bind to morphine receptors in brain tissue. All three have analgesic properties, but β-endorphin is most potent in this regard (29). They are all contained within the structure of a pituitary hormone, β-lipotropin, but whether it can be considered their parent compound is unsettled. Neural localization of the enkephalins and β-endorphin is not coincident. β-Endorphin is found in high concentrations in the pituitary gland, primarily the intermediate lobe. Enkephalins are present in the pituitary gland in only very small concentrations but are found throughout the brain including the hypothalamus (29). Nerve terminals for enkephalin ending in the external layer of the median eminence have been described with a morphology similar to that of the hypophysiotropic neurons (7,17). These opioid peptides release prolactin when administered intracranially, with β-endorphin being most potent (31).

Vasoactive intestinal polypeptide (VIP) (Table 5) was originally isolated from intestinal tissues. Administered systemically, it produces hyperglycemia, hypotension, and water excretion by the gut (24). More recently it was found in the brain with high concentrations present in the hypothalamus (7,17). Unlike the other neuropeptides, there is evidence that it may act directly on the pituitary gland to affect prolactin secretion. It has been found in hypophyseal stalk plasma in higher concentrations than in peripheral blood, suggesting that it is a secretory product of the median eminence (26). Moreover, although it does not alter prolactin secretion when added alone to pituitaries *in vitro,* when mixed with dopamine it antagonizes the effect of dopamine to inhibit prolactin release (18).

The potential importance of this observation—if it is confirmed—is that one cannot rule out a substance acting as a hypophysiotropic factor simply because it alone does not alter hormone release from isolated pituitaries. A re-examination of all of the neurotransmitters and neuropeptides that are thought to affect prolactin secretion indirectly may be required in light of this finding.

Control of Prolactin Secretion

The best-established action of prolactin is that it stimulates breast growth and development as well as milk secretion (Fig. 7). As a corollary, the best characterized stimulus for prolactin release is suckling of the nipple by the baby. Estrogens secreted by the ovaries and placenta during pregnancy also stimulate prolactin secretion in part by an action directly on the pituitary gland and in part by acting directly on the hypothalamus. The relatively low levels of estrogens secreted by the ovaries during the menstrual cycle are insufficient to stimulate baseline prolactin secretion but do increase the amount of prolactin secreted in response to evocative stimuli such as TRH or stress. Stressful stimuli such as surgery and many other lesser stimuli stimulate the secretion of prolactin

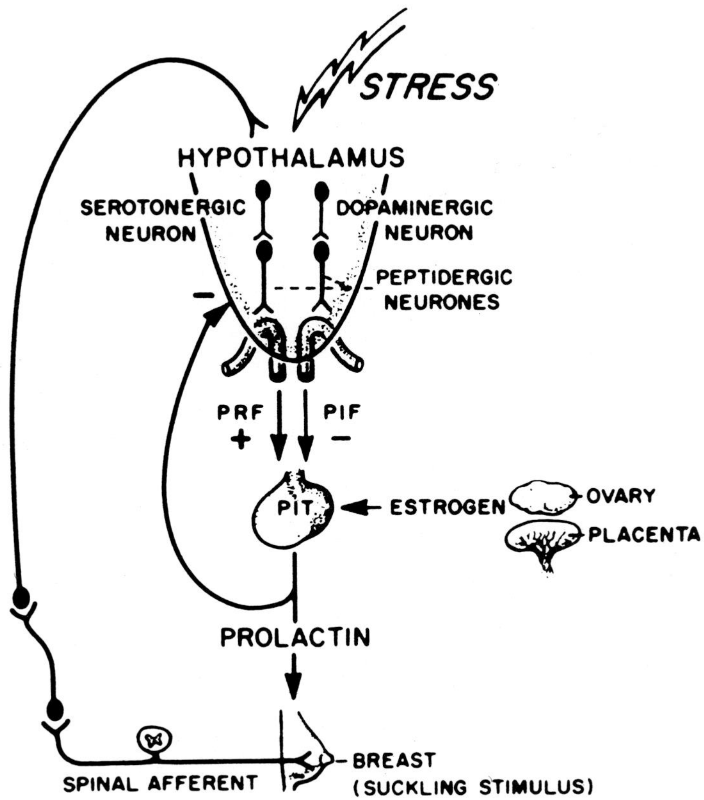

FIG. 7. Control of prolactin secretion. Hypothalamic factors—PIFs and PRFs—regulate prolactin secretion. Exteroceptive neural stimuli (e.g., suckling the nipple and stress) impinge on the hypothalamus to stimulate prolactin release. Estrogens from the ovary and placenta act at the pituitary to increase its sensitivity to prolactin-releasing stimuli and at the hypothalamus (not indicated). Prolactin may inhibit its own secretion via an action on the hypothalamus. (From ref. 20.)

(11). This is enigmatic because prolactin is not known to play a role in those metabolic and behavioral processes that "protect" an organism against stress. Finally, there is evidence that prolactin may inhibit its own secretion via a short-loop feedback action (Fig. 7). The importance of this mechanism in the economy of prolactin secretion is unsettled but appears to be a chronic, rather than an acute, mechanism.

The identity of the hypophysiotropic factors, neurotransmitters, and neuropeptides involved in the reflex pathways for prolactin release subserving the stimuli of suckling, stress, estrogens, and prolactin itself are unknown. For instance, although it seems clear that dopamine is a physiologic PIF—tonically inhibiting prolactin secretion—it is not yet clear whether it plays a dynamic role in the control of prolactin secretion, i.e., whether the secretion of dopamine is altered by suckling, stress, estrogens, or prolactin itself. Similar uncertainties exist about TRH. Likewise, whether neurotransmitters and neuropeptides function in the dynamic regulation of prolactin secretion remains unknown.

Clearly, it will be a formidable experimental task to elucidate which of the PIFs and PRFs, which of the neurotransmitters, and which of the neuropeptides are involved in the reflex release of prolactin in response to suckling, for example. Indeed it is mystifying why a plethora of control substances would be needed for a seemingly simple neuroendocrine reflex such as suckling-induced release of prolactin. Whatever the final answer turns out to be, it seems likely that untangling this complex control system will be necessary before we can specify the specific derangement(s) that lead to the excessive prolactin secretion observed in the amenorrhea–galactorrhea syndrome.

ACKNOWLEDGMENTS

Supported by research grants (HD 07066 and HD 04312) from the National Institute of Child Health and Human Development, NIH, USPHS.

REFERENCES

1. Anastasi, A., Erspamer, V., and Bucci, M. (1971): Isolation and structure of bombesin and alytesin, two analogous active peptides from the skin of the European amphibians Bombina and Alytes. *Experientia,* 27:166–167.
2. Arimura, A., and Schally, A. V. (1977): Prolactin release inhibiting and stimulating factors in the hypothalamus. In: *Hypothalamic Peptide Hormones and Pituitary Regulation,* edited by J. C. Porter. Plenum Press, New York.
3. Ben-Jonathan, N., Oliver, C., Weiner, H. J., Mical, R. S., and Porter, J. C. (1977): Dopamine in hypophysial portal plasma of the rat during the estrous cycle and throughout pregnancy. *Endocrinology,* 100:452–458.
4. Boyd, A. E., III, Sanchez-Franco, F., Spencer, E., Patel, Y. C., Jackson, I. M. D., and Reichlin, S. (1978): Characterization of hypophysiotropic hormones in porcine hypothalamic extracts. *Endocrinology,* 103:1075–1083.
5. Brown, G. M., Seeman, P., and Lee, T. (1976): Dopamine/neuroleptic receptors in basal hypothalamus and pituitary. *Endocrinology,* 99:1407–1410.
6. Carraway, R., and Leeman, S. E. (1976): Characterization of radioimmunoassayable neurotensin in the rat. *J. Biol. Chem.,* 251:7045–7052.
7. Elde, R., and Hökfelt, T. (1978): Distribution of hypothalamic hormones and other peptides in the brain. In: *Frontiers in Neuroendocrinology,* edited by W. F. Ganong and L. Martini. Raven Press, New York.
8. Enjalbert, A., Moos, F., Carbonell, L., Priam, M., and Kordon, C. (1977): Prolactin inhibiting activity of dopamine-free subcellular fractions from rat mediobasal hypothalamus. *Neuroendocrinology,* 24:147–161.
9. Everett, J. W. (1954): Luteotrophic function of autografts of the rat hypophysis. *Endocrinology,* 54:685–690.
10. Ferland, L., Labrie, F., Jobin, M., Arimura, A., and Schally, A. V. (1976): Physiological role of somatostatin in the control of growth hormone and thyrotropin secretion. *Biochem. Biophys. Res. Commun.,* 68:149–156.
11. Frantz, A. G. (1973): The regulation of prolactin secretion in humans. In: *Frontiers in Neuroendocrinology,* edited by W. F. Ganong and L. Martini. Oxford University Press, New York.
12. Fuxe, K. (1964): Cellular localization of monoamines in the median eminence and the infundibular stem of some mammals. *Z. Zellforsch.,* 61:710–724.

13. Gibbs, D. M., and Neill, J. D. (1978): Dopamine levels in hypophysial stalk blood in the rat are sufficient to inhibit prolactin secretion in vivo. *Endocrinology,* 102:1895–1900.
14. Greibrokk, T., Hansen, J., Knudsen, R., Lam, Y., Folkers, K., and Bowers, C. Y. (1975): On the isolation of a prolactin inhibiting factor (hormone). *Biochem. Biophys. Res. Commun.,* 67:338–344.
15. Guillemin, R. (1978): Biochemical and physiological correlates of hypothalamic peptides: The new endocrinology of the neuron. In: *The Hypothalamus,* edited by S. Reichlin, R. J. Baldessarini, and J. B. Martin. Raven Press, New York.
16. Harris, G. W. (1955): *Neural Control of the Pituitary Gland.* Arnold, London.
17. Hökfelt, T., Elde, R., Fuxe, K., Johansson, O., Ljungdahl, A., Goldstein, M., Luft, R., Efendic, S., Nilsson, G., Terenius, L., Ganten, D., Jeffcoate, S. L., Rehfeld, J., Said, S., de la Mora, M. P., Possani, L., Tapia, R., Teran, L., and Palacios, R. (1978): Aminergic and peptidergic pathways in the nervous system with special reference to the hypothalamus. In: *The Hypothalamus,* edited by S. Reichlin, R. J. Baldessarini, and J. B. Martin. Raven Press, New York.
18. Kato, Y., Iwasaki, Y., Iwasaki, J., Abe, H., Seino, Y., Yanaihara, N., and Imura, H. (1978): Prolactin release by vasoactive intestinal polypeptide in rats. In: *Abstracts of the Endocrine Society.*
19. MacLeod, R. M. (1976): Regulation of prolactin secretion. In: *Frontiers in Neuroendocrinology,* edited by L. Martini and W. F. Ganong. Raven Press, New York.
20. Martin, J. B., Reichlin, S., and Brown, G. M. (1977): *Clinical Endocrinology.* Davis, Philadelphia.
21. Neill, J. D., Patton, J. M., Dailey, R. A. Tsou, R. C., and Tindall, G. T. (1977): Luteinizing hormone releasing hormone (LHRH) in pituitary stalk blood of rhesus monkeys: Relationship to level of LH release. *Endocrinology,* 101:430–434.
22. Plotsky, P. M., Gibbs, D. M., and Neill, J. D. (1978): Liquid chromatographic-electrochemical measurement of dopamine in hypophysial stalk blood of rats. *Endocrinology,* 102:1887–1894.
23. Quijada, M., Illner, P., Krulich, L., and McCann, S. M. (1973/74): The effect of catecholamines on hormone release from anterior pituitaries and ventral hypothalami incubated in vitro. *Neuroendocrinology,* 13:151–163.
24. Reichlin, S. (1978): Introduction. In: *The Hypothalamus,* edited by S. Reichlin, R. J. Baldessarini, and J. B. Martin. Raven Press, New York.
25. Rivier, C., Rivier, J., and Vale, W. (1978): The effect of bombesin and related peptides on prolactin and growth hormone secretion in rats. *Endocrinology,* 102:519–522.
26. Said, S. I., and Porter, J. C. (1978): Vasoactive intestinal polypeptide (VIP): Evidence for secretion into hypophyseal portal blood. *Fed. Proc.,* 37:482.
27. Schally, A. V. (1978): Aspects of hypothalamic regulation of the pituitary gland. *Science,* 202:18–28.
28. Terry, L. C., Martin, J. B., Willoughby, J. O., and Brazeau, P. (1976): Antiserum to somatostatin prevents stress-induced inhibition of growth hormone (GH) in the rat. *Fed. Proc.,* 35:3173.
29. Uhl, G. R., Childers, S. R., and Snyder, S. H. (1978): Opioid peptides and the opiate receptor. In: *Frontiers in Neuroendocrinology,* edited by W. F. Ganong and L. Martini. Raven Press, New York.
30. Vale, W. (1976): Application of adenohypophyseal cell cultures to neuroendocrine studies. In: *Hypothalamus and Endocrine Functions,* edited by F. Labrie, J. Meites, and G. Pelletier. Plenum Press, New York.
31. Vale, W., Rivier, C., and Brown, M. (1977): Regulatory peptides of the hypothalamus. *Annu. Rev. Physiol.,* 39:473–527.
32 Villarreal, J. A., Rivier, J., and Brown, M. (1978): Evidence for a bombesin-like substance in hypothalamus: Chemical and immunological characterization. In: *Abstracts of the Endocrine Society.*

Clinical Management of Pituitary Disorders,
edited by G. T. Tindall and W. F. Collins.
Raven Press, New York © 1979.

3

Pathology of Pituitary Tumors and Value of Frozen Section Diagnosis

Yoshio Takei

Department of Pathology and Laboratory Medicine, Emory University School of Medicine, Atlanta, Georgia 30322

A diversity of tissue elements, including endocrine, neuroectodermal, vascular, meningeal, and skeletal structures are arranged in close proximity to the sella turcica. Any one of these tissue elements can give rise to a variety of mass lesions that may cause abnormalities of the sella and which may be confused with primary pituitary tumors. Various disorders presenting as "pituitary mass lesions" are listed in Table 1. In this chapter the pathology of the more important lesions included in Table 1 is discussed with special emphasis on differential diagnosis, followed by a discussion of the value of frozen section diagnosis.

TABLE 1. *Differential diagnosis of "pituitary mass lesions"*

Neoplastic disorders	Nonneoplastic disorders
A. Pituitary origin	A. The "empty sella" syndrome
1. Adenomas of adenohypophysis	B. Nonneoplastic cysts
2. Craniopharyngiomas	1. Arachnoid cysts
3. Tumors of neurohypophysis	2. Rathke's pouch cysts
4. Carcinomas	3. Mucocele
5. Sarcomas	C. Aneurysms and other vascular malformations
B. Nonpituitary origin	D. Inflammatory disorders
1. Meningiomas	1. Abscesses
2. Gliomas of hypothalamic region	2. Granulomatous infections
3. Chordomas	3. "Allergic" hypophysitis
4. Dermoid and epidermoid cysts	E. "Pituitary apoplexy"
5. Teratomas and teratoid tumors including germinomas	
6. Lipomas	
7. Hemangioblastomas	
8. Lymphoproliferative disorders	
9. Tumors of skeletal origin	
10. Metastases	

NEOPLASTIC DISORDERS—PITUITARY ORIGIN

Adenomas of Adenohypophysis

Pituitary adenomas have been estimated to account for 10% of intracranial tumors. However, this figure has increased during recent years owing to advanced diagnostic techniques in endocrinology and neuroradiology combined with transsphenoidal microsurgery. In our neuropathology laboratories, which process approximately 200 tumors of the central nervous system each year, more than 30% have been pituitary adenomas during the past 3 years. Concurrently, the size of pituitary adenomas removed surgically and examined histologically became smaller, thus requiring improved technical and diagnostic neuropathologic skills. Since complex endocrine abnormalities of the patients are now well worked up and functional aspects of the tumor are emphasized, classification of the pituitary adenoma passed solely on cytologic morphology is inadequate.

Current Status of Classification

Traditionally these adenomas have been divided according to their tinctorial properties into three types: chromophobic, eosinophilic (or acidophilic), and basophilic adenomas. The chromophobic type was regarded to have no endocrine function. The eosinophilic type was considered to be a growth hormone (GH)-secreting tumor because of its frequent association with acromegaly, whereas the basophilic type, usually associated with Cushing's disease, was supposed to secrete adrenocorticotropic hormone (ACTH). Although the latest World Health Organization (WHO) classification of brain tumors continues this tradition (55), it has become apparent that this classification is unsatisfactory because of its failure to reflect precise function–morphology relationships. As in any oncological nosology, classification of the pituitary adenomas appropriately begins with studies of the cells in the normal adenohypophysis.

Currently there are seven hormones generally accepted as separate substances in the normal adenohypophysis. These consist of GH, prolactin, ACTH, melanocyte-stimulating hormone (MSH), thyroid-stimulating hormone (TSH), follicle-stimulating hormone (FSH), and luteinizing hormone (LH). However, as to the exact correlation of each hormone with its production site (i.e., cell types), combined studies with immunohistology and electron microscopy appear to agree only in the description of three types of cells, i. e., GH-, prolactin-, and TSH-secreting cells. Although seemingly well established in animal experiments, the "one cell–one hormone" theory cannot be applied to ACTH-MSH- or FSH-LH-producing cells in humans (30,43).

During recent years numerous investigators have attempted to delineate the function–morphology relationship of hormone-producing tumors utilizing immunofluorescence techniques and electron microscopy. Among the adenomas, GH-secreting, prolactin-secreting, and perhaps ACTH-MSH-secreting types are common and well documented (20,30,43). There have been scattered reports on more uncommon TSH-secreting adenomas (53), FSH-LH-secreting adenomas

(12,32), and those producing FSH (56) or LH (15) alone. However, the "one cell–one hormone" theory appears to be less certain with regard to some instances of adenoma compared to the normal adenohypophysis, since tumors producing both GH and prolactin (19,20,58) or combinations of TSH and prolactin (14) or FSH and prolactin (9) have been described.

Function–morphology correlation, the main issue in the taxonomy of the pituitary adenoma, is a difficult task particularly when dealing with patients who exhibit endocrine abnormalities. This is especially so when these result from neoplasms that produce endocrine properties. One fundamental fact in general oncology that is often disregarded is that a neoplasm is not just a clump of abnormally prolific cells; it is a newly formed tissue that contains parenchymal cells as well as stromal elements. Without supporting stroma, no neoplasm can grow. Therefore the function of a few representative tumor cells may not necessarily represent that of the neoplasm as a whole. It must also be remembered that it is almost impossible to identify a given cell as neoplastic or normal when it is in isolation such as when viewed under the electron microscope, especially in a benign pituitary adenoma.

Studies attempting to correlate clinical history, laboratory findings, and morphologic analysis including immunofluorescence techniques and electron microscopy have improved our understanding of the various types of pituitary adenoma, thereby contributing to a more acceptable classification. However, these sophisticated methods may not be readily available to the general medical community at present. Special staining techniques (e.g., Brooke's carmoisine or Herlant's erythrocin) may yield capricious results depending on the fixative used or technique employed. Fluorescence microscopy is becoming increasingly popular, but it may be difficult to obtain pertinent antibodies for pituitary adenomas. Electron microscopy facilities are usually located only at larger medical centers. The only consistently available methods are hematoxylin–eosin (HE) and periodic acid–Schiff (PAS) stains. Taking all of the above factors into consideration, the most practical classification at present would be a compromise between the contemporary concepts and the traditional, readily available techniques.

Practical Classification of Pituitary Adenomas

Nonfunctioning Adenomas

Nonfunctioning adenomas usually cause signs of a space-occupying lesion. Most of these tumors are "chromophobic adenomas," but they may be slightly or partly "eosinophilic" on HE preparations. The PAS stain is negative.

Oncocytomas

Oncocytomas are frequently recognized as "eosinophilic adenomas" with HE stain. PAS is essentially negative, but occasionally there may be scattered positive cells. Electron microscopy is the only way to make the exact diagnosis (30). According to Kovacs et al. (25), oncocytes arise from adenohypophyseal cells;

this transformation is gradual, not being restricted to one particular cell type. It is interesting to note in this regard that the patient with oncocytoma by Rollet et al. (37) showed galactorrhea and hyperprolactinemia.

Functioning Adenomas

GH-secreting adenomas

Acromegaly is the presenting clinical feature of GH-secreting adenomas, and these tumors correspond to the "eosinophilic adenomas." In our experience, however, the tumors frequently appear "chromophobic" with HE stain. Sometimes they show partial eosinophilia and thus may be called "mixed adenomas;" but the PAS stain is always negative.

Prolactin-secreting adenomas

Prolactin-secreting adenomas may result in the Forbes–Albright syndrome or may be asymptomatic. In the latter instance they would be regarded as nonfunctioning adenomas unless immunofluorescence or electron microscopic studies were carried out to demonstrate the hormone-secreting character of the tumor cells (26). Over 70% of these adenomas are "chromophobic adenomas," and the remainder would be labeled either "eosinophilic adenomas" or "mixed adenomas" on HE preparations. The PAS stain is negative in all cases.

GH–prolactin-secreting adenomas

The GH–prolactin-secreting adenoma is a true example of a mixed adenoma and has been recognized since Davidoff (11) reported in 1926 that 4% of his patients with acromegaly had galactorrhea. Studies reveal this type of adenoma to be composed of two types of cell: GH-secreting and prolactin-secreting (19, 20,58). With the HE stain this type of adenoma may be regarded as "eosinophilic," "chromophobic," or "mixed," but the PAS stain is negative.

ACTH–MSH-secreting adenomas

Giving rise to Cushing's disease, the ACTH–MSH-secreting adenoma is relatively easy to identify because of a strong PAS reaction in the tumor cells in most cases. HE preparations may show "basophilic adenomas," but cells may be "eosinophilic" or even "chromophobic" depending on how the stain is done. A clinically silent tumor of this type has been reported (28). Pituitary adenomas in Nelson's syndrome also belong to this type (27).

TSH-secreting adenomas

The TSH-secreting adenoma is a rare tumor as judged by the few reported cases (53). It appears that there are two types of TSH-secreting tumor (30).

The first type is associated with hyperthyroidism of relatively short duration, and the second is seen in patients with congenital or longstanding severe thyroid insufficiency. In the normal adenohypophysis, TSH-secreting cells are basophilic and PAS-positive, but many of the TSH-secreting tumors reported in the literature were labeled "chromophobic adenomas" although some were "basophilic adenomas," whereas "mixed basophilic-eosinophilic adenomas" or even "eosinophilic adenomas" have been described (30). In addition, a pituitary adenoma producing TSH and prolactin and composed of two cell types ultrastructurally has been reported (14).

FSH–LH-secreting adenomas

The FSH–LH-secreting adenoma is an extremely rare tumor. Almost all of the reported cases have been labeled "chromophobe adenomas" (56), although in the normal adenohypophysis FSH–LH-secreting cells are basophilic and PAS-positive (43). Demura (12) reported a case that was composed of 90% "chromophobic" and 10% slightly "eosinophilic," and Luboshitzky and Barzilan (32) described a case of "chromophobic adenoma." FSH and LH secretion was demonstrated in tissue culture of the tumor cells by the former authors and in the cerebrospinal fluid (CSF) by the latter. In addition, a case of "chromophobic adenoma" producing FSH and prolactin has been described (9).

Histologic Appearances of Pituitary Adenomas

In the older pathology textbooks, classification of the adenomas was based on histomorphologic appearances, e.g., diffuse, papillary, sinusoidal. This method of classification has no value because the histologic appearances do not reflect the biologic behavior of the tumors. However, it is important from the point of view of histopathologic diagnosis to be familiar with the microscopic appearances of the adenomas.

Diverse Histologic Appearance of Pituitary Adenoma

As shown in Fig. 1 through 4, adenomas of the adenohypophysis may show a diversity of appearance which may mimic neoplasms of different cytogenesis, often resulting in misdiagnosis. This possibility is especially important when a rapid frozen section is performed *(vide infra).* In our experience malignant lymphomas (Figs. 4A,B) and some meningiomas (Figs. 3C,D and 8) are the most likely lesions to create occasional problems.

Calcification in Pituitary Adenomas

In general, primary calcification in pituitary adenoma is a relatively uncommon occurrence (6,31,57). When it is detectable radiologically, other tumors (e.g.,

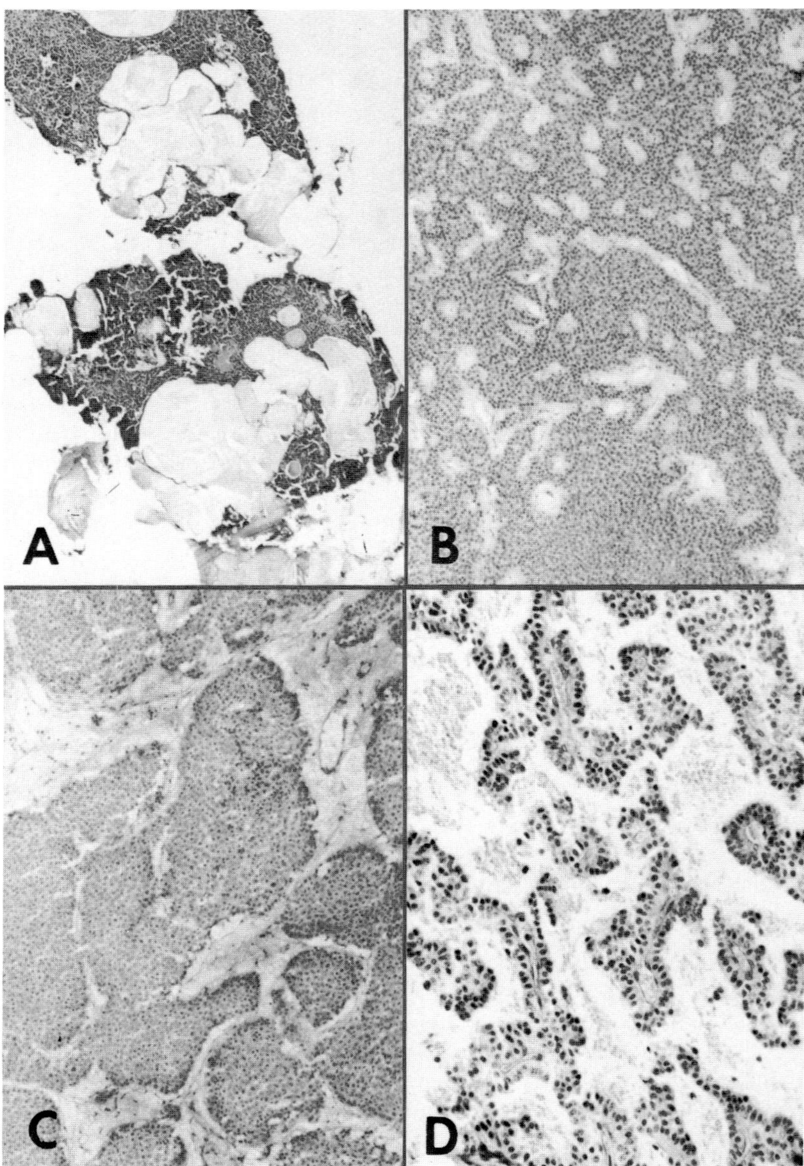

FIG. 1. Pituitary adenomas. **A:** Large cystic areas in a minute specimen from a 30-year-old female with Forbes-Albright syndrome. ×38. **B:** Sheets of cells and mottlings of tumor vessels from a 39-year-old female with a nonfunctioning adenoma. ×60. **C:** Lobular pattern created by thicker perivascular connective tissue in a 47-year-old male with a nonfunctioning adenoma. ×60. **D:** Interstitial hemorrhages bring out papillary structures in a 28-year-old with a nonfunctioning adenoma. ×150.**A–D:** HE.

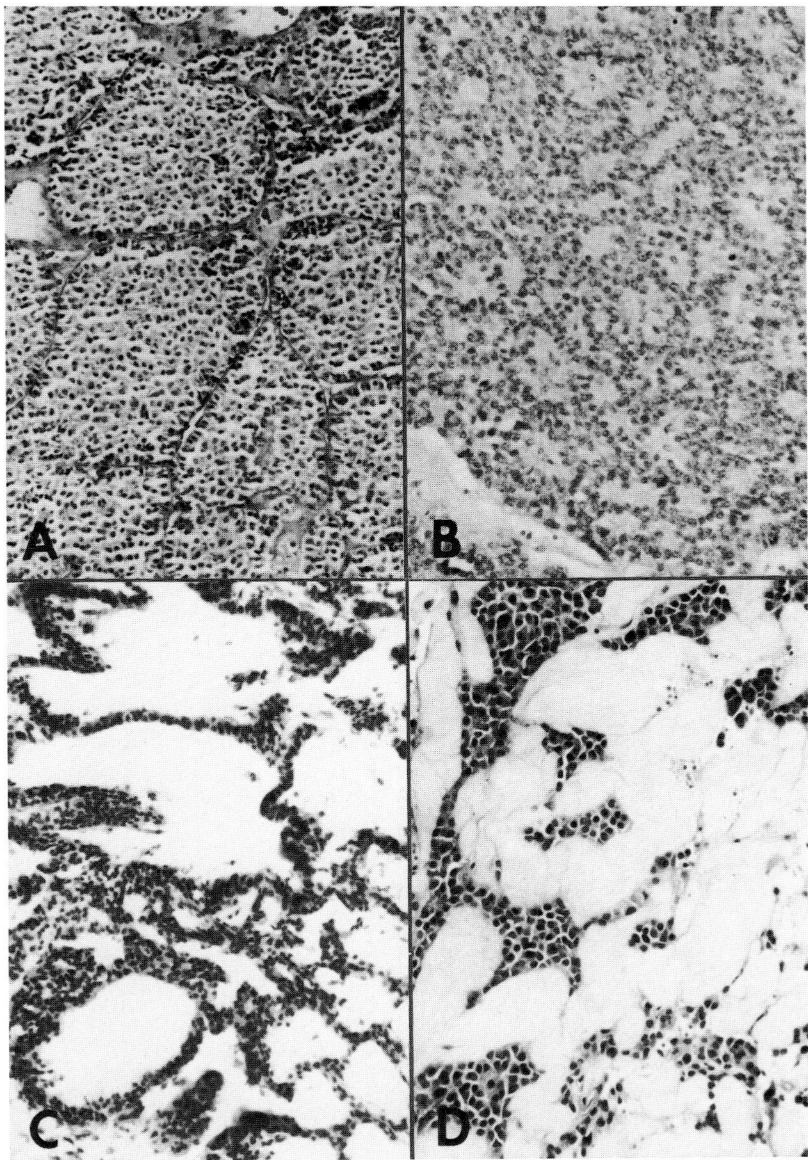

FIG. 2. Pituitary adenomas. **A:** Sinusoidal pattern resembling a chemodectoma in a 65-year-old male with a nonfunctioning adenoma. **B:** Rosette-like pattern may be mistaken for a medulloblastoma, as shown in this 42-year-old female with a nonfunctioning adenoma. **C:** Festoon-like pattern mimicking a yolk sac tumor in a 35-year-old male with acromegaly. **D:** Clumps of tumor cells embedded in an amyloid-like substance reminiscent of a skeletal neoplasm in a 28-year-old female with Forbes-Albright syndrome. **A–D:** HE. ×150.

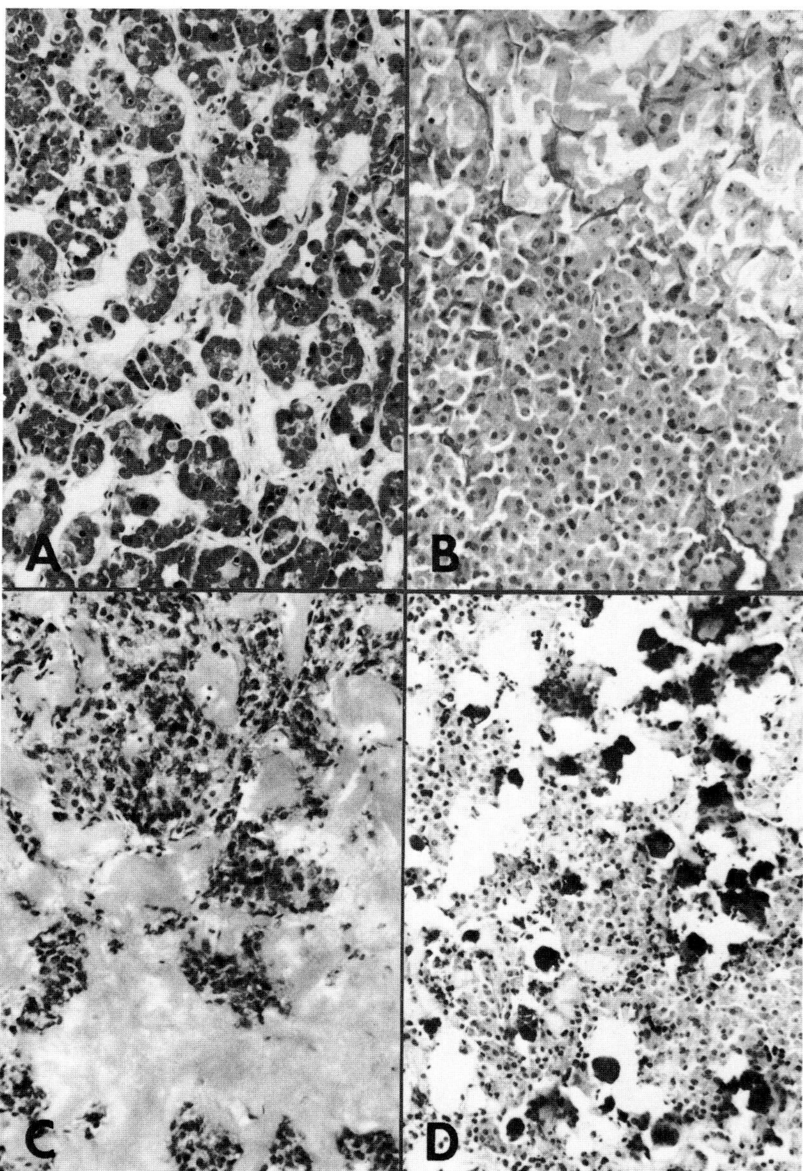

FIG. 3. Pituitary adenomas. **A:** Exaggerated tubular structures made up by eosinophilic cells in a 41-year-old female with Forbes–Albright syndrome. **B:** Two types of eosinophilic cells opposed to each other in a 56-year-old male with acromegaly and a high prolactin level. **C:** Grouping tendency in a sea of fibrous stroma reminiscent of a meningioma in a 47-year-old female with partial hypopituitarism. **D:** Massive calcospherites similar to psammoma bodies of a meningioma in a 28-year-old with Forbes–Albright syndrome. **A–D:** HE. ×150.

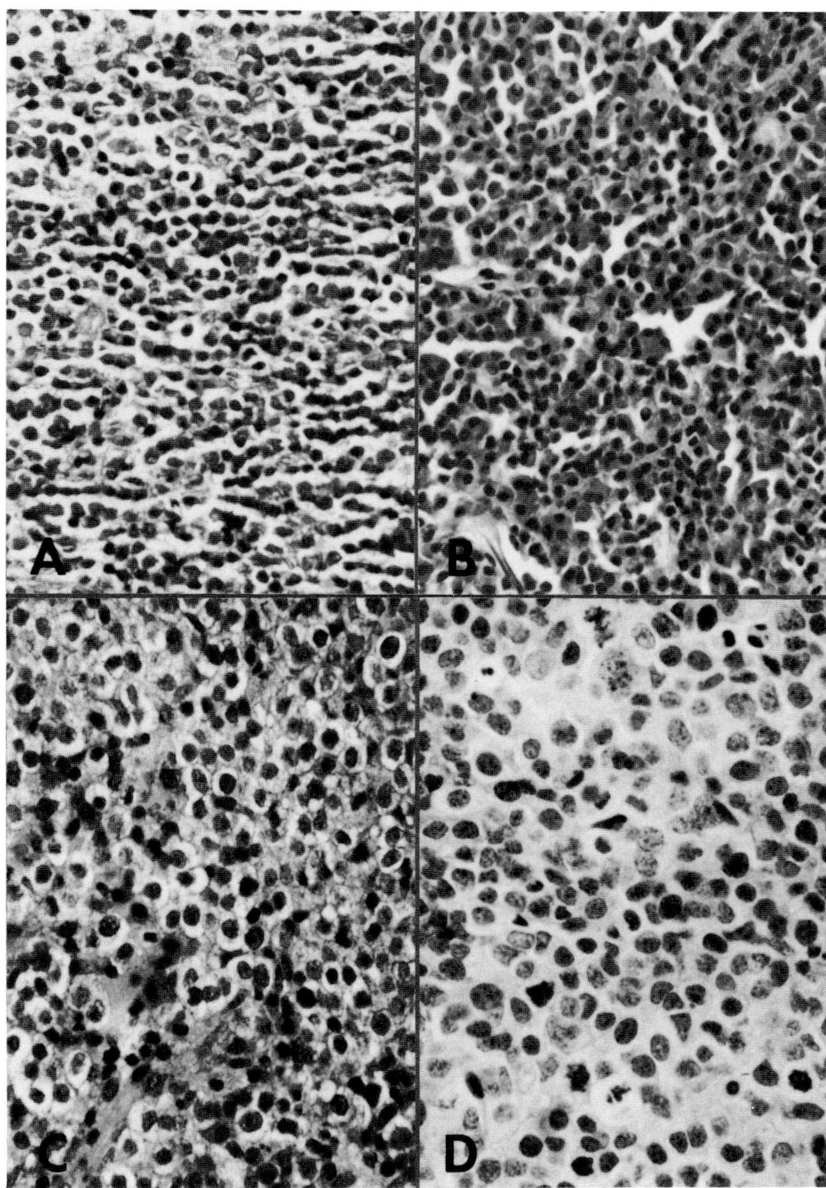

FIG. 4. Pituitary Adenomas. **A:** Sheets of small cells difficult to distinguish from a malignant lymphoma in a 68-year-old male with a nonfunctioning adenoma. **B:** This photograph of a plasmacytoma in the skull base of a 38-year-old male looks more like that of a pituitary adenoma than the tissue in **A. C:** Perinuclear halo (characteristic of oligodendroglioma), which is also seen in pituitary adenomas, appears in this 71-year-old female with a nonfunctioning adenoma. **D:** There are at least five to seven mitotic figures in the field from this pituitary carcinoma in a 38-year-old male. **A–D:** HE. **A–C:** ×380. **D:** ×150.

craniopharyngioma, teratoma) should be considered in the differential diagnosis. Histologically, calcified concretions (calcospherites) are typically spherical, showing concentric lamination, or they may represent irregular aggregates of smaller concretions (Fig. 3D). They may be mistaken for the psammoma bodies of a meningioma. In our experience, calcospherites are more common in prolactin-secreting adenomas.

Spontaneous Infarction or Hemorrhage

The pituitary gland is an uncommon site for spontaneous hemorrhage or infarction, a situation most likely to occur during pregnancy. Rarely adenomas undergo similar pathologic change, a condition referred to as "pituitary apoplexy" (34,41). On histologic examinations, one should examine carefully for neoplastic cells. This is particularly important when a frozen section is performed in acute cases, because specimens received from surgery often consist only of blood clot or necrotic debris. On the other hand, surgical specimens from cases of remote episodes usually show many cholesterol crystals and foreign-body giant cells (Fig. 5), bringing craniopharyngioma into the differential diagnosis.

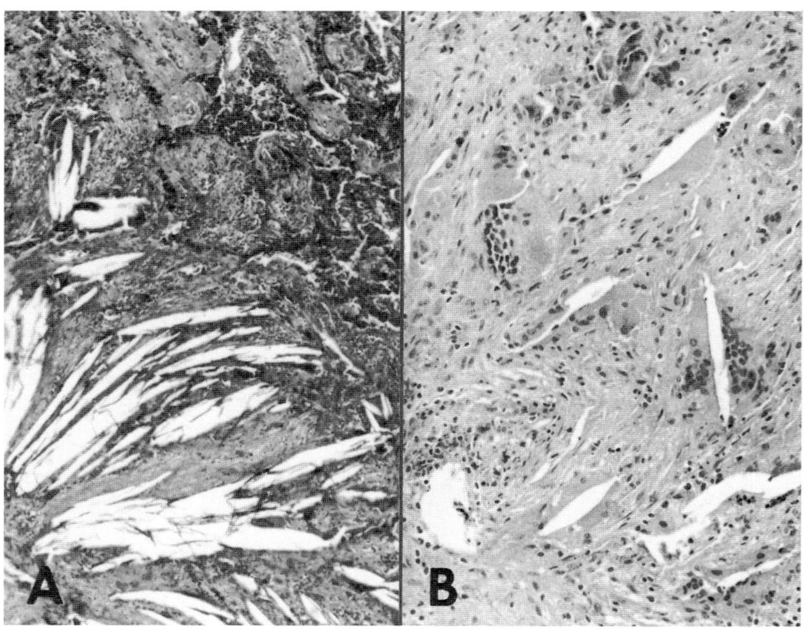

FIG. 5. Clefts of cholesterol crystals accompanied by foreign-body-type giant cells and granulomatous inflammation, histologic evidence of remote pituitary "apoplexy." These lesions can occur within adenomas **(A)** as well as adenohypophyses bearing no tumor **(B)**. **A:** A 26-year-old male with acromegaly. HE. ×60. **B:** A 39-year-old female with hypopituitarism. HE. ×150.

Radiation Changes and Malignancy

Surgically removed specimens of pituitary adenomas that have received previous irradiation usually exhibit, in addition to bizarre anaplastic-appearing tumor cells, vascular fibrosis and calcification and varying degrees of interstitial fibrosis (Fig. 6A). Whereas these altered mesenchymal elements may provide the anlagen for sarcomas (1,18,36), usually wild-looking adenoma cells are worrisome for the examining pathologist in terms of malignancy. Malignant adenomas or adenocarcinomas of the adenohypophysis are rare (30). Several textbooks require the presence of remote metastases in order to make the diagnosis of carcinoma (5,40). However, granting the fact that some adenomas have aggressive, invasive behavior even though they are histologically benign, this definition may be academically correct, but most certainly it is not practical to wait until metastasis is discovered. Based on our own experience with two cases as well as careful analysis of the case reported by Solitaire and Jatlow (46), it is believed that the number of mitoses in a microscopic field may be used as a parameter to determine malignancy of pituitary adenomas (Fig. 4D). Cellular atypicality, as bizarre as it may be in radiation effect, is often found in nonmalignant adenomas, whereas mitotic figures are rare occurrences, even in postirradiation specimens.

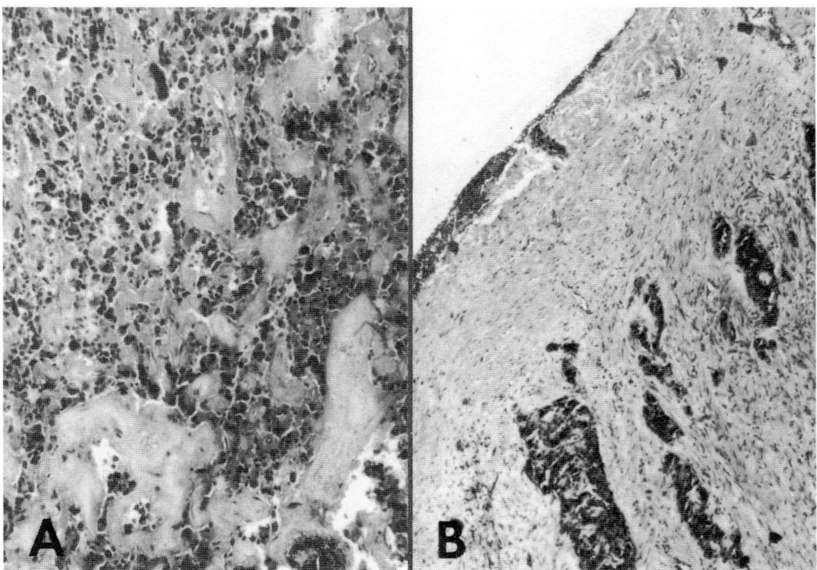

FIG. 6. A: Bizarre, anaplastic-looking cells, interstitial fibrosis, and calcification in fibrosed vessels, which are common findings in postirradiation cases. Mitoses are rare in this 35-year-old male with a nonfunctioning adenoma. HE. ×150. **B:** Adenoma infiltrations in this fibrous capsule could be identified in frozen sections from a 32-year-old female with Forbes–Albright syndrome. HE, frozen. ×60.

Extrasellar Location of Pituitary Adenomas

Intracerebral pituitary adenomas with normal sella turcica have been reported (8,38). These rare lesions may be mistaken for a primary brain tumor (e.g., ependymoma) on routine histologic examination. However, diagnosis can be confirmed by electron microscopy.

Another example, perhaps more common than intracerebral location, is extension of the adenoma into the nasal cavities (42,48). Although most of the cases represent extension of a sella tumor, some might present as nasal polyps without any radiological abnormality in the sella turcica, thus creating a difficult differential diagnosis.

Tumors of the Neurohypophysis

The neurohypophysis provides the site of origin for rare neuroectodermal neoplasms (40). Usually gliomas involving the infundibulum are simply an extension of hypothalamic or chiasmatic tumors. Dysgenetic mislocations of neural tumors in the adenohypophysis with or without endocrine hyperfunction have been reported (22,54).

Granular cell tumors, sometimes referred to as choristoma, occur rarely in

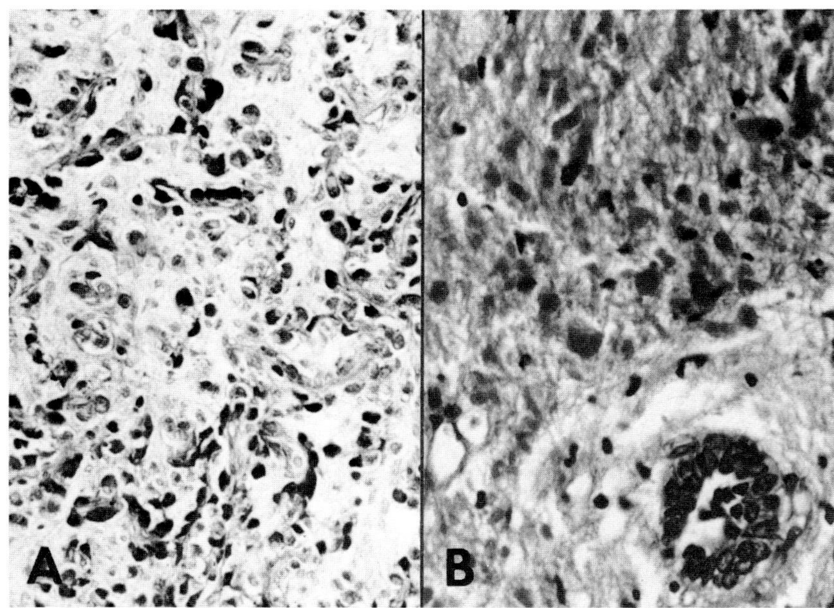

FIG. 7. A: Granular cell tumor of the neurohypophysis with PAS-positive, diastase-resistant granules in eosinophilic cytoplasm from a 58-year-old female. PAS. ×150. **B:** Craniopharyngioma in the lower right evoking gliosis with florid Rosenthal fiber formations in a 20-year-old male. HE. ×150.

the neurohypophysis. These tumors are composed of nonepithelial cells packed with coarse to fine eosinophilic granules which are PAS-positive and diastase-resistant (Fig. 7A). Ultrastructurally the granules are composed of cytosegresomes of lysosomal origin similar to those of granular cell tumors found elsewhere in the body. Although some investigators consider the origin of these granular cells to be the pituicytes (30), since similar ultrastructure may be observed in glial tumors (39,50), the exact origin of these cells is yet to be determined.

Craniopharyngioma

Craniopharyngioma, which arises from squamous epithelium of the remnants of the hypophyseal duct, comprises about 3% of all intracranial tumors. Craniopharyngiomas are usually in a suprasellar location, often with intrasellar, retrosellar, or parasellar extensions. Rarely they may be confined to an intrasellar location (30). Varying degrees of endocrine dysfunction may occur as a result of this tumor (23,24). Histologically, hypothalamic invasion by the tumor usually evokes an astroglial reaction with florid Rosenthal fiber formation (Fig. 7B). Depending on sampling of the surgical specimen, this reactive change may be mistaken for a pilocytic astrocytoma.

NEOPLASTIC DISORDERS—NONPITUITARY ORIGIN

Meningioma

Meningiomas may originate in the area of the tuberculum sellae and characteristically cause hyperostosis in the juxtasellar region. Psammoma bodies or whorl formation may be seen in some specimens, but as already mentioned the former may be mistaken for calcospherites of pituitary adenomas (Fig. 3D). Similar to other mesothelial neoplasms, meningioma cells may be arranged in sheets, often mimicking pituitary adenomas (Fig. 8).

Miscellaneous Tumors

Tumors of germ cell origin in an intracranial location appear to occur most commonly among the Japanese (52). Germinomas homologous to those occurring in the testis or ovary may arise in a suprasellar region; and although the lesion may extend into the sella, it is rarely confined to the intrasellar location (3,16). Although diabetes insipidus is the most common presenting symptom, various hormonal disturbances may also occur (52). Although rare, when precocious puberty is associated with a sellar lesion, choriocarcinoma, which produces human chorionic gonadotropin (hCG), should be considered in the differential diagnosis. Among rarer germ cell tumors in the sellar region is the yolk sac tumor (51), a lesion usually associated with elevated CSF and/or serum level of alpha-fetoprotein.

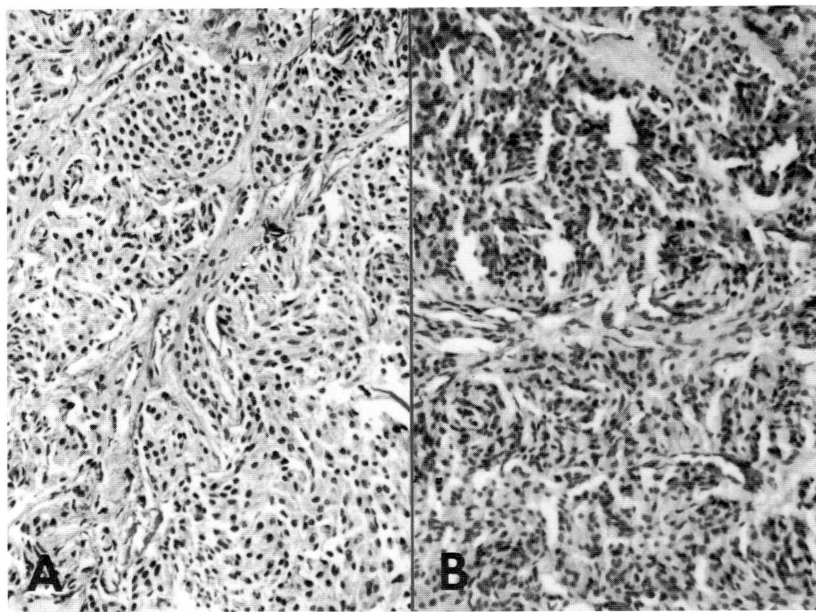

FIG. 8. These sections demonstrate the close resemblance between meningioma and pituitary adenoma. **A:** Slightly eosinophilic cytoplasm and epithelial type of cellular arrangements in a sellar meningioma from a 68-year-old male. **B:** Whorling tendency in a nonfunctioning adenoma from a 44-year-old female. **A** and **B:** HE. ×150.

The cranial chordomas are typically located in the proximity of the sella and should be taken into account in the differential diagnosis. Primary intrasellar chordoma has been recognized (33). Some other rare tumors that may occur in the sellar or parasellar area include plasmacytoma (44), hemangioblastoma (10), melanoma (45), and intrasellar epidermoid cyst (47).

NONNEOPLASTIC DISORDERS

"Empty Sella" Syndrome

The "empty sella" syndrome has been well documented in detail. A pituitary adenoma may coexist with an "empty" sella, particularly in cases with hyperfunctional endocrinopathy (4,7,13,35,49).

Inflammatory Disorders

Granulomatous meningitis may extend to an intrasellar location. Intrasellar abscesses have been described on several occasions (2,17). Histopathologically the necrotic nature and cellular reactions place these lesions in the differential diagnosis with pituitary infarction or "apoplexy." Although a suspected specimen should be sent for culture of organisms, the diagnosis may be established by frozen section during operation.

The "allergic" type of lymphocytic hypophysitis, although rare, usually causes hypopituitarism (21,29). Histopathological diagnosis of this lesion is difficult, particularly when distinguishing it from malignant lymphomas.

VALUE OF FROZEN SECTION DIAGNOSIS

In general the purpose of a rapid frozen section procedure is to identify the histology of the tissue removed at the time of operation so the surgery may be most effective. Speed and accuracy are imperative for the pathologist, and the surgeon should recognize the limitations. Sampling error, poor tissue preservation, and inadequate technique including sectioning and staining are frequent causes for uncertainty. Additionally, the size of tissue sent for frozen section is usually very small. In transsphenoidal microsurgery for pituitary lesions, one should expect to perform frozen section examinations on a specimen less than 1 mm in greatest diameter. Thus a combination of technical skill and comprehensive knowledge of pathology of the pituitary is necessary to enhance the value and accuracy of frozen section diagnosis.

Technique

It is important to keep the specimens moist. The tissue should be placed on a flat piece of rubber glove and then wrapped in a towel with the identification label attached. After taking a small sample for electron microscopy, the specimen is ready to be frozen in a cryostat. The temperature in the cryostat must be kept at −20°C. A small stage or mount comprised of an embedding medium for frozen sections is prepared on a chuck inside the cryostat and then frozen. After freezing, sections are cut at 3 or 4 μm thickness. It is important to cut the sections thin because of the minute pieces of tissue with which one must work. A sharp knife is important. Gauze sponges are kept cold in the cryostat, so the knife edge can be wiped clean after each cut without changing its temperature. Slides are stained with HE and toluidine blue (0.7% solution).

Merits of Frozen Section Diagnosis in Cases of Pituitary Tumors

As shown in Figs. 1 through 4, pituitary adenomas exhibit different histologic appearances. Considering the minute size of the specimens, there are many pitfalls in differential diagnosis, which were already cited above. In our experience, the most useful area for identifying tumor cells arising from endocrine epithelium is in the periphery of the specimen (Fig. 9D).

The identification of a microadenoma and the border between adenoma and the normal gland is important for aiding the neurosurgeon in his efforts to remove all adenomatous tissue and for preserving uninvolved gland. The histologic difference between adenoma and normal gland tissue may be subtle at times, but (a) sudden destruction of normal glandular architecture and (b) abnormally homogeneous cellular population are two important characteristics for establishing the diagnosis (Figs. 9A,B and 10). Cytoplasmic characteristics

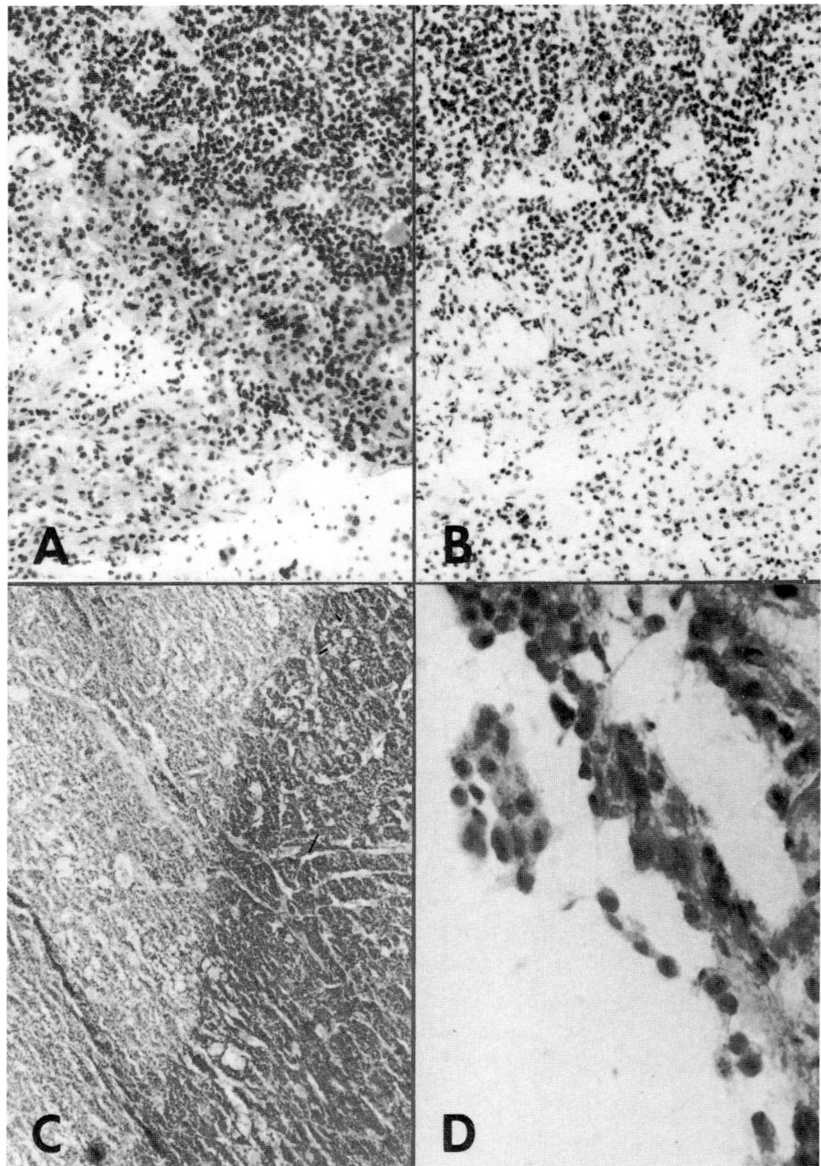

FIG. 9. Examples of frozen sections. **A,B:** There is an apparent difference in cellularity and cytoarchitecture between the adenoma *(upper parts)* and adjacent normal gland *(lower parts)* seen with both HE **(A)** and toluidine blue **(B)** stains in frozen sections. The patient was a 28-year-old female with Forbes–Albright syndrome. ×150. **C:** This is *not* a "mixed" adenoma. The right portion of this section was left in eosin solution 30 sec longer than the left portion. This simply makes the right portion "eosinophilic" and the left portion "chromophobic." The patient was a 42-year-old male with a nonfunctioning adenoma. HE frozen. ×38. **D:** Epithelial characteristics of pituitary adenoma cells are most easily identified at the edges of this frozen section tissue from a 47-year-old male with a nonfunctioning adenoma. HE frozen. ×380.

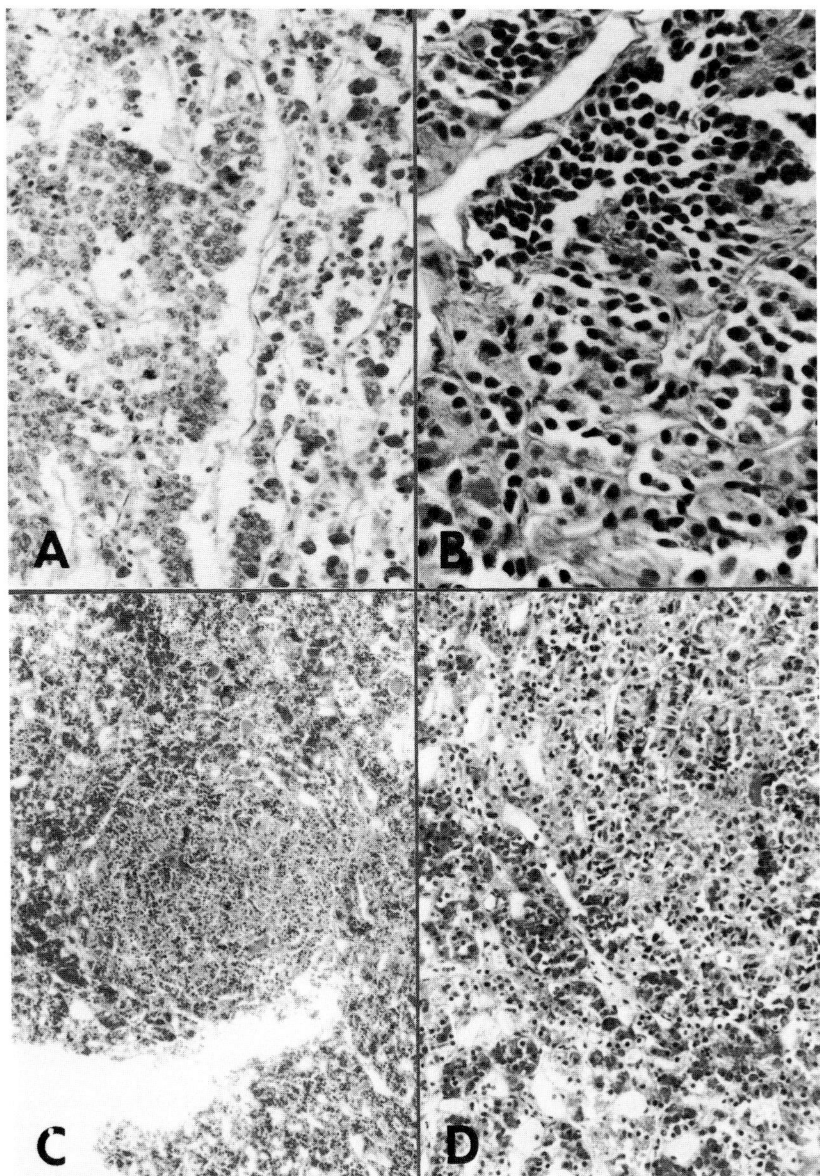

FIG. 10. Identification of a microadenoma and the tumor–normal gland border. **A:** In paraffin sections the border is relatively easy to identify in this 49-year-old female with a nonfunctioning adenoma. Tumor is on the left, normal tissue on the right. HE. ×150. **B:** Even a supermicroadenoma as seen in the upper center exhibits an abnormal cell population and sudden interruption of normal cytoarchitecture in this 28-year-old with Forbes–Albright syndrome. HE. ×380. **C,D:** In frozen sections these changes may be very subtle. A 0.3-mm microadenoma is seen in the center of the lower power view **(C)** and the right upper part with higher magnification **(D)** in this 32-year-old female with Forbes–Albright syndrome. HE, frozen. **C:** ×96. **D:** ×240.

should not be overemphasized, as an abnormality in the tissue pattern is more important than cytologic appearances. Calling tissue "chromophobic" or "eosinophilic" on frozen sections is more habitual than practical since one can easily change the staining attitude of the cells depending on the length of time the slide remains in the staining solutions (Fig. 9C). Identification of capsule infiltration by the adenoma may also be useful information for the neurosurgeon (Fig. 6B). This task might require multiple sectioning from the same block.

ACKNOWLEDGMENT

The author wishes to express his gratitude to Susi Schwarz, Chief Neuropathology Technologist, for valuable technical assistance.

REFERENCES

1. Amine, A. R. C., and Sugar, O. (1976): Suprasellar osteogenic sarcoma following radiation for pituitary adenoma: Case report. *J. Neurosurg.,* 44:88–91.
2. Arseni, C. (1975): Intrasellar abscess. *Neurochirurgia (Stuttg),* 18:207–213.
3. Banna, M., Schatz, S. W., Molot, M. J., and Groves, J. (1976): Primary intrasellar germinoma. *Br. J. Radiol.,* 49:971–973.
4. Bar, R. S., Mazzaferri, E. L., and Malarkey, W. B. (1975): Primary empty sella, galactorrhea, hyperprolactinemia and renal tubular acidosis. *Am. J. Med.,* 59:863–866.
5. Burger, P. E., and Vogel, F. S. (1976): *Surgical Pathology of the Nervous System and Its Coverings.* Wiley, New York.
6. Chambers, A. A., Lukin, R., and Tsunekawa, N. (1976): Calcification in a chromophobe adenoma: Case report. *J. Neurosurg.,* 44:623–625.
7. Check, J. H., Rakoff, A. E., Goldfarb, A. F., and King, L. C. (1977): Amenorrhea-galactorrhea associated with the empty-sella syndrome. *Am. J. Obstet. Gynecol.,* 128:688–689.
8. Clifford, J. R., and Echols, D. H. (1973): Extrasellar extension of a pituitary adenoma in a patient with a normal-sized sella turcica and impaired vision from an atheromatous carotid artery: Case report. *J. Neurosurg.,* 39:398–401.
9. Cunningham, G. R., and Huckins, C. (1977): An FSH and prolactin-secreting tumor: Pituitary dynamics and testicular histology. *J. Clin. Endocrinol. Metab.,* 44:248–253.
10. Dan, N. G., and Smith, D. E. (1975): Pituitary hemangioblastoma in a patient with von Hippel-Lindau disease: Case report. *J. Neurosurg.,* 42:232–235.
11. Davidoff, L. M. (1926): Studies in acromegaly. III. The anamnesis and symptomatology in one hundred cases. *Endocrinology,* 10:461–483.
12. Demura, R. (1977): FSH and LH secreting pituitary adenoma. *J. Clin. Endocrinol. Metab.,* 45:653–657.
13. Domingue, J. N., Wing, S. D., and Wilson, C. B. (1978): Coexisting pituitary adenomas and partially empty sellas. *J. Neurosurg.,* 48:23–28.
14. Duello, T. M., and Halmi, M. S. (1977): Pituitary adenoma producing thyrotropin and prolactin: An immunocytochemical and electron microscopic study. *Virchows Arch.* [*Pathol. Anat.*], 375:255–265.
15. Geller, S., Ayme, Y., Kandelman, M., Grisoli, F., and Scholler, R. (1976): Micro-adénome hypophysaire à LH: Une nouvelle entité nosologique? *Ann. Endocrinol. (Paris),* 37:281–282.
16. Ghatak, N. R., Hirano, A., and Zimmerman, H. M. (1969): Intrasellar germinoma: A form of ectopic pinealoma. *J. Neurosurg.,* 31:670–675.
17. Goldhammer, Y., Smith, L., and Yates, B. M. (1974): Mycotic intrasellar abscess. *Am. J. Ophthalmol.,* 78:478–484.
18. Gonzalez-Vitale, J. C., Slavin, R. E., and McQueen, J. D. (1976): Radiation induced intracranial malignant fibrous histiocytoma. *Cancer,* 37:2960–2963.
19. Gudya, H., Robert, F., Colle, E., and Hardy, J. (1973): Histologic, ultrastructural, and hormonal

characterization of a pituitary tumor secreting both HGH and prolactin. *J. Clin. Endocrinol. Metab.,* 36:531–547.

20. Horvath, E., and Kovacs, K. (1976): Ultrastructural classification of pituitary adenomas. *Can. J. Neurol. Sci.,* 3:9–21.
21. Hume, R., and Roberts, G. H. (1967): Hypophysitis and hypopituitarism. *Br. Med. J.,* 2:548–550.
22. Jakumeit, H. D., Zimmerman, V., and Guiot, G. (1974): Intrasellar gangliocytomas: Report of four cases. *J. Neurosurg.,* 40:626–630.
23. Jenkins, J. S., Gilbert, C. J., and Ang, V. (1976): Hypothalamic-pituitary function in patients with craniopharyngiomas. *J. Clin. Endocrinol. Metab.,* 43:394–399.
24. Korsgaard, O., Lindholm, J., and Rasmussen, P. (1976): Endocrine function in patients with suprasellar and hypothalamic tumors. *Acta Endocrinol. (Kbh),* 83:1–8.
25. Kovacs, K., Horvath, E., and Bilbao, J. M. (1974): Oncocytes in the anterior lobe of the human pituitary gland: A light and electron microscopy study. *Acta Neuropathol. (Berl),* 27:43–53.
26. Kovacs, K., Horvath, E., Corenblum, B., Sirek, A. M. T., Penz, G., and Ezrin, C. (1975): Pituitary chromophobe adenomas consisting of prolactin cells: A histologic, immunocytological and electron microscopic study. *Virchows Arch.* [*Pathol. Anat.*], 366:113–123.
27. Kovacs, K., Horvath, E., Kerenyi, N. A., and Sheppard, R. H. (1976): Light and electron microscopic features of a pituitary adenoma in Nelson's syndrome. *Am. J. Clin. Pathol.,* 65:337–343.
28. Kovacs, K., Horvath, E., Bayley, T. A., Hassaram, S. T., and Ezrin, C. (1978): Silent corticotroph cell adenoma with lysosomal accumulation and crinophagy: A distinct clinicopathologic entity. *Am. J. Med.,* 64:492–499.
29. Lack, E. E. (1975): Lymphoid "hypophysitis" with end organ insufficiency. *Arch. Pathol.,* 99:215–219.
30. Landolt, A. M. (1975): Ultrastructure of human sella tumors: Correlations of clinical findings and morphology. *Acta Neurochir. (Wien) (Suppl),* 22:1–167.
31. Landolt, A. M., and Rothenbuhler, V. (1977): Pituitary adenoma calcification. *Arch. Pathol. Lab. Med.,* 101:22–27.
32. Luboshitzky, R., and Barzilan, D. (1978): Suprasellar extension of tumor associated with increased cerebrospinal fluid activity of LH and FSH. *Acta Endocrinol. (Kbh),* 87:673–684.
33. Mathews, W., and Wilson, C. B. (1974): Ectopic intrasellar chordoma: Case report. *J. Neurosurg.,* 40:260–263.
34. Mohanty, S., Tandon, P. N., Banerji, A. K., and Prakash, B. (1977): Hemorrhage into pituitary adenomas. *J. Neurol. Neurosurg. Psychiatry,* 40:987–991.
35. Molitch, M. E., Hieshima, G. B., Marcovitz, S., Jackson, I. M. D., and Wolpert, S. (1977): Coexisting primary empty sella syndrome and acromegaly. *Clin. Endocrinol. (Oxf),* 7:261–263.
36. Powell, H. C., Marshall, L. F., and Ignelzi, R. J. (1977): Post-irradiation pituitary sarcoma. *Acta Neuropathol. (Berl.),* 39:165–167.
37. Rollet, J., Guinett, P., Girod, C., Trouillas, J., and Cune, M. (1975): Un cas d'adénome oncocytaire de l'hypophyse avec galactorrhée et hyperprolactinémie. *Ann. Endocrinol. (Paris),* 36:221–222.
38. Rothman, L. M., Sher, J., Quencer, R. M., and Tenner, M. S. (1976): Intracranial ectopic pituitary adenoma: Case report. *J. Neurosurg.,* 44:96–99.
39. Rubinstein, L. J., and Herman, M. M. (1972): A light and electron microscopic study of a temporal-lobe ganglioglioma. *J. Neurol. Sci.,* 16:27–48.
40. Russell, D. S., and Rubinstein, L. J. (1971): *Pathology of Tumours of the Nervous System,* 3rd ed. Arnold, London.
41. Sachdev, Y., Everd, D. C., and Hall, R. (1976): Spontaneous pituitary necrosis. *Br. Med. J.,* 1:942.
42. Sadick, M. K., Nagori, M. A., and Jafarey, N. A. (1974): Chromophobe adenoma of the pituitary gland masquerading as bilateral nasal polypi—report of a case. *J. Laryngol. Otol.,* 88:169–173.
43. Saeger, W. (1975): Licht- und elektronenmikroskopische Untersuchungen zur Klassifikation von Hypophysenadenomen. *Z. Krebsforsch.,* 84:108–128.
44. Sanchez, J. A., Rahman, S., Strauss, R. A., and Kaye, G. I. (1977): Multiple myeloma masquerading as a pituitary tumor. *Arch. Pathol. Lab. Med.,* 110:55–56.

45. Scholtz, C. L., and Siu, K. (1976): Melanoma of the pituitary: Case report. *J. Neurosurg.*, 45:101–103.
46. Solitaire, G. E., and Jatlow, P. (1967): Adenohypophysial carcinoma: Case report. *J. Neurosurg.*, 26:624–632.
47. Steimlé, R., Jaequet, G., Carbillet, J. P., Bouneville, J. F., Aganani, G., Dakar, A., Abdul-Razzak, A., and Schwager, J. C. (1977): Kyste épidermöide intra-sellaire. *Acta Neurochir. (Wien),* 38:285–291.
48. Summers, G. W. (1976): Nasal obstruction caused by a pituitary chromophobe adenoma. *Laryngoscope,* 86:1718–1721.
49. Sutton, T. J., and Vezina, J. L. (1974): Co-existing pituitary adenoma and intrasellar arachnoid invagination. *Am. J. Roentgenol. Radium Ther. Nucl. Med.,* 122:508–510.
50. Takei, Y., Mirra, S. S., and Miles, M. L. (1976): Eosinophilic granular cells in oligodendrogliomas. *Cancer,* 38:1968–1976.
51. Takei, Y., Mirra, S. S., and Miles, M. L. (1977): Primary intracranial yolk sac tumor: Report of three cases and an ultrastructural study. *J. Neuropathol. Exp. Neurol.,* 36:618.
52. Takeuchi, J., Handa, H., and Nagata, J. (1978): Suprasellar germinoma. *J. Neurosurg.,* 49:41–48.
53. Tolis, G., Bird, C., Bertrand, G., and Ezrin, C. (1978): Pituitary hyperthyroidism: Case report and review of the literature. *Am. J. Med.,* 64:177–181.
54. Ule, G., and Widelich, F. W. (1976): Neurosekretorisches Ganglienzell-Choristom in der Adenohypophyse. *Acta Neuropathol. (Berl),* 36:81–84.
55. World Health Organization (1977): *Histologic Classification of Tumours of the Central Nervous System.* Outline distributed in the International Society News by the American Association of Neuropathologists.
56. Woolf, P. D., and Schenk, E. A. (1974): An FSH-producing pituitary tumor in a patient with hypogonadism. *J. Clin. Endocrinol. Metab.,* 38:561–576.
57. Zahra, M., and Sengupta, R. P. (1977): An unusual case of chromophobe adenoma with conspicuous calcifications. *Acta Neurochir. (Wien),* 38:279–283.
58. Zimmerman, E. A., Defendini, R., and Franz, A. G. (1974): Prolactin and growth hormone in patients with pituitary adenomas: A correlative study of hormone in tumor and plasma by immunoperoxidase technique and radioimmunoassay. *J. Clin. Endocrinol. Metab.,* 38:577–585.

Clinical Management of Pituitary Disorders,
edited by G. T. Tindall and W. F. Collins.
Raven Press. New York © 1979.

4

Electron Microscopy of Human Pituitary Tumors

Francoise Robert

Department of Pathology, Notre-Dame Hospital and University of Montreal, Montreal H2L 4K8, Canada

Until recently the exclusive use of the photonic microscope for identification of pituitary adenomas had been the occasion of many errors in interpretation and diagnosis. Adequate fixation, essential for the preservation of cytoplasmic granules, was difficult to attain. Special stains were technically arduous and gave variable results. The increasingly frequent utilization of the electron microscope has been rapidly recognized as a major breakthrough in the precise diagnosis of adenomas. More recently immunoperoxidase techniques have been used at the electron microscopic level thus permitting the subcellular localization of hormones in the human pituitary (44,53). The application of ultrastructural immunocytochemical methods to the study of pituitary adenomas opens a challenging new field in pathology (36,50,60,73).

Since 1971 we have performed ultrastructural examinations on 297 pituitary adenomas. We used the immunoperoxidase technique of Sternberger for the identification of hormones in the secretory granules (72). Our material is presented in Table 1.

TABLE 1. *Classification of 297 pituitary adenomas*

Adenoma	No.
Hormone secreting adenomas	
Prolactin-secreting adenomas	132
Growth hormone-secreting adenomas	95
ACTH–MSH-secreting adenomas	21
Thyrotropin-secreting adenoma	1
Growth hormone- and prolactin-secreting adenoma	1
Total:	250
Endocrine inactive adenomas	
Undifferentiated cell adenomas	33
Oncocytomas	14
Total:	47

HORMONE-SECRETING ADENOMAS

The hormone-secreting adenomas, by far the largest group in our series, are characterized by a clinical and/or biological syndrome of hypersecretion of a pituitary hormone. Many of these tumors are microadenomas measuring less than 10 mm (17,60).

Prolactin-Secreting Adenomas

In recent years prolactin-secreting adenomas have been recognized as the most frequent pituitary tumors (1,17). In this study our material includes 112 women and 20 men. The fine structure of these adenomas was characteristic and was similar in women and men.

The tumor cells contained scarce dense spherical or irregular secretory granules that usually reached a maximum diameter of 500 to 600 nm. In four cases where the immunoperoxidase technique for prolactin was performed at the ultra-

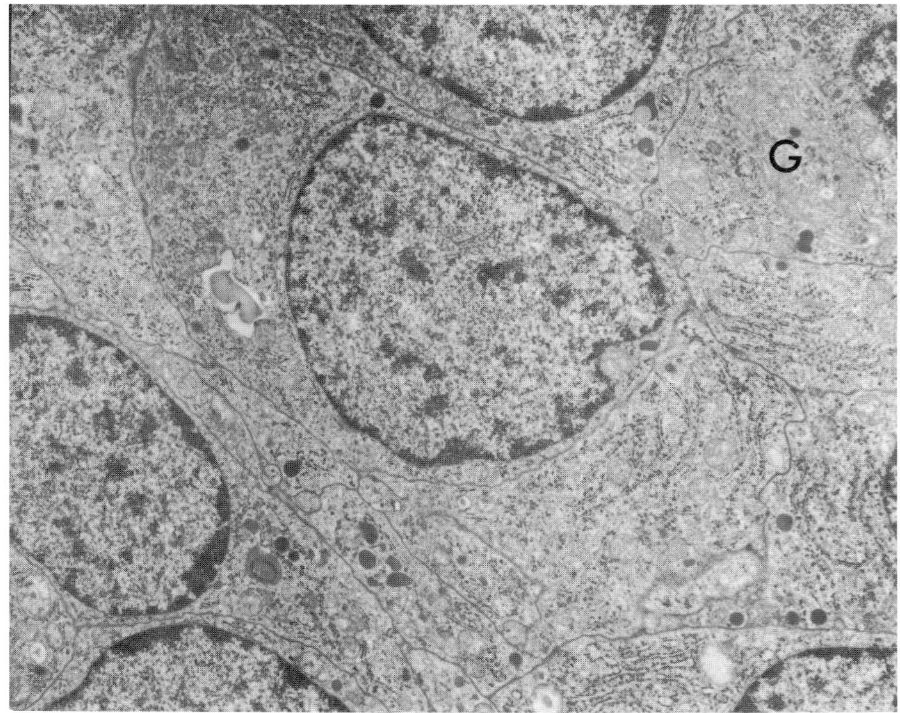

FIG. 1. Prolactin-secreting adenoma in a man [case 8 (in all figures the case number refers to the number in Hardy's series)]. The cells contain scarce pleomorphic secretory granules and abundant rough endoplasmic reticulum. The cell on the right has a prominent Golgi complex (G). ×7,000.

structural level, we found that the secretory granules stained with antiprolactin serum. Scattered throughout the cytoplasm they were also seen as progranules in the saccules of the Golgi apparatus. Misplaced exocytosis (19) or their release by extrusion on the lateral cell membranes of adjacent tumor cells was found in half of the cases (59).

The rough-surfaced endoplasmic reticulum was well developed, forming typical parallel arrays at the periphery of the cytoplasm sometimes with formation of nebenkerns or concentric whorls. The Golgi apparatus was always prominent, sometimes occupying as much as one-third of the cytoplasm. Immature secretory granules were frequently seen in its saccules (Figs. 1 through 3). Microfilaments were infrequently found. Mitochondria were usually normal but sometimes showed nonspecific myelin figures (59). Except for the amount of secretory granules which may occasionally be more impressive (20,52), most reports in the literature are in agreement with our findings (11,12,20,24,27,28,31,38,41, 43,56,70,75,78). By comparison with ultrastructural studies of prolactin cells during lactation in several animal species, we concluded that the adenomatous prolactin cells show signs of great secretory activity (59). The tumor cells have

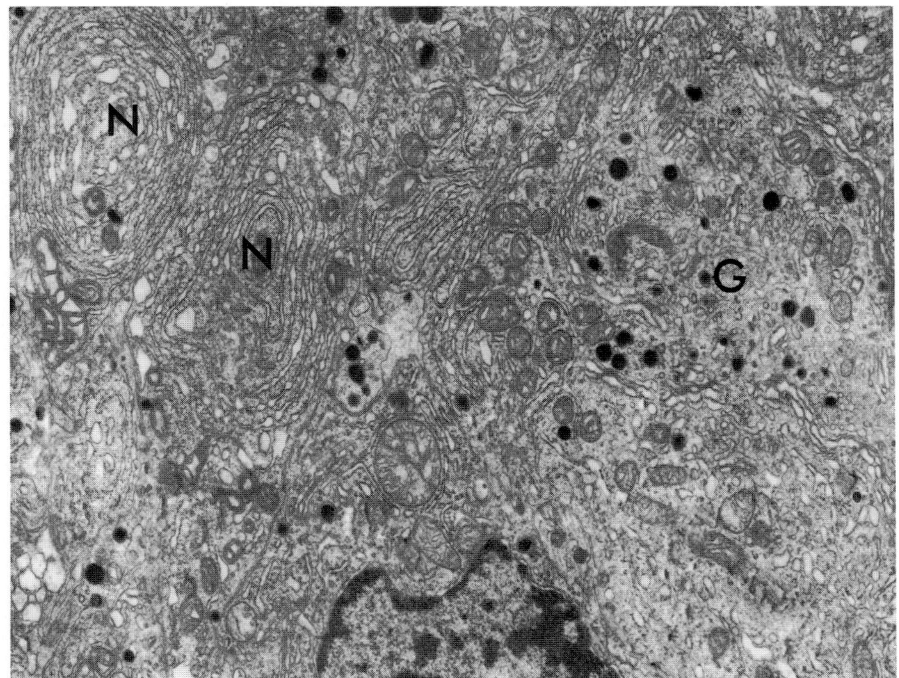

FIG. 2. Prolactin-secreting adenoma (case 110). The rough endoplasmic reticulum forms nebenkerns (N). The prominent Golgi area on the right contains secretory granules (G).

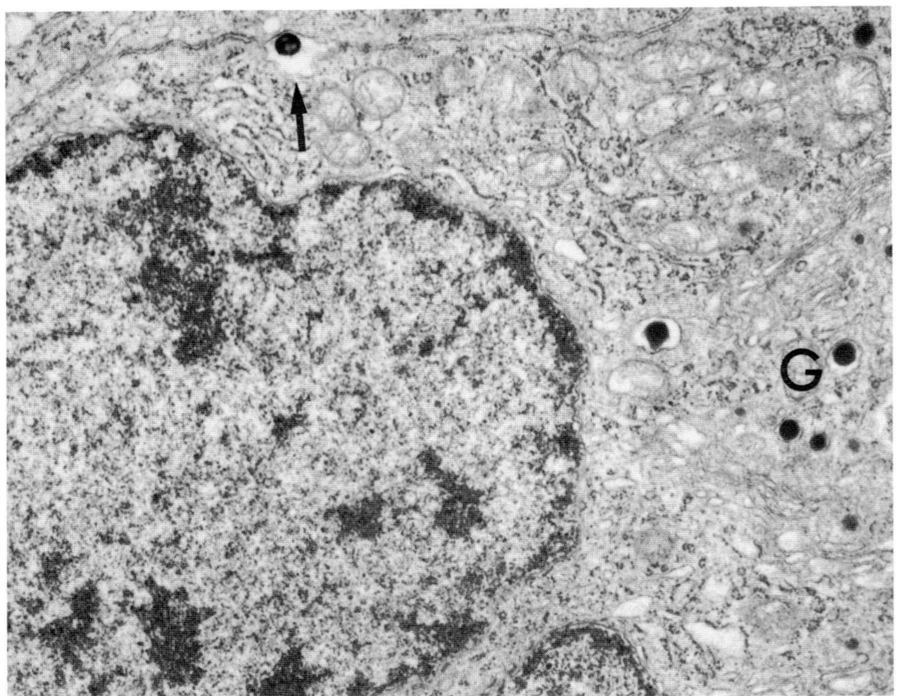

FIG. 3. Prolactin-secreting adenoma (case 78). Note the misplaced exocytosis *(arrow)* and part of the Golgi complex (G). ×17,500.

been described as similar to prolactin cells in women during the postpartum period as well as in estrogen-treated males (15), thus corresponding to "stimulated" prolactin cells.

Growth-Hormone-Secreting Adenomas

In contrast to the homogeneous ultrastructural aspect of the prolactin-secreting adenomas, marked variations exist in the group of growth hormone (GH)-secreting adenomas. On the basis of the number of secretory granules, we divided our 95 GH-secreting adenomas into three subgroups (Table 2).

TABLE 2. *Ultrastructural classification of GH-secreting adenomas*

Adenoma	No.
Densely granulated adenomas	54
Sparsely granulated adenomas	28
Mixed adenomas	13
Total:	95

Densely Granulated Adenomas

The subgroup consisting of 54 cases of densely granulated adenomas is the largest of the three. The tumor cells closely resemble normal somatotrophs (28,58,68). They are round or polyhedral and closely apposed. The nuclei are more or less ovoid and are usually located in the center of the cells. Large secretory granules mostly around 500 nm are numerous. The Golgi complex is prominent, and progranules may be seen within its saccules. Rough endoplasmic reticulum, appearing as parallel arrays, is seen at the periphery of the cells (Fig. 4). Mitochondria are usually present in moderate number, but they may be numerous, suggesting oncocytic transformation. Microfilaments have been found as bundles or spherical aggregates in 15 of 54 cases.

Sparsely Granulated Adenomas

Twenty-eight cases belong to the subgroup of sparsely granulated adenomas. Nuclear pleomorphism is marked with bizarre, often crescent-shaped, single or multiple nuclei capping a spherical aggregate of microfilaments. The Golgi

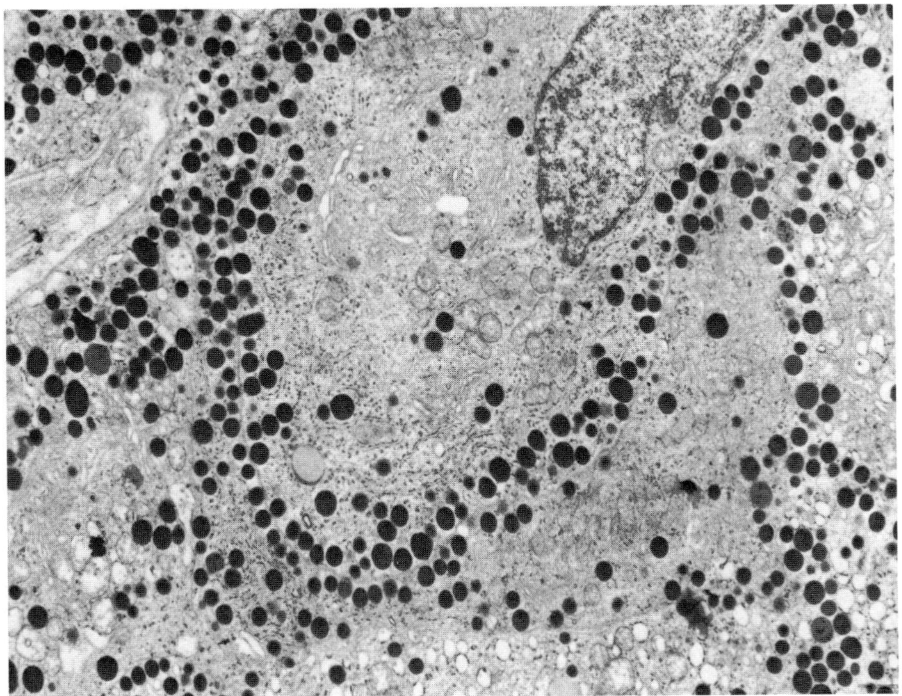

FIG. 4. Densely granulated GH-secreting adenoma (case 154). The cells contain many large secretory granules. The Golgi areas and the parallel arrays of rough endoplasmic reticulum are well seen. The cells contain many mitochondria. ×7,600.

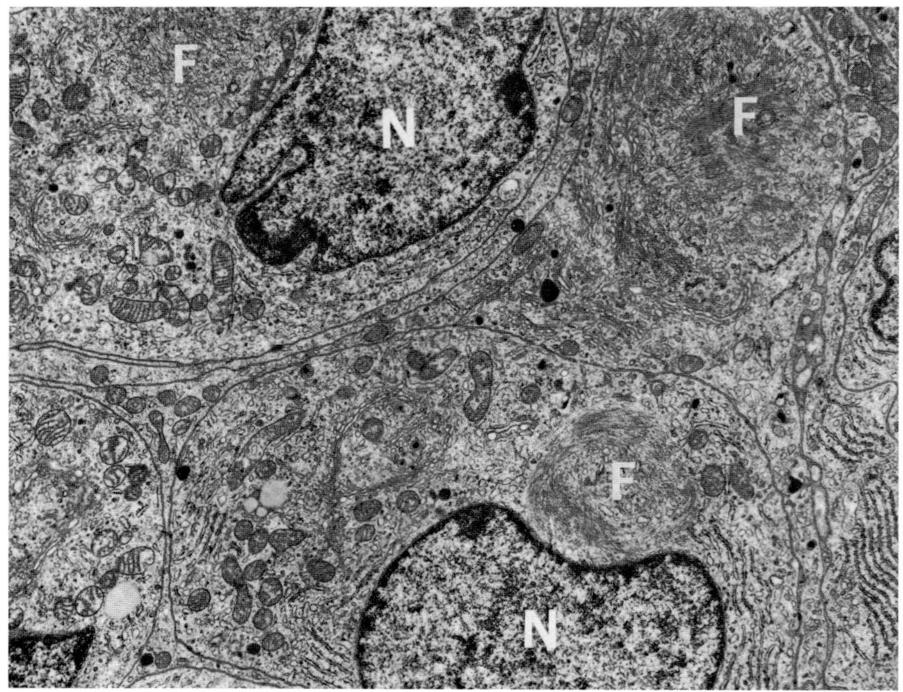

FIG. 5. Sparsely granulated GH-secreting adenoma (case 83). Spherical aggregates of microfilaments (F) are found close to irregular eccentric nuclei (N). Large secretory granules are very scarce. A few very small ones may be seen. ×7,000.

apparatus, closely related to the microfilaments, is well developed. Long parallel rows of rough endoplasmic reticulum are seen at the periphery of the cytoplasm. Scarce secretory granules consist of large ones reaching a diameter of 500 nm often scattered among the microfilaments and small ones in the 100 to 150 nm range. The latter are often aligned along the cell membranes. Mitochondria appear normal (Fig. 5). In this subgroup filament accumulations are extremely frequent, occurring in 22 of 28 cases.

Although some isolated cases of sparsely granulated adenomas in acromegaly have been reported in the literature (57,74), these two subgroups with their distinct ultrastructural features have been recognized in most descriptions (20,23,31,33,40,46,49,58,69).

Mixed Adenomas

Well-granulated and sparsely granulated cells coexist in mixed adenomas. Here again, spherical masses of microfilaments are frequent, having been found in 8 of 13 cases (Fig. 6). In two cases with immunostaining, we found that the secretory granules contained GH.

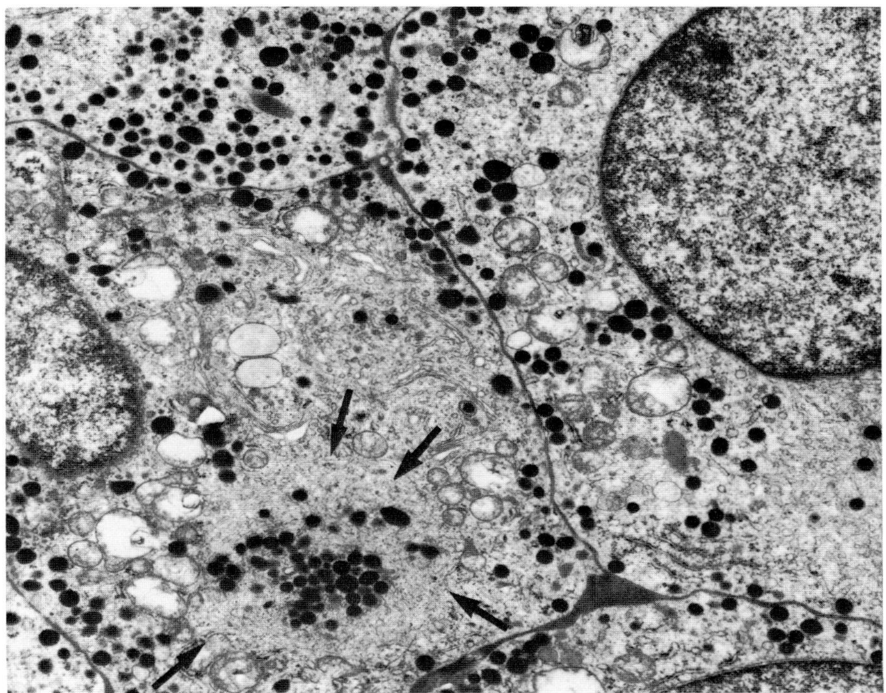

FIG. 6. Mixed GH-secreting adenoma (case 58). The cells are well granulated in this area of the tumor. A filamentous aggregate containing secretory granules is present in one cell *(arrows)*. ×10,500.

Comment

The spherical intracytoplasmic filamentous aggregates first referred to in the French literature (57) and well described 2 years later (4) are highly specific for acromegaly (32). Their occurrence indicates tumoral GH cells or GH precursors (28). A recent review has not yet elucidated their morphogenesis and significance (21).

A study of the ultrastructural aspect of the tumors in relation with their macroscopic classification as previously described (58) is summarized in Table 3. The densely granulated adenomas, which make up the bulk of our microadeno-

TABLE 3. *Ultrastructural aspect of GH-secreting adenomas in relation to macroscopic classification*

	Enclosed adenomas		Invasive adenomas	
Ultrastructural subgroup	Microadenomas	Adenomas	Local	Diffuse
Densely granulated adenomas	15	33	6	0
Sparsely granulated adenomas	0	18	5	5
Mixed adenomas	3	7	2	1

mas, have never been found in diffuse invasive adenomas. On the other hand, the sparsely granulated adenomas have not been seen in microadenomas; yet they are frequent in diffuse invasive adenomas. This finding indicates a more aggressive behavior on the part of the poorly granulated tumor cells in acromegaly.

ACTH–MSH-Secreting Adenomas

Our material consists of 14 cases of Cushing's disease and 7 of Nelson's syndrome. In 11 patients there were microadenomas measuring 2 to 9 mm. The tumor cells were polyhedral or spherical, sometimes elongated. The central nuclei were either round or indented, and showed clumping of chromatin and prominent nucleoli.

There is considerable variation in the size of the secretory granules from one case to the other (48,49,55). In our series they varied between 200 and 700 nm (60). They were spherical or slightly irregular, sometimes varying in electron density and more or less numerous (42). Their tendency for lining up along the cell membranes is well known (3,9,10,20,29,31,49,62). With immuno-

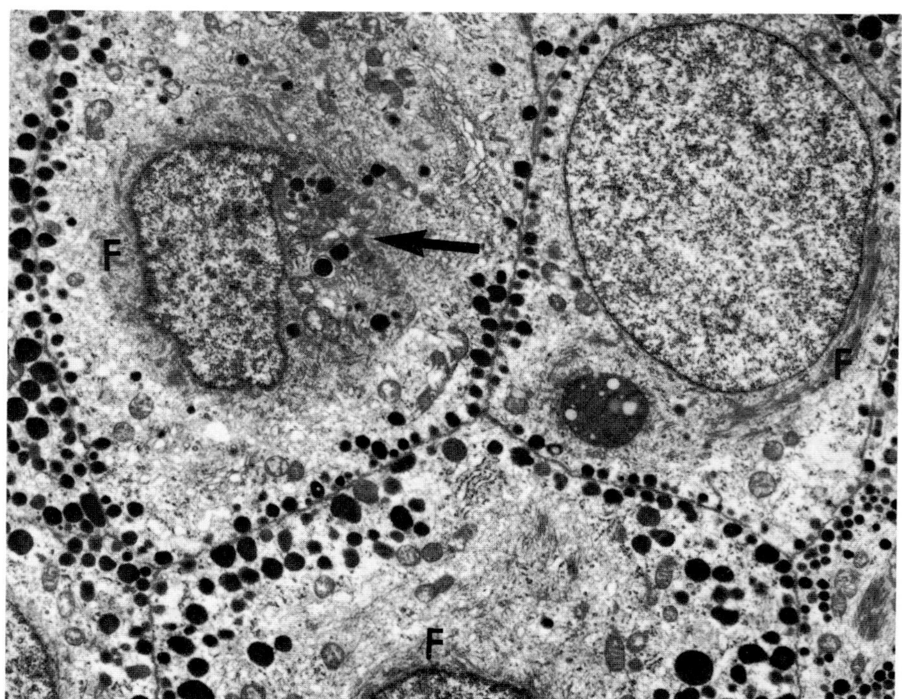

FIG. 7. ACTH–MSH-secreting adenoma (case 21). Three cells contain perinuclear microfilaments (F) entrapping secretory granules and mitochondria in the cell on the left *(arrow)*. The secretory granules are irregular and large, and are located along the cell membranes. ×7,000.

histochemical techniques applied at the electron microscopic level, in three cases we found that the secretory granules were heavily stained with the antiserum to ACTH. In one case the granules also contained β-LPH (60).

The most prominent ultrastructural feature was the presence of bundles of microfilaments averaging 70 Å in diameter encircling the nucleus and sometimes extending into large areas of the cytoplasm. They often entrapped secretory granules and other organelles (Fig. 7). The arrangement of these microfilaments around the nucleus and their somewhat smaller diameter made them quite different from those found in GH-secreting adenomas (20,28,30). On the other hand, they are similar to those seen in Crooke's cells (7,22,30,54,80). Although the significance of the microfilaments remains obscure (30), we suggest that they may act as a web preventing the release of ACTH (60).

The rough endoplasmic reticulum consisting of short parallel arrays, sometimes dilated, is seldom prominent. Ribosomes and polysomes are numerous. The Golgi apparatus, moderately developed, may contain progranules in its saccules. Mitochondria are usually few and appear normal. One case in our series (case 31) showed an increased number of large abnormal mitochondria containing lamellar structures (Fig. 8).

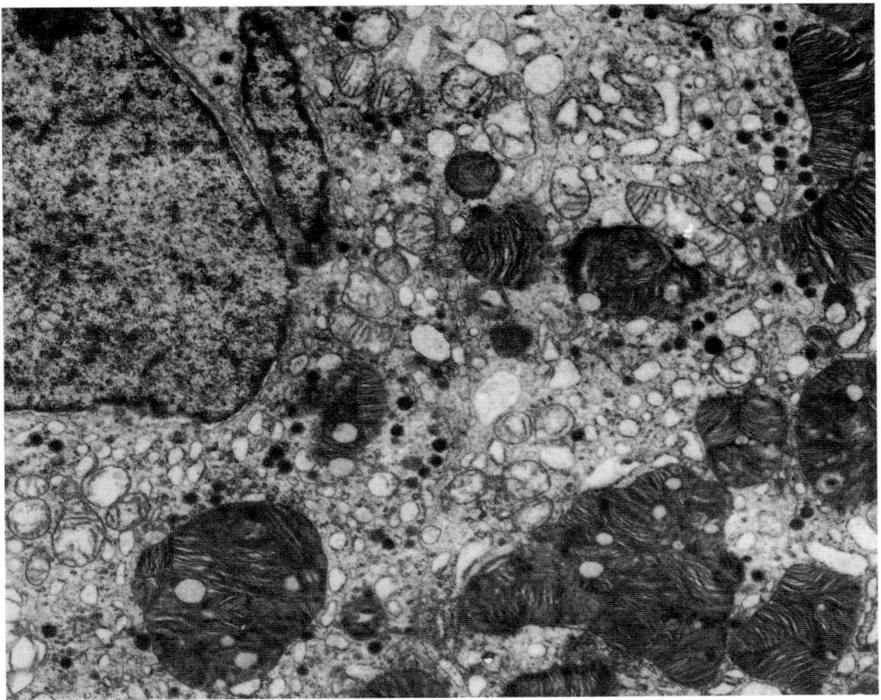

FIG. 8. ACTH–MSH-secreting adenoma (case 31). Part of one cell whose nucleus is surrounded by microfilaments shows large abnormal mitochondria filled with lamellar structures. ×11,600.

We were not able to find any basic differences in the ultrastructure of adenomas in Cushing's disease and Nelson's syndrome. Although microfilaments were reported as not abundant in cases of Nelson's syndrome (20,28), they were prominent in one of our cases (60).

Thyrotropin-Secreting Adenoma

Although thyrotropin-secreting adenomas may be secondary to longstanding hypothyroidism or accompanied by hyperthyroidism and elevated TSH serum levels, their seldom-described ultrastructural features appear to be similar (8, 18,28,39,45,66). In one case we studied a patient who presented with spontaneous hyperthyroidism and elevated TSH in the blood. The tumor cells were angular and contained a variable number of small secretory granules in the 100 nm range, sometimes scattered along the cell membranes. Many cells had a large Golgi area containing progranules (Fig. 9). Mitochondria were abundant and showed a close relation with short parallel structures of rough endoplasmic reticulum which frequently surrounded them (Fig. 10). The capillaries within the tumor had a fenestrated endothelium containing numerous tubular bodies.

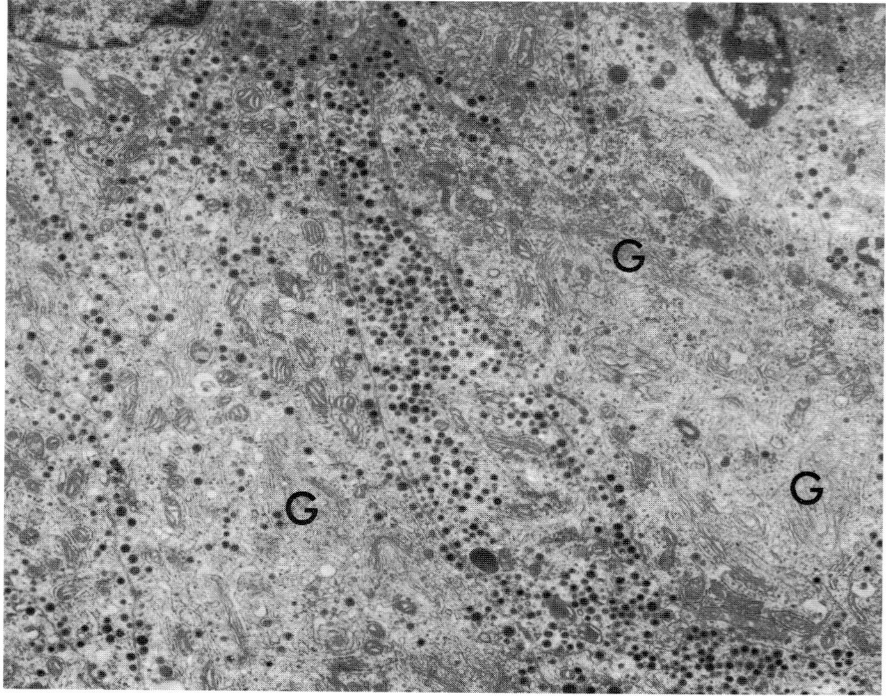

FIG. 9. Thyrotropin-secreting adenoma. The cells are elongated and angular, and contain very small secretory granules. The Golgi areas are prominent (G). ×7,000.

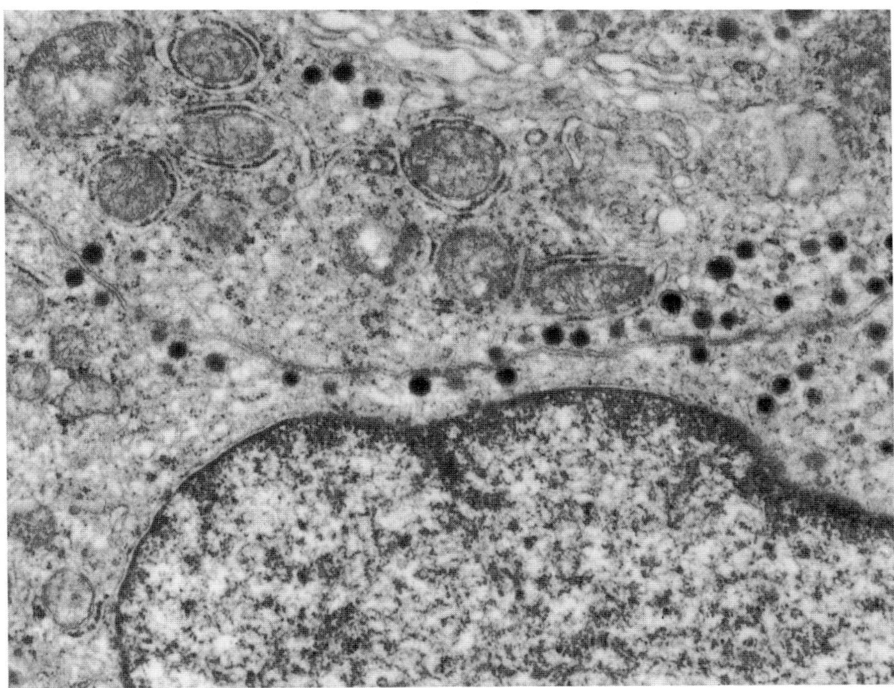

FIG. 10. Thyrotropin-secreting adenoma. A higher magnification shows the relationship between the mitochondria and the rough endoplasmic reticulum that surrounds them. ×25,000.

Tubular inclusions in the endothelial cells were previously reported in a similar type of adenoma (6) as well as in pituitary tumors associated with acromegaly (37).

GH- and Prolactin-Secreting Adenoma

One case in our series fulfills all the requirements for an adenoma that secretes more than one hormone. In this patient there was elevation of GH and prolactin, and incubation of the tumor showed active synthesis of both hormones. The morphologic examination of the tumor revealed a mixture of somatotrophs and lactotrophs at the optic microscopic as well as the ultrastructural levels (13). Since this report six more cases have been described; but although the patients' elevated GH levels had resulted in acromegaly, definite biological or laboratory evidence of prolactin hypersecretion was provided in only two cases (5).

ENDOCRINE-INACTIVE ADENOMAS

Endocrine-inactive adenomas, which do not produce biological and/or clinical signs of hormonal secretion, usually become symptomatic when their size becomes such as to produce hypopituitarism and/or chiasmatic compression.

Undifferentiated Adenomas

The largest group of these tumors consisted of 33 cases of undifferentiated adenomas. The tumors were comprised of small, usually polygonal cells sometimes attached to one another by long intercellular junctions. Secretory granules were scarce, usually small, measuring 100 to 250 nm, and often lying at the periphery under the cell membrane (Fig. 11). In 14 cases large secretory granules measuring up to 600 nm were also seen. The rough endoplasmic reticulum consisting of short profiles was well developed in one-fourth of our cases, and the Golgi areas were prominent in 16 cases sometimes containing progranules in their saccules (Fig. 12). The mitochondria were dense, rod-shaped, and not numerous. In 13 cases, however, they appeared definitely increased in number while retaining their normal appearance. This feature suggests that the tumor cells were undergoing oncocytic transformation. Lysosomes were usually present but seldom prominent.

This ultrastructural picture is similar to that of the chromophobe adenomas of Schelin (69) and other authors (41,67,81) as well as to that of some 32 cases described by Landolt (31) as endocrine-inactive adenomas with secretory

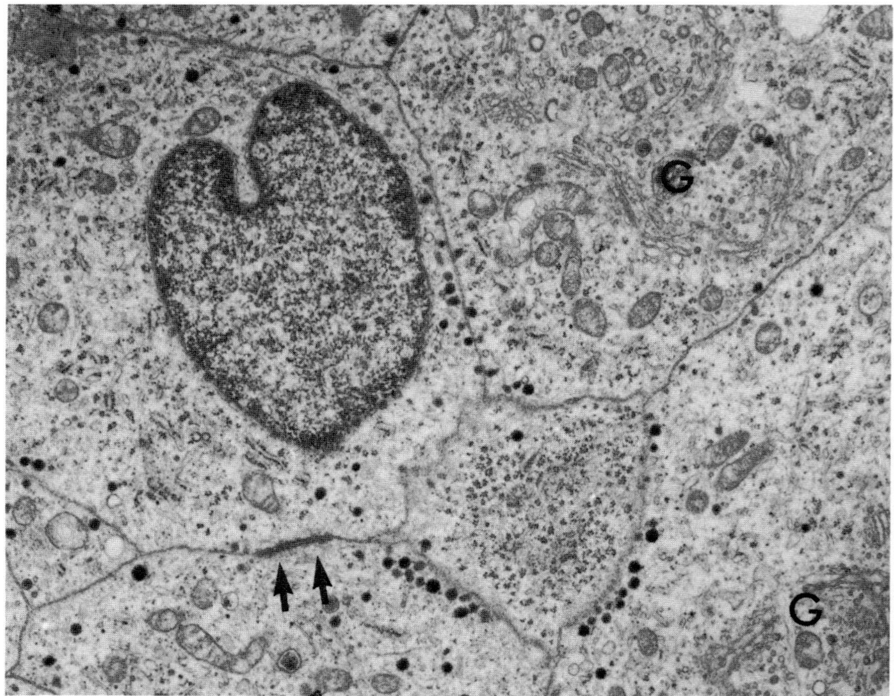

FIG. 11. Undifferentiated adenoma (case 67). The small polyhedral cells contain scarce small secretory granules. There is a long intercellular junction on the left *(arrows)*. Two cells have a prominent Golgi complex (G). ×11,625.

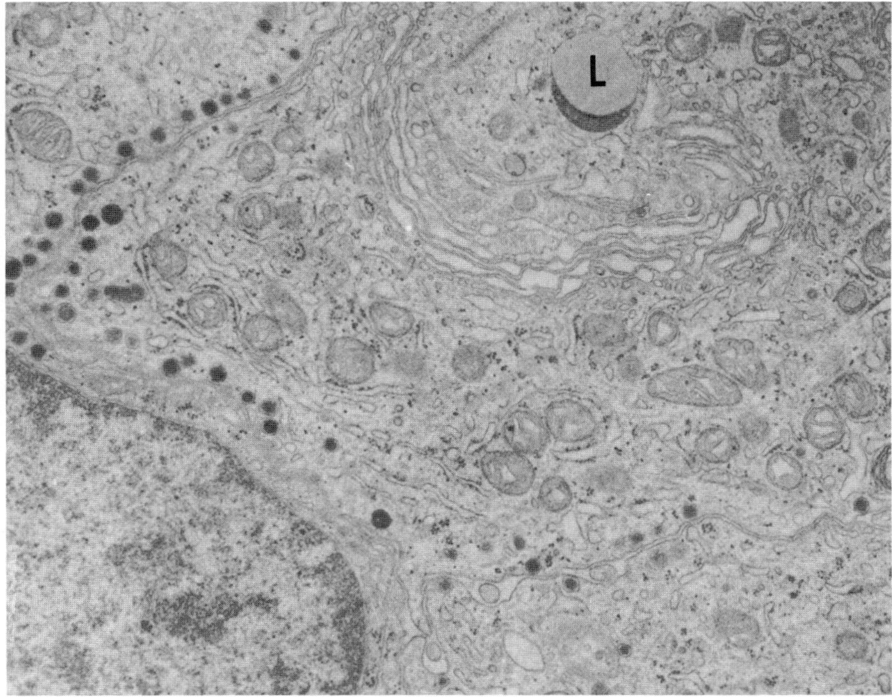

FIG. 12. Undifferentiated adenoma (case 64). A well-developed empty Golgi area is close to a lysosome (L). The small secretory granules lie along the cell membranes. ×17,500.

granules. They have been called inactive "chromophobic" adenomas (14,79) and more recently "undifferentiated cell" adenomas (20,28,71). The well-developed endoplasmic reticulum and Golgi complex indicate that these cells are active in protein synthesis (14,47,64,65,81).

Oncocytomas

Oncocytomas, tumors consisting exclusively of oncocytes (16), were recently described in the pituitary gland (25,35). Since then many other cases have been reported (2,20,28,31,32,34,61,63,64,77,79). These tumors are characterized by the presence of numerous tightly packed mitochondria filling the cytoplasm. We found that the secretory granules are usually very small with a few large ones, and that the other organelles are similar to those found in undifferentiated adenomas (Fig. 13).

Although oncocytes had been found in various organs (76), they were only recently identified in the normal anterior pituitary (26,51). The possibility of some type of mitochondrial disease has been raised (76), but the basic defect for the oncocytic transformation of adenohypophyseal cells remains unknown.

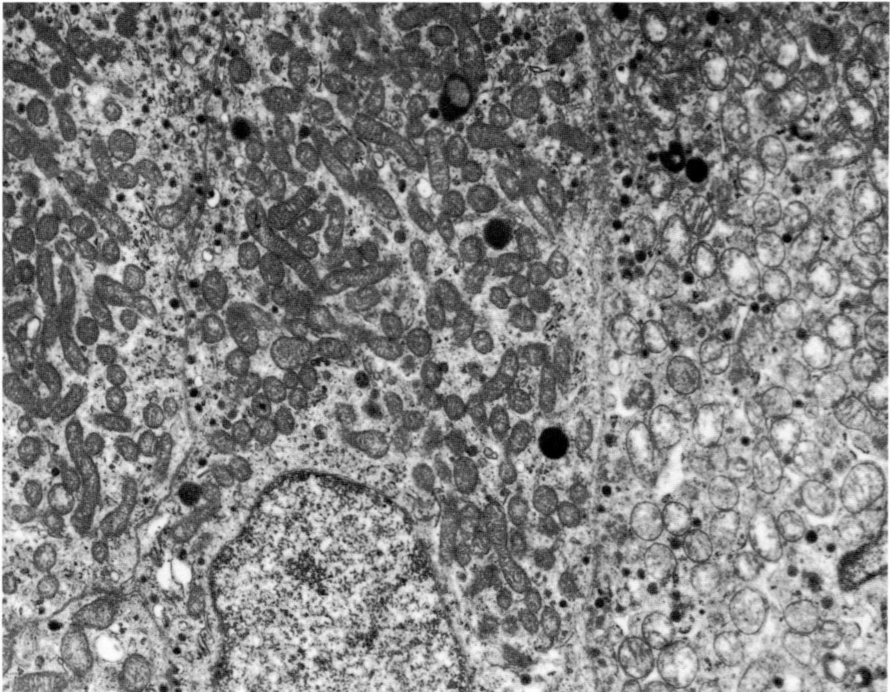

FIG. 13. Oncocytoma (case 98). The cells are filled with mitochondria. Very small secretory granules are seen, as are a few large ones. ×11,600.

As we have seen oncocytic changes in a few cases of acromegaly and in one case of Cushing's disease, it is possible that on some occasions the oncocytic tumor cells are hormonally active (64). Oncocytomas arising from GH cells have been reported (23).

Immunocytochemical studies have been performed in two cases. On one undifferentiated adenoma, no staining was seen with antiserum to ACTH and prolactin. The other case, an oncocytoma, remained unstained when exposed to antiserums to ACTH, prolactin, and thyrotropin.

DISCUSSION

A classification combining the ultrastructural features and the hormonal secretion of pituitary adenomas has proved practical. The size of the secretory granules may show considerable variation within a group or even a subgroup and therefore appears to be an unreliable parameter for classification when used alone. However, by combining the amount, shape, location, and diameter of secretory granules with other ultrastructural findings, a rather distinctive image may be obtained for each group of pituitary adenomas.

With immunocytochemical techniques, it becomes usually feasible to identify the hormone contained in the secretory granules of secreting adenomas. In the case of the endocrine-inactive adenomas, however, the nature of the secretion elaborated by the adenomatous cells remains unknown.

No definite relation has yet been established between the amount of secretory granules found within tumor cells and the serum level of the abnormally secreted hormone. It is now well known and accepted that the prolactin-secreting adenomatous cells are usually scarcely granulated unless modified by previous treatment.

In acromegaly the poorly granulated cells appear to have more aggressive behavior as they are often present in diffuse invasive adenomas. In other types of tumor, however, we have not found any ultrastructural differences between the invasive adenomas and the more benign enclosed adenomas.

SUMMARY

The ultrastructural examination of 297 pituitary adenomas included 250 secreting adenomas and 47 endocrine-inactive tumors. There were 132 prolactin-secreting adenomas with 112 tumors in women and 20 in men. These tumors showed a typical ultrastructural aspect with scarce secretory granules frequently undergoing exocytosis, a prominent rough endoplasmic reticulum, and a large Golgi area containing immature granules.

On the basis of the number of secretory granules, we placed 95 GH-secreting adenomas into three groups. The densely granulated tumors, found in 54 cases, were the most numerous in our series. The most interesting feature was the presence of juxtanuclear spherical aggregates of microfilaments, which were especially common in the sparsely granulated and the mixed tumors. The poorly granulated cells appear to be more aggressive in their behavior, being often present in diffuse invasive adenomas.

No basic ultrastructural differences were found in 14 adenomas in Cushing's disease and 7 tumors in Nelson's syndrome. There was marked variation in the size of the secretory granules in these tumors. The specific ultrastructural finding was the presence of perinuclear microfilaments in the tumor cells.

Thirty-three endocrine-inactive adenomas were comprised of small polyhedral cells containing mostly small secretory granules. In half of these cases the Golgi apparatus was well developed. Fourteen oncocytomas showed numerous closely packed mitochondria filling the cytoplasm of the tumor cells.

REFERENCES

1. Antunes, J. L., Housepian, M., Frantz, A. G., Holub, D. A., Hui, R. M., Carmel, P. W., and Quest, D. (1977): Prolactin-secreting pituitary tumors. *Ann. Neurol.,* 2:148–153.
2. Bauserman, S. C., Hardman, J. M., Schochet, S. S., and Earle, K. M. (1978): Pituitary oncocytoma: Indispensable role of electron microscopy in its identification. *Arch. Pathol. Lab. Med.,* 102:456–459.

3. Bilbao, J. M., Kovacs, K., Horvath, E., Higgins, H. P., and Horsey, W. J. (1975): Pituitary melanocorticotrophinoma with amyloid deposition. *Can. J. Neurol. Sci.,* 2:199–202.
4. Cardell, R. R., Jr., and Knighton, R. S. (1966): The cytology of a human pituitary tumor: An electron microscopic study. *Trans. Am. Microsc. Soc.,* 85:58–78.
5. Corenblum, B., Sirek, A. M. T., Horvath, E., Kovacs, K., and Ezrin, C. (1976): Human mixed somatotropic and lactotropic pituitary adenomas. *J. Clin. Endocrinol. Metab.,* 42:857–863.
6. Curé, M., Trouillas, J., Lheritier, M., Girod, C., and Rollet, J. (1972): Inclusions tubulaires dans une tumeur hypophysaire. *Nouv. Presse Med.,* 1:2309–2311.
7. DeCicco, F. A., Dekker, A., and Yunis, E. J. (1972): Fine structure of Crooke's hyaline change in the human pituitary gland. *Arch. Pathol.,* 94:65–70.
8. Duello, T. M., and Halmi, N. S. (1977): Pituitary adenoma producing thyrotropin and prolactin. *Virchows Arch.* [*Pathol. Anat.*], 376:255–265.
9. Foncin, J. F., Billet, R., and Le Beau, J. (1972): A propos des tumeurs hypophysaires extensives à sécrétion corticotrope (étude ultrastructurale). *Ann. Endocrinol. (Paris),* 33:449–454.
10. Foncin, J. F., and Le Beau, J. (1963): Etude en microscopie optique et électronique d'une tumeur hypophysaire à fonction adrénocorticotrope. *C. R. Soc. Biol.,* 157:249–252.
11. Friesen, H., Webster, B. R., Hwang, P., Guyda, H., Munro, R. E., and Read, L. (1972): Prolactin synthesis and secretion in a patient with the Forbes-Albright syndrome. *J. Clin. Endocrinol. Metab.,* 34:192–199.
12. Guinet, P., Girod, C., Pousset, G., Trouillas, J., and L'Hermite, M. (1973): Un cas d'adénome à cellules à prolactine: Dosage de prolactine, étude au microscope électronique, résultats post-opératoires. *Ann. Endocrinol. (Paris),* 34:407–417.
13. Guyda, H., Robert, F., Colle, E., and Hardy, J. (1973): Histologic, ultrastructural and hormonal characterization of a pituitary tumor secreting both HGH and prolactin. *J. Clin. Endocrinol. Metab.,* 36:531–547.
14. Hachmeister, U. (1973): Ultrastructural aspects of endocrine activity in "chromophobic" pituitary adenomas. *Acta Endocrinol.* [*Suppl*] *(Kbh),* 173:153.
15. Hachmeister, U., Fahlbusch, R., and Werder, K. von (1972): Ultrastructural identity of pituitary adenoma cells in Forbes-Albright syndrome and adenohypophyseal pregnancy cells. *Acta Endocrinol.* [*Suppl*] *(Kbh),* 159:42.
16. Hamperl, H. (1962): Benign and malignant oncocytoma. *Cancer,* 15:1019–1027.
17. Hardy, J., Beauregard, H., and Robert, F. (1978): Prolactin-secreting pituitary adenomas: transsphenoidal microsurgical treatment. In: *Progress in Prolactin. Physiology and Pathology,* Vol. 2, edited by C. Robyn and M. Harter, pp. 361–370. Elsevier North-Holland, Amsterdam.
18. Horn, K., Erhardt, F., Fahlbusch, R., Pickardt, C. R., Werder, K. von, and Scriba, P. C. (1976): Recurrent goitre, hyperthyroidism, galactorrhea and amenorrhea due to a thyrotropin and prolactin-producing pituitary tumor. *J. Clin. Endocrinol. Metab.,* 43:137–143.
19. Horvath, E., and Kovacs, K. (1974): Misplaced exocytosis: Distinct ultrastructural feature in some pituitary adenomas. *Arch. Pathol.,* 97:221–224.
20. Horvath, E., and Kovacs, K. (1976): Ultrastructural classification of pituitary adenomas. *Can. J. Neurol. Sci.,* 3:9–21.
21. Horvath, E., and Kovacs, K. (1978): Morphogenesis and significance of fibrous bodies in human pituitary adenomas. *Virchows Arch.* [*Zellpathol.*], 27:69–78.
22. Ketelbant-Balasse, P., Herlant, M., and Pasteels, J. L. (1973): Modifications hypophysaires dans un cas d'hypercorticisme para-néoplasique. *Ann. Endocrinol. (Paris),* 34:743–752.
23. Kinnman, J. (1973): *Acromegaly: An ultrastructural analysis of 51 adenomas and a clinical study in 80 patients treated by transanthrosphenoidal operation.* Norstedt and Söner, Stockholm.
24. Kovacs, K. (1977): Morphology of prolactin producing adenomas. *Clin. Endocrinol. (Oxf) (Suppl),* 6:71s.
25. Kovacs, K., and Horvath, E. (1973): Pituitary "chromophobe" adenoma composed of oncocytes: A light and electron microscopic study. *Arch. Pathol.,* 95:235–239.
26. Kovacs, K., Horvath, E., and Bilbao, J. M. (1974): Oncocytes in the anterior lobe of the human pituitary gland: A light and electron microscopic study. *Acta Neuropathol. (Berl),* 27:43–53.
27. Kovacs, K., Horvath, E., Corenblum, B., Sirek, A. M. T., Penz, G., and Ezrin, C. (1975): Pituitary chromophobe adenomas consisting of prolactin cells: A histologic, immunocytological, and electron microscopic study. *Virchows Arch.* [*Pathol. Anat.*], 366:113–123.
28. Kovacs, K., Horvath, E., and Ezrin, C. (1977): Pituitary adenomas. *Pathol. Annu.,* 12:341–382.

29. Kovacs, K., Horvath, E., Kerenyi, N. A., and Sheppard R. H. (1976): Light and electron microscopic features of a pituitary adenoma in Nelson's syndrome. *Am. J. Clin. Pathol.,* 65:337–343.
30. Kovacs, K., Horvath, E., Stratman, I. E., and Ezrin, C. (1974): Cytoplasmic micro-filaments in the anterior lobe of the human pituitary gland. *Acta Anat. (Basel),* 87:414–426.
31. Landolt, A. M. (1975): Ultrastructure of human sella tumors. *Acta Neurochir. (Wien) (Suppl),* 22:1–167.
32. Landolt, A. M. (1978): Progress in pituitary adenoma biology: results of research and clinical applications. In: *Advances and Technical Standards in Neurosurgery,* edited by H. Krayenbuhl, Vol. 5, pp. 3–49. Springer-Verlag, New York.
33. Landolt, A. M., and Hosbach, H. U. (1974): Biological aspects of pituitary tumors as revealed by electron microscopy. *Pathologica,* 66:413–436.
34. Landolt, A. M., and Kistler, G. S. (1978): Morphology of chromophobe adenomas. In: *Treatment of Pituitary Adenomas,* edited by R. Fahlbusch and K. von Werder, pp. 154–171. Thieme, Stuttgart.
35. Landolt, A. M., and Oswald, U. W. (1973): Histology and ultrastructure of an oncocytic adenoma of the human pituitary. *Cancer,* 31:1099–1105.
36. Landolt, A. M., and Rothenbühler, V. (1978): Extracellular growth hormone deposits in pituitary adenoma. *Virchows Arch. [Pathol. Anat.],* 378:55–65.
37. Landolt, A. M., Ryffel, U., Hosbach, H. U., and Wyler, R. (1976): Ultrastructure of tubular inclusions in endothelial cells of pituitary tumors associated with acromegaly. *Virchows Arch. [Pathol. Anat.],* 370:129–140.
38. Le Beau, J., and Foncin, J. F. (1972): Contribution à l'étude ultrastructurale des adénomes à prolactine. *Ann. Endocrinol. (Paris),* 33:353–356.
39. Leong, A. S. Y., Chawla, J. C., and Teh, E. C. (1976): Pituitary thyrotropic tumour secondary to long-standing primary hypothyroidism. *Pathol. Eur.,* 11:49–55.
40. Lewis, P. D., and Van Noorden, S. (1972): Pituitary abnormalities in acromegaly. *Arch. Pathol.,* 94:119–126.
41. Lewis, P. D., and Van Noorden, S. (1974): "Nonfunctioning" pituitary tumors: A light and electron microscopical study. *Arch. Pathol.,* 97:178–182.
42. McCarthy, K. S., Bredesen, D. G., and Vogel, F. S. (1978): Neoplasms of the anterior pituitary. *Neurosurgery,* 3:96–104.
43. Mirouze, J., Jaffiol, C., Mary, P., Baldet, P., and Monnier, L. (1969): Deux syndromes originaux: "Aménorrhée-Galactorrhée" par tumeur hypophysaire: discussion anatomoclinique: etude ultrastructurale de l'un d'eux. *Ann. Endocrinol. (Paris),* 30:810–821.
44. Moriarty, G. C. (1973): Adenohypophysis: ultrastructural cytochemistry: A review. *J. Histochem. Cytochem.,* 21:855–894.
45. Mornex, R., Tommasi, M., Curé, M., Farcot, J., Orgiazzi, J., and Rousset, B. (1972): Hyperthyroïdie associée à un hypopituitarisme au cours de l'évolution d'une tumeur hypophysaire sécrétant T.S.H. *Ann. Endocrinol. (Paris),* 33:390–396.
46. Nieuwenhuyzen Kruseman, A. C., Bots, G. T. A. M., Lindeman, J., and Schaberg, A. (1976): Use of immunohistochemical and morphologic methods for the identification of human growth hormone-producing pituitary adenomas. *Cancer,* 38:1163–1170.
47. Oliva, H., Navarro, V., and Obrador, S. (1966): Microscopía electrónica de los adenomas cromófobos de la hipófisis. *Acta Neurochir. (Wien),* 14:141–153.
48. Olivier, L., Vila-Porcile, E., Peillon, F., and Racadot, J. (1972): Etude en microscopie électronique des grains de sécrétion "basophiles" dans les cellules hypophysaires tumorales de la maladie de Cushing. *C R Soc. Biol.,* 166:1591–1595.
49. Olivier, L., Vila-Porcile, E., Racadot, O., Peillon, F., and Racadot, J. (1975): Ultrastructure of pituitary tumor cells: a critical study. In: *The Anterior Pituitary,* Vol. 7, edited by A. Tixier-Vidal and M. G. Farquar, pp. 231–276. Academic Press, New York.
50. Osamura, R. Y., Watanabe, K., Tekamoto, A., Hirakawa, K., Kawano, N., and Morii, S. (1978): Male prolactin-secreting pituitary adenomas in humans studied with peroxidase-labelled antibody method. *Acta Endocrinol. (Kbh),* 88:643–652.
51. Paiz, C., and Hennigar, G. R. (1970): Electron microscopy and histochemical correlation of human anterior pituitary cells. *Am. J. Pathol.,* 59:43–73.
52. Peake, G. T., McKeel, D. W., Jarret, L., and Daughaday, W. H. (1969): Ultrastructural histologic, and hormonal characterization of a prolactin-rich human pituitary tumor. *J. Clin. Endocrinol. Metab.,* 29:1383–1393.

53. Pelletier, G., Robert, F., and Hardy, J. (1978): Identification of human anterior pituitary cells by immunoelectron microscopy. *J. Clin. Endocrinol. Metab.,* 46:534–542.
54. Porcile, E., and Racadot, J. (1966): Ultrastructure des cellules de Crooke observées dans l'hypophyse humaine au cours de la maladie de Cushing. *C R Acad. Sci.,* 263:948–951.
55. Racadot, J., Vila-Porcile, E., Olivier, L., and Peillon, F. (1975): Electron microscopy of pituitary tumors. *Prog. Neurol. Surg.,* 6:95–141.
56. Racadot, J., Vila-Porcile, E., Peillon, F., and Olivier, L. (1971): Adénomes hypophysaires à cellules à prolactine: Etude structurale et ultrastructurale: corrélations anatomocliniques. *Ann. Endocrinol. (Paris),* 32:298–305.
57. Racadot, J., Olivier, L., Porcile, E., De Greye, C., and Klotz, H. P. (1964): Adénome hypophysaire de type mixte avec symptomatologie acromégalique. II. Etude au microscope optique et au microscope électronique. *Ann. Endocrinol. (Paris),* 25:503–507.
58. Robert, F. (1973): L'adénome hypophysaire dans l'acromégalie-gigantisme: Etude macroscopique, histologique, et ultrastructurale. *Neurochirurgie (Suppl),* 19:117–162.
59. Robert, F., and Hardy, J. (1975): Prolactin-secreting adenomas: A light and electron microscopical study. *Arch. Pathol.,* 99:625–633.
60. Robert, F., Pelletier, G., and Hardy, J. (1978): Pituitary adenomas in Cushing's disease: A histologic, ultrastructural and immunocytochemical study. *Arch. Pathol. Lab. Med.,* 102:448–455.
61. Rollet, J., Guinet, P., Girod, C., Trouillas, J., and Curé, M. (1975): Un cas d'adénome oncocytaire de l'hypophyse avec galactorrhée et hyperprolactinémie. *Ann. Endocrinol. (Paris),* 36:221–222.
62. Saeger, W. (1973): Zur Ultrastruktur der Hypophyseadenome beim Cushing-Syndrom nach Adrenalektomie. *Virchows Arch.* [*Pathol. Anat.*], 361:39–50.
63. Saeger, W. (1975): Vergleichende licht- and elektronenmikroskopische Untersuchungen an onkocytären Hypophysenadenomen. *Virchows Arch.* [*Pathol. Anat.*], 369:29–44.
64. Saeger, W., Breuer, H., and Lüdecke, D. (1975): Morphological and functional classification of pituitary adenomas. *Acta Endocrinol.* [*Suppl*] *(Kbh),* 193:89.
65. Saeger, W., Breuer, H., and Lüdecke, D. (1976): Zur Definition und Differentialdiagnose chromophober Hypophyseadenome Licht- und elektronenmikroskopische Untersuchungen. *Beitr. Pathol.,* 157:367–390.
66. Samaan, N. A., Osborne, B. M., Mackay, B., Leavens, M. E., Duello, T. M., and Halmi, N. S. (1977): Endocrine and morphologic studies of pituitary adenomas secondary to primary hypothyroidism. *J. Clin. Endocrinol. Metab.,* 45:903–911.
67. Schechter, J. (1973): Electron microscopic studies of human pituitary tumors. I. Chromophobic adenomas. *Am. J. Anat.,* 138:371–386.
68. Schechter, J. (1973): Electron microscopic studies of human pituitary tumors. II. Acidophilic adenomas. *Am. J. Anat.,* 138:387–400.
69. Schelin, U. (1962): Chromophobe and acidophil adenomas of the human pituitary gland: A light and electron microscopic study. *Acta Pathol. Microbiol. Scand.* [*Suppl*], 158:1–80.
70. Schroffner, W. G. (1976): Prolactin-secreting pituitary tumor in early adolescence: Hormonal and electron microscopical studies. *Arch. Intern. Med.,* 136:1164–1168.
71. Sirek, A. M. T., Corenblum, B., Horvath, E., Rewcastle, B., Ezrin, C., and Kovacs, K. (1976): A new look at pituitary adenomas: Structure elucidating function. *Can. Med. Assoc. J.,* 114:225–229.
72. Sternberger, L. A. (1972): The unlabeled-antibody-peroxydase and the quantitative immunomethods in light and electron immunohistochemistry. In: *Techniques of Biochemical and Biophysical Morphology,* edited by I. D. Glick and R. M. Rosenbaum. Wiley-Interscience, New York.
73. Tani, E., Kawamura, Y., Ametani, T., Handa, H., Imura, H., and Kato, Y. (1969): Immunocytochemistry of acidophil granules of human pituitary. *Arch. Neurol.,* 20:634–643.
74. Tomiyasu, U., Hirano, A., and Zimmerman, H. M. (1973): Fine structure of human pituitary adenoma. *Arch. Pathol.,* 95:287–292.
75. Tournaire, J., Guinet, P., Bachelot, I., Pousset, G., Pallo, D., Sassolas, G., Trouillas, J., and L'Hermite, M. (1974): Les adénomes à prolactine (a propos de 9 observations personelles). *Otolaryngol. Neurol. Ophthalmol.,* 46:303–320.
76. Tremblay, G. (1969): The oncocytes. *Met. Arch. Exp. Pathol.,* 4:121–140.
77. Trouillas, J., Curé, J., Lheritier, M., Girod, C., Guinet, P., Tommasi, M., Goutelle, A., and Allegre, C. E. (1975): L'oncocytome hypophysaire est-il une entité? Discussion anatomo-clinique à propos de trois observations personelles. *Lyon Med.,* 234:25–35.

78. Trouillas, J., Curé, M., Lheritier, M., Girod, C., Pallo, D., and Tourniaire, J. (1976): Les adénomes hypophysaires avec aménorrhée-galactorrhée ou galactorrhée isolée: De la cellule à prolactine normale à la cellule à prolactine adénomateuse; étude microscopique photonique et ultrastructurale avec corrélations anatomo-cliniques dans 11 observations personnelles. *Lyon Med.,* 236:359–375.
79. Trouillas, J., Curé, M., Lheritier, M., Guichard, Y., and Girod, C. (1974): Essai de classification cytofonctionelle de 19 adénomes hypohysaires d'après des données histologiques, immunocytochimiques, biométriques ultrastructurales. *Otolaryngol. Neurol. Ophthalmol.,* 46:223–236.
80. Wagermark, J., and Wersäll, J. (1968): Ultrastructural features of Crooke's changes in pituitary basophil cells. *Acta Pathol. Microbiol. Scand.,* 72:367–375.
81. Zambrano, D., Amezua, L., Dickmann, G., and Franke, E. (1968): Ultrastructure of human pituitary adenomata. *Acta Neurochir. (Wien),* 18:78–94.

Clinical Management of Pituitary Disorders,
edited by G. T. Tindall and W. F. Collins.
Raven Press, New York © 1979.

5

Diagnostic Roentgenology of Pituitary Lesions

Edward R. Laws Jr. and O. Wayne Houser

Departments of Neurologic Surgery and Diagnostic Radiology (Neuroradiology), Mayo Clinic, Mayo Medical School, Rochester, Minnesota 55901

The pituitary gland lies in one of the most protected sites in the human body, with the sella turcica and its surrounding structures forming a secure and complex compartment for the pituitary. The developmental anatomy of this area is important, as the distortions that occur in these bony structures in the presence of pituitary tumors reflect the origin and metabolism of the various bony structures which join to fashion the base of the skull. It is also important to realize that bone, in general, is constantly undergoing a process of absorption and reformation, and that this turnover also is affected by the presence of pituitary pathology.

The earliest published radiograph of a confirmed pituitary adenoma appeared in Harvey Cushing's 1909 article reporting a case of acromegaly referred by Dr. C. H. Mayo and operated on successfully via a transsphenoidal approach (3). This was a lateral skull film of poor quality, but it showed obvious erosion of the sella. The introduction of ventriculography and pneumoencephalography by Walter Dandy provided a valuable tool for the assessment of suprasellar extension of pituitary tumors. Although cerebral angiography was widely used in neurologic diagnosis, until recently it was of little importance in the evaluation of pituitary lesions, the plain skull film and air studies being the mainstays of radiologic diagnosis.

A number of technologic advances coincided with advances in endocrinologic diagnosis and sophistication in concepts of pituitary pathology. Multidirectional polytomography permits detailed evaluation of the bony sella. Magnification–subtraction techniques applied to angiography permit the detection of microadenomas within even a normal-sized sella. Computerized tomography of the head is capable of demonstrating extra- and intrasellar tumors, and its resolving capabilities will undoubtedly improve steadily. Videofluoroscopic X-ray image intensifiers allow intraoperative monitoring of surgery performed for these lesions.

With the advent of accurate assays for many pituitary hormones and increasing awareness of pituitary disorders on the part of the medical community, radiologic studies play an important complementary role in diagnosis. The occasional pituitary microadenoma is diagnosed on clinical endocrinologic grounds alone, with a normal radiologic evaluation.

Although pituitary adenoma is by far the most common cause of radiologic abnormalities of the sella turcica, it is always prudent to consider a differential diagnosis. Other tumors that may cause sellar changes include craniopharyngioma, meningioma, chiasmal glioma, germinoma, myeloma, cholesteatoma, fibrous dysplasia, and metastases. Cysts have been encountered, including arachnoid cysts, Rathke's cleft cysts, and various forms of "empty sella." Inflammatory lesions may occur, e.g., mucocele or granuloma. Finally, it is important to realize that aneurysms may simulate a pituitary tumor.

PLAIN SKULL FILMS

In evaluation of plain skull films, a systematic approach is helpful (11). The basic anatomy of the skull should be noted (2,14). The sphenoid sinus and its development profoundly affect the sella (8). The sphenoid sinus encasing the sella may be completely or partially pneumatized, or not pneumatized at all. The normal sphenoid sinus may have numerous chambers, and its septation may distort the floor of the sella, simulating asymmetries produced by tumors. The sella itself may vary in shape, from round to oval to flat. The shape of the sella may be influenced by the basal angle and the distance to the sella along the frontal base. The quality of bone may affect the quality and reliability of plain skull films, and osteoporosis or sclerosis may accompany pituitary lesions.

The extrasellar structures at the base should be evaluated in detail. The sphenoid sinus may contain a mass lesion or fluid. The clivus may be eroded or expanded by a lesion such as a chordoma. The floor of the anterior fossa may be sclerosed or "blistered" by a meningioma. Bone may be expanded by fibrous dysplasia; optic foramina may be enlarged or asymmetrical; calcifications or metastatic deposits may be present.

In the evaluation of the sella, the most obvious pathologic change is gross enlargement (17). Erosion and destruction of part or all of the sella may occur as well (Figs. 1 and 2). A number of changes may affect the sellar floor: "double" floor, erosion, blistering, slanting, or straightening. The dorsum sellae may be straightened by intrasellar tumors and shortened by suprasellar masses. The clinoids may be affected by erosion or by undercutting and enlargement of the chiasmatic sulcus resulting in the so-called "J-shaped" sella. Intrasellar calcification may occur normally or in association with craniopharyngiomas, pituitary adenomas (4), or carotid aneurysms.

POLYTOMOGRAPHY OF THE SELLA

Tomograms offer a detailed evaluation of many features seen on the plain skull films (12,14–16). A precise assessment of the shape and volume of the

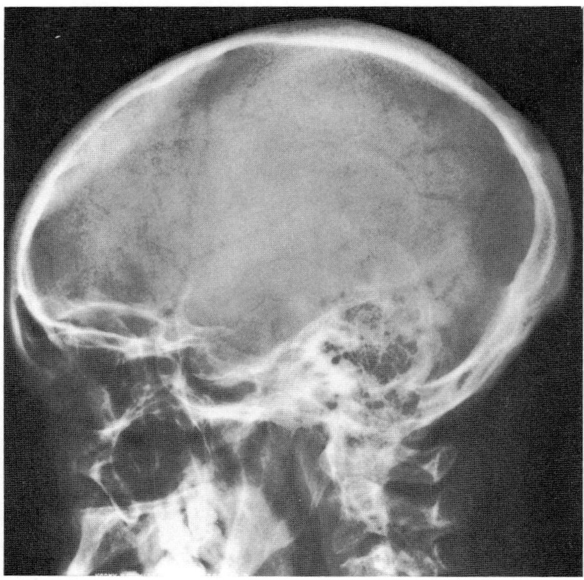

FIG. 1. Left lateral skull film. Large nonfunctioning pituitary adenoma. The sella is eroded, and the dorsum is absent.

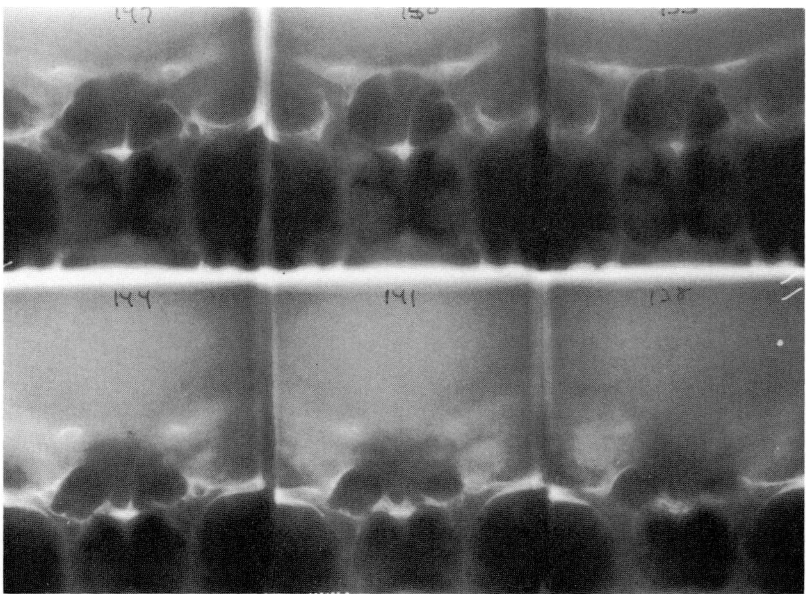

FIG. 2. Same case as Fig. 1. AP polytomography showing destruction of the sellar floor.

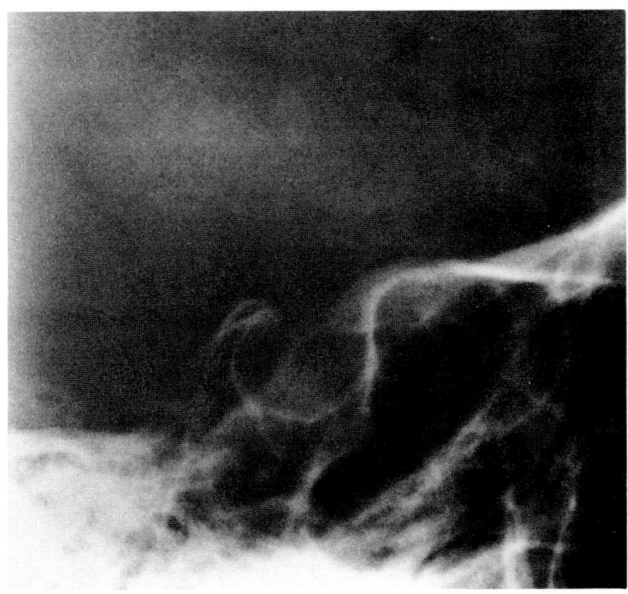

FIG. 3A. Prolactin-secreting pituitary microadenoma. Right lateral skull film showing double floor of sella.

sella becomes possible. The thickness and integrity of the sellar walls can be evaluated, along with their symmetry (Figs. 3–7). Focal changes in the form of blistering and erosion are more readily appreciated, as are calcifications within the sella. Tomography is very useful for assessing the shape and symmetry of the clinoids and for detecting early erosion of these structures. Changes in the dorsum sellae (e.g., straightening, amputation, or erosion) may be readily confirmed by tomography.

CEREBRAL ANGIOGRAPHY

If for no other reason, angiography is important for detecting carotid artery aneurysms, which may simulate or coexist with pituitary lesions (5,18). Angiography may also define other abnormalities in the carotids (6), e.g., tortuosity or atheromas.

A number of angiographic features characterize large pituitary adenomas (1). These include displacement or distortion of the cavernous segments of the carotid arteries and elevation of the A-1 segments of the anterior cerebral arteries (Fig. 8). Changes in finer vessels may be detected with the use of magnification–subtraction techniques (13). These include hypertrophy and proliferation of the meningohypophyseal trunk, the presence of capsular branches, and elevation of the circuminfundibular plexus. Tumor stains may be visualized, even in very small microadenomas (Fig. 9). Angiography may demonstrate pathologic alter-

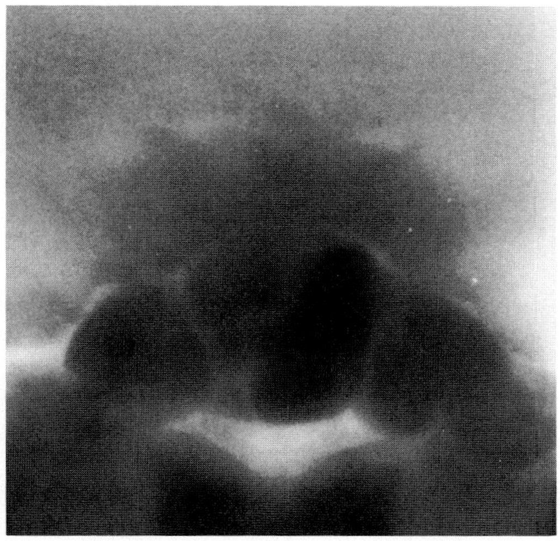

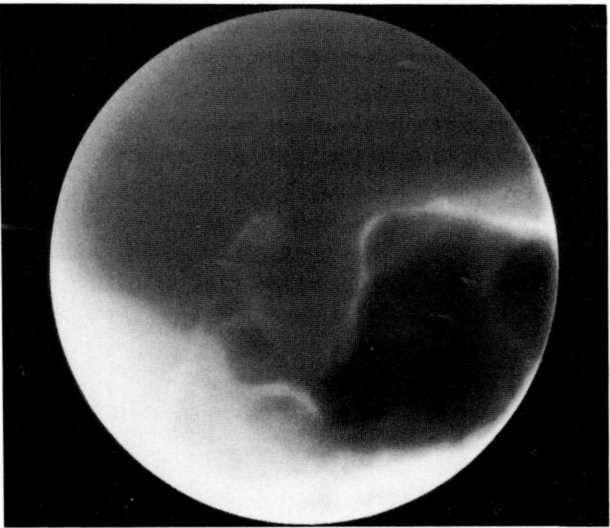

FIG. 3B and C. Prolactin-secreting pituitary microadenoma. **B** *(top):* AP polytomograms. Tumor erodes floor of sella on the right. **C** *(bottom):* Lateral polytomogram.

ations in the posterior pituitary gland, including hypervascularity, elongation, compression, or displacement.

PNEUMOENCEPHALOGRAPHY

Air studies have played a less important role since the advent of CT scanning, and now are of major importance only in the demonstration of the empty sella

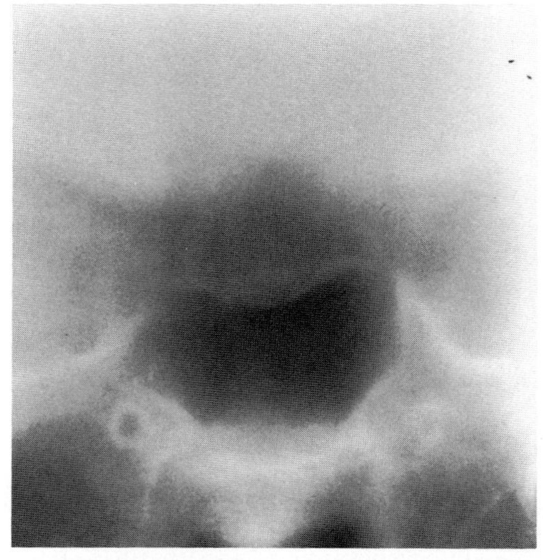

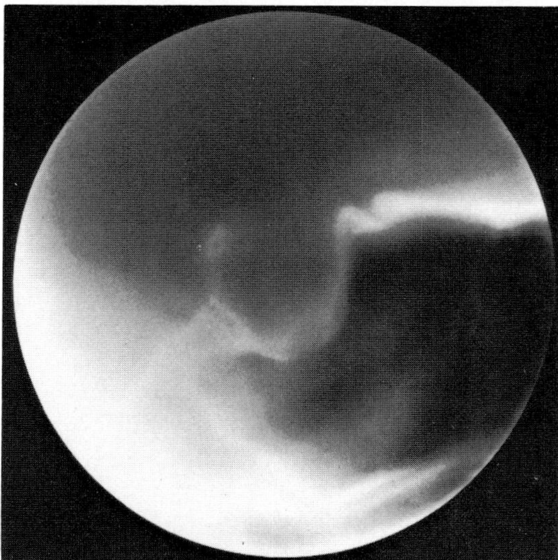

FIG. 4. Prolactin-secreting pituitary microadenoma. PA and right lateral polytomography. Note erosion and expansion of sellar floor.

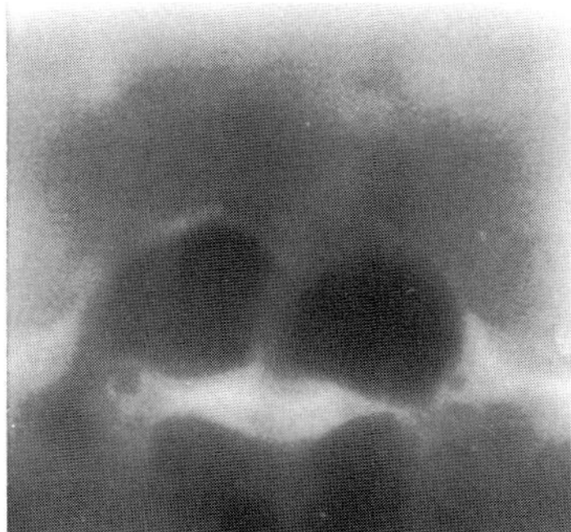

FIG. 5A. Acromegaly—pituitary microadenoma. AP polytomogram.

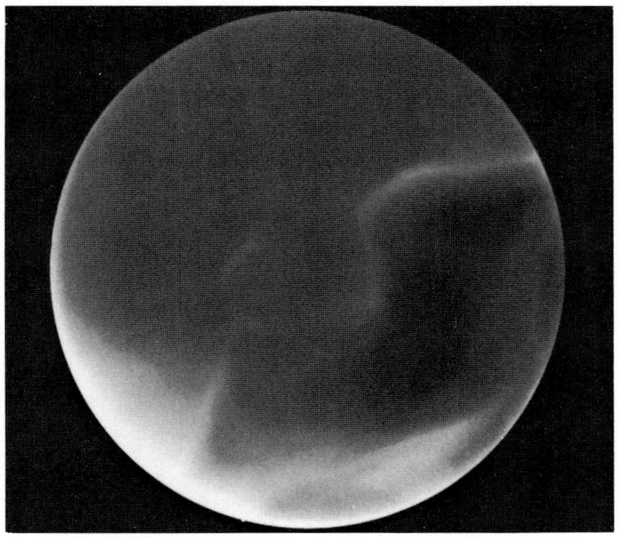

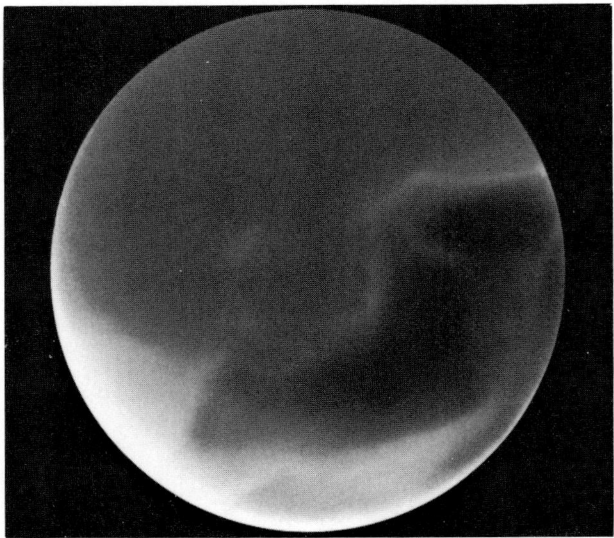

FIG. 5B. and C. Acromegaly—pituitary microadenoma. Right lateral polytomograms. Note "blistering" of the floor of the sella.

(Fig. 10). In addition to demonstrating the configuration and extent of suprasellar lesions, the pneumoencephalogram can outline the diaphragma sellae, and occasionally a microadenoma may be suspected when there is asymmetry of an intrasellar arachnoid diverticulum (10). The intraoperative use of pneumoencephalography monitored by the image intensifier (7,9) can be very helpful in the removal of tumors with suprasellar extension.

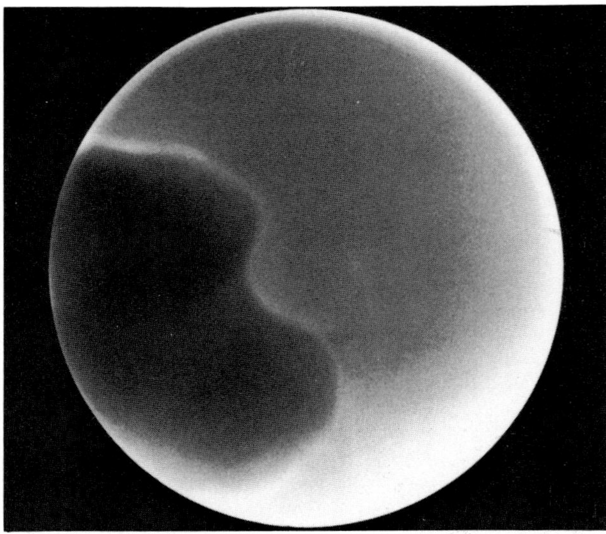

FIG. 6. Cushing's disease—pituitary microadenoma. Left lateral polytomogram. Except for osteoporosis, the study is normal.

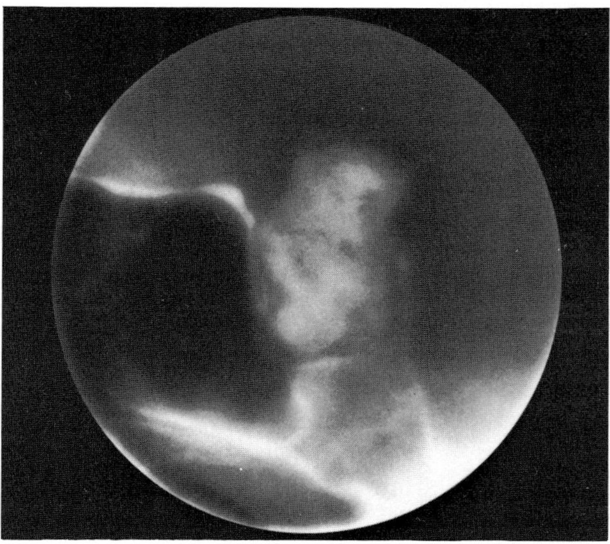

FIG. 7. Craniopharyngioma—left lateral polytomogram.

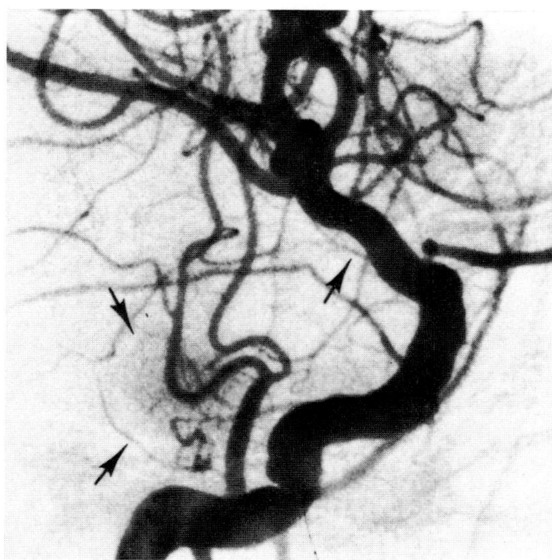

FIG. 8. Large nonfunctioning pituitary adenoma. Magnification–subtraction right lateral carotid arteriogram. Arrows indicate capsular vessels.

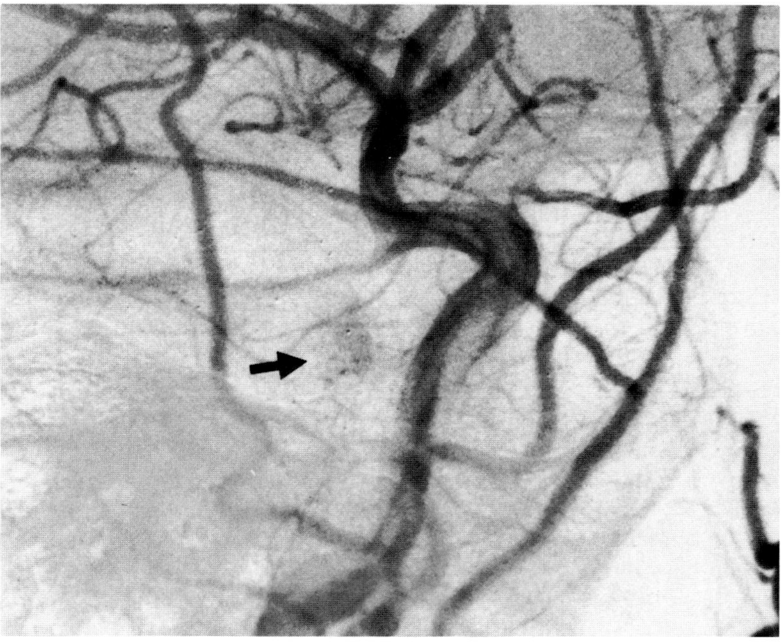

FIG. 9. Cushing's disease—pituitary microadenoma. Magnification–subtraction right carotid arteriogram. Arrow indicates mottled intrasellar tumor stain.

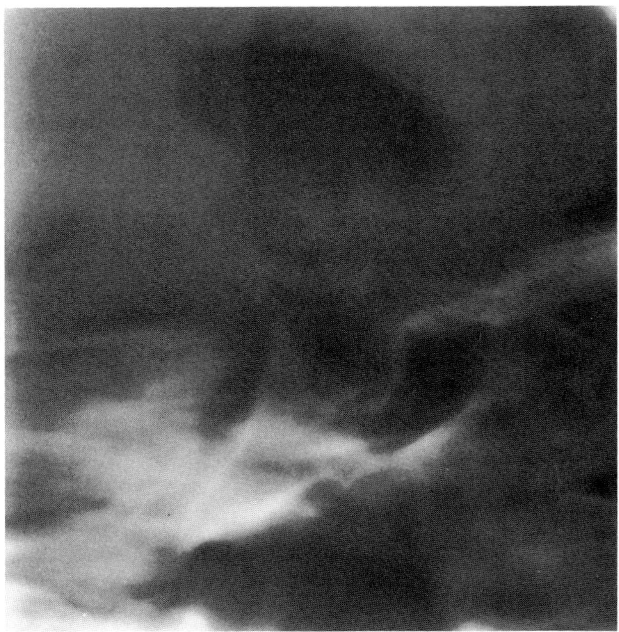

FIG. 10. Empty sella. Right lateral pneumoencephalogram.

COMPUTERIZED TOMOGRAPHY (CT SCAN)

The great appeal of CT scanning lies in the simple and noninvasive nature of the method. Scans demonstrate suprasellar anatomy, cisterns, and tumor masses. The bony sellar and parasellar structures can be evaluated by the CT scan, and with the use of contrast enhancement intrasellar lesions can frequently be detected (Figs. 11 and 12). As techniques of CT scanning improve, the utility of this method for the study of pituitary tumors will increase.

SELECTION OF APPROPRIATE STUDIES

The following represent suggested guidelines for the selection of roentgenographic studies in specific pituitary tumors:

1. *"Nonfunctioning" adenomas:* These tumors usually present with enlarged sella and mass effect. Appropriate studies include:
   A. Plain skull films.
   B. Polytomography.
   C. Angiography. This procedure is done to exclude aneurysm and may show carotid anomalies, tumor blush, and suprasellar extension.

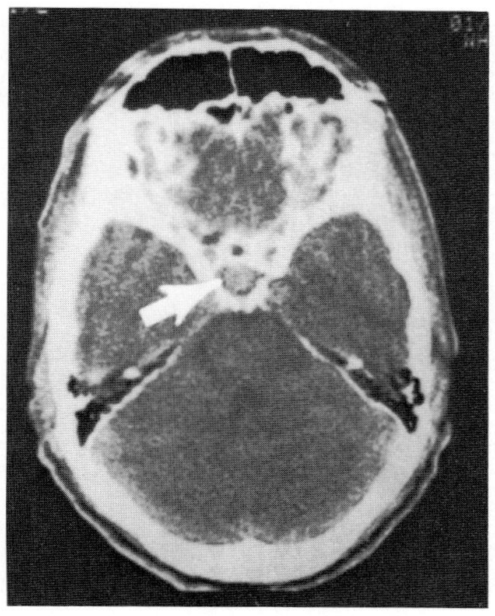

FIG. 11. Acromegaly, intrasellar pituitary adenoma. CT scan with contrast enhancement demonstrating intrasellar tumor.

D. Pneumoencephalography. This is performed intraoperatively to delineate intracranial extension of tumor and its removal under fluoroscopy.
E. CT scan with contrast.

2. *Prolactin adenomas:* These tumors are usually intrasellar adenomas. About 10% of our series have some suprasellar extension. Studies include:
A. Plain skull films.
B. Polytomography.
C. Angiography. This test, which may reveal tumor blush, is not considered mandatory in most cases.
D. Pneumoencephalography. Routine PEG is not considered mandatory in

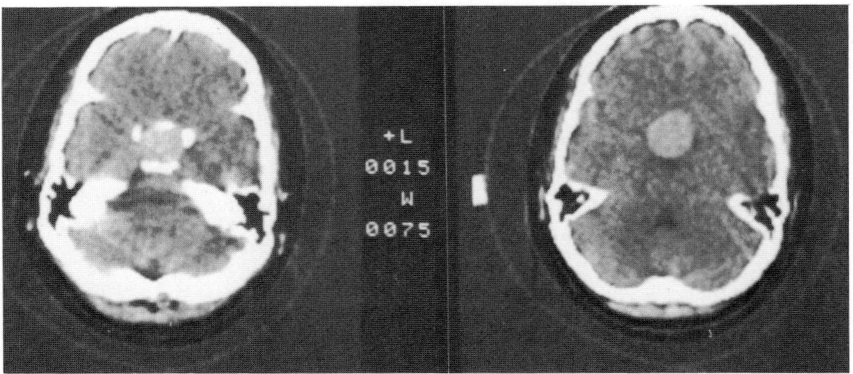

FIG. 12. Nonfunctioning pituitary adenoma. CT scan with contrast enhancement.

most cases. Intraoperative PEG is done when significant suprasellar component is present.

E. CT scan with contrast. This may be helpful but is not considered mandatory in most cases.

3. *Acromegaly (hGH adenomas):* In our experience, most of these tumors have been intrasellar; about 10% have suprasellar extension, and approximately 34% have "invasive" characteristics. Studies include:
   A. Plain skull films.
   B. Polytomography.
   C. Angiography. This procedure is useful but not considered mandatory in most cases.
   D. Pneumoencephalography. This test is not considered mandatory in most cases. Intraoperative PEG is done when significant suprasellar component is present.
4. *ACTH adenomas* (Cushing's disease and Nelson–Salassa syndrome): The majority of these tumors are intrasellar, and those in Cushing's disease may be difficult to demonstrate definitively by preoperative studies. Recommended studies include:
   A. Plain skull films.
   B. Polytomography. These studies may show osteoporosis and either erosion or invasion, particularly in Nelson–Salassa syndrome.
   C. Angiography. In addition to features mentioned for the other functioning tumors, an angiographic tumor stain may be the only radiologic diagnostic feature in a case of Cushing's disease (these stains were seen in 68% of our cases).
   D. Pneumoencephalography. As with acromegalic patients, this test is not considered mandatory in most cases, and intraoperative PEG may be performed when a significant suprasellar component is present.

These guidelines will undoubtedly change as endocrinologic and radiologic diagnostic tests improve, but such studies will continue to be indispensable in the preoperative analysis of pituitary adenomas.

CONCLUSION

Intelligently planned, carefully interpreted radiologic studies are an integral part of the evaluation of pituitary disorders. Such studies help make possible accurate diagnosis and successful surgical management.

REFERENCES

1. Baker, H. L., Jr. (1972): The angiographic delineation of sellar and parasellar masses. *Radiology,* 104:67–78.
2. Bergland, R. M., Ray, B. S., and Torack, R. M. (1968): Anatomical variation in the human pituitary gland and adjacent structures in 225 human autopsy cases. *J. Neurosurg.,* 28:93.

3. Cushing, H. (1909): Partial hypophysectomy for acromegaly with remarks on the function of the hypophysis. *Ann. Surg.,* 50:1002–1017.
4. Deery, E. M. (1929): Note on calcification in pituitary adenomas. *Endocrinology,* 13:455–457.
5. Dussault, J., Plamondon, C., and Volpe, R. (1969): Aneurysms of the internal carotid artery simulating pituitary tumours: Report of two cases. *Can. Med. Assoc. J.,* 101:785–790.
6. Epstein, B. S., and Epstein, J. A. (1968): The angiographic demonstration and surgical implications of imbedding of the carotid syphons by a large pituitary adenoma. *Am. J. Roentgenol. Radium Ther. Nucl. Med.,* 104:162–167.
7. Guiot, G., Rougerie, J., and Hertzog, E. (1958): L'utilization de l'amplicateur de brillance en neurochirurgie. *Sem. Hop. Paris,* 12:689–695.
8. Hammer, G., and Rådberg, C. (1961): The sphenoidal sinus: An anatomical and roentgenologic study with reference to transsphenoidal hypophysectomy. *Acta Radiol. (Stockh),* 56:401–422.
9. Hardy, J., and Wigser, S. M. (1965): Trans-sphenoidal surgery of pituitary fossa tumors with televised radiofluoroscopic control. *J. Neurosurg.,* 23:612–619.
10. Kaufman, B. (1968): The "empty" sella turcica—a manifestation of the intrasellar subarachnoid space. *Radiology,* 90:931–941.
11. Mahmoud, M. E. S. (1958): The sella in health and disease. *Br. J. Radiol. (Suppl),* 8:1–100.
12. McLachan, M. S. F., Wright, A. D., and Doyle, F. H. (1970): Plain film and tomographic assessment of the pituitary fossa in 140 acromegalic patients. *Br. J. Radiol.,* 43:360–369.
13. Powell, D. F., Baker, H. L., Jr., and Laws, E. R., Jr. (1974): The primary angiographic findings in pituitary adenomas. *Radiology,* 110:589–595.
14. Renn, W. H., and Rhoton, A. L., Jr., (1975): Microsurgical anatomy of the sellar region. *J. Neurosurg.,* 43:288–298.
15. Vezina, J. L., and Maltais, R. (1973): La selle turcique dans l'acromégalie—étude radiologique. *Neurochirurgie (Suppl 2),* 19:35–56.
16. Vezina, J. L., and Sutton, T. J. (1974): Prolactin-secreting pituitary adenomas: Roentgenologic diagnosis. *Am. J. Roentgenol. Radium Ther. Nucl. Med.,* 120:46–54.
17. Weisberg, L. A., Zimmerman, E. A., and Frantz, A. G. (1976): Diagnosis and evaluation of patients with an enlarged sella turcica. *Am. J. Med.,* 61:590–596.
18. White, J. C., and Ballantine, H. T., Jr. (1961): Intrasellar aneurysms simulating hypophyseal tumors. *J. Neurosurg.,* 18:34–50.

Clinical Management of Pituitary Disorders,
edited by G. T. Tindall and W. F. Collins.
Raven Press, New York © 1979.

6

Neuroradiographic Evaluation of Pituitary Gland Tumors

James C. Hoffman Jr.

Department of Radiology, Section of Neurovascular Radiology, Emory University School of Medicine, Atlanta, Georgia 30322

Recent advances in transsphenoidal microsurgical techniques and progress in the ability to assay anterior pituitary gland hormones have changed the requirements of radiographic evaluation of lesions of the pituitary gland. Because small pituitary tumors can be suspected earlier, it has become necessary for the radiologist to detect and determine the position of these tumors with neuroradiographic techniques (9). The two most important radiographic methods for evaluating the pituitary fossa and gland are multidirectional tomography of the sella and computed tomography. Because of the importance of the latter techniques the indications for angiography and pneumoencephalography have changed. The purpose of this chapter is to present what we consider the appropriate radiographic evaluation of a patient with a suspected pituitary tumor and the expected yield from the various radiographic techniques.

PRIMARY RADIOGRAPHIC TECHNIQUES

The initial evaluation of a patient suspected of harboring a pituitary tumor should include the standard anterior–posterior (AP) and lateral plain skull films. These films allow an overall assessment of the size and configuration of the sella and the skull in general. The degree of development of the sphenoid sinus can be determined from these films. Calcification in the sella or suprasellar area can be detected. Multidirectional tomography of the sella should be included in the initial evaluation of a patient suspected of having a pituitary tumor. The tomograms should be done at 1-mm intervals in the lateral plane and 2-mm intervals in the AP plane. The lateral tomograms should cover both sides of the sella, and they are adequate if both anterior clinoids are visualized on the tomograms. The tomograms are necessary to detect the bony changes of small adenomas that are 1 cm or less in size. These are the microadenomas that often are not detected on plain films of the sella. In the series of 140 microadenomas reported by Robertson and Newton (5), 50% of the patients had a normal size and appearance of the sella on routine plain films; however, on thin-section tomography abnormalities of the sella were demonstrated in all but three patients.

Because of the complex development of the sella turcica and sphenoid sinus, the detection of abnormal subtle changes in the sella can be difficult and there is some overlap between the normal and abnormal (6). A prominent carotid sulcus can cause apparent asymmetry of the sella on plain films; however, the tomograms demonstrate that there is no abnormality of the sella (Fig. 1). Many physicians consider that the double floor sella seen on lateral skull films is abnormal; however, some asymmetry of the sella floor can be within the range of normal. Lateral skull films made when there is improper positioning of the patient's head may cause apparent asymmetry of the sella and a false double floor (Fig. 2). Asymmetrical development of the sphenoid sinus (e.g., expansion of one side) may cause a double contour of the floor of the sella on lateral films (Fig. 3). Tomography readily detects this asymmetrical development.

The normal tomogram of the sella should demonstrate an intact lamina dura that is uniform in thickness, and there should be no focal areas of erosion or bulging. Both sides of the sella should be compared on the lateral tomograms

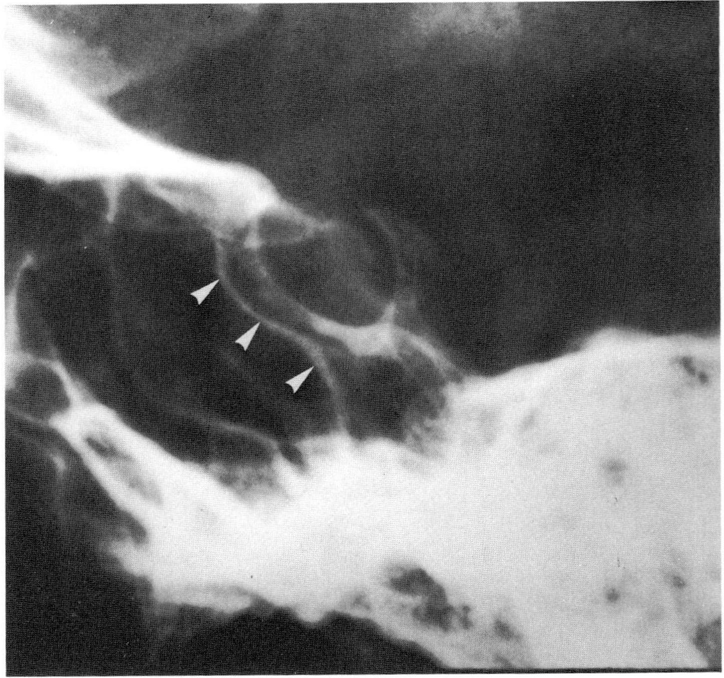

FIG. 1. Lateral view of sella showing a prominent carotid sulcus *(arrowheads).*

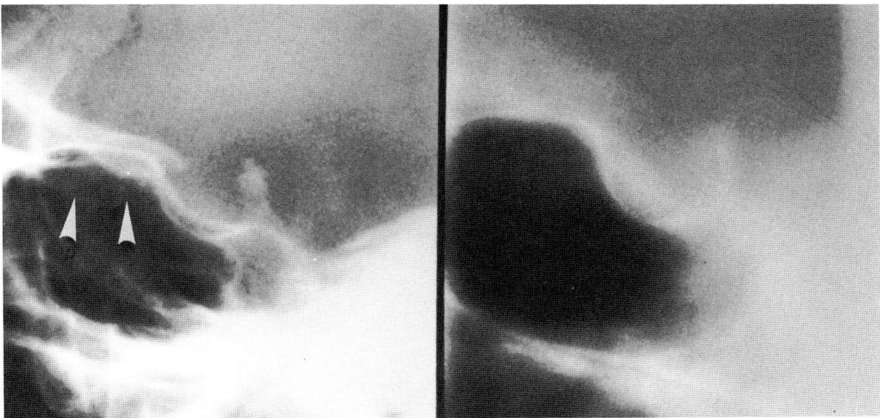

FIG. 2. Poorly positioned lateral view of the skull. **Left:** Double floor sella on lateral view. Note the asymmetry of anterior clinoids *(arrowheads).* **Right:** Lateral tomogram demonstrating normal sella.

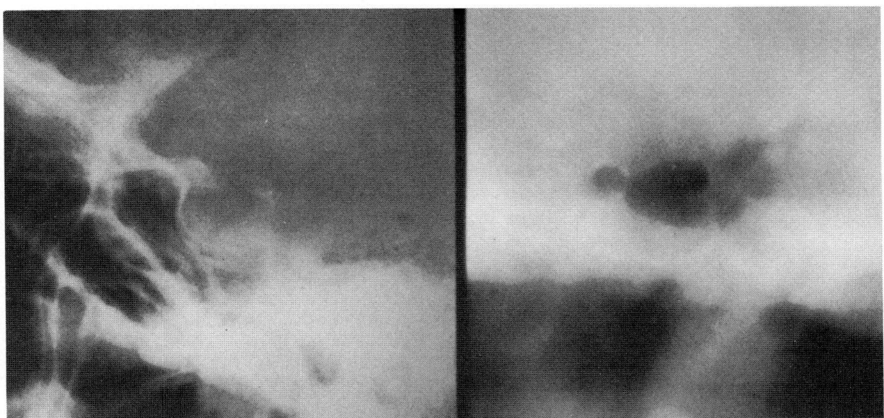

FIG. 3. Asymmetrical development of the sphenoid sinus. **Left:** Lateral view of the skull showing double floor sella. **Right:** AP tomographic cut demonstrating asymmetrical development of the sphenoid sinus.

to detect any asymmetry. The small adenomas show a localized expansion of the sella usually along the anterior–inferior margin (Fig. 4). Erosion of the lamina dura along the anterior–inferior edge of the sella can also be detected in small adenomas (Figs. 5 and 6). Microadenomas may cause asymmetrical ballooning of the sella; therefore, the sides of the sella should be compared on the tomograms to detect this asymmetrical ballooning (Fig. 7). If there is a slope of more than 3 mm on the AP view, this should be considered abnormal and the expansion of the sella should be confirmed on the lateral tomograms.

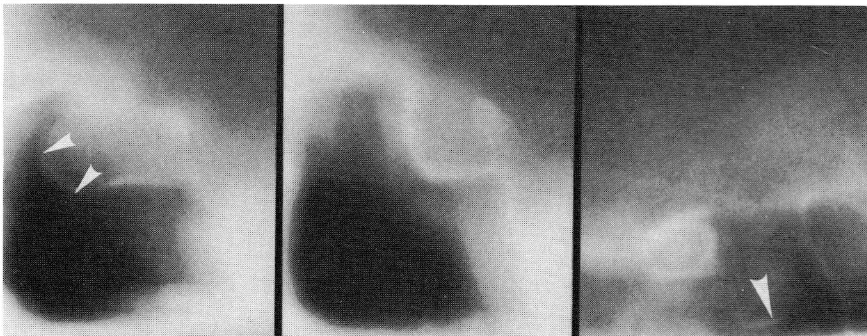

FIG. 4. Focal bulge from small secreting adenoma. **Left:** Lateral tomograms showing focal bulge anteriorly *(arrowheads).* **Center:** Normal left side of sella. **Right:** AP tomogram demonstrating focal bulge in lateral aspect of the floor of the sella *(arrowhead).*

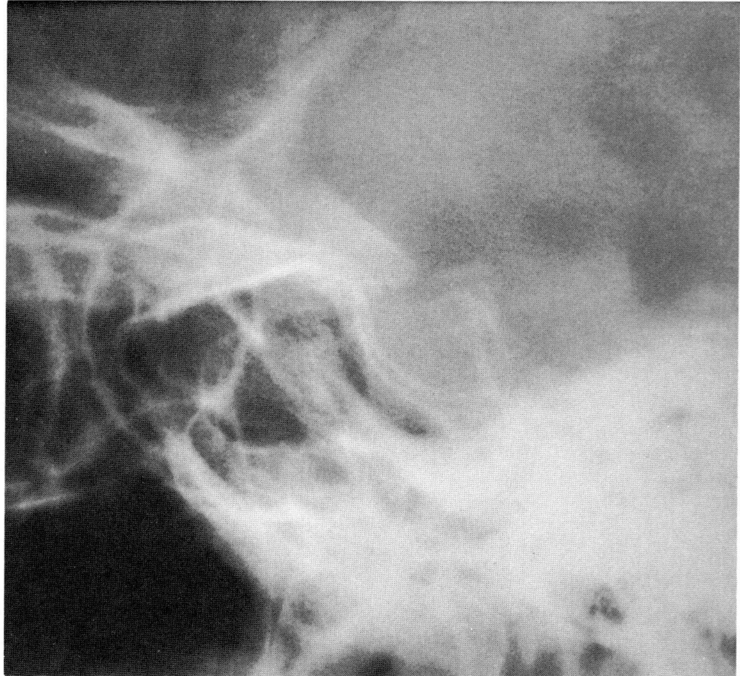

FIG. 5. Microadenoma with normal lateral view of the sella.

Frequently the changes of the adenoma are demonstrated only on the lateral and not on the AP tomograms (5). The location of the sellar changes bears no relationship to the histologic type of the adenoma; however, it does help the neurosurgeon localize the adenoma before and during surgery.

If the plain films show sella destruction, the tomograms frequently are helpful

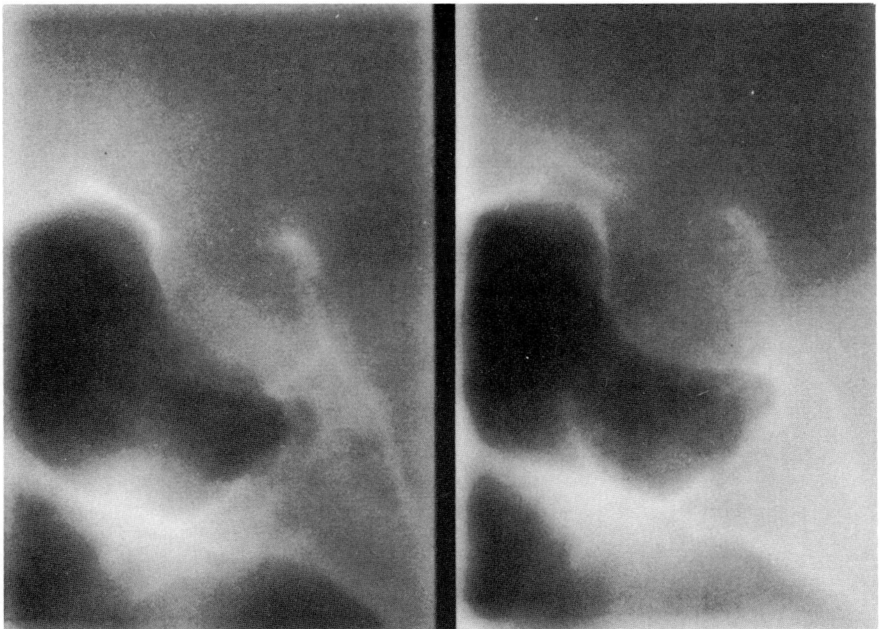

FIG. 6. Secreting microadenoma. **Left:** Focal erosion of the lamina dura on the right side of the sella. **Right:** Tomographic cut demonstrating a normal left side of sella.

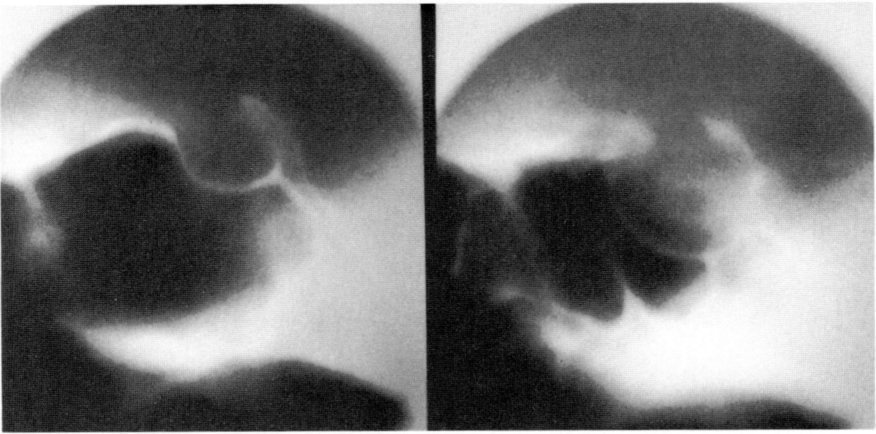

FIG. 7. Ballooning of the sella from a microadenoma. **Left:** Normal left side of sella. **Right:** Ballooned right side of sella.

in detecting whether the sella is destroyed, either by an adenoma within the sella or by extension of tumor from the nasopharynx and/or clivus. The tomograms may also show tumor extension into the sphenoid sinus from a large adenoma (Fig. 8).

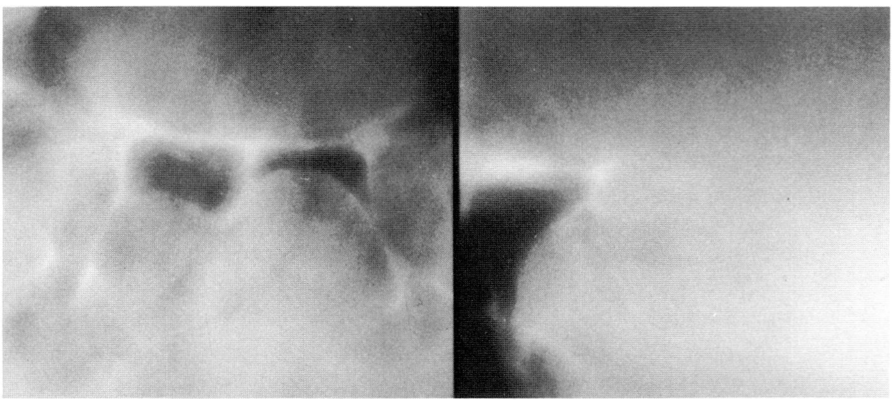

FIG. 8. AP and lateral tomographic cuts demonstrating tumor within the sphenoid sinus and destruction of the floor of the sella.

Despite good quality AP and lateral multidirectional tomography, there have been many reports of patients with pituitary tumors associated with hyperprolactinemia (amenorrhea–galactorrhea syndrome), acromegaly, and Cushing's disease with normal sella tomograms (7,8). With the increasing use of meticulous technique in obtaining the tomograms, however, the number of cases in which adenomas are not detected on the tomographic studies should decrease.

COMPUTED TOMOGRAPHY (CT SCAN)

The newest radiographic modality for evaluating the pituitary gland and sella contents is computed tomography (CT scan). The routine CT scan is done with the slices made at an angle of 15° to 25° from the canthomeatal line. In order to demonstrate better the anatomy of the suprasellar and sellar region, we altered this technique and obtained the scans parallel to the canthomeatal line. Thin-section tomograms using 5- to 8-mm cuts should be done. If thin-section cuts are not available, overlapping cuts should be made through the sella and suprasellar cistern. Noncontrast and contrast enhancement studies using a minimum of 30 g iodine given intravenously for enhancement should be obtained routinely. Coronal scans are valuable for detecting the degree of suprasellar extension of tumor and identifying the empty sella syndrome.

The normal suprasellar cistern can be visualized in approximately 85% of cases. The cistern usually has a configuration of a five-pointed crown (Fig. 9); however, this configuration may vary depending on the angle of the slices (3,10). Pituitary tumors may extend in several directions including into the sphenoid sinus (Fig. 10), the suprasellar area, and/or laterally into the temporal fossa (Fig. 11). More rarely, there is posterior extension into the interpeduncular fossa and onto the clivus. The CT scan can demonstrate the amount of extension

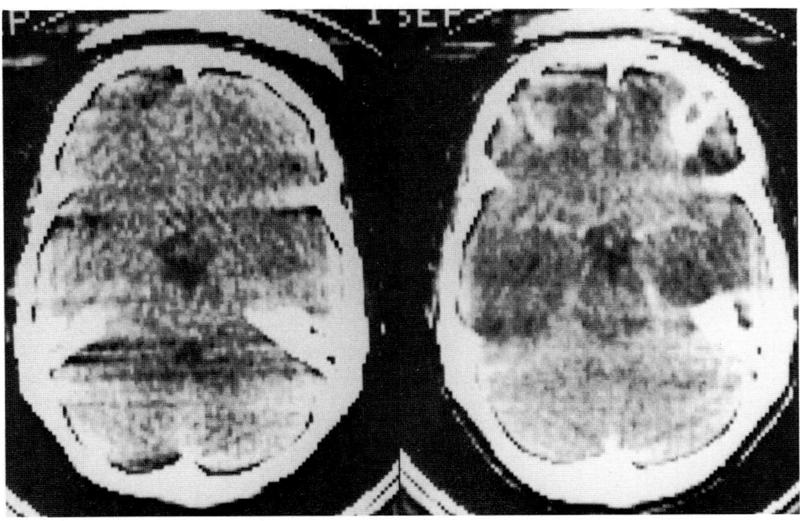

FIG. 9. Normal configuration of the suprasellar cistern. **Left:** Without contrast. **Right:** With contrast.

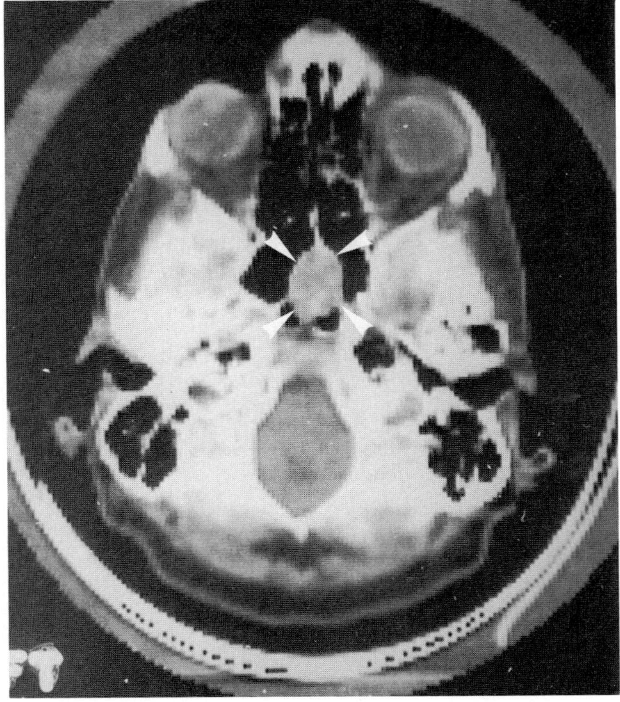

FIG. 10. CT scan demonstrating tumor within the sphenoid sinus *(arrowheads).*

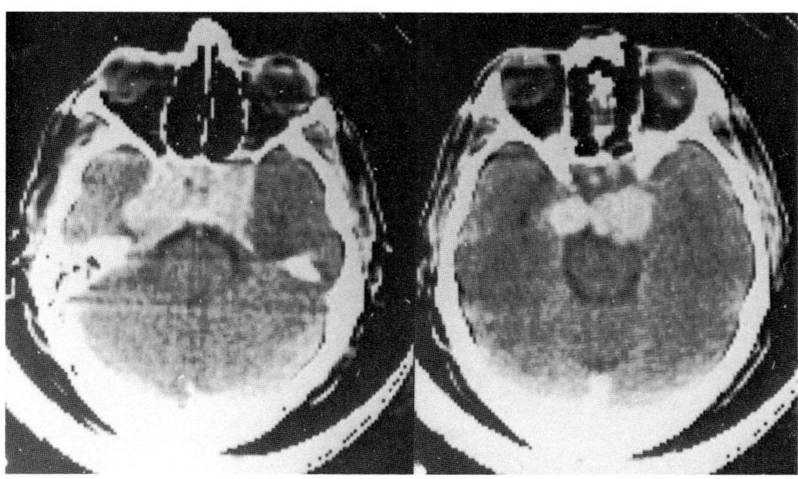

FIG. 11. CT scan following infusion of contrast media showing suprasellar and lateral extension of a nonsecreting tumor.

into these various regions. When evaluating the CT scan it is helpful to have either the lateral skull film or the tomograms available so the level of the CT scan slices can be determined. We have been unable to demonstrate adenomas smaller than 1 cm on the CT scan with any consistency. Bony erosion of the pituitary fossa may be detected on CT scan; however, multidirectional tomography remains the primary procedure for evaluating bony changes. The usual pituitary adenoma is manifested on the noncontrast CT scan as an area of increased density in the suprasellar cistern. The mass lesion may cause either total obliteration or distortion of the cistern. Following contrast enhancement the adenomas usually blush intensely, and the full extent of the tumor may then be detected (3) (Fig. 12). Lucent areas within the lesion probably representing small areas of necrosis and cyst formation as well as occasional calcification may be seen. Hemorrhage into the pituitary gland can also be identified on the CT scan (Fig. 13). When there is a suprasellar extension it is usually necessary for the tumor to have expanded approximately 5 mm above the diaphragma sella before it can be detected on the CT scan. When there is suprasellar extension it may be difficult to differentiate pituitary adenomas from other mass lesions such as meningioma, aneurysm, and hypothalamic glioma (1) (Fig. 14 and 15). In this situation cerebral angiography and/or pneumoencephalography are usually necessary to make the distinction.

We have had some difficulty confirming the diagnosis of empty sella syndrome on the CT scan. Because of partial volume averaging of the sphenoid sinus the horizontal sections may show areas of decreased density in the sella that have the appearance of empty sella syndrome. Although coronal scans are helpful

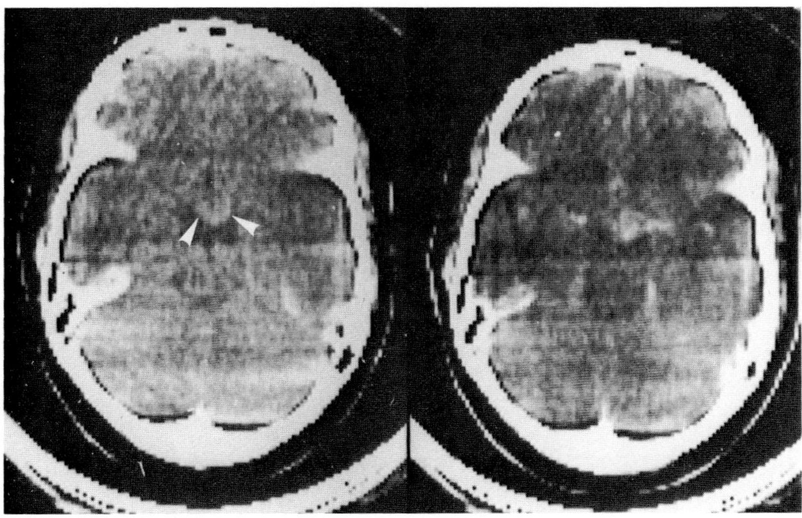

FIG. 12. Chromophobic adenoma. **Left:** Small tumor within the suprasellar cistern *(arrowheads).* **Right:** Enhancement of tumor following infusion of contrast media.

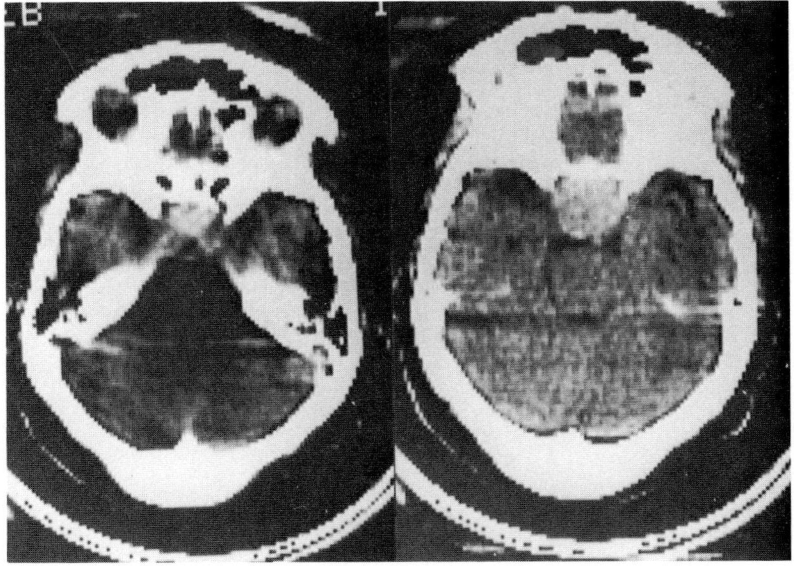

FIG. 13. Hemorrhage within a pituitary tumor. **Left:** CT scan done without contrast media, demonstrating an area of increased density within the sella compatible with hematoma. **Right:** Suprasellar extension of the area of increased density.

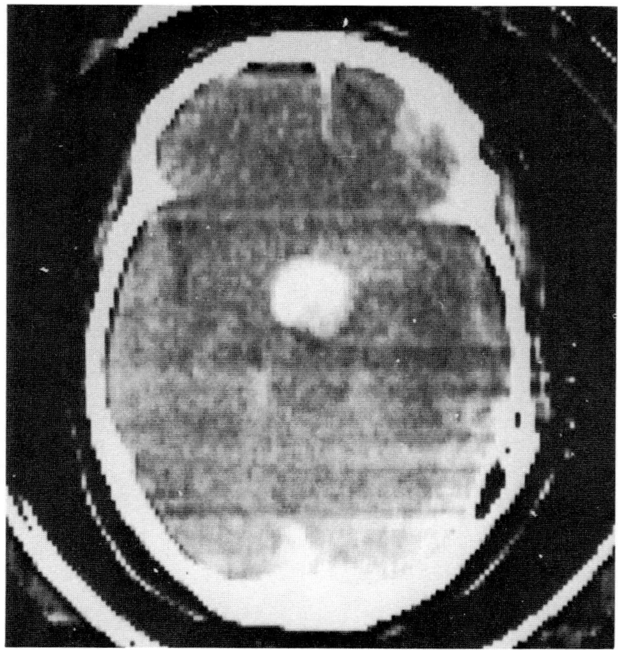

FIG. 14. CT scan done following infusion of contrast media demonstrating an enhancing lesion in the suprasellar cistern that proved to be a hypothalamic glioma.

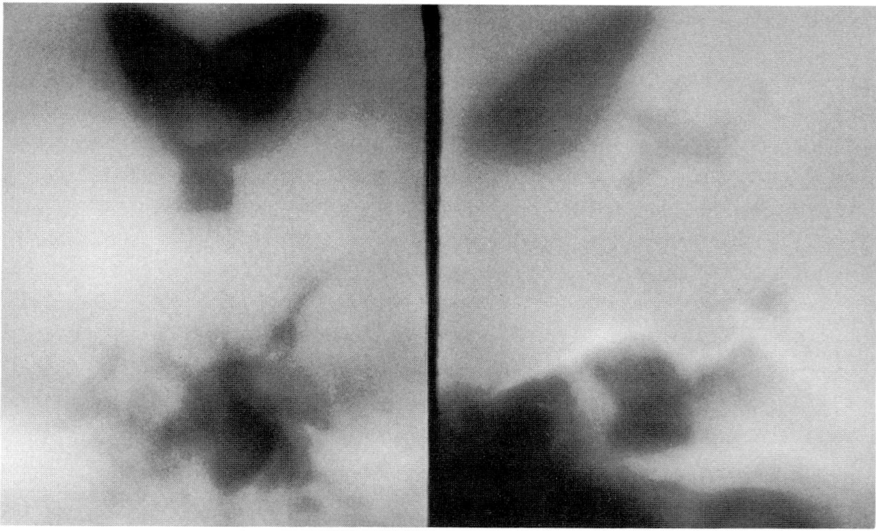

FIG. 15. Hypothalamic glioma. **Left:** AP tomographic cut of pneumoencephalogram. **Right:** Lateral tomogram.

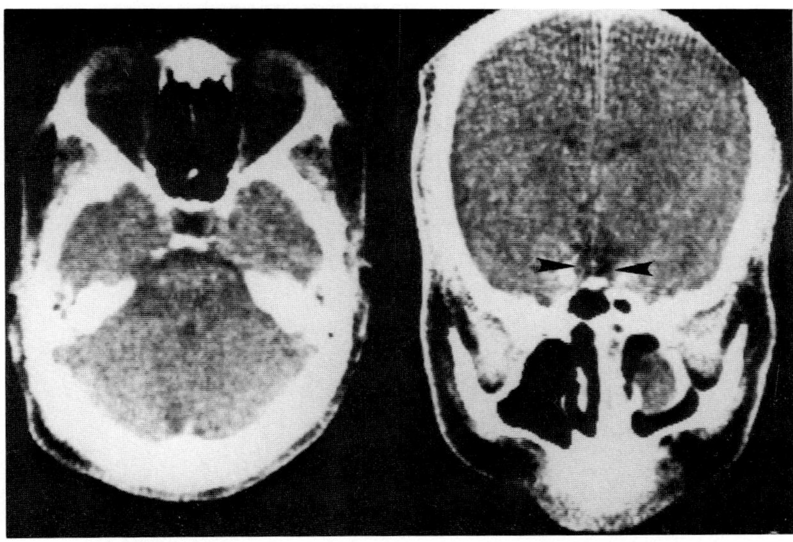

FIG. 16. Empty sella syndrome. **Left:** Horizontal CT scan demonstrating a low-density area within the sella. **Right:** Coronal scan shows a low-density area extending into the sella *(arrowheads).*

for confirming the diagnosis of empty sella syndrome (Fig. 16), pneumoencephalography remains the procedure of choice for evaluating this entity.

CEREBRAL ANGIOGRAPHY

Because of advances made in CT scanning and thin-section multidirectional tomography of the sella, the indications for cerebral angiography have changed. Small microadenomas have been demonstrated with angiography (4); however, we believe that multidirectional tomography of the sella can better demonstrate the bony changes of these lesions. The tomograms do not have the morbidity associated with angiography and are not as technically difficult to perform. Although angiography and cavernous sinus venography have been used to demonstrate lateral extension of adenomas, it is our opinion that the CT scan can better demonstrate lateral spread. We do not believe angiography is indicated in the patient with a secreting microadenoma. These patients should be evaluated with multidirectional tomography and computed tomography. Patients who have nonsecreting adenomas should be studied by angiography to rule out the possibility of an aneurysm or a lesion other than the adenoma causing the sella enlargement. Adenomas may encase the carotid artery, and this can also be determined from the angiogram.

PNEUMOENCEPHALOGRAPHY

The degree of suprasellar extension of pituitary tumors is best demonstrated on the pneumoencephalogram. The position of the anterior third ventricle and optic chiasm may also be well shown. With the advent of CT scanning and the use of coronal scanning, this indication for pneumoencephalography has diminished in importance. However, pneumoencephalography remains the procedure of choice for displaying the empty sella syndrome (Fig. 17). The pneumoencephalogram should also be performed in patients who have unexplained compression of the optic chiasm. It should be remembered that even if air enters the sella during pneumoencephalography the patient may still harbor a small adenoma, as shown by reports in the recent literature in which a hypersecreting microadenoma occurred in association with an empty sella syndrome (2).

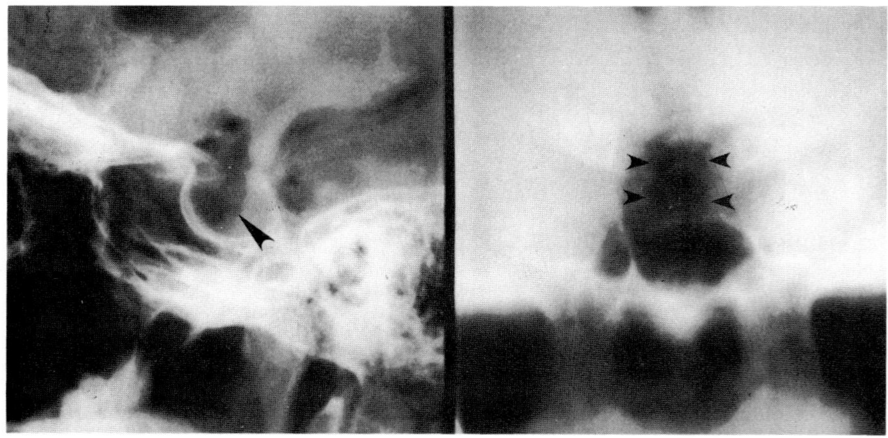

FIG. 17. Empty sella. **Left:** Lateral view on pneumoencephalogram demonstrating air within the sella *(arrowhead).* **Right:** AP tomographic cuts demonstrating air extending into the sella *(small arrowheads).*

REFERENCES

1. Davis, K. R., Taveras, J. M., Roberson, G. H., and Ackerman R. H. (1976): Some limitations of computed tomography in the diagnosis of neurological diseases. *Am. J. Roentgenol. Radium Ther. Nucl. Med.,* 127:111–123.
2. Domingue, J. N., Wing, S. D., and Wilson C. B. (1978): Coexisting pituitary adenomas and partially empty sellas. *J. Neurosurg.,* 48:23–28.
3. Leeds, N. E., and Naidich, T. P. (1978): Computerized tomography in the diagnosis of sellar and parasellar lesions. *Sem. Roentgenol.,* XII:121–135.
4. Powell, D. F., Baker, H. L., Jr., and Laws, E. R. (1974): The primary angiographic findings in pituitary adenomas. *Radiology,* 110:589–595.
5. Robertson, W. D., and Newton, T. H. (1978): Radiologic assessment of pituitary microadenomas. *Am. J. Roentgenol. Radium Ther. Nucl. Med.,* 131:489–492.

6. Swanson, H. A., and du Boulay, G. (1975): Borderline variants of the normal pituitary fossa. *Br. J. Radiol.,* 48:366–369.
7. Tindall, G. T., McLanahan, C. S., and Christy, J. H. (1978): Transsphenoidal microsurgery for pituitary tumors associated with hyperprolactinemia. *J. Neurosurg.,* 48:849–860.
8. Tyrrell, J. B., Brooks, R. M., Fitzgerald, P. A., Cofoid, P. B., Forhsam, P. H., and Wilson, C. B. (1978): Cushing's disease—selective transsphenoidal resection of pituitary microadenomas. *N. Engl. J. Med.,* 298:753–758.
9. Vezina, J. L., and Sutton, T. J. (1974): Prolactin-secreting pituitary adenoma. *Am. J. Roentgenol. Radium Ther. Nucl. Med.,* 120:46–54.
10. Wiggli, U., and Benz, U. F. (1978): Normal computed tomography anatomy of the suprasellar subarachnoid space. *Radiology,* 128:65–70.

Clinical Management of Pituitary Disorders,
edited by G. T. Tindall and W. F. Collins.
Raven Press, New York © 1979.

7

Clinical and Endocrinologic Evaluation of Patients with Suspected Pituitary Tumors

James H. Christy

Department of Medicine (Endocrinology), Emory University School of Medicine, Atlanta, Georgia 30322

During the past decade, a revolutionary trend has occurred in the diagnosis and treatment of pituitary tumors. The availability of hormone determinations by radioimmunoassay, together with better understanding of hypothalamic–pituitary physiology, advances in neuroradiological techniques, and the expanding use of transsphenoidal microsurgery have made possible earlier diagnosis and more effective treatment. As a result of these advances, it is now possible to diagnose and remove a pituitary tumor when it is no larger than 5 mm in diameter and before it has caused significant impairment of general pituitary function or chiasmal compression. In the wake of these developments, obscure clinical syndromes such as galactorrhea/amenorrhea in otherwise asymptomatic patients have assumed new meaning with the finding of hyperprolactinemia, subtle abnormalities of the sella, and surgically proved pituitary microadenomas which previously would have been undetected until mass effects or clinically obvious pituitary dysfunction had occurred.

These developments have created new challenges for the clinician. He must be able to recognize the subtleties as well as the gross anatomic or hormonal effects of pituitary tumors to determine those patients who should undergo full-scale testing of pituitary structure and function, and to interpret properly the meaning of test results.

Pituitary function testing is extremely important, not only to confirm clinically suspected pituitary/target organ dysfunction but also to identify clinically inapparent abnormalities in growth hormone reserve or prolactin secretion. Results of testing are extremely useful in making therapeutic decisions especially in asymptomatic patients with abnormal sellas or in those with suspected pituitary hypersecretion and normal sellas. Finally, pre- and posttreatment testing aids in assessing the effects of therapy on pituitary function.

CLINICAL EVALUATION

Endocrinologic evaluation of patients with suspected pituitary tumors begins with recognition of clinical manifestations that reflect hypothalamic, trophic, or target hormone deficits or excess. By a systematic consideration of basic hypothalamic/pituitary/target organ physiology, a scheme can be developed which identifies the hormonal effects of a pituitary tumor through the corresponding clinical manifestations (Table 1). Although considerable diagnostic information can be obtained from clinical evidence of hormonal abnormalities, there is a growing number of patients in whom the only manifestations of pituitary tumor are headaches, visual disturbances, or the fortuitous finding of a sella abnormality on skull X-rays obtained for an unrelated reason (head trauma, sinusitis, etc.).

PITUITARY FUNCTION EVALUATION

The endocrine testing protocol, which varies among institutions, should be comprehensive enough to evaluate the various pituitary/target organ axes, to determine prolactin and growth hormone reserve, and to assess posterior lobe function. A recommended protocol for evaluation is cited in Table 2.

ANTERIOR PITUITARY FUNCTION TESTS

Gonadotropin–Gonadal Axis

Insufficiency of the gonadotropin-gonadal axis is reflected by decreased levels of follicle-stimulating hormone (FSH), luteinizing hormone (LH), and the corresponding sex steroid (testosterone or estradiol), each of which can be determined by radioimmunoassay. In the context of testing for abnormalities associated with pituitary tumor, further studies are not necessary unless it is critical to determine if hypothalamic disease is responsible for the deficiencies noted in the screening tests. In that event gonadotropin-releasing hormone (GnRH) stimulation (3) can be used, although at the time of this report it is not available for general clinical use. Moreover, failure to respond to GnRH does not necessarily differentiate between hypothalamic and pituitary dysfunction since prolonged GnRH deficiency may impair pituitary responsiveness to exogenously administered hormone.

Clomiphene citrate is also helpful for testing gonadotropin reserve if peripheral blood sex steroid levels are not markedly decreased (14). This agent inhibits the negative feedback effect of sex steroids on the hypothalamic/pituitary axis and causes a significant elevation of LH and FSH in normal individuals presumably through provocation of GnRH. In patients with pituitary tumors, failure of FSH and LH to rise after clomiphene administration indicates only that a defect is present in the hypothalamic/pituitary gonadotropin axis, but it does not identify the anatomic site of the deficiency. This requires the use of GnRH.

TABLE 1. *Clinical manifestations of pituitary tumors*

		Clinical manifestations	
Hypothalamic factor	Pituitary hormone	Deficiency	Excess
Gonadotropin-releasing hormone (GnRH)	Gonadotropin	Male: ↓ Libido, impotence, infertility ↓ Testicular size ↓ Body hair Female: Amenorrhea, infertility ↓ Breast size ↓ Areolar puffiness	No manifestations in adults Precocious puberty in children
Thyrotropin-releasing hormone (TRH)	Thyrotropin	Hypothyroidism: cold intolerance, weight gain, slow mentation, ↓ memory, waxy sallow skin, prolonged relaxation phase DTRs	Thyrotoxicosis
Corticotropin-releasing factor (CRF)	Adrenocorticotropin	Adrenal insufficiency: weakness, postural hypotension, ↓ body hair In stress: shock, hypothermia	Cushing's disease
Growth-hormone-releasing factor (GRF)	Somatotropin	None in adult, except ↓ FBS Dwarfism in children	Acromegaly
Prolactin-inhibitory factor (PIF) Prolactin-stimulating factor (PSF)	Prolactin	Inability to lactate	Galactorrhea/amenorrhea
Melanotropin-inhibitory factor (MIF)	Melanotropin	Decreased pigmentation	Hyperpigmentation
Vasopressin	Vasopressin	Diabetes insipidus	Syndrome of inappropriate ADH (rare)

FBS, fasting blood sugar. ADH, antidiuretic hormone. DTRs, deep tendon reflexes.

TABLE 2. *Minimal tests of endocrine function in patients with suspected pituitary tumor*

Pituitary hormone	Test for hormone deficiency	Test for hormone excess
Gonadotropin (FSH–LH)	Serum FSH, LH estradiol (females) or testosterone (males); when available, GnRH stimulation	Same
Thyrotropin (TSH)	TSH, T_4, FT_4, TRH stimulation	Same
Adrenocorticotropin (ACTH)	Serum cortisol, 24-hr urinary steroids; if both low, metyrapone test	Dexamethasone suppression and metyrapone test
Growth hormone (GH)	Glucagon or L-DOPA provocative test	Glucose suppression
Prolactin (PRL)	CPZ provocative test; TRH provocative test (if no response to CPZ)	CPZ provocative; L-DOPA suppression
Vasopressin (ADH)	Simultaneous urine and serum osmolality after 8–12 hr of water restriction	Same without water restriction + BUN and serum and urinary Na

(FSH) follicular-stimulating hormone. (LH) luteinizing hormone. (GnRH) gonadotropin-releasing hormone. (T_4) total thyroxine. (FT_4) free thyroxine. (TRH) thyrotropin-releasing hormone. (CPZ) chlorpromazine. (BUN) blood urea nitrogen.

Thyrotropin–Thyroidal Axis

Thyroid function is assessed by radioimmunoassay determination of serum thyroxine [preferably as free T_4 and serum thyroid-stimulating hormone (TSH)]. A low T_4 without elevation of TSH (greater than 10 μU/ml) is highly suggestive of deficient TSH reserve, but it does not establish whether the source is a deficient thyrotropin-releasing hormone (TRH) mechanism in the hypothalamus or lack of pituitary response to TRH. This distinction can be made by the intravenous injection of TRH (500 μU) which does not provoke a rise in TSH levels if the pituitary gland is at fault but does cause a delayed and sometimes exaggerated TSH response if there is deficient hypothalamic TRH reserve (9).

Adrenocorticotropin–Adrenal Axis

The minimal data necessary to evaluate pituitary–adrenal axis function is an early morning serum cortisol and a 24-hr urine 17-hydroxycorticosteroid and 17-ketosteroid determination. If the patient has no postural hypotension, normal serum cortisol level, and normal 24-hr urinary steroid excretion, it can be assumed, for practical purposes, that adrenocorticotropin (ACTH) reserve is normal. However, if either of these parameters is suggestive of deficiency, attempts should be made to test ACTH reserve. A plasma ACTH assay would be helpful, but without manipulative testing it is not always a reliable indicator because of technical difficulties in the test procedure and overlap in levels of patients with normal and low reserve. It is reasonable, therefore, to test ACTH reserve indirectly with metyrapone in those patients who exhibit borderline adrenal function (15). This substance inhibits 11β-hydroxylation, hence, conversion of 11-deoxycortisol (compound S), a biologically inactive steroid, to cortisol (compound F), the biologically active steroid. If the ACTH–adrenal axis is intact, inhibition of 11β-hydroxylation results in increased ACTH release, which is reflected by an increase in the serum 11-deoxycortisol. If any component of the axis is deficient, there will be little or no rise in the serum 11-deoxycortisol following metyrapone administration; but in the patient suspected of having a pituitary tumor, hypothalamic or pituitary dysfunction can be implicated. The test is performed simply by obtaining a baseline serum 11-deoxycortisol and serum cortisol at 8:00 A.M. the morning before, and at 8:00 A.M. the day following oral administration of metyrapone 30 mg/kg at midnight. If the pituitary–adrenal axis is intact, the postmetyrapone serum 11-deoxycortisol will be greater than 10 μg/100ml. If ACTH reserve is impaired, the serum 11-deoxycortisol will rise slightly and correspond roughly to the fall in serum cortisol, which must be demonstrated to validate the test.

Growth Hormone Reserve

In testing for growth hormone (GH) reserve, there is no peripheral target organ hormone that can be used to determine the appropriateness of a feedback relationship. The blood glucose, to some extent, serves this purpose since low blood sugar stimulates, and a high blood sugar inhibits, growth hormone release. A low serum growth hormone level in the presence of a low fasting blood glucose would constitute good evidence for deficiency of growth hormone reserve; however, since this particular combination is rarely seen in patients with pituitary tumors, and because of the overlap which exists between the fasting growth hormone level of normal individuals and growth hormone-deficient patients, a provocative test must be done. Several provocative agents are available, including insulin, glucagon, arginine, and in more recent years L-DOPA (5,21). The insulin test is still considered the standard by which all others are measured, but it may pose some risk to patients who have low adrenal reserve. Glugacon, on the other hand, is safer and for practical purposes almost as reliable as insulin for testing growth hormone reserve. The test is simple and is performed by determining the fasting serum growth hormone levels before and 120 and 150 min after the intramuscular injection of 1 mg glucagon. A rise of growth hormone greater than 5 ng/ml constitutes a normal response. Some investigators suggest pretreatment with estrogen to enhance the response, but this is not usually necessary. To ensure greater accuracy in the testing of growth hormone reserve (since some normal individuals show no response to glucagon) L-DOPA can be used as an adjunctive test for growth hormone reserve.

Prolactin Reserve

Like growth hormone, prolactin (PRL) does not relate to a specific target organ hormone, and prolactin levels of the deficient patient overlap with the lower range of normal, making it necessary to utilize a provocative substance to determine prolactin reserve. Unlike most of the other major hormones of the anterior hypophysis, prolactin is primarily under the control of a hypothalamic inhibitory factor (PIF), which is released in response to dopamine stimulation from higher centers of the brain. There is some evidence to suggest that the PIF is dopamine (12). A prolactin-stimulatory factor also exists, but its precise role in regulating prolactin secretion is uncertain (11).

When testing for prolactin deficiency, which is more of a problem in degenerative disease than in tumors of the pituitary gland, TRH stimulation is the most efficient procedure for determining prolactin reserve. After intravenous injection of a 500-μg bolus of TRH, a normal response is a peak prolactin value of 20 ng/ml for males and 40 ng/ml for females (17). Chlorpromazine, which inhibits PIF, can also be used to assess prolactin reserve (17). Low baseline levels of prolactin with failure to respond to chlorpromazine is good evidence for deficiency of prolactin secretion by the lactotrophs of the anterior pituitary gland. Autonomous secretion of prolactin by tumor or interruption of the PIF pathway also results in poor response to chlorpromazine, but in these instances the baseline prolactin level is usually elevated.

The chlorpromazine test entails determination of fasting serum prolactin levels before and 60, 120, and 180 min after intramuscular injection of 50 mg chlorpromazine. A normal response is an increment of two to three times the baseline value.

POSTERIOR PITUITARY FUNCTION TESTS

Vasopressin Reserve

Disruption of the neurohypophyseal regulation of water metabolism causes diabetes insipidus, a condition present in approximately 10% of patients with untreated pituitary tumors. Deficiency of vasopressin results in loss of urine-concentrating ability, polyuria, polydipsia, hyposthenuria, and hypertonic contraction of the plasma volume. The screen for vasopressin reserve is relatively simple (13). As yet a serum or urinary antidiuretic hormone (ADH) assay is not generally available, but this function can be reliably assessed through indirect means. Simultaneous serum and urine osmolalities are obtained before and after 8 to 12 hr of water deprivation. If diabetes insipidus is suspected clinically, the test should not extend beyond 8 hr. If diabetes insipidus is present, the urine osmolality will be greater than 295 mOsm/kg and the urine osmolality less than 250 mOsm/kg. Expressed in another way, the urine/serum ratio after water deprivation is less than 1 in diabetes insipidus and greater than 2 if vasopressin reserve and renal function are normal.

HYPERSECRETION ASSOCIATED WITH PITUITARY TUMORS

Growth Hormone Excess

Excessive secretion of growth hormone by a pituitary tumor causes acromegaly in the adult and gigantism in the prepubertal individual. The clinical features are usually sufficient for diagnosis, but confirmation should be obtained with growth hormone determinations before and 1, 2, and 3 hr following an oral glucose load (100 g). If the tumor is autonomous there will be less than 50% reduction of the serum growth hormone at the nadir of response in 60 to 80% of patients. Normal suppressibility, however, will be demonstrated in 20 to 30% of patients, suggesting at least partial control of tumor secretion by hypothalamic influences (4).

Adrenocorticotropin Excess

Hypersecretion of ACTH is clinically expressed by the typical manifestations of hypercortisolism or Cushing's syndrome. This problem is examined in greater detail in chapter 12 of this volume. Pituitary ACTH excess, the most common source of hypercortisolism, is caused by a pituitary adenoma containing aggregates of ACTH-secreting cells (1,7,8,19). The simplest screening procedure is the overnight dexamethasone suppression test, performed by determining the early morning serum cortisol level before and the morning after the patient receives dexamethasone (1 mg) orally at midnight (18). A normal response is a serum cortisol level of less than 5 μg/100 ml (usually less than 2 μg/100 ml) after dexamethasone administration. Patients with Cushing's syndrome display little suppressibility, and in most the cortisol level remains above 5 μg/100 ml. If nonsuppressibility is demonstrated with the screening test, a 48-hr dexamethasone suppression test should be done (dexamethasone 0.5 mg orally every 6 hr; daily 24-hr urine specimens are required for 17-hydroxycorticosteroid and 17-ketosteroid determinations during the test period). Failure of the urinary steroids to be suppressed by more than 50% of the control values is indicative of hypercortisolism (20). To confirm that the source of hypercortisolism is pituitary ACTH excess, a metyrapone test is done (20). Metyrapone is administered orally in a dose of 750 mg every 6 hr for two consecutive days with daily 24-hr urine specimens collected for 17-hydroxycorticosteroid and 17-ketosteroid determinations. A twofold or greater rise in the urinary steroids during the metyrapone test is indicative of Cushing's disease or ACTH-secreting pituitary adenoma. Failure of the urinary steroids to rise indicates the presence of an autonomously secreting adrenal tumor or an ectopic ACTH-producing tumor.

Prolactin Excess

Hyperprolactinemia is reported to be present in approximately 70% of patients with pituitary tumors (6,10). It may not cause symptoms in some patients, but galactorrhea/amenorrhea are commonly seen in others (16). A repeatedly elevated serum prolactin (greater than 25 ng/ml) indicates hypersecretion due to autonomous production of prolactin by the pituitary tumor or loss of control of prolactin secretion due to disruption of PIF pathways at some point between the hypothalamus and the pituitary gland. Nonpituitary tumor-related causes of hyperprolactinemia include drugs (phenothiazines, tricyclic antidepressants, reserpine) and primary hypothyroidism. These factors, of course, must be excluded before the search for pituitary tumor begins. The chlorpromazine (CPZ) test is then utilized mainly to confirm that the elevated prolactin levels are related to abnormal prolactin secretion rather than a simple variation of normal. Failure of prolactin to rise two to three times the baseline value is the characteristic response in the presence of virtually all pituitary tumors, whether their mechanism of action is related to autonomous secretion or disruption of the PIF pathways. Because this pattern of nonresponsiveness of prolactin to CPZ is so consistently demonstrated in patients with pituitary tumors (with only one false-positive and no false-negative responses in over 100 patients tested at this institution) we now consider the CPZ test one of the most reliable means of determining the presence of a pituitary tumor or other space-occupying lesion involving the sella.

L-DOPA also can be used for evaluating excessive prolactin secretion in patients with suspected pituitary tumors. Its mechanism of action is probably through the intracerebral conversion of L-DOPA to dopamine, which stimulates secretion of PIF by the hypothalamus. A direct inhibitory effect of L-DOPA on pituitary prolactin secretion has not been excluded (2). Regardless of which mechanism is predominant, L-DOPA, when given to normal controls as a single dose of 0.5 g orally, causes an 80% or greater reduction in serum prolactin levels over a 3-hr period (17). Unfortunately, approximately 50% of patients with pituitary tumors also show a similar response to L-DOPA, thus reducing its usefulness as a diagnostic aid in the evaluation of hyperprolactinemia.

A discussion of the galactorrhea/amenorrhea syndrome associated with pituitary tumors is covered in chapter 15.

INDICATIONS FOR DEFINITIVE TREATMENT

In the past, the need for definitive treatment was determined by the presence of clinically obvious mass or hormonal effects of the suspected pituitary tumor. With the technological advances of the past decade and the availability of transsphenoidal microsurgery, it is no longer necessary, or advisable, to await development of chiasmal compression or multiple hormonal deficits before definitive treatment is initiated. With the proved safety and efficacy of transsphenoidal microsurgery, the main issue to be resolved now is the selection of minimal criteria that would be acceptable as indications for surgery. In the view of the author, it seems reasonable to consider surgery in any patient who has two or more of the following: (a) sella asymmetry, focal enlargement, erosion, or generalized enlargement; (b) pituitary hypersecretion; (c) one or more deficiencies in pituitary function; and (d) persistent galactorrhea/amenorrhea syndrome or persistent asymptomatic hyperprolactinemia unrelated to exogenous factors or primary hypothyroidism.

POSTOPERATIVE EVALUATION OF PITUITARY FUNCTION

Evaluation of pituitary function should be done no earlier than 10 days after surgery in order to avoid confusing test results. The same protocol of testing used before surgery is again instituted at this period. Only in this way will it be known if pre-existing pituitary dysfunction has been corrected by surgery or if surgery itself has created any deficits. After surgery (or any definitive treatment) the patient should have periodic follow-up.

REFERENCES

1. Bigos, S. T., Robert, F., Pelletier, G., and Hardy, J. (1977): Cure of Cushing's disease by transsphenoidal removal of microadenoma from a pituitary gland despite a radiographically normal sella turcica. *J. Clin. Endocrinol. Metab.,* 45:1251–1260.
2. Birge, C. A., Jacobs, L. S., Hammer, C. T., and Daughaday, W. H. (1970): Catecholamine inhibition of prolactin secretion by isolated rat adenohypophysis. *Endocrinology,* 86:120–130.
3. Coscia, M., Fleischer, P. K., Brown, L. P., and Desiderio, D. (1974): The effect of synthetic LH levels in pituitary disease. *J. Clin. Endocrinol. Metab.,* 38:83–88.
4. Cryer, P. E., and Daughaday, W. H. (1969): Regulation of growth hormone secretion in acromegaly. *J. Clin. Endocrinol. Metab.,* 29:386–393.
5. Eddy, R. L., Gilliland, P. F., Ibarra, J. D., McMurry, J. F., and Thompson, J. Q. (1974): Human growth hormone release; comparison of provocative test procedures. *Am. J. Med.,* 56:179–185.
6. Franks, S., Jacobs, H. S., and Nabarro, J. D. N. (1975): Studies of prolactin secretion in pituitary disease. *J. Endocrinol.,* 67:55.
7. Ganguly, A., Stachfield, J. B., Roberts, T. S., West, C. D., and Tyler, F. H. (1976): Cushing's syndrome in a patient with an empty sella turcica and microadenoma of the adenohypophysis. *Am. J. Med.,* 60:306–309.
8. Hardy, J. (1975): Trans-sphenoidal microsurgical removal of pituitary micro-adenoma. *Prog. Neurol. Surg.,* 6:200–216.
9. Hershman, J. M. (1974): Clinical application of thyrotropin-releasing hormone. *N. Engl. J. Med.,* 290:886–890.
10. Jacobs, H. S. (1976): Prolactin and amenorrhea. *N. Engl. J. Med.,* 295:954–956.
11. Kolodny, H. D., and Sherman, L. (1974): Laboratory aids in the diagnosis of pituitary tumors. *Ann. Clin. Lab. Sci.,* 4:67–86.
12. MacLeod, R. M. (1976): Regulation of prolactin secretion. In: *Frontiers in Neuroendocrinology,* Vol. 4, edited by L. Martini and W. F. Ganong, pp. 169–194 Raven Press, New York.
13. Miller, M. T., Dalakos, A. M., Fellerman, H., and Streeten, D. H. P. (1970): Recognition of partial defects in antidiuretic hormone secretion. *Ann. Intern. Med.,* 73:721–729.
14. Santen, R. J., Leonard, J. M., Sherins, R. J., Gandy, H. M., and Paulsen, C. A. (1971): Short and long term effects of clomiphene citrate on the pituitary-testicular axis. *J. Clin. Endocrinol. Metab.,* 33:970–979.
15. Spark, R. F. (1971): Simplified assessment of pituitary-adrenal reserve. *Ann. Intern. Med.,* 75:717–723.
16. Spark, R. F., Pallotta, J., Naftolin, F., and Clemens, R. (1976): Galactorrhea-amenorrhea syndromes: Etiology and treatment. *Ann. Intern. Med.,* 84:532–537.
17. Tolis, G., Goldstein, M., and Friesen, H. G. (1973): Functional evaluation of prolactin secretion in patients with hypothalamic-pituitary disorders. *J. Clin. Invest.,* 52:783–788.

18. Tyler, F. H., and West, C. D. (1972): Laboratory evaluation of disorders of the adrenal cortex. *Am. J. Med.,* 53:664–672.
19. Tyrrell, J. B., Brooks, R. M., Fitzgerald, P. A., Cofoid, P. S., Forsham, P. H., and Wilson, C. B. (1978): Cushing's disease: Selective transsphenoidal resection of pituitary microadenomas. *N. Engl. J. Med.,* 298:753–758.
20. Weiss, E. R., Rayyis, S. S., Nelson, D. H., and Bethune, J. E. (1969): Evaluation of stimulation and suppression tests in the etiological diagnosis of Cushing's syndrome. *Ann. Intern. Med.,* 71:941–949.
21. Wieland, R. G., Hallberg, M. C., and Zorn, E. M. (1973): Growth hormone response to intramuscular glucagon. *J. Clin. Endocrinol. Metab.,* 37:329–330.

Clinical Management of Pituitary Disorders,
edited by G. T. Tindall and W. F. Collins.
Raven Press, New York © 1979.

8

Evaluation of the Patient With an Asymptomatic Enlarged Sella Turcica

Earl A. Zimmerman

Department of Neurology, College of Physicians and Surgeons, Columbia University, New York, New York 10032

A specialist interested in clinical neuroendocrinology is often asked how to evaluate and manage an apparently asymptomatic patient with an enlarged sella turcica. This situation frequently arises when an abnormal sella is found on routine skull X-rays after head injury or during the evaluation of common neurological complaints such as headaches or dizziness. A review of the X-rays with the radiologist reveals that the sella is definitely abnormal rather than being a variant of normal. That these patients should be evaluated further is indicated by a recent study of 75 such patients at the Neurological Institute of New York (24). Significant pathology was found in about 50%, and a definite diagnosis was made in more than 80%. An intrasellar tumor was found in 36% and an empty sella syndrome in 33%; 17% had an extrasellar neurological process. The results of such studies are always influenced by patient selection, and the relatively high incidence of neurological disease in this series probably reflects referral to a neurological service. Nevertheless, this study provides a useful guide to the work-up and an indication as to what might be found (Table 1).

PRIMARY EMPTY SELLA SYNDROME

Primary empty sella syndrome is a common disorder with more than 250 cases reported (10). Primary empty sella refers to untreated patients, whereas secondary empty sella is applied to those who have had previous surgery or radiotherapy. The majority of the patients with primary empty sella have been middle-aged overweight women who are frequently hypertensive. Complaints of headache are common and usually longstanding. The patients generally do not have endocrine symptoms. Several patients in a number of studies have had cerebrospinal fluid (CSF) rhinorrhea (10,23), which in many was associated

TABLE 1. *Clinical and radiological findings in lesions causing sellar abnormalities*

Finding	Empty sella	Intrasellar tumor	Extrasellar process
History			
1. Neurological symptoms			
A. Headache	50%	Most	All, pulsatile
B. Visual	Usually not	Common	Frequently
C. Diplopia	No	Occasional	Yes
D. Rhinorrhea	Some	Uncommon	Occasional
2. Endocrine			
A. Amenorrhea	Usually not	Half	Half
B. Galactorrhea	Usually not	Some	Some
C. Weight gain	Usually not	Some	Some
D. Cold intolerance	Usually not	Occasional	Occasional
E. Polyuria	Rare	Usually not	More likely
Physical examination			
1. Visual fields and/or acuity	Usually normal	Abnormal 50%	May be abnormal depending on cause
2. Cranial nerve paresis	Normal	Occasionally: III, VI, less often V	Often
Tomograms sella			
1. Enlarged, normal shape	70%	7%	About 40%
2. Abnormal shape	30%	93%	About 60%
Endocrine			
1. Inadequate growth hormone response to hypoglycemia	Common	Common	Common
2. i.v. ACTH test	Normal	May be decreased	May be decreased
3. Urinary steroids	Normal	May be decreased	May be decreased
4. Gonadotropins	Normal	May be decreased	May be decreased
5. Thyroid hormones	Normal	May be decreased	May be decreased
6. Prolactin elevated	Rare cases	67%	Some
Isotope scan	Normal	Occasionally abnormal	Often abnormal
EEG	Normal	Normal	Abnormal
CSF			
1. Protein increased	Normal	Often	Often
2. Pressure increased	10%	No	Often
Arteriogram			
1. Abnormal	Occasionally helpful	Helpful in a third	More than half

with active pseudotumor cerebri. Weisberg et al. (23) and Jordan et al. (10) report the incidence of headache and CSF rhinorrhea to be about 10%.

Except for obesity and possibly hypertension, the physical examination is normal. Papilledema is present in those patients with pseudotumor cerebri. Formal visual field testing has been normal in most cases. Six cases of field defects and/or optic atrophy with loss of visual acuity have been reported (2,14,16,25). Improvement was reported in some cases after surgical elevation of the chiasm ventrally displaced in the sella (25), after freeing adhesions (14), or after third ventriculostomy at the lamina terminalis (16). As shown by Kaufman et al. (12), the anterior cerebral artery and the chiasm may be displaced downward into the sella. The cranial nerves are usually otherwise normal, although one would anticipate abducens paresis and diplopia in some patients with pseudotumor cerebri. Two patients in the series reported by Neelon et al. (17) complained of trigeminal neuralgia. Eye signs and field defects also occur owing to adhesions in secondary empty sella syndrome after irradiation or surgery for pituitary tumor (13).

Radiographic studies of the sella most often show general enlargement in empty sella syndrome compared to primary intrasellar tumor, where more often an abnormality in shape and particularly erosion of the sella is found. Kaufman et al. (12) note that posterior displacement of the dorsum is most characteristic of an intrasellar process. Focal erosion in our experience is very typical of pituitary adenoma. There are enough exceptions to all of these and other rules to make it necessary to perform pneumoencephalography in the brow-up head-extended position if the clinical setting requires definitive diagnosis. Recent improvements in CT scanning using the body scanner may obviate the need for invasive contrast studies in the future. The results of cerebral arteriography are sometimes helpful for suggesting empty sella when the internal carotid arteries are displaced medially ("kissing carotids") or the anterior cerebral arteries are dislocated inferiorly into the sella. Lateral displacement of the intracavernous carotids can occur in both conditions. The rare but important diagnosis of internal carotid aneurysm giving an X-ray picture of intrasellar tumor can also be detected by arteriography.

Although it is generally considered that some degree of hypopituitarism is found in approximately 30% of patients with an empty sella syndrome (21), usually involving dynamic testing of growth hormone and reduced gonadotropins (4,17), there is a wide variety of opinions on the extent of endocrinopathy in these patients. Jordan et al. (10) found that endocrine testing (ACTH and growth hormone reserves, gonadotropins, thyroid function) was normal in their patients except in one with hyperprolactinemia and hypothyroidism, which was proved surgically to contain a pituitary adenoma. Two patients had primary hypothyroidism as well. Deficiency of ACTH as well as growth hormone reserve was found in some patients by Faglia et al. (8). A number of other studies also showed diminished growth hormone reserve (4,17,24). Although obesity may blunt the growth hormone response (6), failure to lower the glucose adequately with insulin may also produce false-negative results (24). Two patients of Neelon et al. (17) had diminished TSH response to TRH, but others found it to be normal (19,22). Although there has been a tendency to emphasize normality of hypophyseal function in empty sella syndrome, it seems likely that the differences in the results of various studies do not totally reflect differences in either testing procedures or faulty results. Since it is a syndrome, it is likely to be associated with a number of disorders. One of these is the coexistence of a pituitary adenoma with empty sella syndrome. The 27 adenomas reported (Table 2) were undoubtedly discovered because they were hypersecretory. It appears therefore that the incidence of hypersecretory tumor in association with empty sella might be as high as 10% from these data. Since nonsecreting pituitary

TABLE 2. *Pituitary tumors associated with primary empty sella*

Type of tumor	No. of cases	References
Prolactin secreting	12	Domingue et al. (7); Jordan et al. (10); Schaison and Metzger (20)
Growth hormone secreting	14	Domingue et al. (7); Molitch et al. (15); Neelon et al. (17)
Adrenocorticotropin	1	Ganguly et al. (9)

adenomas are at least as common, some "empty sellas" must also be associated with nonfunctional adenomas as predicted by Domingue et al. (7). This real possibility would explain, for example, why one of Neelon's cases had complete and three had partial hypopituitarism (23%). The high incidence of the association of pituitary tumor with empty sella lends further support to the notion that infarction in an adenoma is more important in producing the syndrome (17) than previously considered (7). Neelon et al. (17) summarized their endocrine findings in patients with empty sella and compared them with the results of Nieman et al. (18) in patients with known intrasellar tumor, and thought that the lower incidence of the endocrine abnormalities in empty sella suggested that there was much less endocrine disease in the latter disorder. Neelon et al. (17) found (in primary empty sella) a reduction in growth hormone response in 11 to 22%, gonadotropin loss in 13%, normal ACTH, the TSH response diminished in 9 to 13%, and partial panhypopituitarism in 6 to 17%. In contrast, Nieman et al. (18) found the following in patients with pituitary tumors: a diminution in growth hormone response in 83%, low gonadotropins in 68%, deficient ACTH in 43%, TSH abnormality in 32%, and panhypopituitarism in 30%. One may turn the argument around, however, and say that the data of Neelon et al. (17) show that patients with empty sella are far from normal in terms of endocrine function, although not generally as bad as patients with proved pituitary tumors.

Since most of the tests used do not clearly distinguish between hypothalamic disorders and pituitary adenomas as a cause for endocrine abnormalities, the possibility remains that there is also a disturbance in the hypothalamus or the hypothalamic connections with the pituitary in some cases of empty sella. It remains to be established if the syndrome may cause a disturbance in the portal connections between hypothalamus and pituitary in some of these patients. The stalk is often displaced posteriorly. In addition, the local pressure changes which cause the bony abnormalities in the sella, perhaps due to transmission of CSF pressure from the ventricles via an incompetent diaphragma sella (15), may also cause a functional interruption of the normal dynamics of portal capillary flow. These speculations remain to be proved, but they seem warranted at present since empty sella syndrome remains an enigma and is generally considered a nondisease. However, Busch (5) found some degree of diaphragma sella incompetence in more than half and the full-blown syndrome in 5.5% of autopsies. Bergland et al. (3) found that there was a greater than 5-mm opening in the diaphragma sella in 39% of autopsies, and in 20% the subarachnoid space definitely extended into the sella. Domingue et al. (7) suggest that the incidence of partially empty sella (11) may be lower in prolactin-secreting adenomas (13.3%) and acromegaly (10%) because of the presence of the tumor. Since autopsy studies have shown that some form of empty sella syndrome is present in about a third of the population, it seems unlikely to be much more than an annoyance to those investigating patients with an enlarged sella. Yet the common association with headache without increased intracranial pressure and at least inadequate growth hormone reserve in many patients leaves the possibility open that the syndrome is pathogenic in some cases. In addition, Schaison and Metzger (20) reported two well-established cases of diabetes insipidus with empty sella syndrome and no other obvious cause of the hormone deficiency. Since diabetes insipidus is a manifestation of hypothalamic or upper pituitary stalk disease (Chapter 25), whatever causes empty sella in some cases may also affect vasopressin pathways. This also suggests that not every case of hyperprolactinemia in primary empty sella is due to an associated pituitary adenoma but may be secondary to hypothalamic or upper pituitary stalk disturbance (prolactin is usually <100 ng/ml). Further endocrine tests to differentiate hypothalamic from pituitary disease using releasing factors and other methods are needed in cases of empty sella, especially in patients with mild hyperprolactinemia and/or diabetes insipidus.

INTRASELLAR TUMOR

At least a third of patients presenting with a large sella have an intrasellar tumor, usually a pituitary adenoma. Half have visual complaints (23), although this incidence continues to decrease as clinical acumen and early diagnosis have improved for pituitary adenoma. The common combination of visual and endocrine complaints (most often hypogonadism) provide an early clue during history-taking that there may be a pituitary tumor present. Further evidence can be gained from the physical examination, particularly if there are signs of hypothyroidism (hair loss or delayed relaxation of reflexes) or an indication of excessive secretion of prolactin (galactorrhea on breast manipulation), growth hormone (skin thickening and acral changes), or ACTH (cushingoid features). Careful formal visual field testing, including red objects, establishes abnormalities missed on confrontation (23), as well as disproves the false impression of bitemporal defects or constricted fields due to overhanging eyebrows or hysteria, respectively. Evidence for optic atrophy may be found on fundoscopy, which may be associated with diminished, uncorrectable visual acuity. Infrequently, involvement in cranial nerves III, VI, or sensory V may be found on examination.

Radiological and endocrine testing is discussed in the previous section and in other chapters in this volume. One comment from personal experience concerns the value of multiple blood prolactin determinations for establishing and following therapy of patients with a prolactin-secreting adenoma. Several infertile young women referred for amenorrhea with or without galactorrhea and "classic" changes on sella polytomography for a "microadenoma" (e.g., focal erosion of the anterior floor of the sella) initially had normal or borderline prolactin values (<25 ng/ml). Other endocrine values were normal including gonadotropins, thyroid hormones, and growth hormone response to hypoglycemia. A subsequent series of fasting prolactin determinations resulted in variable values, some normal and others elevated two to seven times normal. Prolactin-containing tumors determined by immunocytochemistry on pathological examination were subsequently obtained during transsphenoidal surgery. Dynamic testing of prolactin with TRH or chlorpromazine is usually not helpful in this situation (14). A single elevated prolactin value, usually <100 ng/ml, can also be seen in a normal individual, perhaps stimulated by the stress of venipuncture. Following tumor removal, serially determined prolactin values can also vary widely from day to day, so results of therapy based on these data require a number of determinations.

EXTRASELLAR LESIONS

Differential diagnosis of lesions causing sella abnormalities should include processes adjacent to but outside the confines of the sella turcica. The sella may be generally enlarged or asymmetrical as found in patients with lesions from other causes, but as in empty sella syndrome it usually lacks the focal erosions seen with pituitary tumor. The endocrine work-up may be indistinguishable from that of a patient with either an intrasellar tumor or empty sella syndrome (24). Major clues to the diagnosis of an extrasellar process, however, are found in the history and neurological examination. Many are secondary to increased intracranial pressure, in which case one would expect a history of an intermittent pulsatile headache present on morning wakening that worsens with activity, diplopia due to abducens paresis, visual obscurations, and nausea and vomiting. All of the patients in our series had characteristic pulsatile headache. A few of these patients had CSF rhinorrhea often associated with pseudotumor cerebri (23). A few others had polyuria; polydipsia; and weight, temperature, and/or psychic disturbances suggesting primary hypothalamic disease (1). Because of their special training the neurologist and neurosurgeon can make a unique contribution when evaluating the large sella since a wide variety of hypothalamic and parasellar lesions can be subtle and varied in their neurological presentations and initially may appear to be empty sella syndrome or pituitary adenoma to other physicians. Even after complete work-up, including contrast procedures, in a small number of cases either the wrong diagnosis or no diagnosis may be made until the correct one declares itself in time after careful follow-up visits.

The catalogue of possible extrasellar diseases is too long and the work-up

TABLE 3. *Extrasellar lesions causing sellar abnormalities*

Lesion	No. of cases
Craniopharyngioma	2
Chordoma	2
Sarcoidosis	2
Obst. hydrocephalus	2
Metastasis	1
Eosinophilic granuloma	1
Atypical pinealoma	1
Parasellar meningioma	1
Pseudotumor	1

From ref. 23.

of each too specific to be described in detail. In our series of 75 patients with abnormal sella, there were 13 cases in whom the lesion responsible for the abnormality was extrasellar in location (23). The list of lesions partially representative of pathology to be expected in this region is shown in Table 3. Notably, gliomas and many other lesions also can occur in this region (1,14).

CONCLUDING REMARKS

A review of the outcome of the evaluation of patients with large sellas reveals that a diagnosis can be made in the majority of cases. The two most common entities are pituitary tumor and empty sella syndrome. An important but smaller group (<20%) have sellar changes due to local or transmitted CSF pressure caused by lesions either above or near the pituitary gland. Often these lesions can be identified by neurological history and examination, and confirmed by the appropriate neurological or neuroradiological tests. A smaller group of undiagnosed asymptomatic patients with normal endocrine and neurological findings probably have an empty sella syndrome that was missed because an adequate pneumoencephalogram could not be performed. New CT scanners may aid in identifying these cases. Patients known to have primary empty sella syndrome, however, must be followed and studied further since this entity is poorly understood. There has been a tendency among physicians to consider it a nondisease, a variant of normal. Although this may be true in some cases, it has become apparent that some of these patients harbor a hypersecreting adenoma (perhaps 10%), and one can suspect that another group will be found to have nonsecreting adenomas as well (approximately 10%). Abnormal growth hormone response to insulin in half the patients in some series and various degrees of hypopituitarism in others suggest hypothalamic stalk or pituitary disease. Progressive visual problems or even diabetes insipidus have occurred in a small number of cases as well, indicating that it is not necessarily a benign condition. The syndrome appears to have a number of causes, some of which remain to be fully defined.

REFERENCES

1. Bauer, H. G. (1954): Endocrine and other clinical manifestations of hypothalamic disease: A survey of 60 cases with autopsies. *J. Clin. Endocrinol. Metab.,* 14:13–31.
2. Berke, J. P., Buxton, L. F., and Kokmen, E. (1975): The "empty" sella. *Neurology (Minneap.),* 25:1137–1143.
3. Bergland, R. M., Ray, B. S., and Torack, R. M. (1968): Anatomical variations in the pituitary gland and adjacent structures in 225 human autopsy cases. *J. Neurosurg.,* 28:93–99.
4. Brisman, R., Hughes, J. E. O., and Holub, D. A. (1972): Endocrine function in nineteen patients with empty sella syndrome. *J. Clin. Endocrinol. Metab.,* 34:570–573.
5. Busch, W. (1951): Die morphologie der sella turcica und ihre beziehungen zur hypophyse. *Arch. Pathol. Anat.,* 320:437–458.
6. Crockford, P. M., and Salmon, P. A. (1970): Hormones and obesity: Changes in insulin and growth hormone secretion following surgically induced weight loss. *Can. Med. Assoc. J.,* 103:147–150.
7. Domingue, J. N., Wing, S. D., and Wilson, C. B. (1978): Coexisting pituitary adenomas and partially empty sellas. *J. Neurosurg.,* 48:23–28.
8. Faglia, G., Ambrosi, G., Beck-Peccoz, P., and Giovanelli, M. (1973): Disorders of growth hormone and corticotropin regulation in patients with empty sella. *J. Neurosurg.,* 38:59–64.
9. Ganguly, A., Stanchfield, J. B., Roberts, T. S., West, C. D., and Tyler, F. H. (1976): Cushing's syndrome in a patient with an empty sella turcica and a microadenoma of the adenohypophysis. *Am. J. Med.,* 60:306–309.
10. Jordan, R. M., Dendall, J. W., and Kerber, C. W. (1977): The primary empty sella syndrome. *Am. J. Med.,* 62:569–580.
11. Kaufman, B., and Chamberlain, W. B., Jr. (1972): The ubiquitous "empty" sella turcica. *Acta Radiol. [Diagn],* 13:413–425.
12. Kaufman, B., Pearson, O. H., and Chamberlain, W. B., Jr. (1973): Radiographic features of intrasellar masses and progressive, asymmetrical non-tumorous enlargements of the sella turcica, the 'empty' sella. In: *Diagnosis and Treatment of Pituitary Tumors,* edited by P. O. Kohler and G. T. Ross, pp. 100–129. Excerpta Medica, Amsterdam.
13. Lee, W. M., and Adams, J. E. (1968): The empty sella syndrome. *J. Neurosurg.,* 28:351–356.
14. Martin, J. B., Reichlin, S., and Brown, G. M. (1977): *Clinical Neuroendocrinology.* Davis, Philadelphia.
15. Molitch, M. E., Hieshima, G. B., Marcovitz, S., Jackson, I. M. D., and Wolpert, S. (1977): Coexisting empty sella syndrome and acromegaly. *Clin. Endocrinol.,* 7:261–263.
16. Mortara, R., and Norrell, H. (1970): Consequences of a deficient sella diaphragm. *J. Neurosurg.,* 32:565–573.
17. Neelon, F. A., Goree, J. A., and Liebovitz, H. E. (1973): The primary empty sella: Clinical and radiographic characteristics and endocrine function. *Medicine (Baltimore),* 52:73–92.
18. Nieman, E. A., Landon, J., and Wynn, V. (1967): Endocrine functions in patients with untreated chromophobe adenomas. *Q. J. Med.,* 36:357–392.
19. Ridgeway, E. C., Kourides, I. A., Kliman, B., Bigos, T., and Maloof, F. (1975): Thyrotropin and prolactin reserve in the empty sella syndrome. *J. Clin. Endocrinol. Metab.,* 41:968–973.
20. Schaison, G., and Metzger, J. (1976): The primary empty sella: An endocrine study of 12 cases. *Acta Endocrinol. (Kbh),* 83:483–492.
21. Schwartz, T. B., and Ryan, W. G. (1978): *The Yearbook of Endocrinology,* p. 27. Yearbook Medical Publishers, Chicago.
22. Snyder, P. J., Jacobs, L. S., Raballo, M. M., Sterling, F. H., Shore, R. N., Utiger, R. D., and Daughaday, W. H. (1974): Diagnostic value of thyrotropin-releasing hormone in pituitary and hypothalamic diseases. *Ann. Intern. Med.,* 81:751–757.
23. Weisberg, L. A., Housepian, E. M., and Saur, D. P. (1975): Empty sella syndrome as a complication of benign intracranial hypertension. *J. Neurosurg.,* 43:177–180.
24. Weisberg, L. A., Zimmerman, E. A., and Frantz, A. G. (1976): Diagnosis and evaluation of patients with an enlarged sella turcica. *Am. J. Med.,* 61:590–596.
25. Wood, J. H., and Dogali, M. (1975): Visual improvement after chiasmapexy for primary empty sella turcica. *Surg. Neurol.,* 3:291–294.

Clinical Management of Pituitary Disorders,
edited by G. T. Tindall and W. F. Collins.
Raven Press, New York © 1979.

9

Pituitary Tumor Management: An Overview

William F. Collins

Department of Neurological Surgery, Yale University School of Medicine, New Haven, Connecticut 06510

The management of pituitary tumors has been controversial since the first attempts at treatment in the latter part of the last century. At first, the controversy revolved around if and how to treat them, since surgery was the only treatment and morbidity and mortality was high. As pituitary surgery evolved and mortality decreased, it became apparent that while surgery was now a viable option, almost all pituitary tumors treated by surgical excision recurred within five years unless radiation therapy was given (1,6). The effectiveness of radiation therapy in controlling the growth of pituitary tumors after surgical decompression led to its use as an initial treatment, with many physicians relegating surgery to those pituitary tumors that had failed to respond to radiation therapy or to cases in which mass effects were so severe that the delay in the effects of radiation therapy might jeopardize life or neurological function (4). The experience of 75 years cannot be ignored, and many cases have demonstrated that one of the best methods to control the proliferative characteristics of a pituitary tumor that causes mass effects is with radiation therapy. My feeling is that radiation therapy is most effective in controlling the growth of pituitary tumors when cystic changes, necrosis, and mass are first treated surgically. It is difficult to prove that such surgical decompression before radiation therapy improves the overall therapeutic statistics, but most series suggest it. Since the mortality with surgical decompression of pituitary tumors that was 10 to 12% in many clinics until a few years ago has dropped to less than 1%, the reason for not decompressing pituitary tumors before giving radiation therapy has become less relevant. Although more than three quarters of a century of experience should have resolved the problem of how to treat pituitary tumors, all except the most recent experience can only be applied to a part of a problem, because with the exception of a relatively small number of growth hormone (hGH)- or adrenocorticotropin (ACTH)-producing tumors, treatment has been confined to large tumors with symptoms of intracranial mass.

Neurosurgery's progress in recent years in lowering mortality with pituitary surgery to almost zero and our endocrine and radiology colleagues' ability to diagnose small pituitary tumors have not only allowed for the diagnosis and treatment of smaller tumors, but have also added to the controversy of the management of these lesions. It has become obvious that some of the controversy is based on lack of knowledge concerning the natural history of pituitary tumors and particularly of small pituitary tumors. In 1936 Costello (2) reported that approximately 23% of patients without known pituitary dysfunction examined at autopsy had pituitary adenoma, and Earle and Dillard (3) recently stated that almost all pituitary glands have foci of hyperplasia. Since it is difficult to differentiate hyperplasia from adenoma grossly or histologically, Earle and Dillard's statement can be interpreted as meaning almost all pituitaries contain adenomas. It is not known if many persons have unrecognized endocrine abnormalities relating to such adenomas or hyperplasia, or whether the incidental finding of pituitary adenoma at autopsy has significance. Perhaps the finding may identify persons who, with the correct stimulus, would develop a proliferative or secretory pituitary tumor capable of causing intracranial compressive symptoms or life-threatening endocrinopathies but who did not receive such a stimulus; in other words, perhaps these foci of hyperplasia or unrecognized adenoma are with some as yet unknown stimuli a cause for endocrinopathic or proliferative intrasellar tumors.

Furth et al. (5), as well as other investigators, have shown that hyperplasia and small adenomas precede the development of autonomous proliferative pituitary tumors when thyroidectomy is performed in or estrogen is given to young animals, suggesting that peripheral endocrine organ abnormalities or excess hormone intake may cause pituitary tumors, either directly or through altered CNS function. However, evidence from series of patients treated with surgery, radiation therapy, or a combination of surgery and radiation therapy suggests that a large portion of clinically recognized pituitary tumors treated following a clinical diagnosis of pituitary adenoma are primary tumors, since proliferative or endocrine aspects can be controlled by treatment confined to the pituitary gland. Recent advances in endocrinology allowing direct measurement of circulating levels of pituitary hormones and in neuroradiology in identifying small changes of the sella turcica and surrounding subarachnoid cisterns may have caused almost an epidemic of clinically diagnosed pituitary tumors. At Yale, there has been about an eightfold increase in the yearly frequency of diagnosed pituitary tumors over the past 20 years, and most of the increase has occurred in the last 5 to 7 years. This increase is in part related to our interest in pituitary surgery but also in part to the identification of prolactin-secreting adenomas and the recognition of the high incidence of pituitary tumors in Cushing's disease. This would suggest that some unrecognized endocrinopathies in the past were caused by the incidental pituitary tumors, but it would still leave the vast majority of adenomas found at autopsy unaccounted for, and it may be giving a false explanation for some environmental stimulus that is causing a part of or most of the recent increased frequency. Estrogens in the diet, birth control pills, widespread use of tranquilizers or other drugs in our culture are just some of the potential causes for an increased incidence of pituitary tumors.

Another problem in the determination of the optimal therapy of pituitary tumors is the fact that with the exception of the rare malignant tumor, pathologists have not been able to determine which adenomas have the potential to produce mass effects. The only evidence concerning the growth potential of pituitary tumors that is accurate enough to base treatment on includes the finding that the tumor is large when first treated or that the growth rate has been documented by radiographic studies over a period of time. Evidence of recent rapid growth or of past growth does determine that mass effects are and will continue to be a problem unless treated. These are not just incidental or interesting aspects of pituitary adenomas, but raise major questions in determining the best way to manage these lesions. With the recognition that too short a period of time has elapsed to evaluate modern methods of diagnosis and treatment of pituitary tumors, I would like to suggest a way of looking at the problem of pituitary adenomas that I think is useful in comparing what is being done with what has been done and that may indicate what information we should have in order to improve the treatment in the future. By dividing clinical problems of pituitary adenomas into those that are caused by (a) mass effects, (b) endocrinopathy of hypersecreting adenomas, and (c) combined mass effects and endocrinopathy, prognosis and, therefore, need for therapy can at least in part be related to past experience, and ongoing treatment can be evaluated as it relates to that experience. With this information, goals of therapy can be defined and methods to obtain maximum benefits with the least risk to the patient can be evolved.

MASS EFFECTS

One problem is to identify clinical symptoms, signs, and findings that determine that a pituitary tumor has the proliferative growth characteristics that result in danger from mass effects now or in the future. It is obvious that a tumor that has caused chiasmatic, third ventricular, or pontine compression has demonstrated that it has the growth potential to act as an intracranial tumor. Does the adenoma that displaces two thirds of the intrasellar structures also have this potential, and if so, what is its rate of growth? Unfortunately, there is not a good answer to this question, and thus far, pathological studies of tumors have not been helpful.

We are presently evaluating ultrastructures of various pituitary tumors; however, our studies, as well as those of other investigators that include scanning electromicroscopic and various light microscopic studies, have not helped clarify questions relating to growth potential. We have approached the problem by assuming that pituitary tumors with significant growth potential to cause mass effects will show one or more of the following characteristics: (a) sella turcica enlargement so that the measurements on standard anterior posterior and lateral skull x-rays exceed 15 mm in depth, 18 mm in maximum anterior posterior diameter, and 15 mm in width, not explained by an empty sella syndrome; (b) destruction of bone adjacent to the sella; (c) more than 5 mm of extrasellar extension.

These arbitrary criteria are and will be evaluated with the passage of time in an attempt to determine whether or not there is a correlation between them and the growth potential of the tumor. All patients with one or more of the above findings receive the recommendation that they have radiation therapy. Not all accept the recommendation. Rationale for this recommendation is that mentioned above, that past experience has shown that 80 to 90% of cases of pituitary tumors with proliferative growth characteristics that cause mass effects will within 5 years of surgical decompression or excision have recurrent mass effects, while with surgical decompression and radiation therapy more than 90% of cases of similar tumors will have control of mass effects (12,15). It should be recognized that in many series, the response of the mass effects of pituitary tumors to radiation therapy alone approaches the response to surgery plus radiation therapy if surgery is performed on those tumors that do not respond to radiation therapy with reduction in mass. It is clear from earlier series that morbidity and mortality are high in pituitary adenomas that have demonstrated proliferative mass effect characteristics and that are not treated adequately. A few series suggest that radical excision with hypophysectomy may improve the end results in large tumors, but since many of these large tumors invade the dura, the cavernous sinus, the diaphragma sella, or the parasellar tissues, the use of x-ray therapy even after radical surgery appears indicated.

In summary, clinical experience indicates that those patients whose pituitary adenomas show proliferative characteristics that cause mass effects should receive radiation therapy, but the diagnosis of pituitary adenoma is not in itself an indication for radiation therapy since the diagnosis does not indicate growth potential of the tumor.

ENDOCRINOPATHIES

The endocrinopathies caused by pituitary tumors cannot be considered as a single problem, because their prognoses extend from severe morbidity and shortening of life expectancy to slight inconvenience or infertility. The need to establish control of the endocrinopathy and the speed with which it should be controlled are determined by the effects of the endocrinopathy on the patient. One extreme is the high morbidity and mortality of patients with ACTH-producing tumors in whom a median survival of 5 years has been demonstrated when hypercortisolism is not controlled (9); the other extreme is the infertility, impotency, or lack of symptoms in hyperprolactinemic patients. The endocrinopathy of excess hGH is intermediate, but its life-shortening effects as well as its high morbidity must be considered in arriving at therapeutic decisions (16).

Cushing's disease is that portion of Cushing's syndrome or hypercortisolism that relates to hypothalamic-pituitary dysfunction. There has been controversy over what portion of these patients have pituitary adenomas and when an adenoma is present whether it is the result of hypothalamic dysfunction or the primary cause of the hypercortisolism syndrome. The incidence of pituitary tumors in Cushing's disease has been reported to be as low as 10% (11) and as high as or greater than 90% (14). The difference reflects in part the criteria for diagnosing pituitary tumor, the lower figure being reported if negative plain X-rays of the sella are assumed to be adequate to rule out pituitary adenoma, and the higher figure resulting from long-term follow-ups or surgical exploration. In our series of pituitary tumors, those tumors associated with Cushing's disease have had the highest incidence of persistent endocrinopathy following surgery, with only two out of ten cases showing control of excess ACTH after 3 years. Eight of the cases received radiation therapy following surgery without controlling the excess production of ACTH. Four of the patients that did not respond had Nelson's syndrome, and two of these four patients had tumors with marked proliferative growth characteristics.

The tumor with mass effects associated with Nelson's syndrome requires radical therapy, because although ACTH-producing tumors are rare, they constitute 30% of malignant pituitary tumors reported in the literature and a significant portion of invasive pituitary tumors (7,10). The patient with persistent ACTH-producing tumors requires complete control of hypercortisolism and control of mass effects of the tumor if present. In those patients without mass effects, if surgical excision of an adenoma has failed, then hypophysectomy is the only pituitary surgery that is effective. If fertility is a factor, then adrenalectomy with radiation of the pituitary may be indicated. The suggestion for radiation therapy reflects the low incidence of pituitary tumor complications reported by Orth and Liddle (8) when therapeutic levels of radiation are given to the pituitary after adrenalectomy.

Wright et al. (16) documented the life-shortening effects of continued circulation of excess hGH, and this, plus the morbidity associated with acromegaly, indicates a need for treatment that completely controls hGH. Although radiation therapy can control the circulating levels of hGH in a significant portion of cases, alleviating much of the morbidity of acromegaly, only excision of the pituitary tumor cures the disease. Neither radiation nor surgery has been conclusively demonstrated to lengthen life, but it can be safely assumed that cure of the disease would be the most likely to do so. The criteria for cure include resting hGH levels between 0 to 4 mg/ml, suppression of hGH with glucose load, reversal of any paradoxic rise in hGH with glucose, absence of hGH response to TRH, and loss of hGH suppression with dopamine agonists. If surgery plus radiation therapy has not controlled hGH, only hypophysectomy or bromocryptine remains as further therapy (13). The following treatment protocol has evolved in our institution for acromegaly, with variations relating to age and general health of the patient. Surgical excision of the pituitary tumor in acromegaly is recommended to all patients whose medical condition permits general anesthesia and transsphenoidal approach to the pituitary. Only a very few patients have had large anterior or lateral extrasellar extensions of their tumor requiring transcranial approach to the mass. Those in the younger group of patients whose disease has not been controlled with pituitary surgery are offered reoperation followed by radiation if control is not attained; those in the older age group, estimated both chronologically and physiologically, are offered radiation therapy followed by hypophysectomy if control is not obtained. Both groups receiving radiation therapy are placed on bromocryptine during the period of time, usually 18 to 24 months, necessary to evaluate radiation therapy effects. If after both forms of treatment, i.e., surgery and radiation, control has not been obtained, then bromocryptine can be continued in order to control circulating levels of hGH. There is too little experience with the drug to know if there is any effect on the proliferative aspects of the tumor.

As mentioned above, the incidence of diagnosing pituitary tumor has increased eightfold in our institution within the past decade, with most of the increase being prolactin-secreting adenomas. While a few of the prolactin-secreting adenomas are diagnosed from the effect of their proliferative growth characteristics on the skull, chiasm, or brain, the vast majority are discovered during work-up for causes of infertility, galactorrhea, or menstrual irregularities. Most of this latter group have either no significant growth potential in the tumor or the tumor has existed too short a time to demonstrate such potential. Although the hypoestrogen states that accompany about half these women with prolactin-secreting adenomas theoretically could lead to the side effects of early menopause, such as osteoporosis and vaginal tissue atrophy, no other significant morbidity or mortality has been demonstrated from the effects of the hyperprolactinemia except for infertility and galactorrhea. Some women, in fact, welcome the infertility. Failure to control hyperprolactinemia in patients with prolactin-secreting adenomas does not, in my judgment, indicate a radical surgical approach or radiation therapy unless mass effects have been demonstrated. Early in our series of transsphenoidal surgery, all patients whose endocrinopathy was not controlled by surgery were treated with radiation therapy. This treatment recommendation was a carry over from the idea that pituitary tumors should be irradiated after surgical decompression in the belief that the laboratory findings indicated persistent proliferative endocrine-active tumor. Significantly, none of the 15 patients with hyperprolactinemia achieved normal serum prolactin values, although most had significant lowering of levels with radiation therapy after failure of surgical therapy. Although this may indicate isolated pituitary stalk damage or hypothalamic damage from surgery and radiation, it also may denote a differential sensitivity to radiation therapy of the prolactin adenoma cell. Presently, we are randomizing patients with prolactin-secreting adenomas diagnosed by sella erosion on polytomography and prolactins above 100 ng/ml and using surgical excision on the tumor in about half the patients. The protocol includes a complete endocrine and neurological evaluation with pneumoencephalography, and if no evidence of mass effects is demonstrated, the patient is randomized to surgical excision and either no treatment or bromocryptine if libido or potency is a problem. In following these patients, repetitive examinations of the sella, visual fields and endocrine function are done. It is difficult, at this point, to know what portion of the patients will have complications associated with no therapy or bromocryptine, but in the first year of following patients with clinical indications of a prolactin secreting adenoma, less than 5% have shown evidence of proliferative growth and/or further marked elevation of prolactin levels. In those patients not accepting randomization, we stress how little is known about prolactin-secreting adenomas of the pituitary and recommend surgical excision of the tumor as early as possible. We do not give radiation therapy to those who fail to attain control of their hyperprolactinemia; rather, we recommend medical treatment if indicated to control symptoms and repetitive endocrine, visual, and x-ray evaluation.

In summary, the clinical problems of the management of pituitary tumors include mass effects, endocrinopathy, and a combination of both. No information is available that will define a pituitary tumor as having proliferative growth characteristics, except the demonstration of its ability to produce a mass. Surgical treatment of pituitary tumors producing mass effects is, in general, unsatisfactory unless combined with radiation therapy. The endocrinopathies produced by secreting pituitary tumors vary both in their clinical significance and in their response to treatment, with ACTH-producing tumors having the highest morbidity and shortening of life expectancy. Growth-hormone-producing tumors are intermediate, and prolactin-producing tumors the least threatening to life. Surgical excision of the secretory adenoma is the best method of controlling the endocrinopathy, with radiation therapy most effective in controlling hGH circulating levels if surgery fails, less effective in controlling the ACTH produced by tumors, and least effective in normalizing hyperprolactinemia. Too little is known to comment on TSH-producing tumors. Modern diagnostic and surgical techniques have allowed earlier and more effective control of the symptoms of pituitary tumor but also have raised questions that may require many years to answer. In the meantime, therapy proven with the passage of time should not be abandoned, and thorough evaluation of patients treated with any or all of the therapies available must be done for extended periods of time if the question as to how best treat pituitary tumors is to be answered.

REFERENCES

1. Bakay, L. (1950): The results of 300 pituitary adenoma operations. *J. Neurosurg.*, 7:240–255.
2. Costello, R. T. (1936): Subclinical adenoma of the pituitary gland. *Am. J. Pathol.*, 12:205–215.
3. Earle, K. M., and Dillard, S. H. (1973): Pathology of adenomas of the pituitary gland. In: *Diagnosis and Treatment of Pituitary Tumors,* edited by P. O. Kohler and G. T. Ross, pp. 3–16. Excerpta Medica, Amsterdam.
4. Fager, C. A., Poppen, J. L., and Takaoka, Y. (1973): Indications for and results of surgical treatment of pituitary tumors by the intracranial approach. In: *Diagnosis and Treatment of Pituitary Tumors,* edited by P. O. Kohler and G. T. Ross, pp. 146–155. Excerpta Medica, Amsterdam.

5. Furth, J., Dent, N. N., Burnett, W. T., and Gadsden, E. L. (1955): The mechanism of induction and the characteristics of pituitary tumors induced by thyroidectomy. *J. Clin. Endocrinol. Metab.,* 15:81–97.
6. Henderson, W. R. (1939): The pituitary adenomata. A follow-up study of the surgical results in 338 cases (Dr. Harvey Cushing's series). *Br. J. Surg.,* 26:811–921.
7. Jefferson, Sir G. (1955): *The Invasive Adenomas of the Anterior Pituitary,* pp. 1–63. University Press of Liverpool, Liverpool.
8. Orth, D. N., and Liddle, G. W. (1971): Results of treatment in 108 patients with Cushing's syndrome. *New. Engl. J. Med.,* 285:243–247.
9. Plotz, C. M., Knowlton, A. I., and Ragan, C. (1952): The natural history of Cushing's syndrome. *Am. J. Med.,* 13:597–614.
10. Rovit, R. L., and Duane, T. D. (1969): Cushing's syndrome and pituitary tumor pathophysiology and ocular manifestation of ACTH secreting pituitary adenoma. *Am. J. Med.,* 46:416–427.
11. Salassa, R. M., Kearns, T. P., Kernohan, J. W., et al. (1959): Pituitary tumors in patients with Cushing's syndrome. *J. Clin. Endocrinol. Metab.,* 19:1523–1539.
12. Sheline, G. E. (1973): Treatment of chromophobe adenomas of the pituitary gland and acromegaly. In: *Diagnosis and Treatment of Pituitary Tumors,* edited by P. O. Kohler and G. T. Ross, pp. 201–216. Excerpta Medica, Amsterdam.
13. Thorner, M. O. (1977): Therapeutic implications of dopaminergic drugs in acromegaly. In: *Clinical Neuroendocrinology,* edited by L. Martini and G. M. Besser, pp. 295–308. Academic Press, New York.
14. Tyrrell, J. B., Brooks, R. M., Fitzgerald, P. B., et al. (1978): Cushing's disease: Selective transsphenoidal resection of pituitary microadenomas. *N. Engl. J. Med.,* 298:753–758.
15. Urdaneta, N., Chessin, H., and Fischer, J. J. (1976): Pituitary adenomas and craniopharyngiomas: Analysis of 99 cases treated with radiation therapy. *Int. J. Radiat. Biol.,* 1:895–902.
16. Wright, A. D., Hill, D. M., Loury, C., and Fraser, T. R. (1970): Mortality in acromegaly. *Q. J. Med.,* 39:1–16.

Clinical Management of Pituitary Disorders,
edited by G. T. Tindall and W. F. Collins.
Raven Press, New York © 1979.

10

Medical Management of Acromegaly

Vijay R. Soman

*Department of Medicine, Yale University School of Medicine,
New Haven, Connecticut 06510*

Acromegaly is a chronic, debilitating, and potentially lethal disease caused by excessive secretion of growth hormone. In 1886 Pierre Marie, a distinguished French physician, published a paper describing two cases of a disorder he called acromegaly (63). Although Marie did not ascribe the disease to any specific anatomic or physiologic cause, he considered the disorder to be a true disease entity and differentiated acromegaly from myxedema and Paget's disease. Minkowski (68) was said to be the first to recognize that an enlargement of the hypophysis was observed in all carefully examined cases of acromegaly. In 1909 Cushing (20) regarded acromegaly as due to glandular hypersecretion of hyperpituitarism, and in 1927 Cushing and Davidoff (21) concluded that the disease was caused by a hyperplastic or adenomatous process of the acidoplastic cells of the pituitary body. In the modern era the following developments may be considered important milestones in the diagnosis and treatment of acromegaly: (a) the demonstration by Hamberger et al. (37) and Ray (78) that complete hypophysectomy, either transsphenoidal or transfrontal, led to rapid reversal of many of the manifestations of the disease; (b) development of radioimmunoassay of growth hormone by Hunter and Greenwood (40); and (c) the promising recent reports that dopaminergic agents such as bromocriptine may be useful for controlling the disease in the majority of patients (14,96) at least on a short-term basis. These studies should provide further impetus for the development of newer pharmacologic agents to control acromegaly.

PATHOGENESIS OF ACROMEGALY

Hypothalamic Versus Pituitary Etiology

The traditional view holds that the primary abnormality in acromegaly is at the level of the pituitary gland. However, there continues to be an ongoing debate regarding hypothalamic versus pituitary origin of acromegaly. Proponents of the hypothalamic etiology of acromegaly believe that the primary hypothalamic dysfunction, probably due to abnormal neurotransmitter regulation, results in a chronic recurrent overproduction of the putative growth hormone-releasing factor that in turn leads to a pituitary tumor secreting excess growth hormone (19,50). Most of the evidence in support of the hypothalamic etiology is of an indirect nature. For instance, in many patients with acromegaly growth hormone secretion is not completely autonomous but is at least partially regulated by various physiologic and pharmacologic stimuli that are believed to be mediated via the hypothalamus (19,50). In this regard the report of Hagen et al. (36), indicating excessive levels of growth hormone-releasing activity in some patients with acromegaly, is of great interest. However, the final proof must await characterization and measurement of the putative growth hormone-releasing factor in acromegaly. In any event, the current weight of evidence seems to favor the primary pituitary etiology of acromegaly. The major argument in favor of primary pituitary etiology is the fact that the growth hormone levels are normalized in the majority of patients with the removal of pituitary tumor and, even more importantly, the demonstration of the reversal of the paradoxical growth hormone response to various stimuli following removal of the pituitary adenoma in carefully studied cases such as that reported by Hoyte and Martin (39).

Acromegaly Due to Nonpituitary Tumors

A distinctly rare but fascinating cause of acromegaly is production of growth hormone-releasing substance or growth hormone-like peptide by nonpituitary tumors in some patients. In patients reported by Dabek (22) and Sönksen et al. (91) acromegaly subsided and abnormal hormone response to glucose tolerance test returned to normal following removal of bronchial carcinoid tumors. Since these investigators were unable to isolate growth hormone in tumor extract of these patients, it has been suggested that acromegaly in these patients was caused by the ectopic secretion of a growth hormone-releasing substance. In this regard studies of Beck et al. (6) provide direct evidence for the ectopic secretion of a growth hormone-releasing substance by demonstrating that extracts of human lung tumors caused release of growth hormone by rat pituitary glands. More recently, Caplan et al. (11) described a fascinating patient in whom acromegaly was cured by removal of an islet cell tumor of the pancreas. These authors postulated that in their patient acromegaly was caused by secretion of growth hormone-releasing substance by the pancreatic tumor.

NATURAL HISTORY OF ACROMEGALY

Although there are no good prospective studies available regarding the natural history of untreated acromegaly, it is generally recognized that the disease is associated with increased morbidity and mortality in affected patients. For example, in 100 cases reported by Evans et al. (30), about 50% of the patients had died before the age of 50 years and 89% by the age of 60 years. In a recent study Wright et al. (99) observed that the number of deaths in their series of 194 patients with acromegaly was almost twice that expected from a general population of a similar structure. With respect to the cause of death, they observed an increased number of deaths due to cardiovascular and respiratory disease in males and to cerebrovascular and respiratory disease in females. Furthermore, increased mortality was found to be associated with hypertension and diabetes. Interestingly, the incidence of deaths due to neoplasm in their acromegalic patients was similar to that of the general population. In addition, treated patients appeared to have reduced mortality compared to the untreated group.

CLINICAL MANIFESTATIONS AND COMPLICATIONS OF ACROMEGALY

Clinical manifestations and complications of acromegaly can be conveniently classified into four groups: (a) effects of excess growth hormone in stimulating tissue growth; (b) metabolic abnormalities due to excess growth hormone; (c) local effects of pituitary tumor; and (d) effects of alterations in other pituitary hormones.

Effects of Growth Hormone on Stimulating Tissue Growth

Effects of growth hormone on tissue growth account for the majority of the commonly recognized overt clinical features of acromegaly. For example, the enlargement of the soft tissue and the tubular bones results in the classic features of prognathism with spacing of the lower teeth and an increase in ring and shoe size. Overgrowth of other tissues and viscera (salivary glands, lungs, heart, and liver) are also commonly found. Increased renal mass is reflected in the increased glomerular filtration rate in these patients. With respect to the visceromegaly in acromegaly, the observations of Sober et al. (87) have important clinical implications. In their series of 57 acromegalics 9 had clinical hepatomegaly, and in 8 of these 9 patients a second disease process accounted for the hepatomegaly. These data indicate that the visceromegaly in these patients should not be automatically attributed to acromegaly per se. Hypertension and cardiac disease occur with increased frequency in acromegaly and are important contributors of morbidity and mortality in this disease (99). It is generally believed that in acromegaly, in addition to atherosclerotic heart disease, a distinct form of cardiomyopathy probably exists (77). However, McGuffin et al. (66) were unable to detect a distinct form of heart disease in their acromegalic population. In a recent study Smallridge et al. (85) reported that echocardiographic abnormalities (asymmetrical septal hypertrophy and left ventricular hypertrophy) are common in acromegaly, particularly in those patients with very high growth hormone levels, and that in many patients this was seen in the absence of overt clinical cardiovascular disease. Acromegaly is a recognized cause of carpal tunnel syndrome, and on occasion it may be a presenting symptom of the disease. O'Duffy et al. (74) reported that 35 of 100 patients with acromegaly had carpal tunnel syndrome. It should be noted that in acromegalic patients symptoms of paresthesias may not always reflect underlying entrapment neuropathies but sometimes may indicate peripheral neuropathy. In a detailed study Low et al. (59) were able to demonstrate evidence of peripheral neuropathy independent of the presence of diabetes in 8 of 11 acromegalics. In addition, some patients, particularly those with longstanding disease, complain of progressive muscle weakness involving mainly the proximal muscle groups. Muscle biopsy in these patients has revealed hypertrophy of type 1 fibers and atrophy of type 2 fibers. These histopathologic changes appeared to correlate better with the duration of the disease rather than with the height of the growth hormone levels (65,71).

Degenerative joint disease is a recognized but poorly understood complication of acromegaly. Clinically it is indistinguishable from that seen in the nonacromegalic patients except for its intensity and early onset in acromegaly (9,26).

Metabolic Abnormalities in Acromegaly

Diabetes

Acromegaly is a recognized cause of secondary diabetes, and the presence of diabetes is known to have a deleterious effect on the prognosis of acromegaly. Diabetes in acromegaly does not result from insulin deficiency, but in fact the glucose intolerance in acromegaly is characterized by hyperinsulinemia and insulin resistance (7). With respect to the etiology of insulin resistance, recent findings indicate that changes in insulin receptor have been implicated in the pathogenesis of insulin resistance in obesity (44) and maturity-onset diabetes (24,75). Recent studies from our laboratory indicate that acromegalic patients exhibit decreased insulin binding to circulating monocytes, and that the decreased insulin receptor concentration in these patients correlates strongly with the decrease in the *in vivo* sensitivity to insulin (89). These observations are supported by our data in patients with isolated growth hormone deficiency (90). In these studies we observed that patients with isolated growth hormone deficiency have increased insulin binding to monocytes, and that growth hormone treatment of these patients led to a fall in insulin binding to monocytes. From these data the following sequence appears likely. The excess growth hormone levels in acromegaly result in hyperinsulinemia with associated decrease in the insulin receptor concentration that is, at least in part, responsible for the insulin resistance, and that with time this results in overt diabetes particularly in those patients with a family history of diabetes.

Lipid Abnormalities

Although growth hormone has been shown to have profound effects on lipid metabolism in various *in vitro* and *in vivo* studies (34,55), observations of Aloia et al. (5) in 24 acromegalic patients failed to reveal a significant incidence of hyperlipidemia in nondiabetic acromegalics. However, in a recent study an increased incidence of hypertriglyceridemia, but not hypercholesterolemia, was noted (73).

Calcium and Phosphorus Metabolism

Acromegaly is traditionally believed to be associated with an increased incidence of osteoporosis. Several recent roentgenographic and densitometric studies, however, failed to detect an increased incidence of osteoporosis in acromegaly (28,70). With respect to the skeletal metabolism, acromegalic patients have an increased total exchangeable calcium pool with an accelerated calcium turnover, increased periosteal apposition, and increased resorption of trabecular bone (4,8). A study by Aloia et al. (2) indicates that the successful treatment of acromegaly may not only lead to the reversal of these changes but may in fact predispose these patients to vertebral compression fractures. Increased serum phosphorus levels are common in acromegaly, and the presence of hyperphosphatemia has been used for many years as an indicator of active acromegaly. Hyperphosphatemia appears to be at least in part due to a direct effect of growth hormone on renal tubular transport of phosphate (16).

Hypertension

The pathogenesis of the increased incidence of hypertension in acromegaly is poorly understood. Although an earlier report by Strauch et al. (92) indicated an increased incidence of aldosterone-producing adenoma in acromegalic subjects, further experience indicates that this is certainly not a common cause of hypertension in the majority of patients. The study of Snow et al. (86) suggests that excess growth hormone in acromegaly results in increased exchangeable sodium pool, which contributes to hypertension and also leads to the low renin activity often reported in these patients. In this regard urinary norepinephrine was reported to be increased in acromegaly (62); however, in a recent study plasma epinephrine and norepinephrine concentrations were found to be normal (17).

Local Effects of Pituitary Tumor

The local effects of pituitary tumor include a wide range of symptoms and signs. The most common, albeit relatively nonspecific, symptom is headache. Headache in acromegalic patients may not only result from the poorly understood local effects of the pituitary tumor but may also be caused by the secondary effects of excess growth hormone on cranial blood vessels and soft tissue. On occasion, previously severe headaches may suddenly remit and be followed by visual loss, indicating that the pituitary adenoma has grown up through the diaphragma sella. Ophthalmologic abnormalities, particularly visual field defects, may be among the initial findings and indicate suprasellar extension of the tumor. The classic abnormality is a bitemporal field defect that may involve the upper or lower field or both. Defects usually appear first in the periphery and are often irregular and unequal in the two eyes. A variety of other defects can be seen (38). Lesions of the anterior chiasm may produce the defect of junctional scotoma. Careful neuro-ophthalmologic examination using simultaneous comparison of colors and using the same size and color objects in two fields may detect early changes (e.g., differences in the intensity or hue of color) when all other tests are normal (60). On occasion paralysis of the III, IV, and VI nerves may be seen with large tumors extending out of the sella turcica into the cavernous sinus and adjacent structures. A rare but catastrophic local complication of pituitary tumor is the syndrome of pituitary apoplexy. Resulting from either infarction or hemorrhagic necrosis of the pituitary tumor, this condition is characterized by an abrupt alteration in consciousness, severe headache, extraocular muscle dysfunction, and visual loss. Taylor et al. (94) described a well-studied subject with acromegaly with diabetes who developed pituitary apoplexy. In this patient pituitary apoplexy resulted in acute reductions in serum growth hormone, cortisol, and thyroxine concentrations along with the onset of diabetes insipidus. Interestingly, the recovery from apoplexy resulted in complete remission of chemical diabetes. In cases reported by Zervas and Mendelson (100), the transnasal operative approach to the pituitary was utilized either for removal of the infarcted tumor or for aspiration of hematoma with survival. In conjunction with surgery, intensive endocrine support is required.

Effects of Alterations in Other Pituitary Hormones

Approximately 25% of acromegalic patients have galactorrhea generally but not necessarily accompanied by moderate elevations in serum prolactin levels. Clinically an increase in serum prolactin does not always correlate with the presence of suprasellar extension of the pituitary tumor. A decrease in libido and overall sexual function (impotence and amenorrhea) is common in acromegaly and is generally due to a decrease in luteinizing hormone (LH) and follice-stimulating hormone (FSH) secretion secondary to a decrease in pituitary gonadotrophs and/or suppression of LH and FSH by hyperprolactinemia in some patients. With respect to thyroid disease, acromegalic patients may have any combination of goiter, hypothyroidism, and hyperthyroidism. Hypothyroidism is generally mild and is a result of decreased TSH reserve. Goiter and hyperthyroidism occur with increased frequency in acromegaly (54). Goiter, at least in some patients, is a result of a direct stimulatory effect of growth hormone on the thyroid gland. The diagnosis of hyperthyroidism in acromegalic patients poses certain difficulties since acromegaly per se is associated with increased basal metabolic rate and increased perspiration; in addition, excess growth hormone has been shown to decrease TSH response to the TRH stimulation test (79), which is used as a sensitive test for the diagnosis of hyperthyroidism. Decreased ACTH reserve with secondary glucocorticoid deficiency is not uncommon with longstanding acromegaly and requires careful testing of ACTH reserve by the standard stimulation tests (insulin–hypoglycemia, vasopressin, and metyrapone test). Although the symptoms of overt diabetes insipidus are absent in the majority of patients when first seen, it is not uncommon to find evidence of partial diabetes insipidus on a carefully done overnight dehydration test such as the protocol employed by Miller et al. (67).

DIAGNOSIS OF ACROMEGALY

Table 1 summarizes the diagnostic protocol used at our institution for acromegaly. In this review, diagnostic problems pertaining to endocrine function tests are emphasized.

Tests of Growth Hormone Secretion

Basal Growth Hormone Measurement

In the majority of patients with longstanding acromegaly, measurement of fasting growth hormone levels on two or three occasions may provide the minimal laboratory confirmation of the diagnosis. However, in this regard it should be noted that various medications (estrogens, clonidine) and, more importantly, physiologic perturbations such as stress and exercise may lead to significant

TABLE 1. *Recommended protocol for work-up of acromegaly*

Endocrine function tests
1. Basal LH, FSH, estrogen, testosterone, and thyroid indices
2. 24-Hour urinary 17-OHCS and 17-ketosteroid
3. Oral glucose tolerance test—glucose and GH
4. TRH stimulation test—TSH, GH, and prolactin[a]
5. Insulin tolerance test—glucose, cortisol, GH[a], and prolactin[a]
6. Metyrapone test[a]
7. Dehydration test for ADH reserve
8. Multiple blood sampling for GH (particularly if there are borderline responses to other tests)

Radiological procedures
1. Polytomes of sella turcica
2. Pneumoencephalogram

Neuro-ophthalmologic evaluation

[a]These measurements and tests are considered optional.

elevations of basal growth hormone levels. In addition, a significant proportion of acromegalic patients have basal growth hormone levels in the borderline zone (5 to 10 ng/ml). For these reasons it is recommended that the diagnosis of acromegaly be confirmed by glucose tolerance test.

Glucose Tolerance Test

It remains the best single test for establishing the diagnosis of acromegaly in the majority of patients. In normal subjects following an oral glucose load (1.75 g/kg), the increase in blood glucose results in at least 50% suppression of basal growth hormone levels with a nadir of < 5 ng/ml. In acromegalic patients the following abnormalities are commonly seen: (a) abnormal (diabetic) blood glucose pattern (30 to 50% patients); (b) less than 50% suppression of basal growth hormone levels with minimal levels > 5 ng/ml; and (c) in some patients (25 to 40%) there is a paradoxical increase in the growth hormone levels. This is exemplified by a patient seen at our institution. As depicted in Fig. 1A, a 38-year-old female (D.S.L.) with features consistent with acromegaly showed a diabetic blood glucose pattern after the oral glucose tolerance test when studied prior to treatment. More importantly, her basal growth hormone levels, which were elevated (15 ng/ml), showed a paradoxical increase to 25 ng/ml. When the patient was restudied 6 months after transsphenoidal surgery, her blood glucose pattern was normalized, and her basal growth hormone levels fell to normal levels (4 ng/ml) and could be suppressed to 1 ng/ml with the oral glucose load.

TRH Stimulation Test

In recent years the thyrotropin-releasing hormone (TRH) stimulation test has gained wide acceptance in the diagnosis of acromegaly. In normal subjects administration of TRH does not result in any change in growth hormone levels, whereas in 60 to 80% of patients with active acromegaly TRH administration causes a paradoxical increase in growth hormone (41,83). It is believed that the neoplastic somatotropes may possess altered receptors resulting in a paradoxical response to various stimuli. The TRH stimulation test has been advocated to assess the activity of the disease such that a continued paradoxical growth hormone response to TRH following treatment of disease has been suggested as indicative of active disease. Our experience with transsphenoidal surgery supports this hypothesis (88). In Fig. 1B, results of the TRH stimulation test before and after treatment in patient D.S.L. are shown. Prior to treatment she exhibited a high basal growth hormone level with a paradoxical increase following a bolus injection of TRH. However, when restudied 6 months after transsphenoidal surgery, her basal growth levels were within normal limits, and she no longer showed a paradoxical response to TRH. Clinically this was accompanied by a significant remission of her disease following surgery.

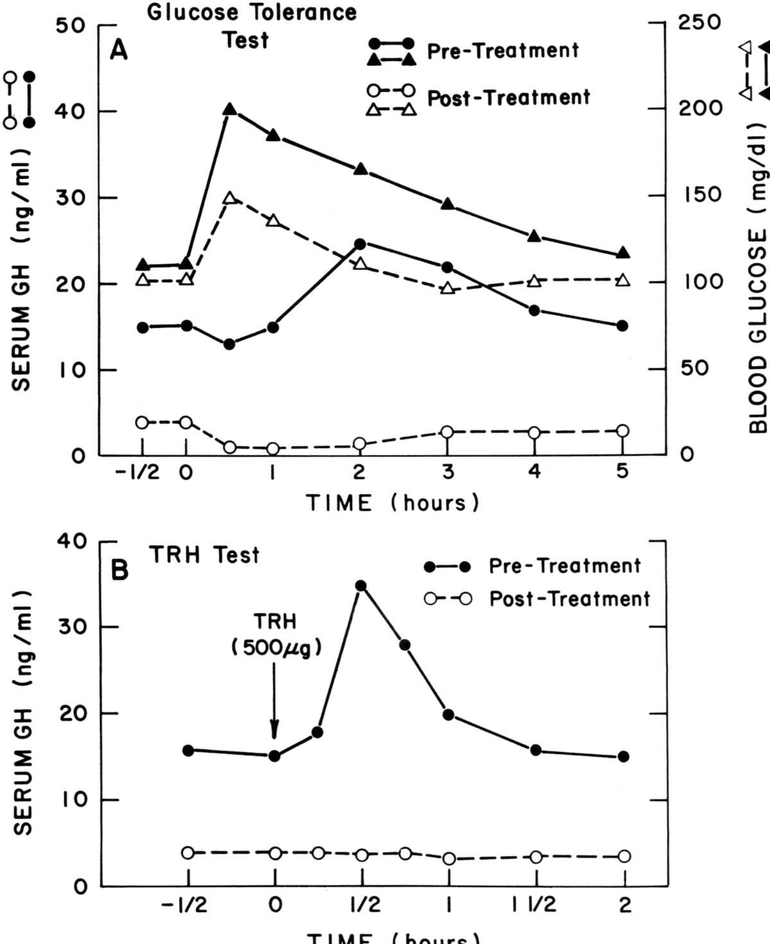

FIG. 1. Oral glucose tolerance test and TRH stimulation test before and 6 months after transsphenoidal pituitary surgery in a 38-year-old acromegalic patient.

Paradoxical Response to Other Agents

In addition to TRH, various other agents such as L-DOPA and luteinizing-hormone-releasing hormone (LRH) have been reported to induce a paradoxical growth hormone response in some patients with acromegaly. In 1973 Rubin et al. (81) and Faglia et al. (31) reported that patients with active acromegaly may show a paradoxical increase in growth hormone after a bolus injection of LRH. In normal subjects LRH fails to alter growth hormone secretion. Further experience with this test indicates that paradoxical response to LRH is seen in a smaller number of patients compared to the TRH response. For example, Ishibashi et al. (42) reported an increase in growth hormone after

LRH administration in only 3 of 22 acromegalic patients. In addition, they observed that in some patients prior administration of bromocriptine may block LRH-induced growth hormone release, whereas it had no effect on TRH-induced growth hormone release, suggesting that the action of LRH on growth hormone release may be modulated by a different mechanism than that of TRH. In this regard, it is of note that the paradoxical growth hormone response is in itself not diagnostic of acromegaly since it has also been reported in other conditions such as chronic renal failure, liver disease, and porphyria (64).

Growth Hormone Stimulation Tests

Various growth hormone stimuli (e.g., insulin-induced hypoglycemia, arginine, and glucagon) elicit a variable growth hormone response in acromegalic patients. In some patients these stimuli cause release of growth hormone, whereas in others they may lead to a paradoxical decrease in growth hormone levels. Clinically, growth hormone stimulation tests generally do not provide significant diagnostic information in the majority of patients.

Multiple Growth Hormone Measurements

In an occasional patient, particularly with early acromegaly, in whom basal growth hormone levels may be borderline elevated and the glucose tolerance test may not be clearly diagnostic, the technique of multiple blood sampling (i.e., every 20 min) for growth hormone measurement may be helpful. A 39-year-old male patient seen by us had features suggestive of early acromegaly, and, as shown in Fig. 2A, a normal glucose tolerance; his basal growth hormone level was 6 ng/ml (upper normal 5 ng/ml) and was suppressed to 3.0 ng/ml following oral glucose load. However, despite a borderline growth hormone response to the glucose tolerance test (Fig. 2B), when growth hormone measurements were done on multiple blood samples the mean growth hormone level was clearly elevated with an absence of sleep-associated growth hormone peak. The mean growth hormone level estimated by this technique also provides a firm baseline for the assessment of therapeutic success.

Other Pituitary Function Tests

In addition to the tests used to establish excess growth hormone secretion, all acromegalic patients should undergo a complete endocrine function protocol to document the adequacy of other pituitary hormones (Table 1). With respect to prolactin secretion, hyperprolactinemia is found in about 30% of patients with acromegaly (33). Hyperprolactinemia in acromegaly is generally moderate (30 to 80 ng/ml) and may result either from the inhibition of the prolactin-inhibiting factor (PIF), particularly in patients with suprasellar extension, or may be secondary to excess prolactin secretion by mixed pituitary adenomas,

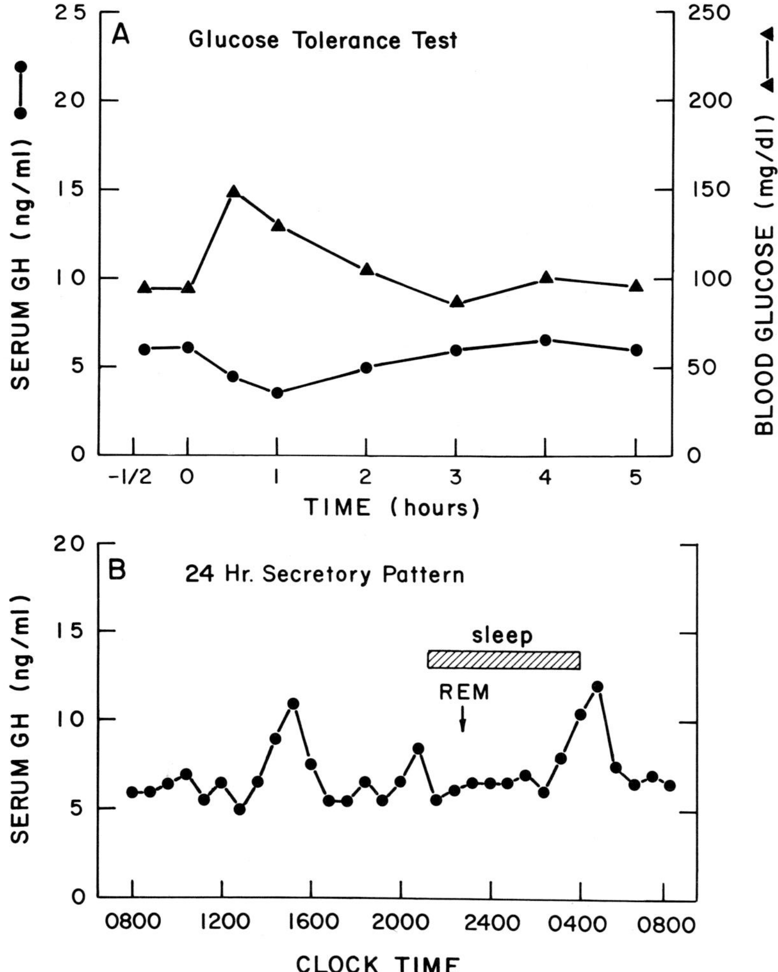

FIG. 2. Oral glucose tolerance test and 24-hr growth hormone secretory pattern in a 39-year-old male with early acromegaly.

as documented by ultrastructural studies reported by Corenblum et al. (15). With respect to the various dynamic tests of prolactin secretion, it appears that the majority of acromegalics with hyperprolactinemia do not exhibit significant blunting of prolactin response to TRH stimulation test (88) in contrast to that reported in patients with prolactin-secreting tumors with galactorrhea–amenorrhea syndrome (47). The integrity of TSH secretion is assessed by the TRH stimulation test. However, as noted earlier, interpretation of this test may be occasionally complicated owing to the recognized suppression of TSH response by excess growth hormone levels. ACTH reserve should be documented by the insulin–hypoglycemia test in conjunction with an additional test, e.g., the vasopressin or metyrapone test. Regarding gonadotropin reserve, the LRH stimulation test has proved to be somewhat disappointing since in clinical situations (e.g., in patients with pituitary and hypothalamic disease) the LRH test does not provide information beyond that obtained by multiple basal LH and FSH levels (69). As emphasized earlier, all patients with acromegaly, irrespective of symptoms of polyuria and polydipsia, should undergo overnight dehydration test to document ADH reserve (67). In patients suspected of having complete diabetes insipidus, the dehydration test should be carried out with great caution to avoid dangerous hypernatremia. In this regard, it should be recognized that the presence of glucocorticoid deficiency may sometimes mask the underlying ADH deficiency. The details of various pituitary function tests are available in various reviews on the subject (12,18,76).

TREATMENT OF ACROMEGALY

Table 2 summarizes various therapeutic modalities employed in the treatment of acromegaly. This review focuses mainly on the medical treatment of acromegaly. Surgical management is discussed by Hardy and Somma in Chapter 11.

Medical (Pharmacologic) Treatment

Until the advent of bromocriptine, the use of various pharmacologic agents to control acromegaly was characterized by initial promise followed by subsequent disappointment.

TABLE 2. *Treatment of acromegaly*

Medical (pharmacologic) treatment
1. Estrogens
2. Medroxyprogesterone
3. α-Adrenergic agents
4. Antiserotonin agents
5. Chlorpromazine
6. Somatostatin
7. Dopaminergic agents (bromocriptine)

Radiation treatment
1. Conventional radiotherapy
2. Heavy-particle radiation: proton beam, alpha particle
3. Implants: yttrium-90, gold-198

Surgical treatment
1. Craniotomy
2. Transsphenoidal, direct vision
3. Stereotactic
   - A. Cryosurgery
   - B. Radiofrequency
   - C. Ultrasound

Estrogens

Estrogen administration is known to decrease signs and symptoms of acromegaly. However, it appears to be effective in only a minority of patients for a relatively short time. Estrogens do not appear to act by lowering the serum growth hormone levels but may work by decreasing somatomedin generation (98).

Medroxyprogesterone

Following the report of Simon et al. (84) that a synthetic progesterone, medroxyprogesterone, blunts the increase in growth hormone following hypoglycemia, Lawrence and Kirsteins reported in 1970 that oral adminstration of medroxyprogesterone resulted in lowered growth hormone levels and decreased clinical symptoms in some patients with acromegaly (51). Subsequent studies, however, showed that the majority of patients failed to show a consistently satisfactory response (43,61). In the studies of Malarkey and Daughaday (61) those patients who responded to medroxyprogesterone still had growth hormone levels that were well above normal; and some patients with relatively low growth hormone levels exhibited a rise in growth hormone during medroxyprogesterone treatment.

α-Adrenergic Agents

α-Adrenergic stimulation leads to stimulation of growth hormone-releasing factor with subsequent growth hormone release from the pituitary. Phentolamine, which is an α-adrenergic antagonist, has been shown to lower growth hormone levels acutely in acromegalic patients (72). Fenfluramine, a derivative of amphetamine, depletes cerebral amine concentration in the hypothalamus and has been shown to decrease growth hormone levels in some acromegalic patients (93). However, at present, a suitable α-adrenergic agent that is effective in the majority of patients is not available.

Antiserotonin Agents

Serotonin acting via the limbic system has a stimulatory effect on growth hormone release. Antiserotonin agents such as metergoline and cyproheptadine have been reported to inhibit both basal and stimulated concentrations of growth hormone in acromegalics (25,32).

Chlorpromazine

In 1971 Kolodny et al. (48) reported that chlorpromazine treatment resulted in a decrease in growth hormone level and improvement in clinical features in a young man with acromegaly. Despite this initial favorable report, in subsequent studies this agent has not proved to be useful in the majority of patients (1,27).

Somatostatin

Isolation and purification of somatostatin generated a great deal of interest in this hormone as a possible cure for acromegaly. It acts at the level of the pituitary and markedly inhibits the release of basal as well as stimulated growth hormone secretion (10). Subsequent studies with this agent, however, pointed out several drawbacks with respect to its clinical use in acromegaly. At present, the available preparations have short half-lives, must be administered parenterally, and inhibit a host of other hormones including insulin, glucagon, gastrin, renin, GIP, and VIP, thereby disturbing the endocrine homeostasis (35). Currently, work is in progress to develop a more specific somatostatin analog with a longer half-life.

Dopaminergic Agents (Bromocriptine)

Growth hormone secretion is regulated by central neurotransmitters, of which dopamine, norepinephrine, and serotonin are considered to be the most important. In normal man, stimulation of dopamine receptors by agents such as L-DOPA, apomorphine, bromocriptine, legotrile, and piribedil results in increased growth hormone secretion. However, in many acromegalic subjects dopamine agonists lead to a paradoxical suppression of growth hormone secretion, as noted first by Liuzzi et al. with the use of L-DOPA (58). The subsequent experience with L-DOPA to control acromegaly on a long-term basis met with little success. However, the development of another dopamine agonist, bromocriptine, by Flückiger and Wagner in 1965 proved to be a major improvement in the medical management of acromegaly.

In 1974 Liuzzi et al. (56) reported on the effects of the acute administration of single doses of bromocriptine to acromegalics. They showed that following a single dose of bromocriptine (2.5 mg), growth hormone levels remained suppressed for a number of hours. Since this initial report several investigators have reported on the long-term use of bromocriptine in acromegaly. In 1975 Sachdev et al. (82) reported results of bromocriptine treatment (6 to 10 months) in 21 acromegalics: 2 patients failed to respond, and in 4 patients mean growth hormone levels were normalized, whereas other patients showed a significant but variable decrease in growth hormone levels. In addition, 2 patients were reported to have "escaped" after 6 months of therapy. Subjective as well as objective improvement was noted in the majority of responders, and carbohydrate tolerance was reported to have improved in all diabetic patients. The results of Cassar et al. (13) are somewhat less encouraging. They treated 12 acromegalics with bromocriptine (7.5 to 30 mg/day) for 6 months and observed that only 4 patients had normalization of growth hormone response to the glucose tolerance test. Further, no obvious improvement in acromegalic features was noted in the majority of patients, whereas glucose tolerance showed improvement in 2 of 4 diabetic subjects. They also noted that increasing the dose of bromocriptine to greater than 20 mg/day did not result in further improvement.

In 1977 Wass et al. (97) reported on the results of bromocriptine treatment in a large series of acromegalic patients. In this study 73 patients with active acromegaly were treated with 10 to 60 mg bromocriptine for 3 to 25 months. These investigators noted clinical improvement in 71 patients and, even more importantly, visual fields were reported to have improved in 2 patients. Among 23 patients with diabetic glucose tolerance tests, the glucose tolerance improved in 87% of patients, with 65% becoming completely normal. Mean circulating growth hormone levels fell by 7 ng/ml in 58 patients (79%) but did not reach normal values, whereas in only 15 patients were growth hormone levels completely normalized.

Recently Eskildsen et al. (29) reported results in 13 acromegalics treated with bromocriptine (30 to 55 mg/day) for 1 to 15 months. They noted a 60% decrease in growth hormone secretion in their patients as reflected by a fall in 24-hr urinary growth hormone excretion. In 10 patients growth hormone excretion was normalized, and one patient showed no response. They also observed significant subjective improvement in the majority of patients and disappearance of glycosuria in 2 diabetic patients. Interestingly, there was a 30% decrease in urinary free cortisol presumably due to the effect of bromocriptine on ACTH secretion in their patients, whereas TSH, LH, and FSH remained unchanged.

In summary, the available data appear to indicate that bromocriptine is an effective treatment for acromegaly with a success rate of 65 to 85%. A great advantage of bromocriptine treatment is that, in contrast to other therapies (e.g., radiation and surgery), it leaves pituitary function intact. However, an important limitation of bromocriptine therapy is that discontinuation of treatment is generally followed by a rapid return of growth hormone to the pretreatment levels in the majority of patients. Therefore bromocriptine is unlikely to be useful as a sole treatment for permanent remission of acromegaly. An important unanswered question is whether bromocriptine can control tumor growth, and in this regard the favorable reports of improvement in visual fields in some patients are encouraging (97). However, at the present time it cannot be recommended for patients with evidence of suprasellar extension. In the majority of patients the optimum dose appears to be 10 to 20 mg/day given in three or four divided doses; in most patients increasing the dose above 20 mg/day does not appear to result in further improvement.

The majority of patients appear to tolerate bromocriptine treatment without significant adverse effects particularly if the dose is kept within 20 mg/day. The reported side effects include nausea, vomiting, constipation, dryness of mouth, hyperkinesis, and alcohol intolerance. An occasional patient may experience more serious side effects, e.g., severe digital spasm and postural hypotension.

An interesting aspect of bromocriptine therapy is that in various studies the overall clinical improvement appears to be significantly greater than would be expected from the extent of the decrease in the growth hormone levels. With respect to the question as to which patients will respond to bromocriptine therapy, Liuzzi et al. (57) suggested that those patients who responded to TRH with a paradoxical increase in growth hormone will respond favorably to bromocriptine. The later experience, however, indicates that this is not true in all patients. Recent studies suggest that there is a good correlation between the acute response of growth hormone to piribedil, a short-acting dopamine agonist, and the long-term success with bromocriptine (95).

At present, bromocriptine appears to be indicated in the following group of patients: (a) those who have had only a partial cure with surgery plus irradiation and in whom second surgery is not desirable; and (b) those in whom it is used as an interim treatment to control the disease when irradiation is employed as a primary mode of treatment. In the latter patients bromocriptine treatment should be stopped at yearly intervals to determine if the radiotherapy has been effective and if it is necessary to continue therapy. Currently bromocriptine is not advocated as a primary treatment of acromegaly.

Radiation Treatment

Conventional external irradiation has been used to treat acromegaly for several decades, and until the resurgence of transsphenoidal pituitary surgery it was the mainstay of treatment in most centers. Regarding the efficacy of conventional radiation, with the widespread use of radioimmunoassay for serum growth hormone, it became apparent that a substantial number of patients with acromegaly continued to have elevated growth hormone levels after conventional radiation treatment. This resulted in a widespread skepticism about the effectiveness of this mode of treatment. However, since then, a number of investigators have reported a relatively favorable experience with conventional radiation. For example, in 1970 Roth et al. (80) reported that conventional radiation treatment resulted in a decrease in serum growth hormone concentration in 19 of 20 patients, and by 1 to 2 years following irradiation the mean decrease in growth hormone levels was 51%. It should be noted, however, that only 35% of their patients had growth hormone levels of 5 ng/ml or less. In 28 acromegalic patients studied by Lawrence et al. (52), 78% had a significant decrease in serum growth hormone levels following conventional radiation and 25% of patients had growth hormone levels of less than 5 ng/ml. In 1974 Aloica et al. (3) reported a similar experience with conventional radiation in their patients. Recently Lamberg et al. (49), in a series of 31 patients followed for 1 to 21 years after conventional radiation treatment, observed that in only 12 patients was serum growth hormone concentration decreased to normal levels and that clinically the disease was found to be still active in 10 patients. An important aspect of conventional radiation therapy is the relative lack of significant side effects. Relatively minor adverse effects include nausea, hair loss, and skin pigmentation particularly when a limited number of radiation ports are used. Hypopituitarism is believed to be relatively uncommon following conventional irradiation. In our experience hypopituitarism is more likely to occur in patients who have undergone prior surgical treatment for their disease. The commonly recommended radiation dose is about 4,000 rads, and it is generally felt that increasing the dose beyond 5,500 rads results in a significant increase in the side effects without a proportionate improvement in the remission rate.

In recent years heavy-particle irradiation (e.g., alpha particle and proton beam therapy) has been used as a method to deliver larger radiation doses to the pituitary tumor. In 1970 Lawrence et al. (53) reported normal growth hormone levels in 27% of 82 acromegalic patients 1 year following heavy-particle irradiation; hormonal treatment for hypopituitarism was required in more than one-fourth of their patients. Kjellberg and Kliman (45) reported that serum growth hormone was normalized in 47% of 62 acromegalic patients treated with proton-beam radiation. In an early series of patients treated with proton-beam therapy, side effects (oculomotor palsies, visual field defects) were appreciable (23). In a follow-up report of 230 acromegalic patients treated by the same group, hormonal replacement for hypopituitarism was required in 10% of the patients (46). At present, the available data are not sufficient to indicate superiority of heavy-particle radiation over conventional radiation in terms of overall benefit in the management of acromegaly.

In summary, conventional external irradiation results in normalization of the serum growth hormone levels in 30 to 40% of acromegalic patients, with a variable improvement in the remaining patients. Because of the relatively low rate of permanent cure with conventional irradiation alone, compared to transsphenoidal resection, it is our practice not to use radiotherapy as a primary treatment unless surgery is contraindicated.

TREATMENT OF ACROMEGALY: GOALS AND RECOMMENDATIONS

All patients with acromegaly should be treated since the disease is clearly associated with increased morbidity and mortality (30,99). Ideally the objectives of successful treatment should include the following:

1. Clinical remission of the disease including various metabolic derangements such as diabetes mellitus.
2. Normalization of growth hormone dynamics as assessed by (a) basal growth hormone levels of < 5 ng/ml; (b) suppression of growth hormone with oral glucose load; and (c) reversal of any paradoxical response of growth hormone to agents such as TRH and L-DOPA.
3. Preservation of pituitary function.

As may be expected, in clinical practice all these goals are achieved in only a minority of patients. In the majority, significant clinical remission of the disease along with basal growth hormone levels of < 5 ng/ml is an achievable and acceptable therapeutic objective. Based on the available data in the literature and our own experience, our current therapeutic recommendations are as follows: In all patients with significant suprasellar extension surgical removal of tumor followed by radiation treatment is indicated. In the majority of these patients the transsphenoidal approach can be employed. In patients with minimal or no suprasellar extension, we recommend transsphenoidal surgery as a first choice. However, if radiation therapy is employed to treat these patients in the future, it can be conveniently combined with bromocriptine treatment until the full effects of radiation are visible, which occasionally takes as long as 3 to 5 years. Patients who fail to respond to radiotherapy are recommended for pituitary surgery. Finally, those patients who fail to be controlled with pituitary surgery plus radiation should be treated with bromocriptine, which often results in a remarkable improvement.

REFERENCES

1. Alford, F. P., Baker, H. W. G., Burger, H. G., Cameron, D. P., and Keogh, E. J. (1974): The secretion rate of human growth hormone. II. Acromegaly, effect of chlorpromazine treatment. *J. Clin. Endocrinol. Metab.,* 38:309–312.
2. Aloia, J. F., Petrak, Z., Ellis, K., and Cohn, S. H. (1976): Body composition and skeletal metabolism following pituitary irradiation in acromegaly. *Am. J. Med.,* 61:59–63.
3. Aloia, J. F., Roginsky, M. S., and Archambeau, J. O. (1974): Pituitary irradiation in acromegaly. *Am. J. Med. Sci.,* 267:81–87.
4. Aloia, J. F., Roginsky, M. S., Jowsey, J., Dombrowski, C. S., Shukla, K. K., and Cohn, S. H. (1972): Skeletal metabolism and body composition in acromegaly. *J. Clin. Endocrinol. Metab.,* 35:543–551.
5. Aloia, J. F., Zanzi, I., and Cohn, S. H. (1975): Absence of an effect of chronic administration of growth hormone on serum lipids. *Metab. Clin. Exp.,* 24:795–798.
6. Beck, C., Larkins, R. G., Martin, T. J., and Burger, H. G. (1973): Stimulation of growth hormone release from superfused rat pituitary by extracts of hypothalamus and of human lung tumors. *J. Endocrinol.,* 59:325–333.
7. Beck, P., Schalch, D. S., Parker, M. L., Kipnis, D. M., and Daughday, W. H. (1965): Correlative studies of growth hormone and insulin plasma concentrations with metabolic abnormalities in acromegaly. *J. Lab. Clin. Med.,* 66:366–379.
8. Bell, N. H., and Bartter, F. C. (1967): Studies of ^{47}Ca metabolism in acromegaly. *J. Clin. Endocrinol. Metab.,* 27:178–184.
9. Bluestone, R., Bywaters, E. G. L., Hartog, M., Holt, P. J. L., and Hyde, S. (1971): Acromegalic arthropathy. *Ann. Rheum. Dis.,* 30:243–258.
10. Brazeau, P., Vale, W., Burgus, R., Ling, N., Butcher, M., Rivier, J., and Guillemin, R. (1973): Hypothalamic polypeptide that inhibits the secretion of immunoreactive pituitary growth hormone. *Science,* 179:77–79.
11. Caplan, R. H., Koob, L., Abellera, R. M., Pagliara, A. S., Kovacs, K., and Randall, R. V. (1978): Cure of acromegaly by operative removal of an islet cell tumor of the pancreas. *Am. J. Med.,* 64:874–882.
12. Carlson, H. E. (1977): In: *Endocrine Pathophysiology: A Patient Oriented Approach,* edited by J. M. Hershman, pp. 9–38. Lea & Febiger, Philadelphia.
13. Cassar, J., Mashiter, K., and Joplin, G. F. (1977): Bromocriptine treatment of acromegaly. *Metab. Clin. Exp.,* 26:539–546.
14. Chiodini, P. G., Liuzzi, A., Botalia, L., Oppizzi, G., Muller, E. E., and Silvestrini, F. (1975): Stable reduction of plasma growth hormone (hGH) levels during chronic administration of 2-Br-α-ergocryptine (CB-154) in acromegalic patients. *J. Clin. Endocrinol. Metab.,* 40:705–708.
15. Corenblum, B., Sirek, A. M. T., Horvath, E., Kovacs, K., and Ezrin, C. (1976): Human

mixed somatrophic and lactotrophic pituitary adenomas. *J. Clin. Endocrinol. Metab.*, 42:857–863.
16. Corvilain, J., Abramow, M., and Bergans, A. (1964): Effect of growth hormone on tubular transport of phosphate in normal and parathyroidectomized dogs. *J. Clin. Invest.*, 43:1608–1613.
17. Cryer, P. E. (1975): Plasma norepinephrine and epinephrine in acromegaly. *J. Clin. Endocrinol. Metab.*, 41:542–545.
18. Cryer, P. E. (1976): *Diagnostic Endocrinology*, p. 8–32. Oxford University Press, London.
19. Cryer, P. E., and Daughday, W. H. (1969): Regulation of growth hormone secretion in acromegaly. *J. Clin. Endocrinol. Metab.*, 29:386–393.
20. Cushing, H. (1909): The hypophysis cerebri: Clinical aspects of hyperpituitarism and of hypopituitarism. *JAMA*, 53:249–255.
21. Cushing, H., and Davidoff, L. M. (1927): In: *Monograph No. 32*. The Rockefeller Institute, New York.
22. Dabek, J. T. (1974): Bronchial carcinoid tumor with acromegaly in two patients. *J. Clin. Endocrinol. Metab.*, 38:329–333.
23. Dawson, D. M., and Dingman, J. F. (1971): Hazards of proton-beam pituitary radiation. *N. Engl. J. Med.*, 282:1434.
24. DeFronzo, R. A., Deibert, D., Hendler, R., Felig, P., and Soman, V. (1978): Direct evidence of insulin resistance in maturity-onset diabetes. *Diabetes (Suppl 2)*, 27:3.
25. Delitala, G., Masala, A., Alagna, S., Devilla, L., and Lotti, G. (1976): Growth hormone and prolactin release in acromegalic patients following metergoline administration. *J. Clin. Endocrinol. Metab.*, 43:1382–1386.
26. Detenbeck, L. C., Tressler, H. A., O'Duffy, J. D., and Randall, R. V. (1973): Peripheral joint manifestations of acromegaly. *Clin. Orthop. Relat. Res.*, 91:119–127.
27. Dimond, R. C., Brammer, S. R., Atkinson, R. L., Jr., Howard, W. J., and Earll, J. M. (1973): Chlorpromazine treatment and growth hormone secretory responses in acromegaly. *J. Clin. Endocrinol. Metab.*, 36:1189–1195.
28. Doyle, F. H. (1967): Radiology of skeleton in endocrine diseases. *Proc. R. Soc. Med.*, 60:1131–1132.
29. Eskildsen, P. C., Svendsen, P. A., Vang, L., and Nerup, J. (1978): Long-term treatment of acromegaly with bromocriptine. *Acta Endocrinol. (Kbh)*, 87:687–700.
30. Evans, H. M., Briggs, J. H., and Dixon, T. S. (1966): In: *The Pituitary Gland*, edited by G. W. Harris and B. T. Donovan, p. 439. University of California Press, Berkeley.
31. Faglia, G., Beck-Peccoz, P., Travaglini, P., Paracchi, A., Spada, A., and Lewin, A. (1973): Elevations in plasma growth hormone concentration after luteinising hormone-releasing hormone (LRH) in patients with active acromegaly. *J. Clin. Endocrinol. Metab.*, 37:338–340.
32. Feldman, J. M., Plonk, J. W., and Bivens, C. H. (1976): Inhibitory effects of serotonin antagonists on growth hormone release in acromegalic patients. *Clin. Endocrinol.*, 5:71–78.
33. Frantz, A. G., Kleinberg, D. L., and Noel, G. L. (1972): Prolactin studies in man. *Recent Prog. Horm. Res.*, 28:527–607.
34. Goodman, H. M. (1965): Early and late effects of growth hormone on the metabolism of glucose in adipose tissue. *Endocrinology*, 76:1134–1140.
35. Guillemin, R., and Gerich, J. E. (1976): Somatostatin, physiological and clinical significance. *Annu. Rev. Med.*, 27:379–388.
36. Hagen, T. C., Lawrence, A. M., and Kirsteins, L. (1971): In vitro release of monkey pituitary growth hormone by acromegalic plasma. *J. Clin. Endocrinol. Metab.*, 33:448–451.
37. Hamberger, C. H., Hammer, G., Norlen, G., and Sjogren, B. (1959): Hypophysectomy in acromegaly. *J. Clin. Endocrinol. Metab.*, 19:1500–1502.
38. Harrington, D. O. (1971): In: *A Textbook and Atlas of Clinical Perimetry*, 3rd ed., pp. 251–298. Mosby, St. Louis.
39. Hoyte, K. M., and Martin, J. B. (1975): Recovery from paradoxical growth hormone responses in acromegaly after transsphenoidal selective adenomectomy. *J. Clin. Endocrinol. Metab.*, 41:656–659.
40. Hunter, W. M., and Greenwood, F. C. (1962): A radioimmunoelectrophoretic assay for human growth hormone. *Biochem. J.*, 85:39p.
41. Irie, M., and Tsushima, T. (1972): Increase of serum growth hormone concentration following thyrotropin-releasing hormone injection in patients with acromegaly and gigantism. *J. Clin. Endocrinol. Metab.*, 35:97–100.

42. Ishibashi, M., Yamaji, T., and Kosaka, K. (1978): Induction of growth hormone and prolactin secretion by luteinising hormone-releasing hormone and its blockade by bromoergocriptine in acromegalic patients. *J. Clin. Endocrinol. Metab.*, 47:418–421.
43. Jackson, I. M. D., and Ormston, B. J. (1972): Lack of beneficial response of serum GH in acromegalic patients treated with medroxyprogesterone acetate (MPH). *J. Clin. Endocrinol. Metab.*, 35:413–415.
44. Kahn, C. R., Neville, D. M., and Roth, J. (1973): Insulin receptor interaction in the obese hyperglycemic mouse: A model of insulin resistance. *J. Biol. Chem.*, 248:244–250.
45. Kjellberg, R. N., and Kliman, B. (1971): Proton-beam therapy. *N. Engl. J. Med.*, 284:333.
46. Kjellberg, R. N., and Kliman, B. (1973): A system for therapy of pituitary tumors. In: *Diagnosis and Treatment of Pituitary Tumors*, edited by P. O. Kohler, and G. T. Ross, pp. 234–252. American Elsevier, New York.
47. Kleinberg, D. L., Noel, G. L., and Frantz, A. G. (1977): Galactorrhea: A study of 235 cases, including 48 with pituitary tumors. *N. Engl. J. Med.*, 296:589–600.
48. Kolodny, H. D., Sherman, L., Singh, A., Kim, S., and Benjamin, F. (1971): Acromegaly treated with chlorpromazine. *N. Engl. J. Med.*, 284:819–822.
49. Lamberg, B. A., Kivikangas, V., Vartianen, J., Raitta, C., and Pelkonen, R. (1976): Conventional pituitary irradiation in acromegaly. *Acta Endocrinol. (Kbh)*, 82:267–281.
50. Lawrence, A. M., Goldfine, I. D., and Kirsteins, L. (1970): Growth hormone dynamics in acromegaly. *J. Clin. Endocrinol. Metab.*, 31:239–247.
51. Lawrence, A. M., and Kirsteins, L. (1970): Progestins in the medical management of active acromegaly. *J. Clin. Endocrinol. Metab.*, 30:646–652.
52. Lawrence, A. M., Pinsky, S. M., and Goldfine, I. D. (1971): Conventional radiation therapy in acromegaly. *Arch. Intern. Med.*, 128:369–377.
53. Lawrence, J. M., Tobias, C. A., Linfott, J. A., Born, J. L., Lyman, J. T., Chong, C. Y., Manougian, E., and Wei, W. C. (1970): Successful treatment of acromegaly: Metabolic and clinical studies in 145 patients. *J. Clin. Endocrinol. Metab.*, 31:180–198.
54. Levin, S. R. (1972): Manifestations and treatment of acromegaly—medical staff conference, University of California, San Francisco. *Calif. Med.*, 116:57–64.
55. Li, C. H., Tanaka, A., and Pickering, B. T. (1964): Human pituitary growth hormone. VII. In vitro lipolytic activity. *Acta Endocrinol.* [*Suppl*] *(Kbh)*, 90:155–162.
56. Liuzzi, A., Chiodini, P. G., Botalla, L., Cremascoli, G., Muller, E. E., and Silvestrini, F. (1974): Decreased plasma growth hormone (GH) levels in acromegalics following CB 154 (2-Br-α-ergocryptine) administration. *J. Clin. Endocrinol. Metab.*, 38:910–912.
57. Liuzzi, A., Chiodini, P. G., Botalia, L., Silvestrini, F., and Muller, E. E. (1974): Growth hormone (GH)-releasing activity of TRH and GH-lowering effect of dopaminergic drugs in acromegaly: Homogeneity in the two responses. *J. Clin. Endocrinol. Metab.*, 39:871–876.
58. Liuzzi, A., Chiodini, P. G., Botalla, L., Cremascoli, G., and Silvertrini, F. (1972): Inhibitory effect of L-DOPA on GH release in acromegalic patients. *J. Clin. Endocrinol. Metab.*, 35:941–943.
59. Low, P. A., McLeod, J. G., Turtle, J. R., Donnelly, P., and Wright, R. G. (1974): Peripheral neuropathy in acromegaly. *Brain*, 97:139–152.
60. Luxenberg, M. N. (1976): In: *The Pituitary: A Current Review*, edited by M. B. Allen and V. B. Mahesh, pp. 331–344. Academic Press, New York.
61. Malarkay, W. B., and Daughday, W. H. (1971): Variable response of plasma GH in acromegalic patients treated with medroxyprogesterone acetate. *J. Clin. Endocrinol. Metab.*, 33:424–431.
62. Marek, J., Horky, K., Kopecka, J., Mestan, J., and Sramkova, J. (1974): Catecholamine excretion in acromegaly. *Endocrinologie*, 63:304–311.
63. Marie, P. (1886): Sur deux cas d'acromegalie; hypertrophie singuliere non congenitale des extremites supericures, infericures et cephalique. *Rev. Med. Paris*, 6:297–333.
64. Martin, J. B. (1973): Neural regulation of growth hormone secretion. *N. Engl. J. Med.*, 288:1384–1393.
65. Mastaglia, F. L., Barwick, D. D., and Hall, R. (1970): Myopathy in acromegaly. *Lancet* 2:907–909.
66. McGuffin, W. L., Sherman, B. L., Roth, J., Gorden, P., Kahn, C. R., Roberts, W. C., and Frommer, P. L. (1974): Acromegaly and cardiovascular disorders: A prospective study. *Ann. Intern. Med.*, 81:11–18.
67. Miller, M., Dalakos, T., Moses, A. M., Fellerman, H., and Streeten, D. H. P. (1970): Recognition of partial defects in antidiuretic hormone secretion. *Ann. Intern. Med.*, 73:721–729.
68. Minkowski, O. (1887): Uber einem Fall von akromegalie. *Klin. Wochenschr.*, 24:371–374.

69. Mortimer, C. H. (1977): In: *Clinical Neuroendocrinology,* edited by L. Martini and G. M. Besser, pp. 213–236. Academic Press, New York.
70. Nadarajah, H., Hartog, M., Redfern, B., Thalassinos, N., Wright, A. D., Joplin, G. F., and Frazer, T. R. (1968): Calcium metabolism in acromegaly. *Br. Med. J.,* 4:797–801.
71. Nagulesparen, M., Trickey, R., Davies, M. J., and Jenkins, J. S. (1976): Muscle changes in acromegaly. *Br. Med. J.,* 2:914–915.
72. Nakagawa, K., and Mashino, K. (1973): Suppressibility of plasma growth hormone levels in acromegaly with dexamethasone and phentolamine. *J. Clin. Endocrinol. Metab.,* 37:238–246.
73. Nikkila, E. A., and Pelkonen, R. (1975): Serum lipids in acromegaly. *Metab. Clin. Exp.,* 24:829–838.
74. O'Duffy, J. D., Randall, R. V., and MacCarty, C. S. (1973): Median neuropathy (carpal-tunnel syndrome) in acromegaly: A sign of endocrine overactivity. *Ann. Intern. Med.,* 78:379–383.
75. Olefsky, J. M., and Reaven, G. M. (1977): Insulin binding in diabetes. *Diabetes,* 26:680–688.
76. Ontjes, D. A., and Ney, R. L. (1972): Tests of anterior pituitary function. *Metab. Clin. Exp.,* 21:159–177.
77. Pepine, C. J., and Aloia, J. (1970): Heart muscle in acromegaly. *Am. J. Med.,* 48:530–534.
78. Ray, B. S. (1960): The neurosurgeon's new interest in the pituitary. *J. Neurosurg.,* 17:1–21.
79. Root, A. W., Snyder, P. J., Razvam, I., DiGeorge, A. M., and Utiger, R. D. (1973): Inhibition of thyrotropin-releasing hormone-mediated secretion of thyrotropin by human growth hormone. *J. Clin. Endocrinol. Metab.,* 36:103–107.
80. Roth, J., Gorden, P., and Brace, K. (1970): Efficacy of conventional pituitary irradiation in acromegaly. *N. Engl. J. Med.,* 282:1384–1391.
81. Rubin, A. L., Levin, S. R., Bernstein, R. I., Tyrrell, J. B., Moacco, C., and Forsham, P. H. (1973): Stimulation of growth hormone by luteinising hormone-releasing hormone in active acromegaly. *J. Clin. Endocrinol. Metab.,* 37:160–162.
82. Sachdev, Y., Gomez-Pan, A., Tunbridge, W. M. G., Duns, A., Weightman, D. R., Hall, R., and Goolamali, S. K. (1975): Bromocriptine therapy in acromegaly. *Lancet,* 2:1164–1168.
83. Samaan, N. A., Leavens, M. E., and Jesse, R. H., Jr. (1974): Serum growth hormone and prolactin response to thyrotropin-releasing hormone in patients with acromegaly before and after surgery. *J. Clin. Endocrinol. Metab.,* 38:957–963.
84. Simon, S., Schiffer, M., Glick, S. M., and Schwartz, E. (1967): Effect of medroxyprogesterone acetate upon stimulated release of growth hormone in man. *J. Clin. Endocrinol. Metab.,* 27:1633–1636.
85. Smallridge, R. C., Rajfer, S., Davia, J., and Schaaf, M. (1978): Acromegaly and the heart: An echocardiographic study. *Clin. Res.,* 26:312A.
86. Snow, M. H., Piercy, D. A., Robson, V., and Wilinson, R. (1977): An investigation into the pathogenesis of hypertension in acromegaly. *Clin. Sci.,* 53:83–91.
87. Sober, A. J., Gorden, P., Roth, J., and AvRuskin, T. W. (1974): Visceromegaly in acromegaly. *Arch. Intern. Med.,* 134:415–417.
88. Soman, V., and Collins, W. F. (1978): Diagnosis and surgical management of acromegaly. In preparation.
89. Soman, V., Deibert, D., and DeFronzo, R. A. (1978): Insulin receptor defect in acromegaly: Correlation with in vivo insulin sensitivity. In preparation.
90. Soman, V., Tamborlane, W., DeFronzo, R., Genel, M., and Felig, P. (1976): Insulin binding and insulin sensitivity in isolated growth hormone deficiency. *N. Engl. J. Med.,* 299:1025–1030.
91. Sönksen, P. H., Ayres, A. B., Braimbridge, M., Corrin, B., Davies, D. R., Jeremiah, G. M., Oaten, S. W., Lowy, C., and West, T. E. T. (1976): Acromegaly caused by pulmonary carcinoid tumors. *Clin. Endocrinol.,* 5:503–513.
92. Stranch, G., Valloton, M. B., Touitou, Y., and Bricaire, H. (1972): The renin-angiotensin-aldosterone system in normotensive and hypertensive patients with acromegaly. *N. Engl. J. Med.,* 287:795–799.
93. Sulaiman, W. R., Johnson, R. H., and Rennie, M. J. (1975): Hormonal and metabolic studies of the action of fenfluramine in normal man, obesity, acromegaly and diabetes mellitus. *Postgrad. Med.,* 51:125–131.
94. Taylor, A. L., Finster, J. L., Raskin, P., Field, J. B., and Mintz, D. H. (1968): Pituitary apoplexy in acromegaly. *J. Clin. Endocrinol. Metab.,* 28:1784–1792.
95. Thorner, M. O. (1977): Therapeutic inplications of dopaminergic drugs in acromegaly. In:

Clinical Neuroendocrinology, edited by L. Martini and G. M. Besser, pp. 295–308. Academic Press, New York.
96. Thorner, M. O., Chait, A., Aitken, M., Benker, G., Bloom, S. R., Mortimer, C. H., Sanders, P., Stuart Mason, A., and Besser, G. M. (1975): Bromocriptine treatment of acromegaly. *Br. Med. J.,* 1:299–303.
97. Wass, J. A. H., Thorner, M. D., Morris, D. V., Rees, L. H., Mason, A. S., Jones, A. E., and Besser, G. M. (1977): Long-term treatment of acromegaly with bromocriptine. *Br. Med. J.,* 1:875–878.
98. Wiedemann, E., and Schwartz, E. (1972): Suppression of growth hormone-dependent human sulfation factor by estrogen. *J. Clin. Endocrinol. Metab.,* 34:51–58.
99. Wright, A. D., Hill, D. M., Lowy, C., and Frazer, T. R. (1970): Mortality in acromegaly. *Q. J. Med.,* 39:1–16.
100. Zervas, N. T., and Mendelson, G. (1975): Treatment of acute hemorrhage of pituitary tumors. *Lancet,* 1:604–605.

Clinical Management of Pituitary Disorders,
edited by G. T. Tindall and W. F. Collins.
Raven Press, New York © 1979.

11

Acromegaly: Surgical Treatment by Transsphenoidal Microsurgical Removal of the Pituitary Adenoma

Jules Hardy and Maurice Somma

Department of Surgery, Service of Neurosurgery, and Department of Medicine, Service of Endocrinology, Notre-Dame Hospital and University of Montreal, Canada

Among the hypersecreting pituitary disorders, acromegaly is a disease produced by a unique cause: a growth hormone (hGH)-hypersecreting adenoma of the pituitary gland. Since no other etiology has yet been demonstrated, the logical treatment consists in complete "exclusion" of the adenoma resulting in normalization of hGH secretion. Ideally the adjacent normal pituitary tissue should remain intact in order to preserve the other pituitary functions.

Optical magnification through the extracranial transsphenoidal open surgical approach (TSS) has permitted clear distinction between normal and pathological tissues (3,4). Selective microsurgical adenomectomy with preservation of the normal gland is possible; thus the ideal aim of treatment can now be attained.

MATERIAL AND METHODS

As of July 1978, 160 patients with active acromegaly have been operated on using the transsphenoidal approach. Reviews of our first 40 and 80 cases have already been published (8,9). The present series consists of 120 cases with clinical and biological pre- and postoperative evaluation. Except for a few cases where the hGH was obtained only during the immediate postoperative period (10 days), the majority of the cases have been followed 1 to 15 years postoperatively. In this series there are 57 females and 63 males. Five patients are less than 20 years of age, including one 5-year-old child; 11 patients are more than 60 years of age.

On the basis of our original classification (8,10) (Fig. 1), 92 patients had an enclosed adenoma—33 within a grade 1 sella, 59 within a grade II sella—and 15 had a suprasellar expansion. Twenty-eight cases had an invasive lesion—

	Radiological classification	No. of Cases	GROUP I UNTREATED (90 cases)	GROUP II PREV. RADIATION (25 cases)	GROUP III PREV. SURGERY (5 cases)
GR. I	ENCLOSED MICROADENOMA (<10 mm)	33	25	8	0
GR. II	ADENOMA (>10 mm)	44	33	10	1
	WITH S.S.E	15	10	4	1
GR. III	INVASIVE ·LOCALISED	16	14	1	2
	WITH S.S.E	5	3	0	1
GR. IV	·DIFFUSE	4	3	1	0
	WITH S.S.E	3	2	1	0
TOTAL		120	90	25	5

FIG. 1. Classification of 120 cases of acromegaly. (S.S.E.) suprasellar extension.

21 in a grade III sella and 7 in a grade IV sella. Among these 28 cases, 8 had a suprasellar expansion. The entire series is divided into three groups as follows: group I, 90 untreated cases; group II, 25 cases previously treated by radiation; and group III, 5 cases previously treated by surgery (Fig. 1). In 72 untreated cases there appeared to be a correlation between the mean levels of hGH and the radiological grading of the sella turcica (Fig. 2).

The transsphenoidal open surgical approach (4–7) was used in all cases of this series. The extent of the surgical excision of the tumor was tailored to the individual case. Our criteria for assessing the extent of surgical excision are described elsewhere (8,9). Eighty-nine cases had a selective total removal (ST), 12 cases a selective subtotal removal (SS), 7 cases a nonselective subtotal removal (NSS), and 12 cases a nonselective total removal (NST), or complete sellar clean-out.

Surgical complications occurred in four cases. One patient died as a consequence of surgery. She was harbouring a grade IV invasive lesion previously treated with radiation. At surgery the tumor was firmly adherent to the walls of the sella turcica and the surrounding vascular structures. Difficult maneuvers to detach the fibrotic scar tissue were unsuccessful and resulted in vasospasm of the left carotid artery with subsequent infarction in the ipsilateral cerebral hemisphere. The patient died 4 months later of pneumonia. One patient had spontaneous profuse bleeding in the sella 10 days after surgery, requiring reopening and successful packing with muscle. One patient had a transitory fourth nerve palsy due to coagulation in the lateral corner of the sella. Another patient

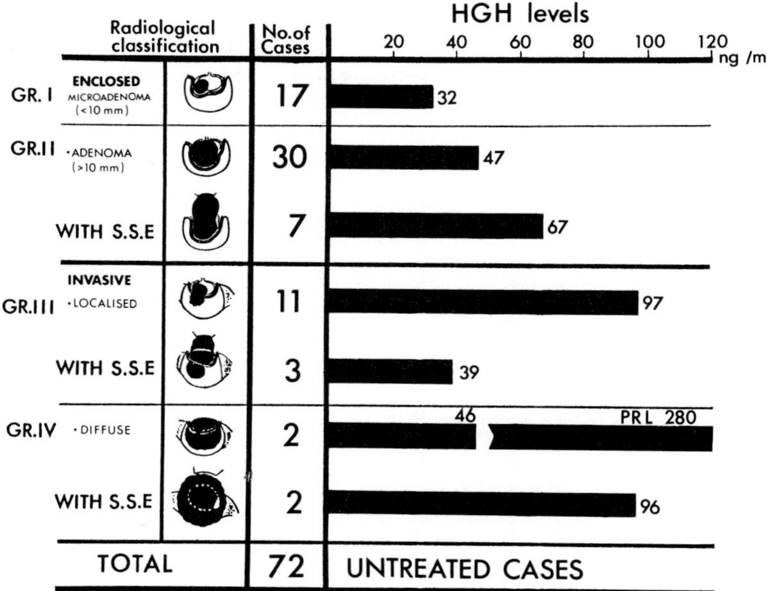

FIG. 2. Correlation between the mean levels of hGH and the radiological classification in 72 untreated cases of acromegaly. One case had also an elevated prolactin level of 280 ng/ml. (S.S.E.) suprasellar extension.

had a postoperative cerebrospinal fluid (CSF) rhinorrhea which was treated successfully by reoperation and duroplasty.

RESULTS

Our criteria for the evaluation of treatment in acromegaly (9) are briefly summarized here. Following treatment, a patient with active acromegaly may be:

Cured—when repeated basal plasma hGH levels have fallen to or below 5 ng/ml. If the plasma hGH is slightly elevated, it should be suppressed below 5 ng/ml under the oral glucose tolerance test (OGTT).

Improved—when the basal plasma hGH levels are significantly reduced by more than 50% of the preoperative levels but still remain above the normal range.

Unchanged—When the plasma hGH levels remain in the same range or have fallen by less than 50% of the preoperative levels.

As for the other pituitary functions, patients are classified as follows:

Unchanged—when the preoperative endocrine functions have not been modified by treatment.

Recovered—when the preoperative endocrine deficits are corrected by treatment.

GROUP I 90 UNTREATED CASES

	Radiological classification		No. of Cases	HGH Cured	HGH Improved	HGH Unchanged	OTHER FUNCTIONS REC.	OTHER FUNCTIONS UNCH.	DEFICIT P.	DEFICIT T.
GR. I	ENCLOSED MICROADENOMA (<10 mm)	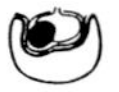	25	21	3	1	5	20	0	0
GR. II	·ADENOMA (>10 mm)	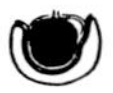	33	27	6	0	5	25	2	1
	WITH S.S.E	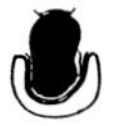	10	8	2	0	2	6	0	2
GR. III	INVASIVE ·LOCALISED	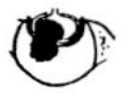	14	12	1	1	2	12	0	0
	WITH S.S.E	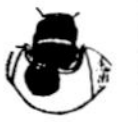	3	2	1	0	0	3	0	0
GR. IV	·DIFFUSE	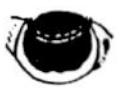	3	0	1	2	0	3	0	0
	WITH S.S.E	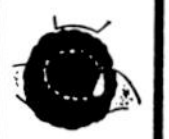	2	1	0	1	0	0	0	2
	TOTAL		90	71	14	5	14	69	2	5

FIG. 3. Results of TSS in 90 previously untreated cases of acromegaly. (S.S.E.) suprasellar extension. (UNCH.) unchanged. (REC.) recovered. (P) partial. (T) total.

Aggravated—when pituitary functions are impaired by treatment. Evaluation may be that of partial or total anterior pituitary insufficiency.

Group I: Previously Untreated Patients

Among the group of 90 patients with acromegaly who were previously untreated, 68 had an enclosed adenoma; 25 of the 68 had a microadenoma. In 43 cases of grade II, 10 had a suprasellar expansion. Twenty-two had an invasive lesion, 5 with a suprasellar expansion. Before treatment, other pituitary functions were normal in 63 patients (70%), whereas 26 (29%) had partial hypopituitarism and 1 had panhypopituitarism. Among these, 6 patients had two operations. Figure 3 indicates that 71 patients (79%) were clinically and biologically cured, 14 were improved (15%), and 5 remained unchanged (6%). Other pituitary functions remained unaltered in 69 cases, whereas 14 patients recovered preoperative partial pituitary insufficiency. Seven patients were aggravated by surgery, 5 in the course of a reoperation producing panhypopituitarism, and 2 unintentionally producing only partial insufficiency. Of the 6 patients who had a second operation, 3 were finally cured. Of the 3 others, 2 were further improved by radiotherapy.

Group II: Previously Treated by Radiation Only

Twenty-five patients (Fig. 4) had previously received radiation therapy ranging from 4,000 to 6,000 rads. The majority of the cases had been treated 2 to 10

GROUP II 25 RADIATION

Radiological classification		No. of Cases	HGH Cured	HGH Improved	HGH Unchanged	OTHER FUNCTIONS REC.	OTHER FUNCTIONS UNCH.	DEFICIT P.	DEFICIT T.
GR. I	ENCLOSED MICROADENOMA (<10 mm)	8	6	2	0	0	8	0	0
GR. II	·ADENOMA (>10 mm)	10	9	1	0	1	5	3	1
	WITH S.S.E	4	3	1	0	0	2	1	1
GR. III	INVASIVE ·LOCALISED	1	1	0	0	1	0	0	0
	WITH S.S.E	0	0	0	0	0	0	0	0
GR. IV	·DIFFUSE	1	0	0	1	0	1	0	0
	WITH S.S.E	1	0	1	0	0	1	0	0
TOTAL		25	19	5	1	2	17	4	2

FIG. 4. Results of TSS in 25 cases of acromegaly previously treated by irradiation only. (S.S.E.) suprasellar extension. See Fig. 3 for abbreviations.

years before surgery. In one patient visual impairment appeared at the end of radiation treatment 3 months before surgery. In another patient acute visual loss occurred during the course of radiotherapy, which was interrupted for emergency surgical decompression. At the time of referral, all patients had persistently elevated hGH; 10 (40%) had normal other pituitary functions, 13 (52%) partial hypopituitarism, and 2 (8%) panhypopituitarism. Therefore in this group of 25 cases, 60% had hypopituitarism before surgery compared with 29% in the group I (untreated) cases. From the radiological point of view, there were 22 enclosed adenomas (4 suprasellar expansions) and 3 invasive lesions (1 suprasellar expansion). Results are summarized in Fig. 4. After transsphenoidal surgery, hGH was normalized in 19 patients (76%). Five were further improved and 1 remained unchanged. The other pituitary functions remained unchanged in 17 cases (68%) whereas 2 patients recovered preoperative partial hypopituitarism. Six were aggravated, 2 voluntarily by total sellar clean-out, producing panhypopituitarism, and 4 had partial hypopituitarism produced by surgery. The patient with a diffuse invasive tumor (IV-B) who had a surgical complication was mentioned above.

Group III: Previously Treated by Surgery

Five patients (Fig. 5) had been previously operated on elsewhere, 3 by the intracranial route and two by TSS. Of these, 3 patients had received further radiation therapy. From the radiological point of view, there were 2 enclosed adenomas (1 suprasellar expansion) and 3 invasive lesions (1 suprasellar expan-

GROUP III PREVIOUS SURGERY (5 cases)

	Radiological classification	No. of Cases	HGH Cured	HGH Improved	HGH Unchanged	Other functions REC.	Other functions UNCH.	Other functions Deficit P.	Other functions Deficit T.
GR. I	ENCLOSED MICROADENOMA (<10 mm)	0	0	0	0	0	0	0	0
GR. II	·ADENOMA (>10 mm)	1	1	0	0	0	1	0	0
	WITH S.S.E	1	0	1	0	0	1	0	0
GR. III	INVASIVE ·LOCALISED	2	2	0	0	0	2	0	0
	WITH S.S.E	1	1	0	0	0	1	0	0
GR. IV	·DIFFUSE	0	0	0	0	0	0	0	0
	WITH S.S.E	0	0	0	0	0	0	0	0
	TOTAL	5	4	1	0	0	5	0	0

FIG. 5. Results of TSS in 5 cases of acromegaly previously treated by surgery. (S.S.E.) suprasellar extension. See Fig. 3 for abbreviations.

sion). Preoperatively 4 were suffering from panhypopituitarism that required complete hormonal replacement therapy, and 1 had partial hypopituitarism. Following transsphenoidal surgery (sellar clean-out), 4 patients were biologically cured (Fig. 5). In one patient previously treated by surgery and radiation therapy resulting in panhypopituitarism, the hGH was still markedly elevated to 339 ng/ml. Following transsphenoidal surgery, the value was reduced to 13.5 ng/ml. This patient is considered improved.

Summary

When compiling all results, regardless of the type of tumor (enclosed or invasive), the existence or absence of a suprasellar expansion, and the previously unsuccessful therapeutic management, the final results of the hGH levels in the three groups of patients are reported in Fig. 6. Ninety-four cases were cured (78%), 20 improved (17%), and 6 remained unchanged (5%). The other pituitary functions (Fig. 7) were not altered in 91 patients (76%), and 16 patients recovered from preoperative partial insufficiency (12%). The other pituitary functions were altered in 13 cases (11%): 6 patients developed partial hypopituitarism and 7 panhypopituitarism after total sellar clean-out (Fig. 7).

COMMENTS

In the treatment of acromegaly, the surgical excision of the secreting pituitary adenoma has the major advantage of producing an immediate fall of

	Radiological classification	No.of Cases	RESULTS ON HGH CURED	IMPROVED	UNCHANGED
GR. I	ENCLOSED MICROADENOMA (<10 mm)	33	27	5	1
GR.II	·ADENOMA (>10 mm)	44	36	8	0
	WITH S.S.E	15	12	3	0
GR.III	INVASIVE ·LOCALISED	16	14	1	1
	WITH S.S.E	5	4	1	0
GR.IV	·DIFFUSE	4	0	1	3
	WITH S.S.E	3	1	1	1
TOTAL		120	94	20	6

FIG. 6. Results on hGH levels in 120 cases of acromegaly. (S.S.E.) suprasellar extension.

hGH hypersecretion, occurring within minutes after removal of the tumor (9).

When the tumor tissue is totally excised, the hgH level is normalized and the patient can often be considered biologically cured on the day of surgery. This is reflected during the immediate postoperative days by obvious clinical changes: weight loss, reduction of the swollen soft tissue in the face, hands, and feet, and a general feeling of well-being.

Subtotal tumor removal often results in similar clinical improvement. However, biological evaluation reveals the persistence of slightly elevated hGH levels. The patients who are classified as biologically improved are often reluctant to undergo further treatment since they feel cured. Several patients in this group have been followed for more than 10 years without significant clinical evidence that the disease has progressed. Recurrence of headaches, perspiration, and arthralgias with persistence of elevated hGH deserves further treatment. If the lesion was enclosed, a second operation is considered.

The only patients who are resistant to surgery are those with a grade IV invasive lesion. Despite extensive excision of the tumor mass, the hGH remains elevated. In these cases radiation therapy may further destroy residual secreting tissue, resulting in clinical and biological improvement, but rarely is a biological cure achieved.

Partial pituitary endocrine insufficiency occurred unintentionally in 6 patients who had a large tumor. Seven patients developed panhypopituitarism as a result of either intentional total sellar clean-out in the course of reoperation or a desperate attempt to cure an invasive lesion. In contrast, the other pituitary functions remained unaltered by surgery in 91 cases (76%). Furthermore, 16 patients (13%) receovered from preoperative partial hypopituitarism.

	Radiological classification		No. of Cases	OTHER PITUITARY FUNCTIONS RECOVERED	UNCHANGED	DEFICIT PARTIAL	TOTAL
GR. I	ENCLOSED MICROADENOMA (<10 mm)		33	5	28	0	0
GR. II	ADENOMA (>10 mm)		44	6	31	5	2
	WITH S.S.E		15	2	9	1	3
GR. III	INVASIVE · LOCALISED		16	3	13	0	0
	WITH S.S.E		5	0	5	0	0
GR. IV	· DIFFUSE		4	0	4	0	0
	WITH S.S.E		3	0	1	0	2
TOTAL			120	16	91	6	7

FIG. 7. Results on other pituitary functions in 120 cases of acromegaly. (S.S.E.) suprasellar extension.

CONCLUSION

The unsuccessful cases encountered in grade IV diffuse invasive lesions are those that present a "stubborn therapeutic challenge" (1). Probably they shorten life expectancy. Fortunately these cases are rare, and earlier diagnosis and treatment will eventually eliminate them. In the meantime, further studies in the enzymatic and molecular biology of the tumor cell membranes are needed to understand better the nature of the invasive lesions that defy all therapeutic procedures so far available.

The cases that improved but were not biologically cured should be reassessed for further treatment. If the lesion was enclosed (grades I and II), identification of residual tumor tissue should be attempted with biopsies. Improvement in the surgeon's experience will provide a higher rate of cure.

Among the patients biologically cured by TSS tumor excision, we must distinguish: (a) Those who are cured with hypopituitarism. For some of these, panhypopituitarism was the *sine qua non* condition to reach a final cure. Partial hypopituitarism occurred infrequently. (b) The patients who have been cured without sustaining any other pituitary hormonal insufficiency. These present a unique opportunity for further understanding the pathophysiology of acromegaly. Patients who have reached a normal basal level of hGH but retain during the immediate postoperative course an abnormal dynamic reaction to the oral glucose tolerance test support the hypothesis of the hypothalamic disturbance of the regulatory factors (2). However, those who remain cured for many years with normal hGH dynamics plead against this hypothesis (8).

In our experience, the persistence of elevated hGH levels after treatment can only be explained by residual adenomatous hypersecreting tissue. Further complete removal provides a biological cure of acromegaly.

REFERENCES

1. Daughaday, W. H. (1970): Acromegaly—a stubborn therapeutic challenge. *N. Engl. J. Med.*, 282:1430–1431.
2. Daughaday, W. H., Cryer, P. E., and Jacobs, L. S. (1973): The role of the hypothalamus in the pathogenesis of pituitary tumors. In: *Diagnosis and Treatment of Pituitary Tumors,* edited by P. O. Kohler and G. T. Ross, pp. 26–34. Excerpta Medica/Elsevier, Amsterdam.
3. Hardy, J. (1969): Transsphenoidal microsurgery of the normal and pathological pituitary. *Clin. Neurosurg.,* 16:185–217.
4. Hardy, J. (1969): Microsurgery of the hypophysis: Subnasal transsphenoidal approach with television magnification and televised radiofluoroscopic control. In: *Microneurosurgery,* edited by R. W. Rand, pp. 87–103. Mosby, St. Louis.
5. Hardy, J. (1971): Transsphenoidal hypophysectomy: Neurosurgical techniques. *J. Neurosurg.,* 34:582–594.
6. Hardy, J. (1973): Transsphenoidal surgery of hypersecreting pituitary tumors. In: *Diagnosis and Treatment of Pituitary Tumors,* edited by P. O. Kohler and G. T. Ross, pp. 18–194. Excerpta Medica/Elsevier, Amsterdam.
7. Hardy, J. (1975): Transsphenoidal microsurgical removal of pituitary microadenoma. In: *Progress in Neurological Surgery,* edited by H. Krayenbuhl, P. E. Maspes, and W. H. Sweet, pp. 200–216. Karger, Basel.
8. Hardy, J., Robert, F., Somma, M., and Vezina, J. L. (1973): Acromégalie-gigantisme: Traitement chirurgical par exérése transsphénoidale de l'adénome hypophysaire. *Neurochirurgie, (Suppl 2),* 19:1–184.
9. Hardy, J., Somma, M., and Vezina, J. L. (1976): Treatment of acromegaly: radiation or surgery? In: *Current Controversies in Neurosurgery,* edited by J. P. Morley, pp. 377–391. Saunders, Philadelphia.
10. Hardy, J., and Vezina, J. L. (1976): Transphenoidal neurosurgery of intracranial neoplasm. In: *Advances in Neurology, Vol. 15: Neoplasia in the Central Nervous System,* edited by R. A. Thompson and J. R. Green, pp. 261–274. Raven Press, New York.

Clinical Management of Pituitary Disorders,
edited by G. T. Tindall and W. F. Collins.
Raven Press, New York © 1979.

12

Cushing's Disease and Nelson's Syndrome

James H. Christy

Department of Medicine (Endocrinology), Emory University School of Medicine, Atlanta, Georgia 30322

Cushing's disease (CD) as we understand it today is a form of endogenous hypercortisolism associated with bilateral adrenal cortical hyperplasia caused by pituitary ACTH hypersecretion (13). It remains debatable whether the primary source of the disease is in the hypothalamus (4,9) or the anterior hypophysis (10,19), but it is now quite clear that pituitary adenomas containing aggregates of ACTH-secreting cells are present in most patients who have the disorder (1,6,10,17,19). It thus seems that the most rational therapeutic approach would be the selective resection of the pituitary adenoma, leaving normal pituitary and adrenal function intact. This has been accomplished with transsphenoidal microsurgery, and the success of this method is now well documented in several large series (1,6,10,17,19). The only question yet to be answered is whether selective removal of the pituitary adenoma results in permanent cure of Cushing's disease. If a pituitary adenoma is the primary source of the problem and complete removal is accomplished, permanent remission should be achieved. If disordered hypothalamic function with inappropriate secretion of corticotropin-releasing factor (CRF) is the cause, however, recurrence of Cushing's disease can be expected in many patients. Only careful, long-term follow-up of patients treated by transsphenoidal microsurgery will resolve the question.

The increasing availability of transsphenoidal microsurgery makes it extremely important to identify accurately those patients with endogenous hypercortisolism due to Cushing's disease in contradistinction to those with Cushing's syndrome due to primary adrenal disease or ectopic ACTH-secreting lesions. To accomplish this, the physician must be thoroughly familiar with the varieties of Cushing's syndrome (Table 1) and able to design an appropriate battery of tests to confirm the presence and determine accurately the source of hypercortisolism. Obviously it would be a serious error in judgment to perform pituitary surgery on a patient with clinically suspected Cushing's disease who in actuality has an adrenal adenoma.

TABLE 1. *Causes of endogenous hypercortisolism (Cushing's syndrome)*

Primary source	Pathology	ACTH secretion	Cortisol secretion	Approximate % patients
Hypothalamus/pituitary (Cushing's disease)	Pituitary adenoma; adrenocortical hyperplasia	Increased	Increased	75
Adrenal	Adrenal adenoma	Decreased	Increased	20
	Adrenal carcinoma	Decreased	Increased	5
Ectopic secretion of ACTH	Carcinoma of lung, pancreas, kidney, thymus, thyroid (medullary); adrenocortical hyperplasia	Markedly increased	Increased	<1

CLINICAL RECOGNITION OF HYPERCORTISOLISM

Most clinicians are thoroughly familiar with the usually quoted classic features of Cushing's syndrome (regardless of etiology): "moon facies," truncal obesity, "buffalo hump," hypertension, thin skin, purple striae, ecchymoses, osteoporosis, amenorrhea and hirsutism in females, glucose intolerance, and emotional disorders. Although these features are suggestive, they are not pathognomonic of hypercortisolism, since many patients with exogenous obesity have the same

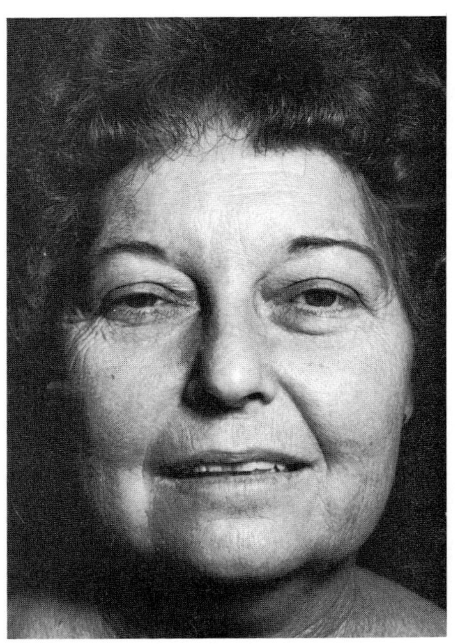

FIG. 1. Wide, rectangular appearance of face in a patient with Cushing's syndrome.

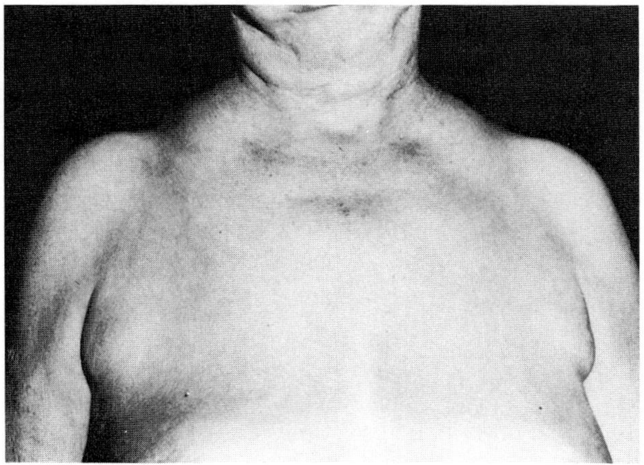

FIG. 2. Supraclavicular fat pad prominence characteristic of Cushing's syndrome.

manifestations. There are two helpful signs, however, localized to the face and supraclavicular areas which are invariably present in hypercortisolism and are useful for determining which patients should undergo screening tests. The face, instead of being round or moon-shaped as popularly described, has a wide, rectangular appearance due to extension of prominent cheek fat pads over the mandible with obliteration of the normal angle between the mandible and the horizonal plane of the chin (Fig. 1). Simple obesity causes a more-rounded appearance of the face with preservation of the angle and the normally sharp chin contours. The supraclavicular fat pads are characteristically prominent in CD and appear as convexities in the region adjacent to the base of the neck (Fig. 2). This peculiar distribution of fat has been present in every patient with endogenous or exogenous hypercortisolism seen at our institution, and is more valuable diagnostically than dorsal nuchal fat pad prominence (buffalo hump), which is inconsistently present. If a patient has either or both of these signs with or without any of the other manifestations of hypercortisolism he should undergo appropriate screening tests before being subjected to more extensive definitive studies.

SCREENING TESTS FOR HYPERCORTISOLISM

All forms of endogenous hypercortisolism are associated with (a) excessive secretion of cortisol that is nonsuppressible with standardized doses of exogenous glucocorticoids, and (b) loss of normal circadian rhythm in ACTH and cortisol secretion. The screening tests therefore should be devised to reflect these abnormalities (18). The preferred tests are listed in Table 2. Although not included in Table 2, measurements of 24-hr urine steroid excretions (17-hydroxysteroids, 17-ketosteroids, free cortisol) can be used in the screen, but these are of greater

TABLE 2. *Screening tests for hypercortisolism*

Test	Cortisol (μg/100 ml) by radioimmunoassay	
	Normal	Hypercortisolism
Morning serum cortisol (8:00 a.m.)	6–18	Usually >18
Evening serum cortisol (8:00 p.m.)	<8	Usually >14
Overnight dexamethasone suppression (serum cortisol at 8:00 a.m. after 1 mg dexamethasone at midnight)	<2	Usually > 8

value when used in the more definitive manipulative tests performed to confirm the presence of hypercortisolism and to establish its source.

DEFINITIVE TESTS FOR HYPERCORTISOLISM

If the clinical and screening laboratory data are strongly indicative of hypercortisolism, definitive tests must be done to confirm the diagnosis and to determine if pituitary hypersecretion of ACTH is the cause. These tests are well standardized (12,14,18,20) and are designed to reflect nonsuppressibility of cortisol secretion as well as responsiveness of ACTH secretion to an inhibitor of cortisol synthesis (metyrapone). Radioimmunoassay of plasma ACTH levels can be done optionally during the manipulative tests, but when used only in baseline studies a single ACTH level may be very misleading since it is often within the normal range in patients with Cushing's disease (1,20). Moreover, the assay is technically difficult and lacks the standardization of some of the other procedures. The preference therefore is to implement a protocol (Table 3) that involves measurement of reliable and simply determined parameters of pituitary/adrenal axis function during 48-hr segments under test conditions in the following sequence: control (48 hr), low-dose dexamethasone (0.5 mg every 6 hr × 48 hr), control (48 hr), and metyrapone (750 mg every 6 hr × 48 hr). Collection of 24-hr urine specimens for the determination of 17-hydroxycorticosteroid (17-OHCS), 17-ketosteroid (17-KS), and creatinine excretion (to confirm the accuracy of the collection and to allow correction for body size) are made daily throughout the entire protocol, and blood is obtained at the end of each test period for measuring serum cortisol and plasma ACTH (optional). Serum 11-desoxycortisol (cpd S) measurement is made only at the beginning and at the end of the metyrapone test period.

The characteristic test results for each type of hypercortisolism are listed in Table 4. It can be seen that in all forms of endogenous hypercortisolism urinary and plasma steroids are not suppressed during low-dose dexamethasone administration; only in patients with Cushing's disease is there a significant rise in the urinary steroids and serum 11-desoxycortisol during the metyrapone test

TABLE 3. *Protocol for evaluation of hypercortisolism*

Date	Day	Medication	24-Hour urinary excretion (mg/24 hr)			Serum cortisol (μg/100 ml)	Serum 11-desoxycortisol (μg/100 ml)	Plasma ACTH (pg/ml)
			17-OHCS	17-KS	Creatinine			
	1	Control	Daily ↓	Daily ↓	Daily ↓	a.m. p.m.		a.m. p.m.
	2	Control						
	3	Dexamethasone 0.5 mg q 6 hr						
	4	Dexamethasone 0.5 mg q 6 hr						
	5	Control				a.m.		a.m.
	6	Control						
	7	Metyrapone 750 mg q 6 hr				a.m.	a.m.	a.m.
	8	Metyrapone 750 mg q 6 hr						
	9	Day 9, a.m., completes protocol				a.m.	a.m.	a.m.

TABLE 4. *Manipulative test results in hypercortisolism*

Condition	24-Hr urinary 17-OHCS or free cortisol, second day		
	Baseline	Low-dose dexamethasone (0.5 mg q 6 hr × 2 days)	Metyrapone (750 mg q 6 hr × 2 days)
Normal	Normal	> 50% Suppression	2–3 × Baseline
Cushing's disease	Normal or ↑	< 50% Suppression	2–3 × Baseline
Adrenal adenoma	Normal or ↑	No suppression	No response or ↓
Adrenal carcinoma	Normal or ↑↑	No suppression	No response or ↓
Ectopic ACTH	↑↑↑	No suppression	No response or ↓

period. The reason for this differential response pattern is that in Cushing's disease the secretion of ACTH is inappropriate for a given plasma level of cortisol, but it is not completely autonomous and may be the result of a disordered hypothalamic/pituitary/adrenal axis in which the set-point of the negative feedback system between cortisol and ACTH is displaced to a higher level (13). Thus inhibition of cortisol synthesis by metyrapone in patients with Cushing's disease results in increased ACTH secretion, hence, increased plasma 11-desoxycortisol levels (greater than 7 ng/100 ml) and increased 24-hr urinary excretion of 17-OHCS and 17-KS (two to three times baseline). The failure of metyrapone to evoke a positive response in patients with nonpituitary sources of hypercortisolism (whether adrenal tumor or extrapituitary ACTH-secreting neoplasm) can be attributed to profound inhibition of normal pituitary ACTH-secreting mechanisms by high levels of cortisol resulting from autonomous secretion of an adrenal tumor or from ectopic ACTH-induced adrenocortical hyperfunction. This inhibition cannot be overcome by the normally potent stimulus of acutely reduced cortisol synthesis. We tested more than 20 patients with endogenous hypercortisolism and never observed false-positive or false-negative responses during the metyrapone test period.

The high-dose dexamethasone suppression test (2 mg every 6 hr × 48 hr) has been deleted from this protocol because of its poor differential value in as many as 15% of patients with Cushing's disease who show no suppressibility of urinary steroid excretion with this or even higher doses of dexamethasone (20). This response is indistinguishable from that obtained in patients with adrenal tumors or ectopic sources of ACTH secretion and necessitates the use of metyrapone for final differentiation.

In summary, the preoperative diagnosis of Cushing's disease rests on the clinical recognition of hypercortisolism, the laboratory findings of incompletely suppressible cortisol hypersecretion, and normal responsiveness of the urinary steroids and serum 11-desoxycortisol during metyrapone administration. If these criteria are satisfied, one can assume that pituitary hypersecretion of ACTH is present and can make a therapeutic decision accordingly.

EVALUATION OF PITUITARY ANATOMY AND FUNCTION

Since the diagnosis of Cushing's disease in a given patient presupposes the presence of a pituitary adenoma, it is reasonable to obtain as much information as possible relating to pituitary structure and function before treatment is initiated. These data are obtained in the manner outlined in Chapter 7 and include the minimal data protocol for testing pituitary function, sella polytomography, CT scan of the head, and visual field tests. Rarely is it necessary to perform pneumoencephalography or carotid arteriography because most pituitary adenomas associated with Cushing's disease are small and confined to the sella. If pneumonencephalography is done, and air is demonstrated in the sella, a pituitary microadenoma is not ruled out since the coexistence of a pituitary tumor and empty sella has been documented in a number of patients (3,5).

Pituitary functional abnormalities unrelated to ACTH hypersecretion are not generally seen, but a few patients have shown evidence of prolactin hypersecretion with or without galactorrhea (1). Even those without hyperprolactinemia show evidence of abnormal prolactin secretory mechanisms as reflected by inadequate prolactin response to chlorpromazine administration, a finding present in most patients with pituitary tumors, regardless of type.

TREATMENT

On the basis of the experience reported by Hardy (6), Salassa et al. (17), and Tyrrell et al. (19), the initial treatment of choice is transsphenoidal microsurgery, provided neurosurgical expertise in the use of this procedure is available. If not, bilateral adrenalectomy combined with conventional pituitary irradiation is quite acceptable, although it necessitates life-long glucocorticoid replacement therapy (16). Heavy-particle or proton-beam irradiation (7,11) of the pituitary gland is effective, but the risk of immediate or delayed impairment of normal pituitary function seems to be higher than with transsphenoidal microsurgery. In the patient considered to be at high risk for surgery because of hypertensive cardiovascular or other medical complications concurrent with Cushing's disease, pituitary irradiation may be the preferred treatment. An alternative would be the use of metyrapone (750 mg every 6 hr) combined with a maintenance dose of glucocorticoid to ameliorate the clinical manifestations of the disease. By this method the patient's general condition may improve sufficiently to allow definitive treatment with surgery. A promising drug that may be used for the same purpose is cyproheptadine, an antiserotonin agent which has been shown to produce clinical and biochemical remission in some patients presumably by suppressing abnormal ACTH secretion (8). The prospect of using cyproheptadine as the sole therapy for Cushing's disease on a long-term basis remains to be explored. Other alternatives include the use of *o,p'*-dichlorodiphenyl-dichloroethane (*o,p'* DDD) and aminogluthemide, but the relative toxicity of these agents limits their use to short-term therapy.

Medical management of the patient undergoing transsphenoidal microsurgery for Cushing's disease is the same as for patients with other types of pituitary tumor. The main concerns are proper corticosteroid coverage and monitoring for diabetes insipidus (2). Hydrocortisone in divided dosage of 300 mg on the day of surgery is gradually tapered over 5 to 7 days to a physiologic dose range of 30 to 40 mg daily. It is advisable to continue physiologic doses of hydrocortisone (or analog equivalent) for 6 to 12 months following surgery because of the usual lag time for recovery of the normal pituitary/adrenal axis. Early discontinuation of the steroid supplement results in extremely severe withdrawal symptoms (nausea, anorexia, weakness, hypotension, and depression) which necessitate reinstitution.

The time required for recovery of normal pituitary/adrenal axis function may be 6 to 12 months or longer (1,10,19). Restitution of normal function is reflected in normal serum cortisol levels, normal circadian periodicity, normal 24-hr urine steroid excretion, and normal suppressibility during low-dose dexamethasone administration.

Other pituitary functions found to be intact before surgery usually remain normal after selective removal of the pituitary adenoma, but this should be confirmed with a repeat of general pituitary function tests 10 days or more after surgery.

NELSON'S SYNDROME

The syndrome of intensive skin pigmentation and varying manifestations of pituitary tumor occurring several years after bilateral adrenalectomy for Cushing's disease was described by Nelson et al. in 1959 (15). Believed initially to be the consequence of unrestrained secretory and proliferative activity of ACTH-secreting cells due to the inadequate negative feedback effect of physiologic corticosteroid replacement therapy, it more than likely represents intensified activity of the pituitary tumor that was present before adrenalectomy. Occurring in approximately 10% of patients treated with bilateral adrenalectomy alone, it is seen much less frequently in patients receiving combined adrenalectomy and pituitary irradiation therapy as initial treatment for Cushing's disease (16).

Extremely elevated plasma ACTH levels (greater than 200 pg/ml) with loss of circadian rhythmicity and failure to suppress with low-dose dexamethasone administration can be demonstrated in most patients. By the time of clinical recognition, the pituitary tumor is usually large and often infiltrative, making definitive treatment mandatory. Unfortunately, complete ablation of the tumor is difficult to achieve with either selective resection or pituitary irradiation. It is recommended, therefore, that these patients receive total hypophysectomy with supplementary pituitary irradiation therapy as indicated by evidence of extrasellar extension of the tumor or continued ACTH hypersecretion following surgery (21).

REFERENCES

1. Bigos, S. T., Robert, F., Pelletier, G., and Hardy, J. (1977): Cure of Cushing's disease by transsphenoidal removal of a microadenoma from a pituitary gland despite a radiographically normal sella turcica. *J. Clin. Endocrinol. Metab.,* 45:1251–1260.
2. Christy, J. H., and Tindall, G. T. (1977): Endocrinologic diagnosis of pituitary tumor: Indications for surgery and pre- and postoperative management. *Clin. Neurosurg.,* 24:151–166.
3. Domingue, J. N., Wing, S. D., and Wilson, C. B. (1978): Coexisting pituitary adenomas and partially empty sellas. *J. Neurosurg.,* 48:23–28.
4. Feldman, J. M. (1975): Cushing's disease: A hypothalamic flush? *N. Engl. J. Med.,* 293:930–931.
5. Ganguly, A., Stanchfield, J. B., Roberts, T. S., West, C. D., and Tyler, F. H. (1976): Cushing's syndrome in a patient with an empty sella turcica and a microadenoma of the adenohypophysis. *Am. J. Med.,* 60:306–309.
6. Hardy, J. (1973): Transsphenoidal surgery of hypersecreting pituitary tumors. In: *Diagnosis and Treatment of Pituitary Tumors,* edited by P. O. Kohler and G. T. Ross, pp. 179–194. Elsevier, New York.
7. Kjellberg, R. N., and Kliman, B. (1973): A system for therapy of pituitary tumors. In: *Diagnosis and Treatment of Pituitary Tumors,* edited by P. O. Kohler and G. T. Ross, pp. 243–252. Elsevier, New York.
8. Krieger, D. T., Amorosa, L., and Linick, F. (1975): Cyproheptadine-induced remission of Cushing's disease. *N. Engl. J. Med.,* 293:893–896.
9. Krieger, D. T., and Glick, S. M. (1972): Growth hormone and cortisol responsiveness in Cushing's syndrome: Relation to a possible central nervous system etiology. *Am. J. Med.,* 52:25–40.
10. Lagerquist, L. G., Meikle, A. W., West, C. D., and Tyler, F. H. (1974): Cushing's disease with cure by resection of a pituitary adenoma: Evidence against a primary hypothalamic defect. *Am. J. Med.,* 57:826–830.
11. Lawrence, J. H., Choung, C. Y., Lyman, J. T., Tobias, C. A., Born, J. L., Garcia, J. F., Manougian, E., Linfoot, J. A., and Connell, G. M. (1973): Treatment of pituitary tumors with heavy particles. In: *Diagnosis and Treatment of Pituitary Tumors,* edited by P. O. Kohler and G. T. Ross, pp. 253–262. Elsevier, New York.
12. Liddle, G. W. (1960): Tests of pituitary-adrenal suppressibility in the diagnosis of Cushing's syndrome. *J. Clin. Endocrinol. Metab.,* 20:1539–1560.
13. Liddle, G. W. (1972): Pathogenesis of glucocorticoid disorders. *Am. J. Med.,* 53:638–648.
14. Liddle, G. W., Estep, H. L., Kendall, J. W., Williams, W. C., and Townes, A. W. (1959): Clinical application of a new test of pituitary reserve. *J. Clin. Endocrinol. Metab.,* 19:875–894.
15. Nelson, D. H., Menkin, J. W., and Thorn, G. W. (1960): ACTH-producing pituitary tumors following adrenalectomy for Cushing's syndrome. *Ann. Intern., Med.,* 52:560–569.
16. Orth, D. N., and Liddle, G. W. (1971): Results of treatment in 108 patients with Cushing's syndrome. *N. Engl. J. Med.,* 285:243–247.
17. Salassa, R. M., Laws, E. R., Jr., and Carpenter, P. C. (1978): Transsphenoidal removal of pituitary microadenoma in Cushing's disease. *Mayo Clin. Proc.,* 53:24–28.
18. Tyler, F. H., and West, C. D. (1972): Laboratory evaluation of disorders of the adrenal cortex. *Am. J. Med.,* 53:664–672.
19. Tyrrell, J. B., Brooks, R. M., Fitzgerald, P. A., Cofoid, P. B., Forsham, P. H., and Wilson, C. B. (1978): Cushing's disease: Selective trans-sphenoidal resection of pituitary microadenomas. *N. Engl. J. Med.,* 298:753–758.
20. Weiss, E. R., Rayyis, S. S., Nelson, D. H., and Bethune, J. E. (1969): Evaluation of stimulation and suppression tests in the etiological diagnosis of Cushing's syndrome. *Ann. Intern. Med.,* 71:941–949.
21. Wilson, C. B., and Dempsey, L. C. (1978): Transsphenoidal microsurgical removal of 250 pituitary adenomas. *J. Neurosurg.,* 48:13–22.

Clinical Management of Pituitary Disorders,
edited by G. T. Tindall and W. F. Collins.
Raven Press, New York © 1979.

13

Neurosurgical Aspects of Cushing's Disease and Nelson's Syndrome

* Charles B. Wilson, ** J. Blake Tyrrell, ** Paul A. Fitzgerald, and *Lawrence Pitts

** Department of Neurological Surgery and **Metabolic Research Unit and Department of Medicine, University of California San Francisco, San Francisco, California 94143*

With his characteristic slavish devotion to detail, Harvey Cushing presented and subsequently published his extraordinary study of basophilic pituitary adenomas (1). Validation of his observations followed long after his death through the fortunate coincidence of two developments: first, conclusive biochemical definition of pituitary-based hypercortisolism became possible, for the first time differentiating this distinct clinical entity from other causes of hypercortisolism (3,4); and second, the evolution of transsphenoidal microsurgery not only provided an effective means of treating the disease but also permitted unequivocal documentation of ACTH-secreting microadenomas as a distinct entity (2). Because it is now possible in one maneuver to detect and remove minute adenomas situated in a pituitary gland of normal dimensions, there has been a revolutionary change in the management of Cushing's disease. Until a superior form of treatment evolves, microsurgical removal of these remarkably occult adenomas offers a high probability of restoring normal pituitary function to patients affected with the disease.

The endocrinologic data from our series of patients was presented separately (5), and the subject at hand is the surgical perspective based on these cases. When faced with a patient carrying the diagnosis of Cushing's disease, the surgeon assumes that the pituitary gland contains an ACTH-secreting adenoma.

PREOPERATIVE EVALUATION FOR TRANSSPHENOIDAL EXPLORATION

In experienced hands the operation requires 2 hr of general anesthesia, and to date transsphenoidal exploration has not been rejected as a form of treatment because of a patient's poor general health. Although many patients are seriously ill in a metabolic sense, most if not all can be prepared adequately for an operative procedure of this magnitude.

To determine the approximate size of an intrasellar adenoma and to define exactly any extrasellar extension, the surgeon requires hypocycloidal polytomograms of the sella and sphenoid sinus and a pneumoencephalogram with polytomographic sections at 2-mm intervals.

Tomograms of the sella may be normal, in which instance the tumor is small (in the range of 5 mm or less), and its location can be determined only by exploring the normal gland. If the sella is enlarged, the point of focal expansion indicates the tumor's position. The degree of sellar enlargement, focal and generalized, provides a reasonable estimate of the tumor's size subject to modification by pneumoencephalographic findings. A surprising number of ACTH-secreting adenomas, small as well as large, penetrate dura and bone to occupy the sphenoid sinus; and although none has extended into the body of the incompletely pneumatized sphenoid, undoubtedly this tumor has the potential to do so. Finally, the surgeon determines the anatomy of the sphenoid sinus and its septations. Because the majority of patients with Cushing's disease have osteoporotic bones as a consequence of longstanding hypercortisolism, the desired detail may not be obtained even with polytomograms taken at 1-mm intervals.

Pneumoencephalography is an unpleasant procedure at best, and at worst it causes headache, vomiting, and incapacitation, sometimes continuing for several days. Sharp definition of the subarachnoid cisterns in direct proximity to a tumor's superior surface affords clear visualization of small suprasellar tumor nodules and, less often, extension of the suprasellar cistern into the sella, a finding that may indicate prior necrosis of the adenoma. Computerized tomographic (CT) scans can demonstrate large suprasellar extensions that deform the subarachnoid cisterns, but the technique does not permit detection of the small and usually eccentric suprasellar extensions more likely to be encountered in Cushing's disease. Recently we used a newly developed water-soluble iodinated contrast medium instead of air, and the same detailed anatomy can be portrayed with minimal morbidity.

In a few cases we omitted pneumoencephalography because the sellar tomograms were normal and the patient's general condition was poor. Carotid angiography was performed on all patients early in our experience, but the discomfort and risk were not justified by the information obtained, and angiography has been eliminated as a routine preoperative test.

OPERATIVE APPROACH FOR TRANSSPHENOIDAL EXPLORATION

The transsphenoidal procedure developed by Hardy is followed without significant modification (2). Because the designated subject is the adenoma whose diameter measures less than 10 mm (i.e., microadenoma), removal of larger tumors is not considered.

At the outset, the surgeon recognizes the difficulties involved when approaching a normal sella. Microadenomas seldom present on the exposed surface of the anterior lobe, and with few exceptions the tumor's location must be determined by entering an apparently normal gland. Adequate exploration for a small tumor requires wide exposure: laterally to the edge of both cavernous sinuses, superiorly to the junction of diaphragma sellae and tuberculum, and inferiorly to the horizontal plane of the sellar floor. In two cases early in our experience, the presence of large dural venous sinuses overlying the gland precluded adequate exploration in a bloodless field, and in both instances the operation was abandoned without opening the dura.

The operative approach is based on a series of 37 adenomas, with completed postoperative testing and follow-up for 4 to 56 months after operation. Microadenomas (diameter 9 mm or less) accounted for 31 tumors, 4 of which had extended beyond the sella: 1 perforated the floor of the sella to present in the sphenoid sinus, 1 extended extradurally beneath the cavernous sinus, and 2 had small suprasellar nodules. The majority of microadenomas (20 of 31) measured 5 mm or less (Table 1). Particular difficulty may be encountered in locating adenomas 3 mm and smaller, the size of 10 tumors in this group. The two smallest tumors, 1.5 and 1 mm, were missed at the time of exploration, and both were identified in serial sections through the totally excised glands.

When the tumor's intrasellar location is known either from tomographic changes or by direct inspection of the exposed anterior lobe, removal follows the technique described by Hardy (2). With no clue to the tumor's location,

TABLE 1. *Size of pituitary adenomas in Cushing's disease*

Size of adenoma (mm)	No. of adenomas
Microadenomas	
1	2
2	5
3	3
4	3
5	7
6	3
7	2
8	3
9	3
Total	31
Macroadenomas	
10	3
15	1
20	1
30	1
Total	6
Grand total	37

the surgeon must make stepwise incisions into the gland. In our series the tumors were distributed almost equally in the lateral lobes and middle of the anterior lobe. Two tumors occupied the pars intermedia and posterior lobe, where the customarily clear delineation of tumor from normal anterior lobe is lacking.

Until an unlocalized tumor is identified, the following steps are carried out in order:

1. A horizontal incision is made completely across the midportion of the anterior lobe, bisecting the gland, to expose the posterior lobe at the depth of the incision.
2. A vertical incision is extended from the gland's upper surface to the sellar floor, first in the midline and then into each lateral lobe.
3. The surface of the gland lying against each cavernous sinus and on the floor of the sella is inspected.
4. The superior surface of the anterior lobe beneath the diaphragma sellae is visualized *if* the preoperative pneumoencephalogram did not conclusively exclude a suprasellar nodule.
5. With the anterior lobe now divided into eight sections, any of the eight sections that are disproportionately large should be incised.
6. Finally, if the patient understands the implications of total hypophysectomy and has agreed beforehand, the pituitary stalk is sectioned and the entire pituitary gland excised and submitted for pathologic examination.

With five exceptions, soft, dull, white to gray adenomas were sharply demarcated from adjacent anterior lobe and dura. Three tumors, each measuring 2 mm, were atypical: the pathologic nature of the tissue was unequivocal, but the appearance suggested a focal area of softening rather than a discrete neoplastic nodule. Two tumors occupied the pars intermedia and posterior lobe, and because of similarities in color as well as texture, these adenomas were removed along with the immediately adjacent posterior lobe.

A curative operation demands strict attention to details. The surgeon must visualize the entire surface of the cavity that remains after gross removal of the adenoma. This may require additional incisions into the overlying anterior lobe; and if the tumor is small and lies posteriorly, adequate visualization often dictates removal of a 2 to 3-mm wedge of normal anterior lobe. Because of its remarkable resiliency and an apparent capacity to re-establish vascular connections when separated into islands by multiple exploratory incisions, the described maneuvers did not impair anterior lobe function, as determined by postoperative testing.

Thorough inspection of the cavity should be carried out under high magnification in a bloodless field. Unless the tumor rests against the cavernous sinus—in which instance the most anterior surface may be obscured by a medial extension of the cavernous sinus across the sella—the tumor's bed can be visualized directly. Mirrors are useful aids for removing macroadenomas, but their use is no substitute for direct inspection.

Frozen sections of grossly normal anterior lobe are not obtained. The demarcation between anterior lobe and tumor is distinct, and anything beyond token sampling with frozen sections is considered unnecessary in view of the small number of recurrences in a large series of endocrine-active adenomas. Perhaps a few clonogenic neoplastic cells penetrate the apparently uninvolved anterior lobe; but if so, present evidence suggests that they are destroyed by alcohol.

Alcohol is used liberally to destroy cells that almost certainly remain in microscopic clusters or sheets. The only contraindication to the use of alcohol is a wide aperture into the subarachnoid space, but this situation arises only rarely when removing small tumors. Alcohol (absolute) is introduced into the cavity with a blunt needle followed by tight packing of the cavity with Gelfoam soaked in alcohol. The latter maneuver restores the cavity to its original size and thereby ensures that the entire surface is exposed to the necrotizing action of alcohol. Irrigation and packing are alternated several times, and finally alcohol-saturated Gelfoam is left within the cavity. Depending on the size and position of the cavity, and therefore the potential for postoperative cerebrospinal rhinorrhea, fat or muscle may be used to pack the tumor cavity. We follow Hardy's technique for closing the sella with nasal septal cartilage.

We detected no clinically significant damage to anterior lobe function as a result of the multiple incisions and prolonged exposure to absolute alcohol during the course of identifying and removing these adenomas. Of 12 patients tested serially following selective removal of microadenomas, 11 have had normal values after conventional pituitary stimulation tests, and the remaining patient had normal values except for a blunted response of growth hormone following L-DOPA stimulation. All premenopausal women are menstruating normally; one became pregnant and delivered a normal child.

RESULTS OF OPERATIONS

The outcome of operations in our first 20 patients was published previously (5). Included in that report were two patients in whom the pituitary gland was not entered because the presence of large dural venous sinuses precluded adequate exploration for a microadenoma. Rather than risk the complications of a potentially inconclusive search under these adverse circumstances, the operation was abandoned.

Disregarding these two cases, intrasellar exploration was carried out in 37 patients between February 1974 and May 1978. Pituitary adenomas were removed in each case. The results of operation in the 31 patients who had microadenomas are shown in Table 2; the period of follow-up ranged from 6 months to 4 years 9 months. Remission was achieved in 28 cases (90%): selective adenomectomy was performed successfully in 25 cases (80%); in three cases the disease

TABLE 2. *Microadenomas: operative results in 31 cases*

Treatment and result	No.	%
Selective removal of adenoma without recurrence	25	80
Adenoma missed, total hypophysectomy	2	
Adenoma removed, subsequent hypophysectomy	1	
Control of disease	28	90
Initial incomplete removal	2[a]	
Initial remission, subsequent recurrence	1	
Failure of operation	3	10

[a] One patient in remission after alpha-particle pituitary irradiation. One patient improved, with subsequent negative re-exploration.

was controlled following total hypophysectomy. Selective removal of a macroadenoma was successful in three cases (50%), and in the other three removal was known to be incomplete at the time of operation.

The details of preoperative testing and follow-up endocrine evaluation were described in the earlier report (5). The results in the present series were judged by the same criteria. Among the entire group there have been no deaths and no serious operative complications.

ANALYSIS OF OPERATIVE FAILURE

The two smallest tumors, 1.5 and 1.0 mm, were missed at exploration, and in all probability some tumors of this size will be missed in the future. Seven tumors either were removed incompletely or recurred after initial correction of hypercortisolism. Three failures (two primary failures and one recurrence) were macroadenomas. The present analysis involves four microadenomas.

In two patients who had undergone what was thought to be complete and selective removal of their 5-mm adenomas, hypercortisolism persisted during the immediate postoperative period. One, a young female, was referred for heavy-particle irradiation. The other, a male medical student, was improved and a year later requested reoperation at which time no additional tumor was identified. Except for mild hypercortisolism he has normal pituitary function and at this point declines further treatment.

The third microadenoma failure was a middle-aged female from whom a 2-mm tumor was removed. She too had persisting hypercortisolism during the early postoperative period; because of alarming hypertension she elected to undergo reoperation and, if no additional tumor could be identified and removed selectively, total hypophysectomy. When no tumor was identified at reoperation, total removal of the anterior and posterior lobes was performed. Serial sections through the excised gland failed to disclose either an adenoma or hyperplasia of ACTH-secreting cells, although this secondary procedure corrected the hypercortisolism.

The fourth patient had a microadenoma that extended beneath the right cavernous sinus, and its location precluded removal under direct vision. Complete removal was considered doubtful, and an effort was made to destroy nonvisualized tumor with alcohol. Although hypercortisolism was corrected when tested 4 months after operation, recurrence was documented within 1 year. In this instance the tumor could not be completely removed because of its position.

DISCUSSION

Transsphenoidal microsurgical removal of the adenomas that cause Cushing's disease has proved to be a therapeutically successful procedure, although the results to date have not resolved the seminal roles of the hypothalamus and adenohypophysis. However, until more specific or selective therapy becomes available, the described operative approach should replace adrenalectomy for the initial management of this condition. The reported results are good, and with further experience improvement is almost inevitable.

Cushing's disease is an uncommon entity, the diagnosis, treatment, and long-term endocrine supervision of which can be (and often are) difficult. The operative identification and removal of the ACTH-secreting adenomas taxes and may exceed the technical virtuosity of experienced surgeons. The preceding factors (i.e., the rarity of Cushing's disease and the technical demands of removing the offending microadenomas) argue forcefully for the selective referral of these patients to surgeons who have had extensive experience in pituitary microsurgery. Obviously, younger surgeons must gain experience in transsphenoidal operations, but that experience can and should be gained while treating the vastly larger number of patients with other endocrine-active and endocrine-inactive pituitary tumors.

The exciting activity in neuroendocrinology and the emerging role of transsphenoidal operations for certain endocrine disorders should be predictive of rapid advances in both fields, and no single group will derive greater benefit than patients affected with Cushing's disease. The state of the art at the time of Cushing's death denied him the satisfaction that comes with confirmation of one's pioneering observations and the honor of eponymic designation.

NELSON'S SYNDROME

With no evidence to the contrary, we assume that every patient with Nelson's syndrome harbors an ACTH-secreting pituitary adenoma, a point of view that finds support in our experience with 19 patients, each of whom underwent operative verification of a tumor. The interval between adrenalectomy and transsphenoidal exploration ranged from 7 months to 18 years. This wide range reflects the unpredictable behavior of the adenomas causing Nelson's syndrome. The indolent course exhibited by many of these tumors has fostered a complacent attitude in some quarters, but such an attitude ignores the extremely aggressive or frankly malignant behavior of a significant minority.

In our series of 19 patients treated by transsphenoidal operation, three died later as a direct result of their tumors, and during the same period a fourth patient died from recurrent tumor following craniotomy and postoperative irradiation. Our current attitude toward the role of transsphenoidal microsurgery in the management of Nelson's syndrome has been influenced by experience with these 19 operations and serial observations of patients who received no treatment for their presumed adenomas.

Ten of the 19 tumors had a diameter of 10 mm or greater, in contrast to the 16% of macroadenomas in the Cushing's disease series. Not surprising was the frequency of visual complaints, three patients presenting with diplopia and an additional two patients with loss of vision. Cavernous sinus involvement in two patients accounted for trigeminal anesthesia.

At the time of operation only five tumors were known to be incompletely removed. The surgeon thought that gross total removal had been achieved in the remaining 14 tumors. Of note is the fact that 6 patients had undergone prior pituitary irradiation and their tumors had no distinguishing gross characteristics.

Using the return of plasma ACTH to normal as the sole criterion of success, only four patients were cured by operation. One of the four died later, and another exhibited panhypopituitarism. One patient who had a minimally elevated plasma ACTH before operation and later died, did not have a postoperative ACTH determination.

Of the 16 living patients, 2 have undergone pituitary irradiation and 1 had a second operation (craniotomy); ACTH levels in all 3 remain elevated. Serial polytomograms of the sella indicated clinically silent growth of several tumors, and in other cases progressive increases in plasma ACTH levels were unaccompanied by radiographic change.

A review of our experience poses two questions: by what criteria should patients with Nelson's syndrome be selected for treatment, and what role does transsphenoidal surgery play in the treatment of those patients selected? We have partial and tentative answers to these questions based on the following presumptions:

1. Nelson's syndrome is produced by a pituitary adenoma capable of ACTH production and progressive growth.
2. A significant but still uncertain proportion of these tumors can exhibit aggressive behavior leading to disability and death.
3. In the majority of tumors, growth is slow and many remain as microadenomas during several years of observation.
4. Failure of ACTH levels to fall to normal following selective removal of microadenomas contrasts with the restoration of normal ACTH after removal of similar tumors in patients with functioning adrenal glands. This difference suggests that the pathology in Nelson's syndrome may involve more than a single discrete adenoma. We have no evidence implicating multiple adenomas,

diffuse corticotropic hyperplasia, or continuing overproduction of a corticotropin-releasing hormone.

Noncontroversial indications for treatment relate to the adenoma as an expanding mass. Any tumor that either attains a diameter of 10 mm or extends beyond the sella should be treated aggressively by irradiation or operation as the first step. If radiation therapy is selected, a decision must be made regarding the appropriate type of radiation to be employed. In chapter 16, Sheline presents data favoring heavy-particle irradiation over megavoltage X-irradiation. However, heavy-particle irradiation is suitable only for adenomas confined to the sella. Tumors with an extrasellar component should be treated by radical transsphenoidal removal with exenteration of the sella unless the extrasellar component is inaccessible. If transsphenoidal removal is selected as the primary treatment of an adenoma that has a diameter of 10 mm or greater, but remains entirely intrasellar, we currently recommend exenteration of the sella in all patients except children. This procedure should be followed by irradiation if the radical approach proves to be unsuccessful.

The management of microadenomas is a subject characterized by strong opinions, controversy, and uncertainty. Many patients go untreated and remain healthy for years. Others are referred for some form of irradiation. Certain patients, after considering the options, elect transsphenoidal removal. Among the latter group, selective removal of the adenoma can be justified in children and informed young adults, but older adults are advised to undergo total hypophysectomy.

Any tumor may, at some time, begin to produce manifestations of an expanding mass; should this occur, a more radical approach is clearly indicated for all patients except the elderly. We anticipate that the incidence of Nelson's syndrome will decrease as bilateral adrenalectomy is abandoned in favor of direct approaches to the pituitary gland.

SUMMARY

In a series of 37 patients referred for the treatment of Cushing's disease, transsphenoidal exploration of the sella disclosed either a focal area of softening with inadequate tissue for histologic examination or an adenoma in all but 2 cases. In these 2 cases total hypophysectomy was performed when exploration disclosed no focal abnormality; on serial sectioning, adenomas measuring 1.5 and 0.5 mm, respectively, were found in the glands of the patients.

Our experience with Nelson's syndrome in 19 patients has been disappointing to the extent that our current recommendation is total hypophysectomy, except in children and possibly in young adults. Although the tumor's behavior following adrenalectomy is unpredictable, it has an aggressive potential that argues for initial radical therapy.

For the purposes of management, it must be assumed that every patient with documented Cushing's disease harbors a pituitary adenoma, the operative removal of which is curative with preservation of normal pituitary function in the majority of cases. It follows that every patient with Nelson's syndrome has a corticotropin-producing tumor, either overt or occult. For reasons that remain unclear, these tumors have a high potential for malignant behavior; consequently the therapeutic approach should be uncompromising unless retention of anterior pituitary function is elected by the patient in full knowledge of the liability for recurrence.

ACKNOWLEDGMENTS

This investigation was supported in part by grants from the Levi J. and Mary C. Skaggs Foundation of Oakland, California; the Susan Greenwall Foundation of New York City; and (at the General Clinical Research Center of the University of California, San Francisco) by funds provided by the Division of Research Resources (RR-79), U.S. Public Health Service.

REFERENCES

1. Cushing, H. (1932): The basophil adenomas of the pituitary body and their clinical manifestations (pituitary basophilism). *Bull. Johns Hopkins Hosp.,* 50:137–197.
2. Hardy, J. (1973): Transsphenoidal surgery of hypersecreting pituitary tumors. In: *Diagnosis and Treatment of Pituitary Tumors,* edited by P. O. Kohler and G. T. Ross, pp. 179–194. American Elsevier, New York.
3. Liddle, G. W. and Shute, A. M. (1969): The evolution of Cushing's syndrome as a clinical entity. *Adv. Intern. Med.,* 15:155–175.
4. Liddle, G. W. (1972): Pathogenesis of glucocorticoid disorders. *Am. J. Med.,* 53:638–648.
5. Tyrrell, J. B., Brooks, R. M., Fitzgerald, P. A., Cofoid, P. B., Forsham, P. H., and Wilson, C. B. (1978): Cushing's disease: Selective transsphenoidal resection of pituitary microadenomas. *N. Engl. J. Med.,* 298:753–758.

Clinical Management of Pituitary Disorders,
edited by G. T. Tindall and W. F. Collins.
Raven Press, New York © 1979.

14

Ophthalmological Aspects of Pituitary Tumors

George S. Stefanis, H. Dwight Cavanaugh, and George T. Tindall

Department of Surgery (Neurosurgery) and Ophthalmology, Emory University School of Medicine, Atlanta, Georgia 30322

The relationship between pituitary tumors and visual impairment was first noted in the late 1800s. Since then therapeutic efforts have focused on operative approaches designed to remove the tumors and thus either restore or preserve vision. Craniotomy was the first operative procedure used in pituitary adenomas, but it carried a prohibitively high morbidity and mortality rate. For this reason, surgeons sought extracranial approaches to the sella such as the transsphenoidal operative technique. This latter method was first used by Schoffler in 1907 and subsequently modified by Cushing, Hirsch, and many others (28). Problems such as infection, lack of magnification, inadequate illumination, and no intraoperative fluoroscopic control plagued these early transsphenoidal operations. About this time, craniotomy was evolving into a relatively safe operation; thus, by 1920 many surgeons had switched to transcranial techniques for pituitary tumors. Subsequently, craniotomy techniques continued to improve but the mortality rate remained at approximately 5%, and complications such as optic pathway damage occurred not infrequently. In the 1960s, the transsphenoidal operation was modernized by making the operating microscope and televised fluoroscopy an integral part of the surgical procedure (14,23). These new additions have eliminated many of the problems early surgeons encountered and gradually, over the past few years, have served to establish the microsurgical transsphenoidal technique as the operative procedure of choice for the treatment of the majority of pituitary tumors.

In this chapter, practical anatomical relationships of the optic chiasm and pituitary gland, possible mechanisms of visual loss with pituitary tumors, and the results of transsphenoidal surgery in patients with visual loss secondary to pituitary adenomas will be discussed.

ANATOMICAL ASPECTS

Pituitary Gland

The pituitary gland is contained in the sella turcica, which is a deep depression in the middle of the intracranial portion of the sphenoid bone. The bony landmarks consist of the tuberculum sella, anteriorly; dorsum sella and posterior clinoids, posterior-laterally; and the anterior clinoid processes, anterior-laterally.

The diaphragm sella is stretched between the anterior and posterior clinoid processes. Through the opening in the diaphragm, which varies considerably in size among individuals, passes the pituitary stalk. The pituitary gland is a

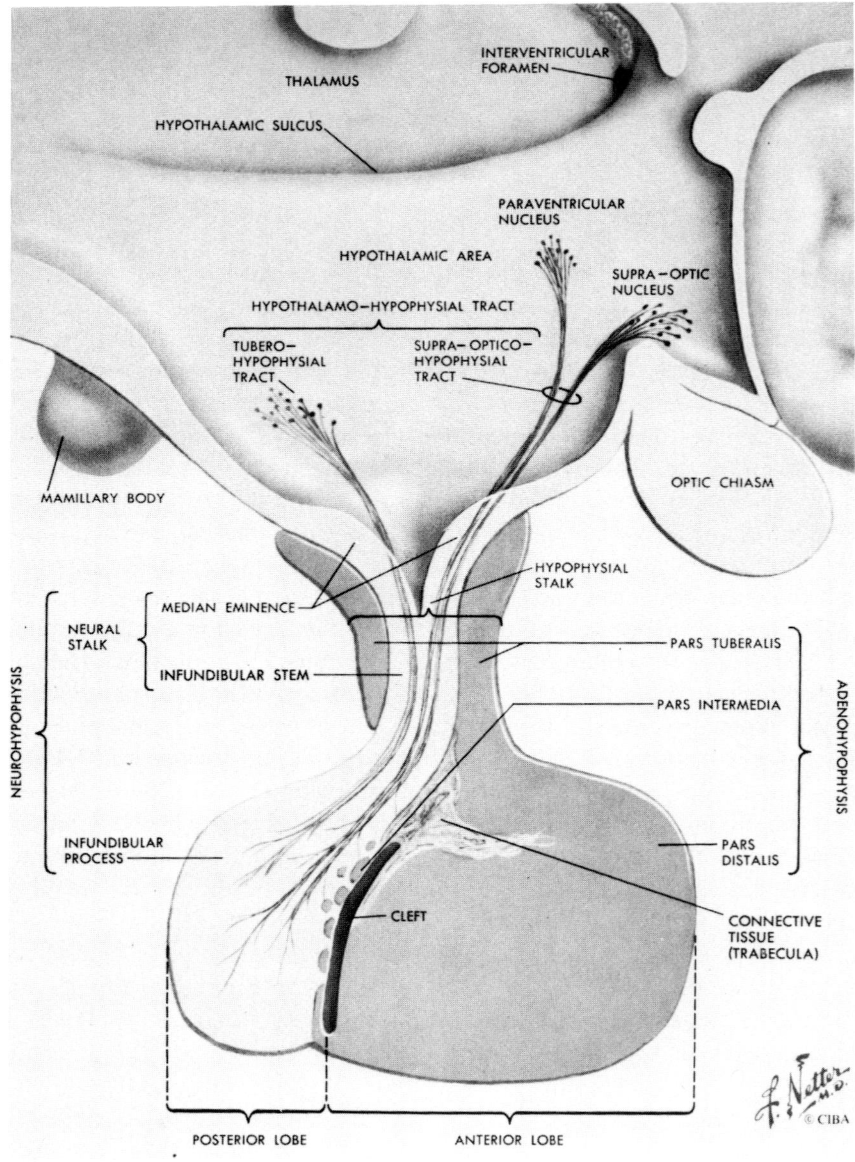

FIG. 1. Anatomy of the pituitary gland. (From ref. 14a.)

small ovoid body with average measurements of 1.2 × 1.0 × 0.5 cm and an average weight of 0.5 to 0.6 g in the adult. On the basis of morphology, embryology, and function, the gland is divided into an anterior (adenohypophysis) and posterior (neurohypophysis) lobe (Fig. 1). The adenohypophysis is derived from the ectoderm of Rathke's pouch of the stomodeum, and the neurohypophysis,

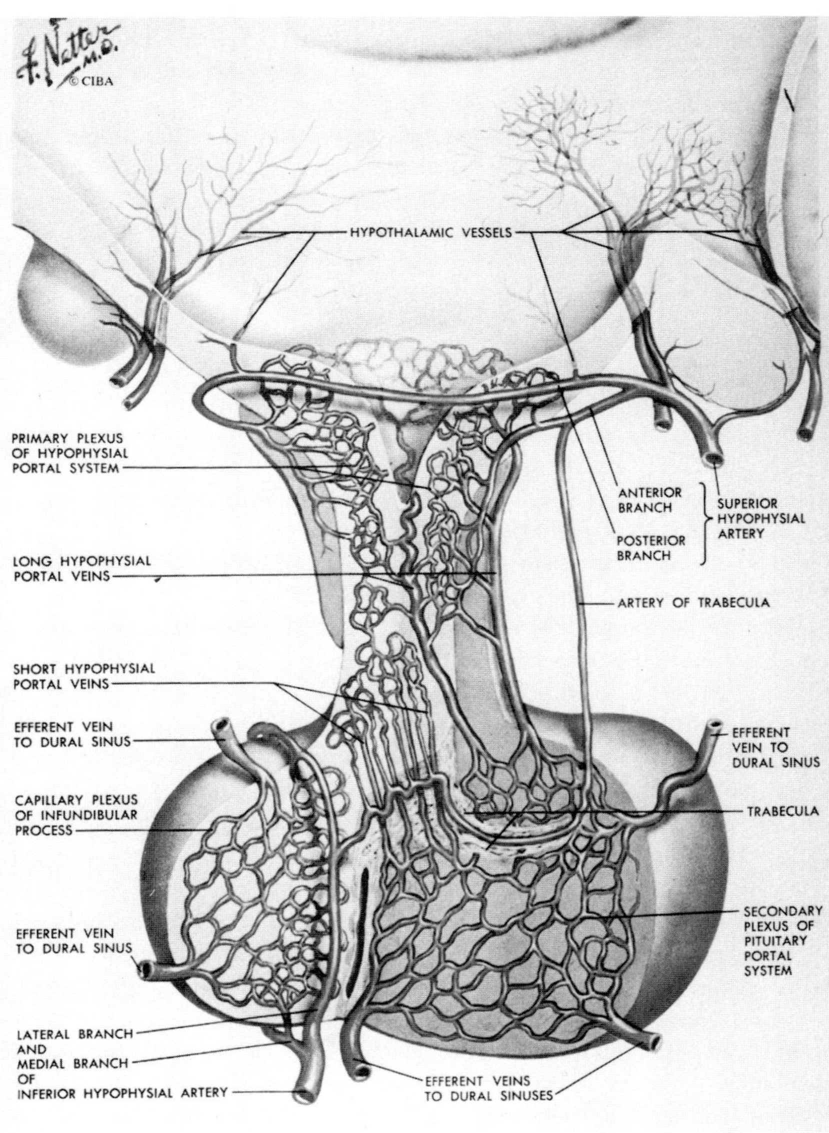

FIG. 2. Blood supply of the pituitary gland. (From ref. 14a.)

from the neural ectoderm of the floor of the forebrain. Functionally, the neurohypophysis consists of the median eminence of the tuber cinereum and the infundibular stem and process. The anterior lobe is divided into the pars tuberalis, which surrounds the distal pituitary stalk, and the pars distalis. Unlike many animal species, the human adenohypophysis does not contain a pars intermedia (20). The adenohypophysis secretes growth hormone (hGH), prolactin (PRL), thyroid-stimulating hormone (TSH), adrenocorticotrophic hormone (ACTH), follicle-stimulating hormone (FSH), luteinizing hormone (LH), and melanocyte-stimulating hormone (MSH). The neurohypophysis releases antidiuretic hormone (vasopressin) and oxytocin, both of which are synthesized in the hypothalamus and then transported and stored in the posterior lobe.

The pituitary gland derives its arterial supply from the inferior and superior hypophyseal arteries, which arise from the intracavernous portion of the internal carotid artery. Usually, the inferior hypophyseal artery supplies the posterior lobe, and the superior hypophyseal artery, the anterior lobe (Fig. 2) (22).

Optic Chiasm

Gross Anatomical Aspects

The optic chiasm, whish is a flattened oblong structure formed by the union of the optic nerves, measures 12 mm in transverse diameter, 8 mm in anterior-posterior diameter, and 4 mm in thickness. The chiasm forms the anterior-inferior wall of the third ventricle, and at this point it is tilted 45° from the horizontal plane. Its anatomical relations superiorly are the lamina terminalis, anterior commissure, and the third ventricle; posteriorly, the pituitary stalk, tuber cinereum, mammillary bodies, and oculomotor nerves; and inferiorly, the diaphragm sella and pituitary gland (Fig. 3). From a clinical viewpoint, the close anatomic relationship between the optic chiasm above and the immediate underlying pituitary gland provides a reasonable explanation for the frequency of visual impairment seen with pituitary tumors that enlarge to the point of producing mass compressive effects. An appreciation of the variability in the position of the chiasm in relation to the underlying gland is also important, particularly since this feature can influence the surgical approach to the pituitary gland if transcranial operative procedures are used (50). In the majority of cases (80%) the chiasm lies directly above the central portion of the diaphragm sella and the gland. However, the chiasm is anteriorly situated and overlies the tuberculum sella in 9% of individuals, in which case it is termed a prefixed chiasm. A postfixed chiasm overlies the posterior clinoids and was found in 11% of Bergland and Ray's series (6). These various positions are shown in Fig. 4. Technical difficulties in the transcranial approach to the pituitary gland is encountered in cases in which the chiasm is prefixed in position, thus markedly obscuring the surgeon's view of the dorsal aspect of the gland.

The position of the chiasm in reference to the pituitary gland and diaphragm sella may also affect the pattern of visual field changes in patients with pituitary

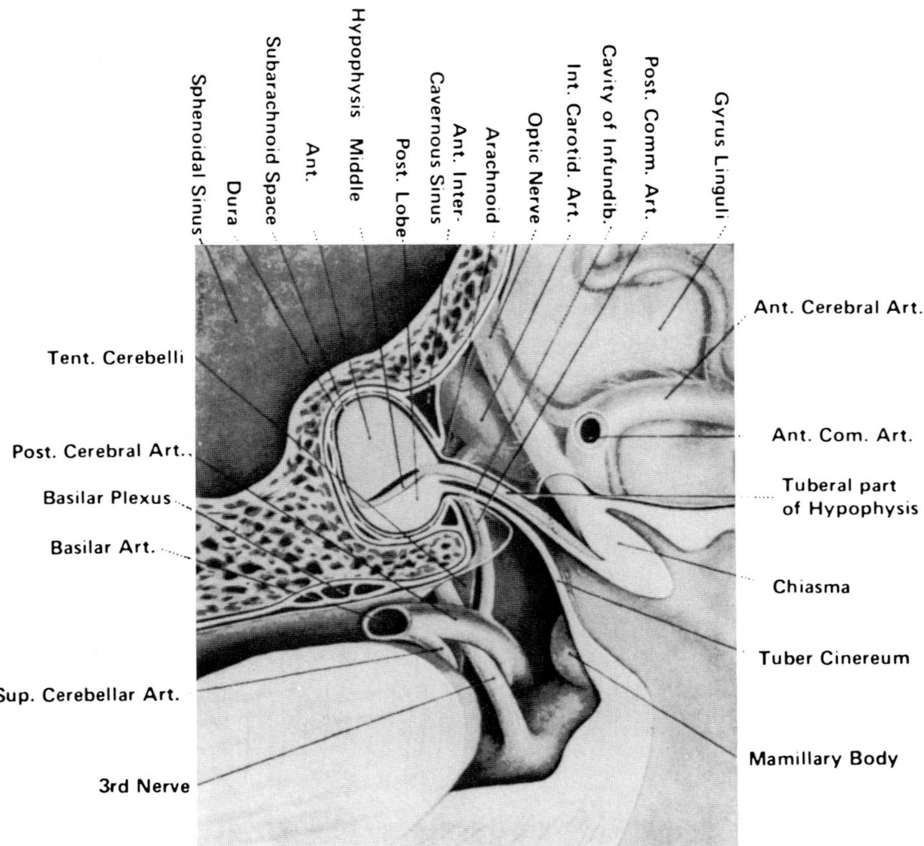

FIG. 3. Diagrammatic median section of hypophysis. (From ref. 64a.)

tumors. For instance, with a prefixed chiasm, an expanding tumor may result in a bitemporal scotomatous hemianopsia rather than the classic superior bitemporal quadrantanopsia as a result of posterior infrachiasmal compression (29). Further, pituitary tumors in patients with a postfixed chiasm involve the junction of the optic nerve with the chiasm and thus may present with the anterior chiasmal syndrome, which consists of an ipsilateral visual field loss and a contralateral superior temporal quadrantanopsia (43).

Microscopic Anatomical Aspects: Nerve Pathways

Optic nerve fibers are classified according to their origins in the retina, and correspond to subdivisions horizontally (upper and lower fields) and vertically

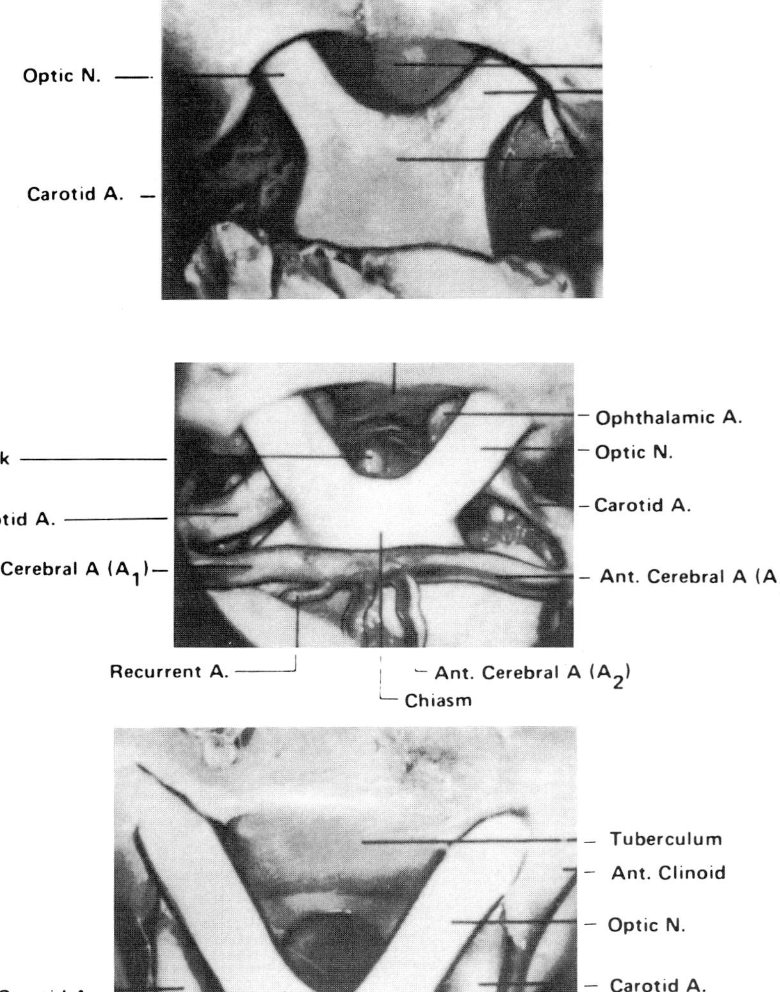

FIG. 4. Superior view of sellar region. **Top:** Prefixed chiasm. **Center:** Normal chiasm. The ophthalmic artery protrudes medial to the right optic nerve. The anterior cerebral arteries pass dorsal to the chiasm. The left recurrent artery arises from the A-1 segment of the left anterior cerebral artery. The pituitary stalk lies between the optic nerves. **Bottom:** Postfixed chiasm. Diaphragma sellae and the pituitary gland removed. The third nerve (CN III) lies to the carotid arteries. (From ref. 50.)

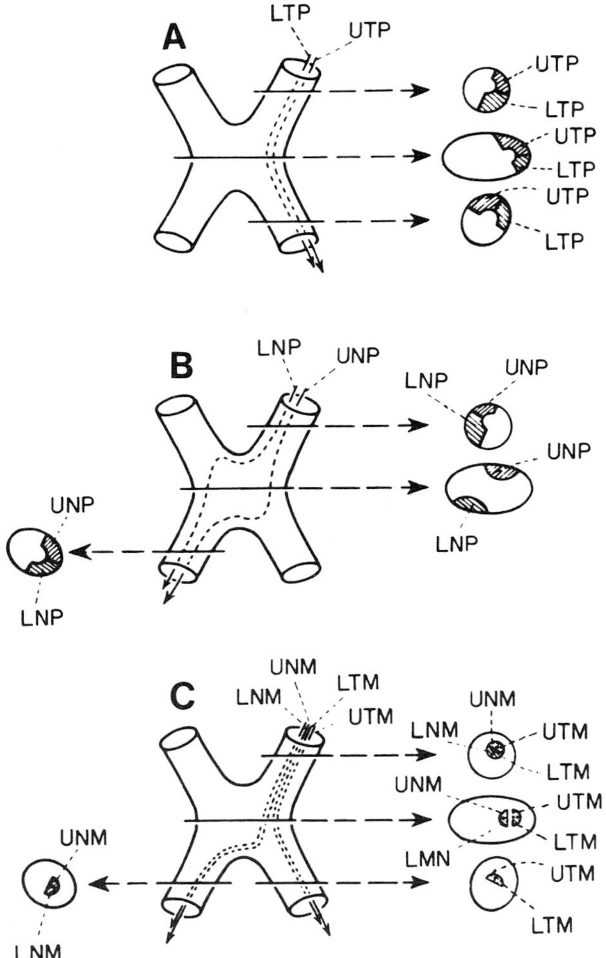

FIG. 5. Distribution of visual fibers in optic chiasma and adjacent parts of optic nerves and optic tracts. **A:** Temporal peripheral fibers. **B:** Nasal peripheral fibers. **C:** Temporal and nasal macular fibers. [Viewed from above, and in cross-section *(arrowed)*]. (UTP) upper temporal peripheral. (LTP) lower temporal peripheral. (UNP) upper nasal peripheral. (LNP) lower nasal peripheral. (UTM) upper temporal macular. (LTM) lower temporal macular. (UNM) upper nasal macular. (LNM) lower nasal macular. (From ref. 66.)

(temporal and nasal fields) through the fovea. These fibers converge on the optic nerve head with the same anatomical arrangement as in the retina, but behind the lamina cribrosa undergo a shift as shown in Fig. 5. Knowledge of the distribution of the visual fibers in the chiasm is essential in understanding the pathophysiology of the chiasmal syndrome and its variations. The temporal fibers, which are uncrossed, traverse the lateral portion of the chiasm in two compact masses (Fig. 6). The nasal peripheral fibers cross the chiasm to form

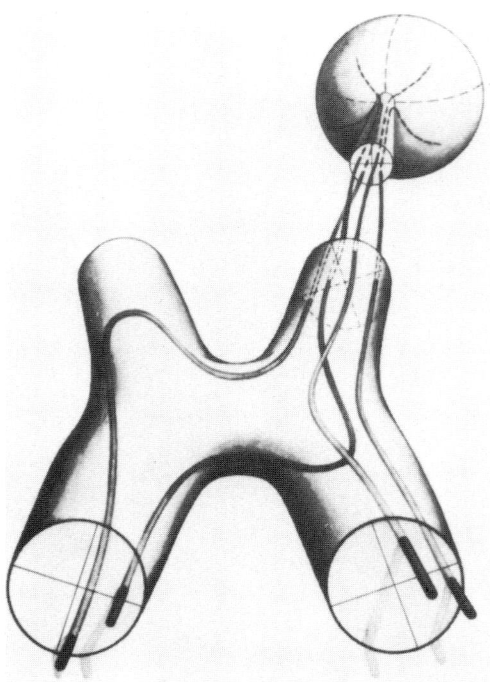

FIG. 6. Stereogram, showing course of fibers in chiasm. Back of retina is pictured. Chiasm is seen as transparency from above. (From ref. 41a.)

two distinct bundles—the upper fibers which lie dorsally and the lower fibers which lie ventrally (66).

Vasculature of the Optic Chiasm

The optic nerves, chiasm, and tract pass through the circle of Willis, coursing below the anterior communicating and anterior cerebral arteries and above the posterior cerebral, basilar, and posterior communicating arteries (7) (Fig. 7). The inferior chiasm is supplied by branches of the anterior superior hypophyseal artery, either by a direct branch or via a peri-infundibular arterial plexus. The superior surface is supplied by branches of the anterior communicating and anterior cerebral arteries. Several investigators have identified a branch from the internal carotid artery to the lateral and inferior aspect of the chiasm to be the only true chiasmal artery to this region (12). The ophthalmic, anterior choroidal, middle cerebral, and posterior communicating arteries usually do not contribute significantly to the vasculature of the optic chiasm.

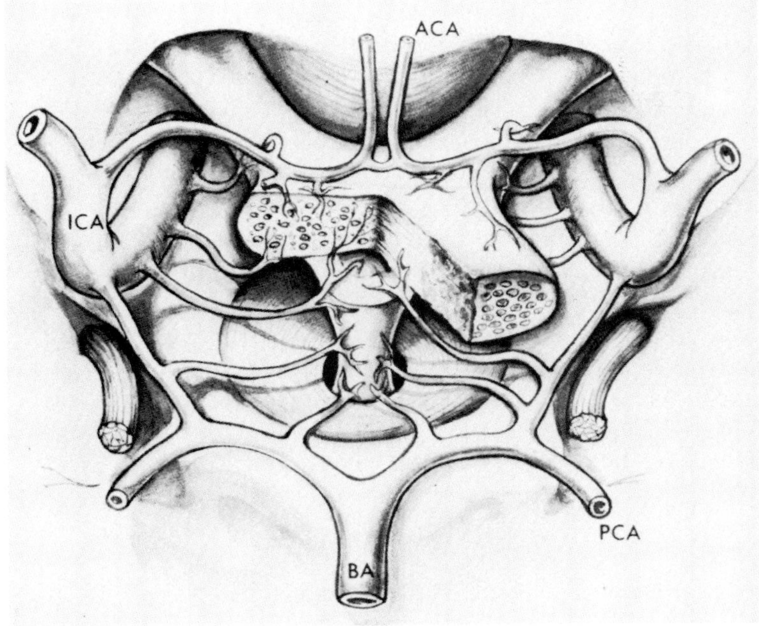

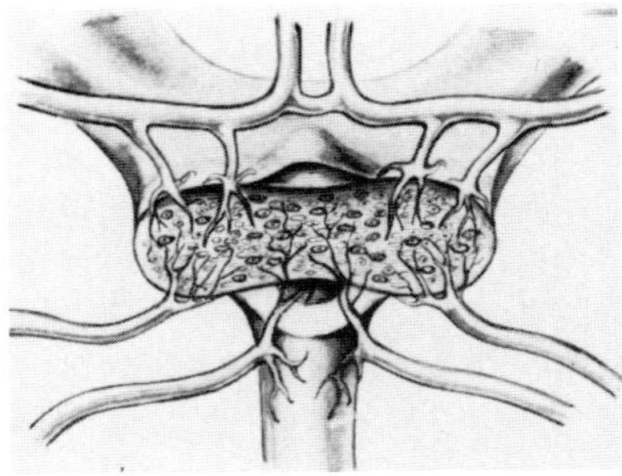

FIG. 7. Illustrations of the visual pathways and their arterial supply. (ACA) anterior cerebral artery. (BA) basilar artery. (ICA) internal carotid artery. (PCA) posterior cerebral artery. (From ref. 7.)

PATHOLOGY AND INCIDENCE OF PITUITARY TUMORS

The reported incidence of pituitary adenomas is approximately one new case per 100,000 population each year (27,48). Over the past several years, this has been a uniform figure in several epidemiologic studies relative to the subject. In recent years, however, there appears to have been a real and significant increase in the incidence of pituitary tumors, particularly in women of child-bearing age. Since 1970 the mean annual incidence per 100,000 women has been 7.1 as opposed to only 0.7 in the same group from 1935 to 1969 (4).

Possible reasons for this increase could be related to refinement in diagnostic endocrinologic testing, to better appreciation of the fact that many infertility problems in women may be caused by small pituitary adenomas, and/or to some change in an environmental factor. One potential factor that conceivably could result in an increased incidence of pituitary adenomas is the widespread use of oral contraceptives; however, to date there are no data showing an established relationship between pituitary adenomas and birth control pills.

The histologic classification of pituitary tumors is based on the three cell types—chromophobe, acidophil, and basophil—found in the adenohypophysis (52). Although in use in many centers, this classification has never had any significance in terms of consistently relating either function or biologic behavior to tumor type. A more practical classification is one that is predicated on function and that divides the adenomas into an endocrinologically active and a nonactive group (34,45). This newer division carries no morphologic significance as does the classical one, but is more useful in clinical practice.

CLINICAL FINDINGS OF PITUITARY TUMORS

The clinical findings of pituitary adenomas can be divided into two groups: (a) detectable abnormalities of endocrine metabolism and (b) mass compressive effects. Pituitary tumors that produce endocrinopathy also occasionally cause mass effects due to progressive growth and extrasellar spread of the tumor, and thus patients with obvious and easily recognized clinical signs of either acromegaly or Cushing's disease should also be evaluated carefully for evidence of visual impairment. The pituitary gland produces many important hormones; thus, either an excess or a deficiency of one or more can usually lead to clinical findings that serve to establish the diagnosis. The clinical presentation of hormone deficiencies and excesses has been well summarized in Chapter 7.

Mass Compressive Effects

Progressive growth of a pituitary adenoma with extrasellar extension can compress surrounding structures and cause clinical findings such as headache, optic pallor, papilledema, bitemporal hemianopsia, extraocular muscle paralysis, decreased visual acuity, and proptosis (60). A dramatic and, fortunately, relatively rare presentation of pituitary tumors is the symptom complex associated with pituitary apoplexy. The most serious and common mass effect is chiasmal compression with resultant visual loss. These various clinical manifestations will be discussed.

Headache

Pain referred to the bifrontal area and around the eye may accompany pituitary adenomas. In most cases, headache is believed to be due to stretching of the diaphragm sella which is innervated by the ophthalmic division of the fifth cranial nerve.

Optic Pallor

The finding of optic pallor may represent ischemia of the optic nerve and may result in optic atrophy with associated visual impairment. Pallor may represent a difficult subjective impression in early cases, and careful comparisons of each disk must be made. Atrophy results from interruption of axoplasmic flow within individual neurons of the optic nerve (40) (see below).

Papilledema

Papilledema, which is due to increased intracranial pressure from obstruction of the third ventricle by a large extension of tumor, is seen infrequently.

Visual Fields

The characteristic visual field defect caused by a pituitary tumor is a bitemporal hemianopsia. In a typical case, the superior temporal quadrants are affected initially, followed thereafter by the inferior temporal quadrants. In instances of progressive chiasmal compression from continued tumor growth, the inferior nasal followed by the superior nasal quadrants are subsequently involved, with resulting blindness. These defects are due to involvement of the crossing and noncrossing fibers in the chiasm (Fig. 8). Since many, if not the majority, of patients currently present with endocrine abnormalities, visual fields are now usually obtained at an earlier stage in tumor development. In these cases bitemporal hemicentral scotomatous hemianopsia is more likely to present as the initial clinical finding (64). Careful visual testing to small red isopters with targets presented bilaterally can provide important evidence for the presence of pituitary tumors. Deficits to red-color testing may precede detectable abnormalities to white or other targets.

Extraocular Palsies

Paralysis of the extraocular muscles is a relatively uncommon manifestation of pituitary adenomas. When present, the oculomotor nerve is the most commonly involved, followed next by the abducens and then the trochlear nerve (42). The internal carotid artery offers some protection to the cranial nerves in the cavernous sinus from expanding pituitary adenomas, but occasionally the nerves are compressed against the edge of the dura at their entry into the cavernous sinus (54). Partial or complete third, sixth, or fourth nerve palsies may result.

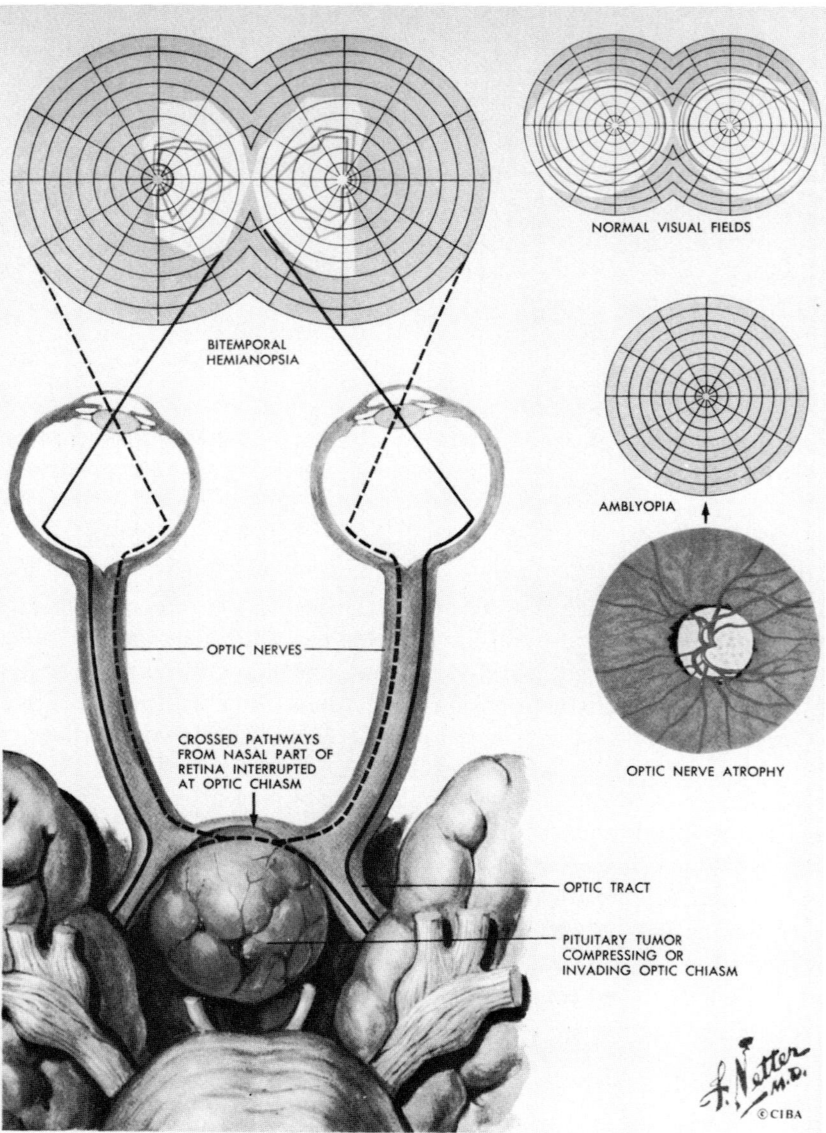

FIG. 8. Interruption of optic chiasmal fibers by pituitary adenoma, and the resultant visual field defect. (From ref. 42a.)

Proptosis

A rare finding of pituitary adenomas, proptosis can occur secondary to tumor extending into the cavernous sinus with resultant vascular congestion (61).

Pituitary Apoplexy

Pituitary apoplexy results from either acute hemorrhagic infarction of or spontaneous hemorrhage into a pituitary tumor, and is manifest clinically by findings such as headache, altered mental status, meningismus, and visual disturbances. The pathogenetic factor implicated is tumor necrosis due to failure of the vasculature to supply the entire tumor. Pituitary apoplexy has been described following pituitary irradiation, as a complication of head injury, during therapy with anticoagulants, and during pregnancy (39). Significant enlargement of the pituitary occurs in pregnancy and is believed to be due to an increase in the cells associated with the secretion of prolactin (15). Normally, this physiologic enlargement does not compress the chiasm, but in the presence of an adenoma, both gland and tumor can rapidly enlarge and possibly result in compressive visual field defects or, more rarely, pituitary apoplexy (59). Surgical intervention is indicated when significant visual defects exist, and the timing of surgery with respect to recovery of visual function is a major consideration in the preoperative planning (9). While several investigators have shown excellent return of visual function in delays of at least 4 days from the time of onset to the time of surgery (62), it is our opinion that the earlier one initiates surgical intervention, the better the prognosis for visual recovery. Clinical studies have implied that the extent of damage to the optic pathways that occurs initially may be the greatest determinant of future reversibility (62).

PATHOPHYSIOLOGY OF VISUAL IMPAIRMENT IN PATIENTS WITH PITUITARY TUMORS

The pathophysiologic mechanism responsible for visual field impairment is not a settled issue, and while many explanations have been proposed, to date the exact mechanism has not been established. Proposed mechanisms include:

Mechanical Compression

Direct Compression

Simple mechanical compression has been implicated by many investigators (32). Direct pressure by the tumor forcefully displaces the optic nerve and chiasm against either the margins of the optic canals or the anterior cerebral arteries which normally cross the optic nerves at their junction with the chiasm. Thus, it could logically be assumed that the vice-like entrapment along with the physiologic pulsations of the anterior cerebral arteries causes a progressive visual impairment. Notching of the chiasm by overlying arteries was reported by Rucker and Kernohan in five patients with pituitary adenomas associated with bitemporal hemianopsia (51).

Tension Theory

Tension theory is based on physical properties of the optic nerves, chiasm, and tracts. Anteriorly, the optic nerves are attached in the optic canals by the dural and arachnoid sheaths. Posteriorly, the lateral fibers are continued into the optic tracts, and their attachment to the midbrain is relatively lax. The medial fibers cross and interweave in the chiasm and have a firm attachment at its posterior edge. It is estimated that up to one-half million nerve fibers from each optic nerve cross one another at angles up to 90° in the chiasm. Upward displacement of the optic nerves and chiasm from an underlying and enlarging pituitary tumor causes tension in these crossing fibers and thus could lead to fiber compression and/or transsection. It has been shown by Sunderland and Bradley that the tensile strength of nerves is dependent on the endoneurial collagen (55). The optic nerves have collagenous septa to support the funiculi, while in the chiasm and optic tracts, the collagen is absent and the support consists of glial tissue. Because of this lack of collagen support for nerve fibers, it is postulated that the optic chiasm is more vulnerable to stretch injury (44).

Interruption of Axoplasmic Circulation

After observing several cases in which restoration of vision occurred promptly following surgical decompression of the optic chiasm, Cushing concluded that there must be a "physiologic block" which can be reversed relatively rapidly with removal of the mass. Assuming that the block would be secondary to either mechanical distortion and/or ischemia provided neither were long lasting in effect (11), he further postulated that the physiologic block might interfere with the conduction of neural impulses at a subcellular level. These observations are consistent with the modern concept of axoplasmic transport, which entails a flow of substance from the nerve cell body to its axonal extensions. In relating this concept to optic pathways, the cells in the retina are the nerve cell bodies and their axonal extensions are the fibers found in the optic nerves and chiasm. Two types of axoplasmic transport have been described. The first consists of a rapid transport which is responsible for movement of substances required at synaptic intervals, such as enzymes required for neurotransmitter synthesis; the second is a slow transport system which maintains and replenishes substances necessary for the structural integrity of the axon (2). Several investigators have observed experimentally that raising intraocular pressure either slows or stops the axoplasmic transport in the optic nerves (3,38). Theoretically, compression of the chiasm by a pituitary tumor could impede axoplasmic transport and cause failure of neural impulses to be transmitted.

Evoked potentials test the ability of a nerve to conduct neural impulses from a peripheral receptor to a central nucleus. Feinsod and associates used visual evoked potentials (VEPs) preoperatively, intraoperatively, and postoperatively in two patients with tuberculum sellae meningiomas and in one patient with a pituitary adenoma. Effective surgical removal of the meningioma and pituitary tumor resulted in significant improvement in VEPs and in visual impairment (16,17). The visual improvement, which occurred in the early postoperative course and which correlated well with the restoration of VEPs to normal shortly after recovery from anesthesia, lends support to the theory of mechanical compression at a subcellular level.

While the compression theories are appealing, they do not explain certain aspects of the chiasmal syndrome, such as the relative resistance of the portion of the chiasm that would produce an altitudinal nasal field loss, which clinical experience has shown to be an uncommon finding. This relative sparing of the upper nasal fibers cannot be explained anatomically or physiologically.

Ischemia

While performing intracranial surgery for a pituitary tumor, Hughes observed that the crossing fibers in the chiasm were gray and fragmented while the lateral bundles appeared normal, pink, and well vascularized (30). He interpreted these findings to be consistent with ischemic rather than mechanical compression as a cause for visual impairment.

Dawson was able to identify only one chiasmal artery, which is a branch from the internal carotid artery and which supplies the lateral and inferior portion of the chiasm (12). The remainder of the chiasm is supplied by a periarterial plexus which varies anatomically among patients. François believes that the ischemic lesions in the chiasm are not due to compression of individual arteries, but arise at the capillary level (18).

Frisen et al. reported a patient with a cystic craniopharyngioma situated beneath the right optic nerve which after several surgical recurrences was connected to a subcutaneous reservoir (19). Symptoms of decreasing visual acuity and visual field changes recurred over 50 times in 1 year and were relieved within seconds by percutaneous drainage of the reservoir. Because of the rapid reversal of symptoms, these workers conjectured that optic nerve ischemia was the most important factor causing visual failure. However, one could also argue that relieving ischemia might have resulted in prompt restoration of axoplasmic flow. This pattern of recovery is not unusual, as case reports in the literature have shown a rapid improvement (i.e., several days to weeks) in visual field impairment following decompression of the chiasm. However, knowledge of ischemic damage in the nervous system makes it unlikely that reduced visual function present for long periods of time would be rapidly reversed following surgical decompression if the pathophysiology were due entirely to long-established ischemia.

DIAGNOSIS

Current endocrinologic and neurodiagnostic evaluation of patients with pituitary tumors is discussed elsewhere in this book (see Chapters 5–8).

Ophthalmological Evaluation

Ophthalmological evaluation is an essential part of assessing patients with suspected pituitary tumors. A specific evaluation protocol follows:

1. Funduscopic examination is important in detecting signs of optic pallor, atrophy, or papilledema. Careful comparisons with white and red-free light should be made between each disk.
2. Snellen's visual acuity testing should be done at a distance and close up to detect any compromise in central vision, and observed deficits should be tested for possible corrective refractive error by an ophthalmologist.
3. Visual fields, both tangent screen and perimetry testing, are necessary in evaluating these patients. We believe that the Goldman perimeter is more accurate than other perimeters because it allows quantification and reproducibility of data collected. Static perimetry may be useful in doubtful cases. Tangent screen testing for small deficits in red-color vision to simultaneously presented targets may detect early cases.

TREATMENT OF PITUITARY TUMORS

During the past 10 to 15 years, the treatment of pituitary adenomas has changed considerably. Until recently, with few exceptions, surgical treatment was reserved for patients with mass effects caused by these tumors, such as decreasing visual acuity and visual field disturbances. However, with the introduction and increasing use of pituitary hormone radioimmunoassays, and with the availability of a safer operative approach, neurosurgeons are now treating tumors because of endocrinopathy in addition to mass effects.

As discussed above, surgical techniques for treating pituitary tumors have varied over the years. Large series of cases have been treated by craniotomy as well as by the transsphenoidal method, and the results in terms of restoring vision will be analyzed and compared below. Currently, for several good reasons, most neurosurgeons use the transsphenoidal microsurgical technique for treating the majority of pituitary tumors, regardless of whether these tumors cause mass effects or endocrinopathy.

During the era of the craniotomy technique, mass effect was the primary indication for surgery. The indications for treating pituitary tumors have changed since the modernization of the transsphenoidal technique. Mass effects caused by pituitary tumors continue to be indications for treatment by the transsphenoidal approach, but they are far outnumbered by cases of endocrinopathy. Also, differences in the technical advancements between the two procedures are significant, because the operating microscope, which is an integral part of the transsphenoidal operation, was not generally available for surgeons using the craniotomy technique. For these reasons, it is difficult to compare the results of treating pituitary tumors by craniotomy versus the transsphenoidal approach. Mortality in the craniotomy series has ranged from 1.2% to 14%, whereas in the transsphenoidal series it has ranged from 1.2% to 5.3%. The recurrence rate in the craniotomy series has ranged from 42% to 48% as opposed to transsphenoidal approach which has been 4% to 8%. However, the follow-up is inadequate for the transsphenoidal approach; consequently, long-term comparative recurrence rates cannot be ascertained (35,49,56).

The advantages of the transsphenoidal approach include an overall comparative decrease in both morbidity and mortality. Also, excellent illuminated magnification provided by the operating microscope afford the surgeon a better opportunity at total tumor removal and less chance of chiasmal damage. The operative time and anesthetic risks have been significantly reduced. Complications such as postoperative subdural or epidural hematomas and frontal lobe contusion, which were seen following craniotomy, have now been eliminated. Cosmetically, the frontal craniotomy often leaves the patient with a scar, while none is visible with the transsphenoidal approach.

However, the transsphenoidal approach is not without complications. CSF rhinorrhea occurs in less than 2% of cases and can lead to meningitis or brain abscess formation. As with transcranial approaches, endocrinologic complications such as postoperative hypopituitarism may occur. Also, postoperative diabetes insipidus, although usually transient, is encountered infrequently. Injury to the structures in the cavernous sinus by the transsphenoidal approach have been reported, and rarely, damage to the hypothalamus, optic nerves, and chiasm may occur (36).

The results of transcranial and transsphenoidal operations with special emphasis on visual status postoperatively from several major series are shown in Table 1. In the patients treated by craniotomy, a significant number showed either improvement or return of normal vision. Seventy percent of Cushing and Walker's patients improved, as did 80% of those of Hemibache and of Guilleance and Caron. Ray and Patterson treated 146 patients with chromophobe adenomas with the transcranial approach. Most of these patients had preoperative visual impairment, and 75% had some degree of endocrine dysfunction. Postoperatively, 80% of the patients had an improvement in visual impairment, and 50% had normal vision restored. Their mortality was only 1.2% (49).

The improvement or normalization of vision in the transsphenoidal group ranges from 41% in Demailly and Guiot's to 77% in Cushing and Walker's series. Using the transsphenoidal approach, Laws et al. operated on 62 patients who had visual impairment associated with pituitary adenomas. Vision improved in 81% of these patients, was unchanged in 11%, and worsened in 5% (35). Thus, it appears that the incidence of postoperative visual improvement is comparable for the two operative approaches. The major difference lies in the large number of patients in whom vision worsened (2% to 26%) following craniotomy compared with the transsphenoidal approach (<5%). Although the optic nerves and chiasm are not visualized during the transsphenoidal operation, it would appear to be at least as effective and certainly less hazardous than the transcanial approach in terms of vision.

TABLE 1. *Results of transcranial and transsphenoidal operations*

Series	Dates	Mortality (%)	Normal/Improved (%)	Unchanged (%)	Worsened (%)
Craniotomy					
Cushing and Walker (11)	1913–1932	4.5	70.5	20.5	9
Bakay (5), Olivocrona (46)	1929–1947	11.4	40.7	33.2	26.2
Tonnis et al. (58)	1933–1952	10.4	62	31	7
Heimbach (25)	1938–1956	9.4	83	12	5
Guillaume and Caron (21)	1941–1957	12.0	83	10	7
Olivocrona (46)	1948–1959	14.0	42.6	43.4	14
Svien et al. (56)	1950–1958	6.8	63.4	15.5	21.1
Ray and Patterson (49)	1950–1969	1.2	80	18	3
Transsphenoidal					
Cushing and Walker (11)	1913–1932	5.3	71.5	24.5	3.8
Demailly and Guiot (14)	1957–1972	1.24	41	41	17.8
Laws et al. (35)	1972–1975	1.4	85.7	14.3	0

Medical Treatment

Medical treatment as primary treatment is often used in patients with endocrinopathy and is not used in patients with mass effects. Bromocriptine, an ergot alkaloid, recently has been approved for use in the United States. In Europe and other countries it has been used to treat patients with amenorrhea-galactorrhea syndrome and acromegaly. The drug lowers prolactin levels by acting directly on the pituitary gland, activating dopamine receptors, and functioning as a prolactin inhibitory factor (59).

Other Treatment Modalities

External Radiation

Conventional irradiation of pituitary tumors is a useful adjunct to surgical therapy in some instances, but in our opinion should not be used as primary and sole treatment. There does not appear to be any large statistically significant series of patients treated with irradiation in whom systematic pre- and posttreatment assessment of vision has been reported.

We do not recommend routine postoperative radiation in patients operated via the transsphenoid approach unless the surgeon feels that a complete removal of the tumor was not accomplished. Irradiation is not without risks. Harris and Levene reported five patients in whom damage to the optic nerves and chiasm occurred, which they attributed to postoperative irradiation (24). Postradiation complications such as cerebral necrosis, hypothalamic damage, and hypopituitarism have also been reported (1,53).

Heavy Particle Irradiation

Bragg peak proton hypophysectomy is another method of treating patients with pituitary adenomas. Kjellberg and Kliman believe that this is the treatment of choice in many pituitary adenomas that are confined to the sella turcica (33). However, complications such as cranial nerve palsies, vertigo, and seizures may occur rarely in patients receiving this therapy (13). The data relating to the effects on visual impairment using this technique are not available.

CASE MATERIAL

Over the past 5 years (1973–1978), a total of 168 patients with pituitary adenomas were treated at Emory University Hospital using the transsphenoidal technique described by Hardy. Of these 168 patients, a total of 58 had impairment in visual acuity and/or visual fields, and they form the basis for this brief analysis.

Preoperative clinical findings are shown in Table 2. Headache was the most common symptom, while 28 patients complained of decreased visual acuity

TABLE 2. *Preoperative clinical findings in 58 patients with pituitary adenomas treated at Emory University Hospital (1973–1978)*

Clinical finding	No. cases
Headache	38
Decrease in visual acuity	28
Impairment in visual field	13
Optic pallor or atrophy	10
Endocrinopathy	33
A–G syndrome	8
Acromegaly	24
Cushing's disease	1

and 13 noted changes in their peripheral vision. These visual complaints were confirmed on ophthalmologic examination and consisted of acuities ranging from near normal to hand motion only, and field defects ranging from bilateral superior temporal quadrantanopsia to bilateral temporal hemianopsias. Optic pallor was present in 10 patients. Endocrinopathy occurred in 33 patients, 24 with amenorrhea-galactorrhea, eight with acromegaly, and one with Cushing's disease. CT scan and polytomography of the sella turcica were positive in 70% and 94%, respectively. As shown in Table 3, following transsphenoidal microsurgical removal of the pituitary tumor, visual acuity returned to normal in four patients and improved in 23, and visual fields returned to normal in eight patients and improved in 29. As would be expected, the greatest deficit in visual acuity and fields occurred in patients with a tumor greater than 1 cm in diameter. Our results are consistent with those reported in other series. We were impressed with the rapid recovery period of visual impairment that occurred in our cases following the use of the transsphenoidal technique. The following case typifies the results seen following the transsphenoidal surgical approach.

Case 1: A 28-year-old man presented to Emory University Hospital on 2/9/78 complaining of headaches and visual problems consisting of occasional blurring of vision and decreased vision in the periphery for 6 weeks' duration.

Physical examination revealed an obese man with scanty facial and pubic hair. The remainder of the general medical examination was normal. Neurological examination revealed a superior bitemporal quadrantanopsia, worse on the left than on the right side (Fig. 9, top). Ophthalmological evaluation revealed a superior bitemporal quadrantanopsia with visual acuity of 20/25 OD and 20/400 OS.

He underwent the routine protocol work-up for a pituitary tumor. The endocrinologic studies revealed a serum prolactin of 26 ng/ml. The CT scan showed a nonenhancible mass in the sella with extension into the sphenoid sinus. Polytomography revealed balloon-

TABLE 3. *Results of surgery*

	Normal	Improved	No change	Worsened
Visual acuity	4	23	28	3
Visual fields	8	29	20	1

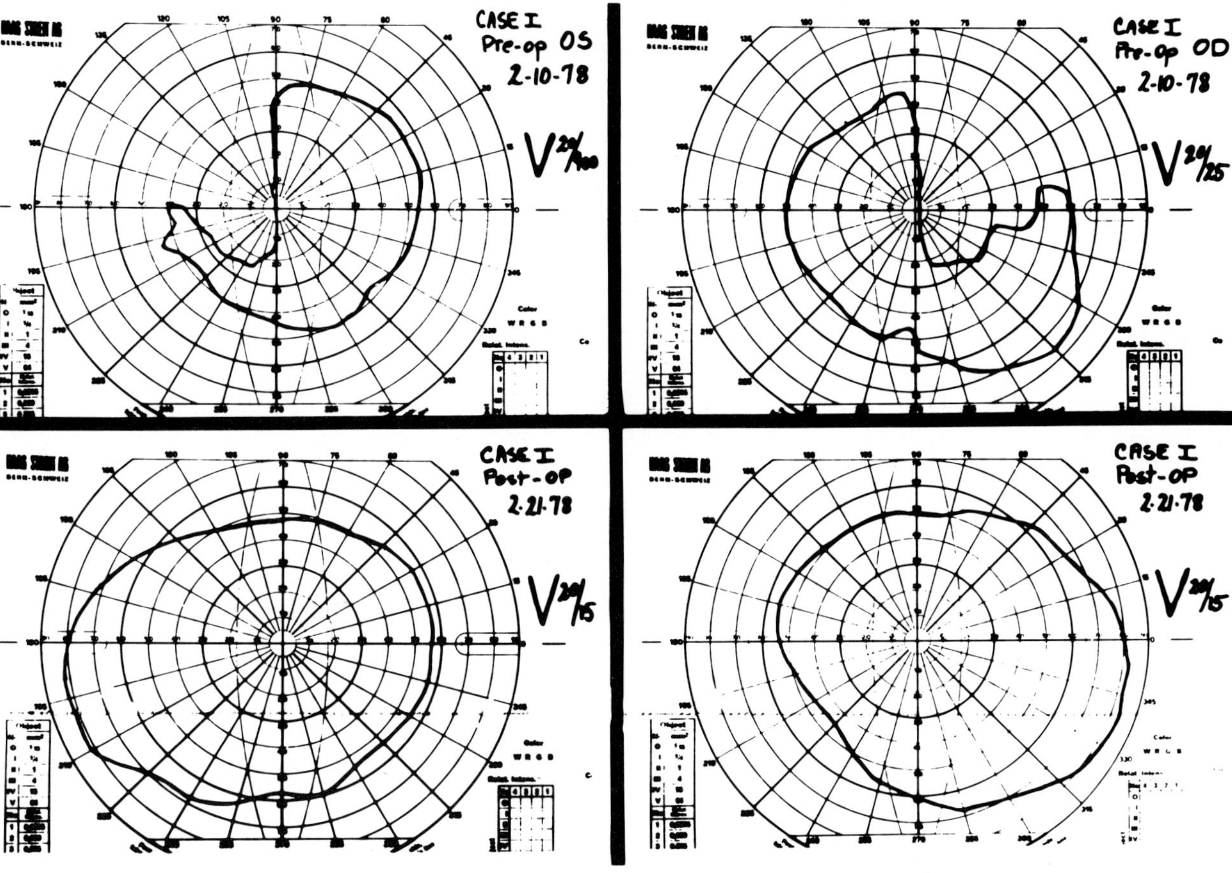

FIG. 9. Visual fields and acuities of patient in case 1. **Top:** Preoperative visual fields. **Bottom:** postoperative visual fields.

ing of the sella with erosion of the sella floor and extension into the sphenoid sinus. An arteriogram showed elevation of the horizontal segment of both anterior cerebral arteries.

Transsphenoidal microsurgical excision of a 20 × 22 mm eosinophilic adenoma was performed on 2/16/78. Subjective improvement in vision occurred by the second postoperative day, and formal ophthalmological evaluation performed on the fifth postoperative day showed a significant improvement in the visual field deficit (Fig. 9, bottom). Visual acuity improved to 20/15 OD and 20/15 OS. The postoperative serum prolactin (10th day) was 5 ng/ml.

EMPTY SELLA SYNDROME

An entity that often presents radiologically similar to a pituitary tumor and that can rarely present with the chiasmal syndrome is the empty sella syndrome (ESS). An empty sella is defined as one that contains a large intrasellar cistern that enlarges the sella turcica and compresses and flattens the normal pituitary gland inferiorly and posteriorly. Rarely, patients may present with headache, blurred vision, endocrinopathy, CSF rhinorrhea, and visual field defects (8). The ESS is characterized radiologically by symmetrical ballooning of the sella, and the diagnosis is confirmed by the appearance of air in the sella on pneumoencephalogram (37).

There are two types: primary and secondary. Primary ESS is thought to be caused by an incompetent diaphragm sellae which allows the pulsatile movements of the CSF to push the chiasmatic cistern into the sella (31). Secondary ESS is seen in patients who have had either pituitary surgery or irradiation. Adhesive arachnoiditis forms around the optic nerves and chiasm following treatment for pituitary adenomas, and these structures can be pulled into the "empty" sella, with visual field defects resulting from the traction. In addition to the above mechanism, it has been postulated that radiation causes vasculitis and occlusion of the small blood vessels supplying the optic chiasm. Several authors have reported cases of secondary ESS with visual field defects in which improvement in vision followed chiasmplexy and filling of the sella with bone chips and muscle (47,63). Mortara and Norrell believed that opening of the lamina terminalis and venting of third ventricular CSF pulsations would prevent downward curvature into the sella (41). Visual field defects may be associated with the primary ESS, but they are very rare. Buchman et al. presented a patient with an enlarged sella, normal pituitary function, and bitemporal superior quadrantanopsia on whom a pneumoencephalogram revealed air in the sella (10). Chiasmplexy has been shown to improve visual field defects in patients with primary ESS (65).

SUMMARY

The pathophysiologic mechanisms for visual impairment that have been discussed, both the theories of mechanical compression and ischemia, may explain certain aspects of visual impairment associated with pituitary tumors, but neither totally elucidates the entire chiasmal syndrome. In our opinion, it appears that a combination of ischemia and mechanical compression at a subcellular level may explain the clinical findings and rapid recovery in patients with pituitary tumors.

The incidence of pituitary tumors appears to be on the increase as is the ability of physicians to diagnose them at an earlier stage. Patients suspected of harboring pituitary adenomas should have early visual, radiologic, and endocrinologic evaluation, and thus permanent visual impairment from chiasmal compression will be seen less often.

We believe that decompression of the chiasm in the presence of visual impairment can be best achieved by the transsphenoidal approach. Its superiority to the transcranial approach becomes evident when one looks at the decreased morbidity and mortality associated with the transsphenoidal approach. In our opinion, the current treatment of choice of pituitary adenomas is the microsurgical transsphenoidal technique.

REFERENCES

1. Aloia, J., and Arehanbeau, J. (1978): Hypopituitarism following pituitary irradiation for acromegaly. *Horm. Res.*, 9:201–207.
2. Anderson, D. (1977): Transport in the retina and optic nerve. In: *Neuro-ophthalmology,* Vol. 9, Ch. 9, edited by J. S. Glaser. L. V. Mosley, St. Louis.
3. Anderson, D., and Hendrickson, A. (1974): Effect of intraocular pressure on rapid axoplasmic transport in monkey optic nerve. *Invest. Ophthalmol.*, 13:771–783.
4. Annegers, J. F., et al. (1978): Pituitary adenoma in Olmsted County, Minnesota. *Mayo Clin. Proc.*, 53:641–643.
5. Bakay, L. (1950): The results of 300 pituitary adenoma operations. (Prof. Herbert Olivercrona's series). *J. Neurosurg.*, 7:240–255.
6. Bergland, R., and Ray, B. (1968): Anatomical variations in the pituitary gland and adjacent structures in 225 human autopsy cases. *J. Neurosurg.*, 28:93–99.
7. Bergland, R., and Ray, B. (1969): The arterial supply of the human optic chiasm. *J. Neurosurg.*, 31:327–333.
8. Berre, J. P. (1975): The empty sella. *Neurology (Minneap),* 25:1137–1143.
9. Berti, G., et al. (1974): Pituitary apoplexy treated by stereotaxic transsphenoidal aspiration. *Cleve. Clin. Q.*, 163:168–178.
10. Buckman, M. T., et al. (1976): Primary empty sella syndrome with visual field defects. *Am. J. Med.*, 61:124–128.
11. Cushing, H., and Walker, C. B. (1915): Distortion of the visual fields in cases of brain tumor. IV Chiasmal lesions with special reference to bitemporal hemianopsia. *Brain,* 37:341–400.
12. Dawson, B. H. (1958): The blood vessels of the human optic chiasma and their relation to those of the hypophysis and hypothalamus. *Brain,* 81:207–217.
13. Dawson, D., and Denginer, J. (1970): Hazards of proton beam pituitary irradiation. *N. Engl. J. Med.*, 282:1134.
14. Demailly, P., and Guiot, G. (1967): Resultats visuels des exereses d' adenomes hypophysaires par voie transsphenoidale. *Arch. Ophthalmol.*, 27:5–34.

14a. Ezrin, C. (1963): *The Pituitary Gland,* Clinical Symposia. CIBA Pharmaceutical Company, Summit, New Jersey.

15. Falconer, M., and Stafford Bell, M. (1975): Visual failure from pituitary and parasellar tumors with favorable outcome in pregnant women. *J. Neurol. Neurosurg. Psychiatry,* 38:919–930.
16. Feinsod, M., and Auerbach, E. (1971): The electroretinogram and the visual evoked potential in two patients with tuberculum sella meningioma before and after decompression of the optic nerve. *Ophthalmologica,* 163:360–368.

17. Feinsod, M., Hoyt, W. F., and Wilson, C. B. (1976): Monitoring optic nerve function during craniotomy. *J. Neurosurg.*, 44:29–31.
18. François, J. (1958): Vascularization of the primary optic pathways. *Br. J. Ophthalmol.*, 42:65.
19. Frisen, L., et al. (1976): Cyclic compression of the intracranial optic nerve. Patterns of visual failure and recovery. *J. Neurol. Neurosurg. Psychiatry*, 39:1109–1113.
20. Gray, H. (1973): *Anatomy of the Human Body*, pp. 186–187. Formur International, St. Louis.
21. Guillaume, J., and Caron, J. P. (1958): Remarques cliniques et chirurgicales relatives aux adenomes hypophysares. *Neurochirurgie*, 4:338–343.
22. Hankinson, J., and Banna, M. (1976): *Pituitary and Parapituitary Tumors*, pp. 5–11. Saunders, Philadelphia.
23. Hardy, J. (1971): Transsphenoidal hypophysectomy. *J. Neurosurg.*, 34:582–594.
24. Harris, J. R., and Levene, M. B. (1976): Visual complications following irradiation for pituitary adenomas and craniopharyngiomas. *Radiology*, 120:167–171.
25. Heimbach, S. B. (1959): Follow-up studies on 105 cases of verified chromophobe and acidophile pituitary adenomata after treatment by transfrontal operation and x-ray irradiation. *Acta. Neurochir. (Wien)*, 7:101–155.
26. Henderson, W. B. (1939): The pituitary adenomata: A follow-up study of the surgical results in 338 cases (Dr. Harvey Cushing's series). *Br. J. Surg.*, 26:811–921.
27. Heshmat, M., et al. (1976): Neoplasms of the central nervous system: Incidence and population selectivity in Washington, D.C. *Cancer*, 38:2135–2142.
28. Hirsch, O. (1952): Symptoms and treatment of pituitary tumors. *Arch. Otolaryngol.*, 55:268–306.
29. Hoyt, W. F. (1969): Correlative anatomy of the optic chiasm. In: *Clinical Neurosurgery*, Ch. 12, edited by R. Ojemann. Williams & Wilkins, Baltimore.
30. Hughes, B. (1958): Blood supply of optic nerves and chiasma. *Br. J. Ophthalmol.*, 42:106–125.
31. Kaufman, B. (1962): The empty sella turcica—A manifestation of the intrasellar subarachnoid space. *Radiology*, 90:931–941.
32. Kayan, A., and Earl, C. J. (1975): Compressive lesions of the optic nerves and chiasm. *Brain*, 98:13–28.
33. Kjellberg, R. N., and Kliman, B. (1976): Treatment of acromegaly by proton hypophysectomy. In: *Current Controversies in Neurosurgery*, edited by T. Morley. Saunders, Philadelphia.
34. Landolt, A. (1975): Ultrastructure of human sella tumors. *Acta Neurochir. (Suppl.)*, 22:1–167.
35. Laws, E. R., et al. (1977): Transsphenoidal decompression of the optic nerve and chiasm. *J. Neurosurg.*, 46:717–722.
36. Laws, E. R. (1975): Complications of transsphenoidal surgery. In: *Clinical Neurosurgery*, Vol. 23, edited by E. Keener. Williams & Wilkins, Baltimore.
37. Lee, W. (1968): The empty sella syndrome. *J. Neurosurg.*, 28:351–354.
38. Levy, N. (1974): The effects of elevated intraocular pressure on slow axonal flow. *Invest. Ophthalmol.*, 13:691–695.
39. Lloyd, M., and Belchete, P. (1977): The clinical features and management of pituitary apoplexy. *Postgrad. Med. J.*, 53:82–85.
40. Lundstrom, M., and Frisen, L. (1977): Atrophy of optic nerve fibres in compression of the chiasm. *Acta Ophthalmol.*, 55:208–216.
41. Mortara, R., and Norrell, H. (1970): Consequences of deficit sellar diaphragm. *J. Neurosurg.*, 32:565–573.
41a. Moses, R. (editor) (1973): *Alder's Physiology of the Eye*, 5th ed. Mosby, St. Louis.
42. Neetens, A., and Selosse, P. (1977): Oculomotor abnormalities in sellar and parasellar pathology. *Ophthalmologica*, 175:80–104.
42a. Netter, F. (1973): *CIBA Series, Vol. 5: Endocrine Glands.* CIBA Pharmaceutical Company, Summit, New Jersey.
43. Newman, M. (1967): The chiasmal syndrome. In: *Clinical Concepts in Neuro-ophthalmology*, edited by A. J. Gay and R. Burde. Little, Brown and Co., Boston.
44. O'Connel, J. E. (1973): The anatomy of the optic chiasm and heteronymous hemianopia. *J. Neurol. Neurosurg. Psychiatry*, 36:710–723.
45. Oliver, L., et al. (1975): *The Anterior Pituitary: Ultrastructure of Pituitary Cells, A Critical Study.* Academic, New York.
46. Olivocrona, H. (1967): The surgical treatment of intracranial tumors. *Handbuch der Neurochirurgie*, Vol. 4, part 4, pp. 1–301. Springer-Verlag, Berlin.

47. Olson, D. R., and Guiot, G. (1972): The symptomatic empty sella: Prevention and correction via transsphenoidal approach. *J. Neurosurg.,* 37:533–537.
48. Percy, A., et al. (1972): Neoplasms of the central nervous system. *Neurology,* 22:40–48.
49. Ray, B., and Patterson, R. H. (1971): Surgical experience with chromophobe adenomas of the pituitary gland. *J. Neurosurg.,* 34:726–729.
50. Renn, W., and Rhoton, A. (1975): Microsurgical anatomy of the sellar region. *J. Neurosurg.,* 43:288–298.
51. Rucker, C. W., and Kernohan, J. W. (1954): Notching of the optic chiasm by overlying arteries in pituitary tumors. *Arch. Ophthalmol.,* 51:161–170.
52. Russell, D., and Rubinstein, L. (1977): *Pathology of Tumors of the Nervous System,* 4th ed. Williams & Wilkins, Baltimore.
53. Shalt, S. M., et al. (1977): Endocrine morbidity in adults treated with cerebral irradiation for brain tumors during childhood. *Acta Endocrinol. (Kbh),* 84:673–680.
54. Simmonds, C. (1962): Ocular palsy in pituitary adenoma. *Bull. Johns Hopkins Hosp.,* 111:72–82.
55. Sunderland, S., and Bradley, R. (1961): Stress-strain phenomenon in human peripheral nerve trunks. *Brain,* 84:102–119.
56. Svien, H. J., et al. (1965): Status of vision following surgical treatment for pituitary chromophobe adenoma. *J. Neurosurg.,* 22:47–52.
57. Thorner, M. O., et al. (1974): Long term treatment of galactorrhea and hypogonadism with bromocriptine. *Br. Med. J.,* 2:419–422.
58. Tonnis, W., Oberdisse, K., and Weber, E. (1950): Bericht uber 264 operierte hypophysemadenome. *Acta Neurochir. (Wien),* 3:113–130.
59. Van Dallen, J. T., and Greve, E. L. (1977): Rapid deterioration of visual fields during bromocriptine induced pregnancy in a patient with a pituitary adenoma. *Br. J. Ophthalmol.,* 61:729–733.
60. Walsh, F. B., and Hoyt, W. F. (1969): *Clinical Neuro-Ophthalmology,* 3rd. ed. Williams & Wilkins, Baltimore.
61. Weinberger, J. (1940): Primary pituitary adenoma and the syndrome of the cavernous sinus. *Arch. Ophthalmol.,* 20:1197–1201.
62. Weiss, M., et al. (1976): Pituitary apoplexy. Therapeutic assessment. *Bull. Los Angeles Neurol. Soc.,* 41:143–147.
63. Welch, K. (1971): Chiasmplexy for the correction of traction on the optic nerves and chiasm associated with their descent into an empty sella. *J. Neurosurg.,* 35:760–763.
64. Wilson, P., and Falconer, M. (1978): Patterns of visual failure with pituitary tumors. *Br. J. Ophthalmol.,* 52:94–110.
64a. Wolff, E. (1968): *Anatomy of the Eye and Orbit.* Saunders, Philadelphia.
65. Wood, J. H., and Dogali, M. (1975): Visual improvement after chiasmplexy for primary empty sella turcica. *Surg. Neurol.,* 3:291–293.
66. Wybar, K. (1977): Chiasmal compression. *Proc. R. Soc. Med.,* 70:307–317.

Clinical Management of Pituitary Disorders,
edited by G. T. Tindall and W. F. Collins.
Raven Press, New York © 1979.

15

Pituitary Tumors Associated With Hyperprolactinemia

George T. Tindall, C. Scott McLanahan, and Alan S. Fleischer

Department of Surgery, Division of Neurosurgery, Emory University, School of Medicine, Atlanta, Georgia 30322

During recent years major progress has been accomplished in the management of pituitary tumors diagnostically and therapeutically (3,21,29,46). This has been due to important advances in endocrinology, neurosurgery, and neuroradiology. In neuroradiology the increasing usage of hypocycloidal polytomography has allowed detection of subtle changes in the sella turcica caused by tumors often <1.0 cm in greatest diameter. Also the widespread use of computerized axial tomography (CT scan) has improved the diagnostic management of these lesions. In neurosurgery increasing use of transsphenoidal microsurgical techniques has made it possible to remove selectively adenomas as small as 3 to 4 mm in diameter, as well as larger lesions, with a low morbidity and essentially no mortality. In endocrinology the measurement of prolactin and growth hormone by radioimmunoassay has contributed significantly to the early detection of pituitary tumors, especially those microadenomas associated with infertility. As a result of this progress, most neurosurgeons have become more aggressive in their attitude toward the treatment of pituitary tumors and currently are operating on patients for the endocrinopathies as well as the mass effects caused by these lesions.

A precise and sensitive radioimmunoassay for prolactin has provided information concerning the regulation of this hormone in physiologic and pathologic states and, further, has been instrumental in disclosing that a significant number of women with secondary amenorrhea (with or without galactorrhea) have small, otherwise asymptomatic pituitary tumors. These tumors, some of which are no more than 5 mm in diameter, either secrete autonomously an excessive quantity of prolactin or otherwise cause an inappropriate release of this hormone from the remaining normal adenohypophysis. The resultant excessive level of serum prolactin is the basic cause for disruption of the normal reproductive cycle.

In this chapter the current clinical, diagnostic, and therapeutic aspects of pituitary tumors associated with hyperprolactinemia are discussed. Additionally, the results of transsphenoidal microsurgical operations on 42 women with amenorrhea–galactorrhea syndrome associated with hyperprolactinemia are presented. Discussion of the results focuses on the completeness of tumor removal, preservation or return of normal pituitary function, return of abnormal levels of prolactin to normal, and improvement in symptoms related to the tumor.

DESCRIPTION OF PROLACTIN

Prolactin is produced by the erythrosinophilic subtype of acidophilic cell in the adenophypophysis (16) and is released into the systemic circulation through the influence of releasing and inhibiting hypothalamic neurohormones (24). It is unique among known pituitary trophic hormones in that the predominant hypothalamic modulator is prolactin-inhibiting factor (PIF), which is required to prevent an unrestrained release of prolactin by the adenohypophysis. Thus pituitary stalk section or certain hypothalamic lesions which interfere with the normal delivery of PIF to the anterior lobe increase serum prolactin (37,42). The prolactin inhibitory mechanism is dopaminergic in nature (7), and some authorities believe that PIF is dopamine (26).

The physiology of prolactin is complex. The only established function of this hormone in humans is the initiation and maintenance of lactation provided the glandular breast tissue has been appropriately primed by the interaction of several other hormones (7). The only clinical impairment resulting from elevated levels of serum prolactin in women is either suppression of, or interference with, the menstrual cycle and ovulation resulting in amenorrhea and infertil-

TABLE 1. *Factors known to affect serum prolactin*

Increased prolactin	Decreased prolactin
General anesthesia	L-DOPA
Surgery	Ergot alkaloids
Stress	Apomorphine
Exercise	
Sleep	
Pregnancy	
Nipple stimulation	
Hypothyroidism	
Hypoglycemia	
Thyroid-releasing hormone (TRH)	
Phenothiazines	
Reserpine	
Methyldopa	
Opiates	

Data from refs. 12 and 15.

ity. In men impotence has been ascribed to elevated levels of prolactin, although this relationship is not definitely established. Spontaneous galactorrhea occurs in about 35% of women with hyperprolactinemia (14) and only rarely in men (9).

Hyperprolactinemia has been identified in a variety of pathologic clinical states (Table 1). In practice, the three most common are the ingestion of certain drugs (particularly phenothiazines), primary hypothyroidism, and pituitary tumors (10,22). Thus in the diagnostic work-up of patients with hyperprolactinemia due to suspected pituitary tumors, it is essential to obtain a detailed history and to perform appropriate tests in order to determine the cause for the elevated serum prolactin.

The clinical significance of serum prolactin measurements is twofold: It serves to identify patients with pituitary tumors, particularly those associated with fertility problems, and it affords a reliable means for following patients with prolactin-secreting pituitary tumors following treatment.

PATHOLOGY

Histologically pituitary tumors are identified as chromophobic, acidophilic, basophilic, and mixed adenomas—the classic morphological differentiation; this classification is now regarded as obsolete by most clinicians, who prefer to differentiate these tumors with respect to function, thus categorizing them as hormone-secreting and nonhormone-secreting varieties. The hormone-secreting pituitary tumors include those producing an excess of growth hormone (gigantism or acromegaly) (6), prolactin (amenorrhea with or without galactorrhea) (2,5,36,43,47), adrenocorticotropin (Cushing's disease) (36), rarely thyrotropin (17) (thyrotoxicosis), and even more rarely a combination of hypersecretory states (17,36,47). To complete the classification, the tumor of Nelson's syndrome should be mentioned. This lesion is a pituitary tumor which develops or becomes symptomatic in a limited number of patients who have had bilateral adrenalectomy for treatment of Cushing's disease. The presence of the tumor, which is usually chromophobic and often invasive, may be associated with intense skin pigmentation (33).

Many pituitary tumors do not secrete excessive levels of trophic hormones, and in most instances these tumors are chromophobic. In our experience those tumors associated with hyperprolactinemia are usually chromophobic, although a significant number are found to be acidophilic. Fortunately, the great majority of pituitary tumors are histologically benign, slow-growing lesions.

Special investigations, including electron microscopic, immunohistochemical, and fluorescence techniques have been used in an effort to define better the ultrastructure, particularly the size and chemical composition of the secretory granules of these tumors and to relate the morphology to clinical findings. Robert and Hardy (35) determined characteristic sizes of granules along with other ultrastructural features among the various types of secreting tumors, correlating them with clinical syndromes but not linking granules to specific hormones by histochemical studies. Kovacs et al. (25) and Zimmerman et al. (47) used immunoperoxidase techniques to label prolactin in tumor tissue obtained from autopsies and from patients with chromophobic adenomas. Interestingly, Zimmerman et al. (47) demonstrated that growth hormone and prolactin can be secreted by the same tumor, which may account in part for the 15 to 20% incidence of hyperprolactinemia among acromegalics.

McCarty et al. (27), who recently reviewed the present state of the art, indicated that special histochemical techniques (i.e., the tetrachrome method of Herlant) and electron microscopy are helpful but not infallible for identifying prolactin-secreting adenomas. The best available description of the prolactin granule is that of an electron-dense spherical or elliptical mass ranging from 200 to 800 μm in diameter (27).

The term "prolactinoma" has been applied to those pituitary tumors that autonomously secrete prolactin (13,22). Currently prolactinoma is the most frequently diagnosed functional pituitary tumor and accounts for approximately 25% of all pituitary tumors (30,32,34). Curiously, prolactin-secreting tumors are usually located in the lateral portions of the pituitary gland (18). Hyperprolactinemia (i.e., prolactin >25 ng/ml) in patients with pituitary tumors may occur as a result of one or more of three possible mechanisms (23). (a) The tumor (i.e., a prolactinoma) autonomously secretes excessive quantities of prolactin. (b) Pressure on the pituitary stalk with resultant interference in the delivery of PIF allows an unrestrained release of hormone by the normal, nontumorous prolactin cells of the anterior lobe. (c) A primary disorder in the hypothalamus involving either diminished secretion of PIF or overproduction of prolactin releasing factor may result in hyperprolactinemia.

In patients with pituitary tumors, it is difficult to identify the underlying mechanism for elevated prolactin levels when the values are only moderately elevated (i.e., >25 ng/ml but <100 ng/ml) as such an elevation can result from compression of the stalk and/or hypothalamus as well as autonomous secretion by a tumor. On the other hand, when the fasting level of prolactin exceeds 150 ng/ml, it almost certainly indicates that the mechanism for hyperprolactinemia is secretion by a functioning adenoma. Although the chlorpromazine (CPZ) test for prolactin reserve has been useful for identifying structural lesions in the vicinity of the stalk and gland, the test has not served to differentiate between the three mechanisms responsible for elevated prolactin levels in patients with pituitary tumors. The response (of serum prolactin levels) to CPZ is blunted or negative in all three situations.

Persistent elevations in prolactin following treatment do not necessarily mean that viable tumor fragments remain. In most cases it seems more likely that the elevations are due to stalk damage either by the tumor and/or the treatment, with resultant interference with the normal delivery of PIF to the adenohypophysis and subsequent unrestrained release of prolactin from the normal gland. In such a case the prolactin levels should continue to fall gradually or remain unchanged, which implies that the stalk is gradually regenerating its capacity to deliver PIF or that it is permanently damaged. On the other hand, if prolactin begins to rise, the implication is that the tumor has recurred and that a residual tumor fragment was probably responsible for the failure of prolactin to return to normal during the immediate postoperative period. Currently serial posttreatment determinations of prolactin probably comprise the most reliable method for determining tumor recurrence and probably rise well in advance of either clinical or other endocrinological findings.

CLINICAL FEATURES

The clinical findings of pituitary tumors can be divided into three categories: mass effects, hormonal deficiencies, and hormonal excesses. Mass effects are most commonly manifested by disturbances in visual acuity, visual field defects (usually bitemporal cuts), cranial nerve palsies (usually oculomotor), and infrequently signs of hypothalamic involvement. The most serious problem is compression of the optic chiasm, which can result in irreversible blindness. Pituitary tumors can also cause various degrees of hypopituitarism, the clinical manifestations of which are summarized in Table 2. In terms of mass effects and hormonal deficiencies produced by compromise of the normal gland, pituitary tumors associated with hyperprolactinemia are no different from other pituitary tumors. On the other hand, the specific clinical manifestation of a pituitary tumor associated with hyperprolactinemia in the female consists of amenorrhea often accompanied by galactorrhea (9); galactorrhea is rarely seen in the male.

Several eponyms have been used to describe varieties of the amenorrhea–

TABLE 2. *Clinical effects of hormone deficiencies*

Hormone	Clinical manifestations
Gonadotropin (LH and FSH)	
Male adult	Decreased libido and impotence; decrease in body hair, size of testicles, and sperm count
Female adult	Amenorrhea; infertility; decrease in breast tissue
Prepubertal males and females	Failure to develop secondary sexual characteristics
Somatotropin	
Adults	Usually no manifestation but occasionally fasting hypoglycemia
Prepubertal children	Retarded general growth and development; dwarfism if it occurs during early childhood
Adrenocorticotropin	Adrenal insufficiency; generalized weakness; postural hypotension
Thyrotropin	Hypothyroidism; cold intolerance; weight gain; sallow skin; slowed mentation
Prolactin	No manifestation in male; loss of lactating ability in females
Melanotropin	Loss of pigmentation
Vasopressin	Diabetes insipidus

galactorrhea syndrome and for the sake of completeness should be mentioned. The Forbes–Albright syndrome applies to patients with amenorrhea–galactorrhea with a radiographically demonstrable pituitary tumor (11). In the Chiari–Frommel syndrome the amenorrhea–galactorrhea follows pregnancy, and in the Argonz–Del Castillo syndrome symptoms are spontaneous, unrelated to a previous gestation, and associated with a normal sella turcica. In view of recent developments, however, particularly the finding that many patients with the amenorrhea–galactorrhea syndrome with radiologically normal sellae are found to have microadenomas, the strict use of these clinical syndromes has come to have little practical clinical value. Rather than attempt to classify a patient with amenorrhea–galactorrhea into one of the eponymic syndromes, we agree with Bohnet et al. (1) that the term "hyperprolactinemic–anovulatory syndrome" is a more practical one.

ENDOCRINOLOGICAL EVALUATION

Endocrine testing in patients with pituitary tumors associated with hyperprolactinemia should include determination of the three pituitary–target organ axes, reserve and suppression tests for prolactin, reserve tests for growth hormone, and evaluation of posterior lobe function. The protocol currently in use at our institution (Table 3) has been valuable not only for detecting small tumors that produce minimal compromise but also, when repeated following treatment, determining if (a) any additional impairment in endocrine function was created, or (b) pituitary endocrine function was restored. The provocative tests for prolactin and growth hormone have proved useful in detecting small tumors and, in fact, have often been a more sensitive indicator of compromise of the pituitary gland than the pituitary–target organ testing. The mechanism for prolactin secretion appears to be quite sensitive and easily disturbed, so that impairment of the normal response to chlorpromazine occurs with tumors as small as 5 mm in diameter. For instance, in a previously reported study (40), 13 patients with pituitary tumors associated with hyperprolactinemia were found to have intact pituitary–target axes, and yet all showed flat or blunted responses following administration of chlorpromazine.

The pituitary–gonadal axis is tested by determining follicle-stimulating hormone (FSH), luteinizing hormone (LH), testosterone (males), and estradiol (females) in serum all by the radioimmunoassay technique. If FSH, LH, and the target organ hormones are within the defined range of normal, the axis is considered to be intact. In the case of postmenopausal women, elevated FSH and LH values are considered normal.

Serum thyroid-stimulating hormone (TSH) and total thyroxine (T_4), both of which are determined by radioimmunoassay, and free thyroxine (FT_4), which is assessed by a modification of the effective thyroxine ratio (ETR) determination, are used to evaluate the pituitary–thyroid axis. If TSH and FT_4 are within the normal range, the axis is considered to be intact. If the FT_4 is low without corresponding elevation of TSH, the axis is considered abnormal.

TABLE 3. *Tests used to assess pituitary endocrine function*

Axis	Test	Normal values	
		Male	Female
Anterior lobe function			
Pituitary–gonadal	Serum FSH	2–15 MIU/ml	5–20 MIU/ml
	Serum LH	1–20 MIU/ml	2–30 MIU/ml
	Serum testosterone	300–1,200 ng/100 ml	20–80 ng/100 ml
	Serum estradiol	1–3 ng/100 ml	2–7 ng/100 ml
Pituitary–thyroidal	Serum total thyroxine (T_4)	4.5–11.5 μg/100 ml	
	Serum free T_4	1.0–2.3 ng/100 ml	
	Serum TSH	<6 μunits/ml	
Pituitary–adrenal	Serum cortisol (a.m.)	6–18 μg/100 ml	
	Urine (24-hr) 17-KS	3–24 mg/24 hr	1–18 mg/24 hr
	Urine (24-hr) 17-OHCS	2.9–12.0 mg/24 hr	1.1–8.6 mg/24 hr
Growth hormone reserve; glucagon or L-DOPA provocative			
Growth hormone suppression: used only in suspected acromegaly			
Prolactin reserve: chloropromazine provocative			
Posterior pituitary function			
Simultaneous serum and urine osmolalities after 8–12 hr of water deprivation			

The pituitary–adrenal axis is assessed by determining serum cortisol and 24-hr urinary 17-ketosteroid (17-KS) and 17-hydroxycorticosteroid (17-OHCS) excretions. If the serum cortisol and urinary steroids are within normal limits and no postural drop in systolic blood pressure can be demonstrated, the axis is considered intact. If the serum cortisol and urinary steroids are low without postural hypotension, the axis is considered borderline low. If all three parameters are low, the axis is considered definitely abnormal. Because of their additional expense and questionable value, the metyrapone test and ACTH determination are not carried out routinely.

Serum growth hormone (hGH) is determined by radioimmunoassay. After obtaining fasting values, hGH reserve is evaluated by determining serum hGH levels 120 and 150 min after intramuscular administration of 1 mg glucagon (8,45). hGH reserve is considered normal if an increment of 5 ng/ml or greater is measured at 120 or 150 min.

Baseline serum prolactin (PRL) is determined by radioimmunoassay, with repeat determinations at 60, 120, 180, and 240 min after injection of chlorpromazine 50 mg i.m. (41). The fasting normal value ranges from 5 to 25 ng/ml. A less than twofold increase at some time after chlorpromazine administration is considered indicative of impairment of reserve if the baseline PRL value is low, and loss of hypothalamic control if baseline is high.

Posterior pituitary function is assessed by determining simultaneous serum and urine osmolalities following 8 to 12 hr of water deprivation, thus providing a measure of antidiuretic hormone (ADH) reserve. The duration of deprivation depends on the clinical severity of diabetes insipidus either before or after surgery. The test is considered valid only if the serum osmolality exceeds 285 mOsm/kg. If urine osmolality is less than twice the serum osmolality after deprivation (assuming normal intrinsic renal function), diabetes insipidus is considered present, and gradations of severity are judged according to the degree by which the ratio was less than 2.

NEURODIAGNOSTIC EVALUATION

The following neuroradiological studies are valuable in the diagnostic evaluation of patients with pituitary tumors:

Routine Skull X-rays and Hypocycloidal Polytomography of the Sella Turcica

Anteroposterior and lateral skull X-rays should be made in all patients with suspected pituitary tumors. The upper limits of normal for the sella turcica are an anteroposterior (AP) diameter of 17 mm, a depth of 14 mm, and a width of 10 to 15 mm (38). A more important X-ray examination, however, and one that should be performed routinely in all patients with suspected pituitary tumors is hypocycloidal polytomography of the sella turcica. This examination shows small areas of erosion and/or asymmetry of the sella turcica, alterations in the clinoid processes, as well as other abnormalities that may not be discernible on routine skull X-rays (44). Polytomography of the sella turcica region should be made in an AP and a lateral projection at 1-mm intervals.

Cerebral Angiography

Cerebral angiography is useful for determining the degree of suprasellar or parasellar extension of a pituitary tumor and, in fact, is probably the most reliable test for assessing the lateral extent of these tumors. An equally important diagnostic application of angiography is to exclude the possibility of an intracranial aneurysm with intrasellar extension. As experience with the CT scanner increases, however, it is likely that it will largely replace angiography for determining the extent of extrasellar extension of pituitary tumors.

Pneumoencephalography

Pneumoencephalography (PEG) has been used reliably in the past to determine the degree of suprasellar extension of the tumor and to exclude the diagnosis of the empty sella syndrome. PEG is superior to cerebral angiography for determining the extent of the suprasellar extension of pituitary tumors. However, the CT scan eventually may also replace PEG for this purpose. At present the most important value of PEG for evaluating patients with suspected pituitary tumors and enlarged sella turcica is to exclude the possibility of the empty sella syndrome. It is important that the physician recognize this condition because it usually is not a surgical problem.

CT Scan

Over the past few years CT scanning of the head justifiably has become the most important neurodiagnostic procedure in patients with suspected intracranial pathology. Performed with and without contrast enhancement, it is also proving to be valuable for identifying suprasellar and parasellar extension of pituitary tumors. A CT scan is now considered a routine part of the evaluation of all pituitary tumors. Ultimately, with continued refinements in technique, it may become accurate for diagnosing the empty sella syndrome.

SELECTION OF ENDOCRINE AND NEURODIAGNOSTIC STUDIES IN PATIENTS WITH SUSPECTED PITUITARY TUMORS ASSOCIATED WITH HYPERPROLACTINEMIA

The diagnostic work-up of a patient with suspected pituitary tumor associated with hyperprolactinemia (i.e., serum prolactin $>$25 ng/ml) has undergone considerable revision in recent years. Thus it seems appropriate to summarize current diagnostic evaluation of these patients. As certain medications (e.g., phenothiazines) cause hyperprolactinemia, their usage should be excluded by careful history. A complete endocrine battery as outlined in Table 3 eliminates another common cause of hyperprolactinemia—i.e., hypothyroidism—and determines whether the response of prolactin to administration of chlorpromazine is normal or inappropriate. As indicated above, complete baseline endocrine studies are also important, serving as a control for comparison with posttreatment values to determine if any endocrine axis was impaired (or improved) by the treatment. AP and lateral hypocycloidal polytomography of the sella turcica is an essential part of the examination. Ophthalmological evaluation for determining visual fields and acuity should be obtained routinely in every patient, as increasing clinical experience indicates that patients with small tumors but no subjective visual complaints often have minimal bitemporal upper quadrantic defects, particularly when tested by a skilled perimetrist using a Goldmann perimeter. As already indicated, a CT scan with and without contrast enhancement is a routine part of the diagnostic evaluation. As already mentioned, PEG has been used in the past to determine the degree of suprasellar tumor extension but now is used primarily to exclude the diagnosis of empty sella syndrome. PEG demonstration of an empty sella syndrome generally indicates a nonsurgical condition and usually concludes the diagnostic evaluation. However, a decision to proceed with pituitary surgery in some of these cases can now be based on clinical and endocrinological findings. Since the empty sella syndrome usually is not associated with endocrinopathy (31) or clinical findings, it can be regarded as an incidental finding. Consequently it is no longer essential to establish its presence or absence in order to make a decision regarding treatment. Thus it is our opinion that PEG, except under unusual circumstances, is seldom indicated in the diagnostic evaluation of these patients. The question of cerebral angiography is more controversial. The primary reason for performing this test has been to exclude the rare occurrence of an intrasellar aneurysm, so it is our opinion that the test is unnecessary in most cases, particularly when the patient is relatively young (<40 years old) and has a small hypersecreting tumor.

THERAPEUTIC OBJECTIVES

Ideally, treatment of a pituitary tumor associated with hyperprolactinemia should achieve the following goals:

1. Eradication of tumor
2. Minimal mortality
3. Low morbidity
4. Relief of symptoms
5. Reduction of hormonal elevations to normal (i.e., prolactin <25 ng/ml)
6. Minimal risk to remaining pituitary endocrine function and a reasonable chance of restoring the impaired function

Although these goals may seem somewhat idealistic, significant advances in therapy for pituitary tumors have been made in recent years, and as a result the goals can now be reached in many cases.

There is little if any controversy regarding the need for definitive therapy of pituitary tumors causing mass effects, particularly chiasmal compression. In this instance, relief of the compression is mandatory to protect vision, and most physicians agree that surgical decompression of the chiasm and removal of the tumor is the most appropriate form of therapy. The majority of these cases can be handled satisfactorily by the transsphenoidal microsurgical technique.

With respect to hyperfunctional tumors, there appears to be a consensus that patients with pituitary tumors secreting ACTH or growth hormone should be treated since the natural history of Cushing's disease and acromegaly entails considerable morbidity and mortality to the patients involved. The controversy in these two disease states is not over the need for treatment but over the form of therapy (proton beam, cryohypophysectomy, transsphenoidal microsurgery) to recommend. On the other hand, there remains a modicum of controversy over whether the small tumor associated with hyperprolactinemia should be treated at all. In these cases the argument could be made that since the clinical findings (amenorrhea, galactorrhea) caused by these tumors do not result in either serious disability or impaired health, there is no rationale for therapy unless the patient wishes to become pregnant. If no immediate treatment is offered, careful clinical follow-up is mandatory to ensure that these tumors do not enlarge significantly and begin to produce mass effects. To our knowledge, there are no reliable tests or other methods to predict reliably, for instance, when a 5-mm tumor will double or triple its size. The natural history of a benign pituitary adenoma, particularly the microadenoma associated with hyperprolactinemia, is not completely known, and the most appropriate treatment for the majority of these patients with microadenoma is still uncertain. Although many of these tumors may lie dormant or even possibly regress over a period of several years, clinical experience indicates that some will become aggressive and ultimately spread beyond the confines of the sella turcica. If such should occur, any of the treatment modalities may fail to eradicate the tumor completely. Also, in patients with small prolactin-secreting tumors but otherwise normal pituitary function, there is a good possibility that removing the tumor while it is still small will restore a normal menstrual pattern without significant risk of damaging the normal residual gland. Thus it is our opinion that, except under unusual circumstances, definitive treatment should be advised in all patients in whom a diagnosis of pituitary tumor has been made with reasonable certainty using currently available endocrinological, neuroradiological, and clinical criteria.

THERAPEUTIC OPTIONS

Practical therapeutic options available to patients with pituitary tumors include medical therapy, proton-beam irradiation, and surgery. Currently, of the three available options—craniotomy, cryohypophysectomy, and transsphenoidal microsurgery—it appears that the transseptal, transsphenoidal microsurgical operation described by Hardy (19,20) is the appropriate method for surgical management of most pituitary tumors. Chief among the advantages of this operative approach is the capability for complete tumor removal with preservation of the pituitary gland and a significant reduction in operative mortality and morbidity compared to other operative approaches, particularly craniotomy (4,21,32,36,40,46).

Medical Therapy

Current medical treatment is aimed at the endocrinopathies caused by pituitary tumors, as presently there is no effective medical treatment for pituitary tumors causing mass effect. The medical therapy of the various tumor types is covered in depth in Chapter 12 (Cushing's disease), Chapter 10 (acromegaly), and Chapter 14 (hyperprolactinemia) of this book, and the reader is referred to these sections for discussions of these subjects.

Heavy-Particle Irradiation

As a means for primary treatment of small pituitary tumors, heavy-particle irradiation appears to be superior to the conventional forms of radiotherapy. Indeed until recently it was used extensively in the treatment of acromegaly. Heavy-particle irradiation, discussed in Chapter 17, is reserved for small tumors located entirely within the sella. Although generally effective as a treatment modality, radiation therapy of any type involves a long delay between treatment and clinical response (i.e., 2 to 4 years). In addition, the use of heavy-particle therapy has an inherent potential for damaging the normal pituitary gland as well as adjacent cranial nerves. Moreover, very expensive equipment accessible to only a few institutions is required, and the method is not suitable for tumors that have suprasellar or parasellar extensions. Regardless of how refined heavy-particle irradiation becomes, it cannot match the precision and completeness of selectively removing small tumors with sparing of the normal pituitary gland that can be accomplished with transsphenoidal microsurgery. Also, there is justifiable concern over the long-term effects of the radiation delivered to the sella region, particularly the potential for later development of malignant tumors in tissues exposed to large amounts of radiation.

Surgery

In our opinion surgery is the best therapeutic option for pituitary tumors that seriously compromise any neighboring structure, notably the optic chiasm. Moreover, based on several recent reports in the literature and our own experience, it appears that surgery (i.e., transsphenoidal microsurgery) is currently also the treatment of choice for tumors that produce endocrinopathy. The low incidence of complications and a negligible mortality rate represent major advantages of the procedure (4,21,32,36,40,46). The transient nature of diabetes insipidus in the few patients who develop this problem is probably due to edema of the pituitary stalk incident to operative manipulation, and the rare occurrence of cerebrospinal fluid (CSF) rhinorrhea is related to the fact that pituitary tumors are separated from the subarachnoid space by the diaphragm sella–pseudocapsule of the tumor. Thus it is possible to remove all gross tumor, spare this covering structure, and never enter the subarachnoid space.

Another outstanding advantage of transsphenoidal surgery over other operative approaches is that gross total removal of most tumors, including those that extend significantly (i.e., 1 to 2 cm) above the upper limits of the sella turcica, can be accomplished with preservation of the pituitary gland in the majority of cases. Not only can pituitary function be maintained, but often certain hormonal functions may be restored following tumor removal. In the authors' opinion, total removal of an adenoma without damaging normal pituitary tissue with an operation that carries a low incidence of complications and rare mortality constitutes a major advance in pituitary tumor surgery.

The use of routine postoperative irradiation following transsphenoidal microsurgical removal of a pituitary tumor is not a settled issue. In those cases where obvious gross total tumor removal is not accomplished, it is our opinion that conventional radiotherapy should be used. However, when all gross-appearing tumor tissue is excised, particularly in patients with tumors <1.0 cm, it seems inappropriate to employ postoperative irradiation.

TECHNIQUE OF TRANSSPHENOIDAL MICROSURGERY FOR PITUITARY ADENOMA

At our institution a modification of Hardy's operation (19,20) is used to perform either hypophysectomy or pituitary tumor removal. The procedure is performed using general anesthesia. The upper lip is retracted and an incision made in the gingival mucosa. After separating the soft tissues from the maxilla and exposing the nasal mucosa, a submucosal dissection plane is developed along one side of the nasal septum as described in a previous report (39). Using this technique, the septum remains intact except posteriorly. After removing the anterior wall of the sphenoid sinus, the operating microscope is brought into the surgical field and the remainder of the operation performed using magnification.

Since many tumors associated with hyperprolactinemia are relatively small, often no larger than 5 mm in diameter, it is important to not damage the pituitary gland during the dural opening. Disruption of the normal appearance and structure of the gland makes it extremely difficult, if not impossible, to detect the subtle differences that exist between normal gland and microadenomas; these must be determined if the surgeon is to remove the tumor successfully and avoid injuring the normal gland. Also, minimal manipulation of the gland improves the chances for preservation of anterior and posterior pituitary lobe function postoperatively. In our experience the prolactin microadenomas are almost invariably located in the lateral portion of the gland. Larger pituitary tumors enlarge and usually erode the floor of the sella turcica, and in such cases tumor commonly extrudes into the operative wound when the floor of the sella is removed and the dura mater opened. Frequently with the larger tumors the pituitary gland is compressed and flattened against the dorsum sella or diaphragma sella. Following either total or subtotal tumor removal, we apply absolute alcohol to the tumor bed for a period of several minutes. Alcohol is used only when the diaphragma sella–tumor capsule is intact thereby forming an effective barrier between the subarachnoid space and the tumor site.

Adipose tissue taken from the abdominal wall is inserted loosely into the tumor bed and sphenoid sinus. Closure of the wound is simple and involves a single catgut suture in the incision in the gingival mucosa. Soft airway tubes are inserted into each nostril to reapproximate the nasal mucosa, and the patient is allowed to recover from anesthesia. The nasal tubes are removed within 24 hr.

CASE MATERIAL AND METHODS

Over a 5-year-period (1973–1978) at Emory University Affiliated Hospitals, a total of 168 patients with pituitary tumors were operated via the transsphenoidal microsurgical approach. Among this group there were 42 women who presented with secondary amenorrhea and who had associated hyperprolactinemia. These 42 cases form the basis for this report. Their ages ranged from 20 to 40 (mean 27.7) years. Amenorrhea had been present for periods ranging from 6 months to 7 years. Thirty-one patients had spontaneous galactorrhea.

RESULTS

Gross total removal was accomplished in every patient. In only one case was it necessary to remove the gland with the tumor. Histologically, the adenoma was classified as chromophobic in 27 cases, eosinophilic in 11 cases, and mixed type in 4 cases.

Amenorrhea was present in every case, galactorrhea in 32, headache in 8, and impairment in visual acuity and/or fields in 5 cases. The relatively low incidence of headache and impairment in vision was attributed to the fact that the majority of tumors were small (i.e., <1.0 cm in greatest diameter).

Effect of Surgery on Amenorrhea, Galactorrhea, and Elevated Prolactin Levels

The preoperative fasting serum prolactin levels, which ranged from 26 to 6,600 ng/ml among the 42 cases, were used to classify the patients into two groups. Group 1 (28 cases) consisted of patients in whom the preoperative fasting prolactin value ranged from 25 to 200 ng/ml; group 2 (14 cases) were those in whom the value was above 200 ng/ml (Table 4). The 10-day post-

TABLE 4. *Polytomography, tumor size, and effects of surgery on amenorrhea, galactorrhea, and elevated prolactin levels (42 patients)*

Group	No. of cases	Post-operative menstrual status		Galactorrhea		Tumor size		10-Day fasting post-op PRL		Sellar polytomography	
		Resumed periods	Persistent amenorrhea	Pre-op	Post-op	< 1 cm	> 1 cm	< 25 ng/ml	> 25 ng/ml	Normal	Abnormal
I: preop fasting PRL 25–200 ng/ml	28	19 (68%)	9	22	4	24 (86%)	4	19 (68%)	9	8 (29%)	20
II: preop fasting PRL > 200 ng/ml	14	4 (29%)	10	10	4	4	10	5 (36%)	9	0	14

transsphenoidal microsurgical basal prolactin level was below 25 ng/ml in 19 (68%) of the 28 patients in group 1. In 6 patients in this group, the values were >25 ng/ml but significantly ($p < 0.05$) below preoperative levels. The mean pre- and postoperative values for these 6 patients were 96 ± 19 (SE) ng/ml and 44 ± 6 ng/ml, respectively. In 2 cases the 10-day postoperative level was higher than the preoperative level. In group 2 patients the 10-day prolactin values were below 25 ng/ml in only 5 (36%) of the 14 patients. Although the values in the remaining 9 patients in group 2 did not return to normal postoperatively, they were nevertheless significantly ($p < 0.025$) less than the preoperative values.

Following transsphenoidal microsurgical tumor removal, 19 (68%) of 28 women in group 1 resumed normal menstrual periods, and 5 subsequently had normal pregnancies and deliveries. On the other hand, only 4 (29%) of 14 patients in group 2 resumed normal periods. These 4 also had a return of the elevated prolactin values to normal postoperatively. Galactorrhea ceased in 18 (82%) of 22 patients in group 1 and in 6 of 10 patients in group 2. In the patients in whom galactorrhea continued, it was usually less in amount postoperatively. All 5 patients with visual impairment experienced noticeable improvement, and vision was not made worse in any patient. Headache was either cured or significantly relieved in 6 of 8 patients with this complaint.

Tumor Size and Sellar Polytomography

There was a close correlation between tumor size and the preoperative prolactin levels. As shown in Table 4, 24 (86%) of 28 patients in group 1 had tumors <1 cm in greatest diameter. In group 2 only 4 of 14 patients had tumors <1 cm in greatest diameter.

The sellar polytomes were interpreted as normal in 8 (29%) of 28 patients in group 1. The decision to operate on these patients despite normal polytomography was based on clinical history, hyperprolactinemia, a flat or blunted prolactin response to chlorpromazine, and the exclusion of other causes of hyperprolactinemia. The polytomes were abnormal in all 14 cases in group 2.

Pituitary Endocrine Function Following Transsphenoidal Microsurgery

Complete preoperative and 10-day postoperative endocrine data as listed in Table 3 were available in 30 of the 42 patients, thus permitting evaluation of the effect of surgery on the pituitary–target organ axes. Prior to surgery, 24 (group A in Table 5) of these 30 patients had intact pituitary–target organ axes. Tumor size was <1.0 cm in 19 of the 24 cases. Following transsphenoidal removal of the tumor, 21 cases maintained intact pituitary function in all three axes. One patient had impaired pituitary–thyroid and pituitary–gonad axes, and 2 patients had impairment in the pituitary–gonad axis postoperatively. In each of the latter 3 patients the tumor was >1.0 cm. There was preoperative impairment in one or more pituitary–target organ axes in 6 (group B in Table 5) of

TABLE 5. *Pre- and postoperative pituitary endocrine function (30 cases)*

Group	No. of cases	Tumor size (cm)		Postoperative status
		<1.0	>1.0	
Group A: pre-op endocrine function intact	24	19	5	Endocrine status intact—21 cases Impairment in pituitary–gonad axis—2 cases Impairment in pituitary–gonad and pituitary–thyroid axis—1 case
Group B: preop endocrine function impaired	6	2	4	Unchanged—1 case Additional impairment—1 case (pituitary–adrenal axis) Improvement in pituitary–gonad axis—3 cases Improvement in pituitary–gonad and pituitary–thyroid axis—1 case

the 30 cases. In 4 of the 6 cases, the tumor size was >1.0 cm. Preoperatively among the 6 cases the pituitary–thyroid axis was impaired in 3 cases, the pituitary–gonad in 6, and the pituitary–adrenal in none. Postoperatively there was return to normal function in the pituitary–thyroid and pituitary–gonad in 1 case and in the pituitary–gonad in 3 cases. Surgery resulted in additional impairment in the pituitary–adrenal axis in 1 case. One case remained unchanged. Thus there was either no change or an improvement in pituitary endocrine function following transsphenoidal microsurgical removal of the tumor in 26 (87%) of the 30 cases.

Repeat prolactin determinations were obtained in 15 patients in group 1 and in 9 in group 2 at intervals ranging from 6 months to 2 years following surgery. We arbitrarily decided that a 15% change in either direction from the 10-day value of prolactin is significant. Patients in whom values remained below 25 ng/ml were considered to show no change. Of 15 group 1 patients, follow-up serum prolactin determinations showed no change in 10, a further decrease in 2, and a significant increase in 2 patients compared to the 10-day value. In one additional case there was a decrease at the 6 to 12-month period, but no change at the 1 to 2-year interval. In the 9 group 2 patients, 3 showed no change, 2 a significant decrease, and 4 a significant increase. It is believed that the elevations in these latter 4 cases are of such magnitude as to indicate the presence of recurrent tumor.

NEURORADIOLOGICAL FINDINGS

As mentioned above, polytomography of the sella turcica was normal in 8 (29%) of 28 patients in group 1. All patients in group 2 had abnormal polytomes. The CT scan was abnormal in 2 cases in group 1 and in 8 of the 14 cases in group 2. Pneumoencephalograms were abnormal in 4 of 9 cases in group 1 and in the one instance in which it was performed in group 2. The abnormality in 3 of the abnormal studies in group 1 consisted of a significant quantity of air in the sella turcica, i.e., an empty sella syndrome that occurred as an incidental finding in association with a pituitary microadenoma. Cerebral angiograms were abnormal in 2 of 6 instances in group 1 and in both cases in which it was performed in group 2.

COMPLICATIONS OF SURGERY

Immediate postoperative complications were relatively few and were benign in nature. There were no deaths, and no patient developed meningitis or CSF rhinorrhea. Temporary diabetes insipidus occurred in 8 patients postoperatively requiring one to five doses of pitressin tannate in oil. Five patients were further treated with clofibrate, a drug which has been found to be effective in treating partial diabetes insipidus (28). All patients subsequently were able to discontinue the drug.

COMMENT

Many neurosurgeons who are experienced in pituitary microsurgery currently hold the attitude that women with the amenorrhea–galactorrhea syndrome associated with hyperprolactinemia due to a pituitary adenoma are candidates for transsphenoidal microsurgery (18,21,40,46). Consistent with this view are the results of the present study, which indicate that a significant number of these women can expect a return of normal menstrual cycling after an operation that is safe and associated with minimal morbidity.

Our results emphasize the important relationship between the preoperative fasting level of prolactin and the surgical outcome. In terms of restoring menses and lowering elevated prolactin levels to normal, the results were much better when the preoperative fasting level of prolactin was below 200 ng/ml. For instance, normal levels of prolactin were obtained in 19 (68%) of 28 cases in group 1 (i.e., preoperative prolactin was 25 to 200 ng/ml) compared to 5 (36%) of 14 patients in group 2 (preoperative prolactin was above 200 ng/ml). Also, 68% of women in group 1 resumed normal periods compared to only 29% in group 2. These findings are comparable to those reported by others. Hardy et al. (21) showed that transsphenoidal microsurgery for pituitary tumors associated with hyperprolactinemia was followed by a return of prolactin levels to normal in 59 (74%) of 80 cases. In 50 (63%) of these 80 cases, menses returned and 29 (36%) patients became pregnant. Similar beneficial results were obtained by Chang et al. (4) who noted return of menses in 16 of 17 women with prolactin microadenomas (<1.0 cm in diameter) and in 2 of 7 women with adenomas larger than 1 cm in diameter.

SUMMARY

Much progress has been made over the past decade in diagnosis and management of patients with pituitary tumors. The headache and characteristic visual loss associated with pituitary tumors in the past have been joined by the usually more subtle symptoms and signs of hypersecreting tumors as indicators for further endocrinologic and neuroradiologic investigation. We believe that the latter two evaluations should be complete and include:

1. Assessment of the status of all three anterior pituitary–end organ axes
2. Dynamic studies of prolactin and growth hormone
3. Assessment of posterior lobe function
4. Plain skull films
5. Hypocycloidal polytomography of the sella in both AP and lateral projections
6. CT scan
7. Other neuroradiologic contrast studies when appropriate (see text)
8. Ophthalmological evaluation of visual fields and acuities

It has been our experience that the more thorough the evaluation of even relatively minor symptoms that can be related to pituitary dysfunction, the higher is the rate of success in definitive diagnosis of the problem, and the easier the management. This has been especially true in the care of the hyperprolactinemic–anovulatory syndrome associated with pituitary tumors as small as 5 mm in diameter. These patients may present with nothing more than infertility but on careful evaluation are found to have: (a) elevated serum prolactin (above 25 ng/ml); (b) a blunted response to the intramuscular administration of chlorpromazine; and (c) in most cases a subtle asymmetry of the floor of the sella seen on polytomography.

Although other therapeutic options are available for patients with small pituitary tumors associated with hyperprolactinemia, we prefer an open transsphenoidal microsurgical approach to the sella with the goal of selective total removal of the adenoma as popularized by Hardy. A series of 42 patients with hyperprolactinemia were managed in this manner at the Emory University Affiliated Hospitals between 1973 and 1978. In general, those whose initial prolactin values were below 200 ng/ml had smaller tumors and were more successfully treated in terms of remission of symptoms and return of normal endocrine function than those patients whose initial prolactin values were above 200 ng/ml. Serial prolactin determinations have also been helpful in the early diagnosis of recurrent tumor, although it is not yet clear which of the available treatment modalities is most valuable in managing recurrent tumor.

It is apparent, however, when considering the entire spectrum of pituitary neoplasia, that especially the small tumors can be treated safely and effectively by the transsphenoidal route. We therefore believe that a careful and complete evaluation of the patient who may often present with only minor complaints is rewarding and justified.

REFERENCES

1. Bohnet, H. G., Dahlen, H. G., Wuttke, W., and Schneider, H. P. G. (1976): Hyperprolactinemic anovulatory syndrome. *J. Clin. Endocrinol. Metab.,* 42:132–143.
2. Boyar, R. M., Kapen, S., Weitzman, E. D., et al. (1976): Pituitary microadenoma and hyperprolactinemia. *N. Engl. J. Med.,* 294:263–265.
3. Boyd, A. E., Reichlin, S., and Turksoy, R. N. (1977): Galactorrhea-amenorrhea syndrome: Diagnosis and therapy. *Ann. Intern. Med.,* 87:165–175.
4. Chang, R. J., Keye, W. R., Young, J. R., et al. (1977): Detection, evaluation and treatment of pituitary microadenomas in patients with galactorrhea and amenorrhea. *Am. J. Obstet. Gynecol.,* 128:356–363.
5. Child, D. F., Nader, S., Mashiter, K., et al. (1975): Prolactin studies in "functionless" pituitary tumors. *Br. Med. J.,* 604–606.
6. Cryer, P. E., Daughaday, W. H., Coxe, W. S., et al. (1975): Diagnosis and therapy of acromegaly. *Arch. Intern. Med.,* 135:338–343.
7. Daughaday, W. H. (1974): The adenohypophysis. In: *Textbook of Endocrinology,* edited by Robert H. Williams, pp. 31–77. W. B. Saunders, Philadelphia.
8. Eddy, R. L., Gilliland, P. F., Ibarra, J. D., et al. (1974): Human growth hormone release: Comparison of provocative test procedures. *Am. J. Med.,* 56:179–185.
9. Finn, J. E., and Mount, L. A. (1971): Galactorrhea in males with tumors in the region of the pituitary gland. *J. Neurosurg.,* 35:723–727.
10. Fluckiger, E. (1972): Drugs and the control of prolactin secretion. In: *Prolactin and Carcinogenisis,* edited by A. R. Boynes and K. Griffiths, pp. 162–171. Alpha Omega Alpha, Publishers.
11. Forbes, A. P., Henneman, P. H., Griswold, G. C., Albright, F., et al. (1954): Syndrome characterized by galactorrhea, amenorrhea and low urinary FSH: Comparison with acromegaly and normal lactation. *J. Clin. Endocrinol. Metab.,* 14:265–271.
12. Fournier, P. J. R., Desjardins, P. D., and Friesen, H. G. (1974): Current understanding of human prolactin physiology and its diagnostic and therapeutic applications: A review. *Am. J. Obstet. Gynecol.,* 118:337–343.
13. Franks, S., Jacobs, H. S., and Nabarro, J. D. N. (1975): Studies of prolactin secretion in pituitary disease. *J. Endocrinol.,* 67:55p.
14. Franks, S., Murray, M. A. E., Jequier, A. M., Steele, S. J., Nabarro, J. D. N., and Jacobs, H. S. (1975): Incidence and significance of hyperprolactinemia in women with amenorrhea. *Clin. Endocrinol.,* 4:597–607.
15. Frantz, A. G. (1978): Prolactinemia. *N. Engl. J. Med.,* 298:201–207.
16. Friesen, H. G., Fournier, P., and Desiardins, P. (1973): Pituitary prolactin in pregnancy and normal and abnormal lactation. *Clin. Obstet. Gynecol.,* 16:25–45.
17. Hamilton, C. R., Jr., Adams, L. C., and Maloof, M. (1970): Hyperthyroidism due to a thyrotropin-producing pituitary chromophobe adenoma. *N. Engl. J. Med.,* 283:1077–1080.
18. Hardy, J. (1973): Transsphenoidal surgery of hypersecreting pituitary tumors. In: *Diagnosis and Treatment of Pituitary Tumors,* edited by P. O. Kohler and G. T. Ross, pp. 179–194. International Congress Series 303. *Excerpta Medica,* Amsterdam.
19. Hardy, J. (1971): Transsphenoidal hypophysectomy. *J. Neurosurg.,* 34:582–594.
20. Hardy, J. (1968): Transsphenoidal microsurgery of the normal and pathological pituitary. *Clin. Neurosurg.,* 16:185–217.
21. Hardy, J., Beauregard, H., and Robert, F. (1978): Prolactin-secreting pituitary adenomas: Transsphenoidal microsurgical treatment. In: *Progress in Prolactin Physiology and Pathology,* edited by C. Robyn and M. Harter, pp. 361–370. North Holland Biomedical Press, Amsterdam.
22. Jacobs, H. S. (1976): Prolactin and amenorrhea. *N. Engl. J. Med.,* 295:954–956.
23. Kleinberg, D. L., Noel, G. L., and Frantz, A. G. (1977): Galactorrhea: A study of 235 cases, including 48 with pituitary tumors. *N. Engl. J. Med.,* 296:589–600.
24. Kolodny, H. D., and Sherman, L. (1974): Laboratory aids in the diagnosis of pituitary tumors. *Ann. Clin. Lab. Sci.,* 4:67–86.
25. Kovacs, K., Corenblum, B., Sirek, A. M. T., Penz, G., and Ezrin, C. (1976): Localization of prolactin in chromophobe pituitary adenomas: Study of human necropsy material by immunoperoxidase technique. *J. Clin. Pathol.,* 29:250–258.
26. MacLeod, R. M. (1976): Regulation of prolactin secretion. In: *Frontiers in Neuroendocrinology,* Vol. 6, edited by L. Martini and W. F. Ganong, pp. 169–194. Raven Press, New York.

27. McCarty, K. S., et al. (1978): Neoplasma of the anterior pituitary. *Neurosurgery,* 3:96–104.
28. Moses, A. M., Howanitz, J., and van Gemert, M. (1973): Clofibrate-induced antidiuresis. *J. Clin. Invest.,* 52:535–542.
29. Naidich, T. P. (1976): Evaluation of sellar and parasellar masses by computed tomography. *Radiology,* 120:91–100.
30. Nasr, H., Mozaffarian, G., Pensky, J., et al. (1972): Prolactin secreting pituitary tumors in women. *J. Clin. Endocrinol.,* 34:505.
31. Neelon, P. A., Gove, J. A., and Lebovitz, H. E. (1973): The primary empty sella: Clinical and radiographic and endocrine function. *Medicine (Baltimore),* 52:73.
32. Nielson, K. D., and Clark, K. (1976): Transsphenoidal microsurgery for selective removal of functional pituitary microadenomas. *Texas Med.,* 72:61–66.
33. Nelson, D. H., Meakin, J. W., and Thorn, G. W. (1960): ACTH-producing pituitary tumors following adrenalectomy for Cushing's syndrome. *Ann. Intern. Med.,* 52:560–569.
34. Pearson, O. H., Brodkey, J. S., and Kaufman, B. (1974): Endocrine evaluation and indication for surgery of functional pituitary adenomas. *Clin. Neurosurg.,* 21:26–38.
35. Robert, F., and Hardy, J. (1975): Prolactin-secreting adenomas: A light and electron microscopical study. *Arch. Pathol.,* 99:625–633.
36. Samaan, N. A., Leavens, M. E., and Jesse, R. H. (1974): Pituitary tumors, recent advances in diagnosis and management. *Texas Med.,* 70:55–62.
37. Sherman, L., and Kolodny, H. D. (1974): The effects of drugs on human hypophysiotrophic functions. In: *Mammary Cancer and Neuroendocrine Therapy,* edited by B. A. Stoll, pp. 369–400. Butterworth, London.
38. Taveras, J., and Wood, E. (1964): *Diagnostic Neuroradiology,* p. 102. Williams & Wilkins, Baltimore.
39. Tindall, G. T., Collins, W. F., and Kirchner, J. A. (1978): Unilateral septal technique for transsphenoidal microsurgical approach to the sella turcica. *J. Neurosurg.,* 49:138–142.
40. Tindall, G. T., McLanahan, C. S., and Christy, J. H. (1978): Transsphenoidal microsurgery for pituitary tumors associated with hyperprolactinemia. *J. Neurosurg.,* 48:849–860.
41. Tolis, G., Goldstein, M., and Friesen, H. G. (1973): Functional evaluation of prolactin secretion in patients with hypothalamic-pituitary disorders. *J. Clin. Invest.,* 52:783–788.
42. Turkington, R. W., Underwood, L. E., and Van Wyk, J. J. (1971): Elevated serum prolactin levels after pituitary stalk section in man. *N. Engl. J. Med.,* 285:707–710.
43. Turkington, R. W. (1972): Secretion of prolactin by patients with pituitary and hypothalamic tumors. *J. Clin. Endocrinol.,* 34:159–164.
44. Vezina, J. L., and Sutton, T. J. (1974): Prolactin-secreting pituitary microadenomas: Roentgenologic diagnosis. *Am. J. Roentgenol. Radium Ther. Nucl. Med.,* 120:46–53.
45. Wieland, R. G., Hallbert, N. C., and Zorn, E. (1973): Growth hormone response to intramuscular glucagon. *J. Clin. Endocrinol.,* 37:329–330.
46. Wilson, C. B., and Dempsey, L. C. (1978): Transsphenoidal microsurgical removal of 250 pituitary adenomas. *J. Neurosurg.,* 48:13–22.
47. Zimmerman, E. A., Defendini, R., and Frantz, A. G. (1974): Prolactin and growth hormone in patients with pituitary adenomas: A correlative study of hormone in tumor and plasma by immunoperoxidase technique and radioimmunoassay. *J. Clin. Endocrinol.,* 38:577–585.

Clinical Management of Pituitary Disorders,
edited by G. T. Tindall and W. F. Collins.
Raven Press, New York © 1979.

16

Conventional Radiation Therapy in the Treatment of Pituitary Tumors

Glenn E. Sheline

Department of Radiation Oncology, University of California, San Francisco, California 94143

Historically, radiation therapists have classified pituitary tumors as eosinophilic adenomas (producing acromegaly), basophilic adenomas (thought to cause Cushing's disease), and nonfunctional chromophobic adenomas. Improved diagnostic studies—endocrinologic, neuroradiographic, and histopathologic—have made such a classification obsolete. Newer fixation and staining methods and electron microscopy have shown that thyroid-stimulating hormone (TSH), growth hormone (hGH), adrenocorticotropic hormone (ACTH), prolactin, follicle-stimulating hormone (FSH), and luteinizing hormone (LH) are secreted by specific types of cells which by earlier staining methods would have been termed acidophilic, basophilic, or chromophobic. Tumors producing excessive quantities of each of these pituitary hormones have been reported. Many, perhaps 70%, of those tumors that prior to the prolactin assay would have been diagnosed as nonfunctioning chromophobic adenomas are now known to secrete prolactin and produce hyperprolactinemia. Although there still are pituitary tumors with no known function, there is doubt regarding the existence of a true chromophobic adenoma (24). Due to lack of hormone storage, functional tumors may have granules that are few, small, and difficult to identify.

The effects of pituitary tumors and the results of their treatment depend on the hormones produced and on mass effects associated with extrasellar extension. Thus it is necessary to consider these tumors according to the presence or absence of endocrine activity as well as the degree of extrasellar extension with its secondary effects due to pressure on, or invasion of, surrounding structures. Relatively small tumors with little or no mass effect other than perhaps minimal distortion of the sella can cause acromegaly, Cushing's disease, or hyperprolactinemia. Acromegaly and rarely Cushing's disease, however, may result from moderately large tumors; in the older radiotherapy literature, tumors large enough to produce visual field deficits were reported in as many as 40 to 45% of acromegalic patients. Hyperprolactinemia is often associated with large tumors with substantial mass effects. Small tumors are diagnosed primarily because of hypersecretion, whereas larger ones may display mass effects and/or functional abnormalities. In the following presentation, response of function and of mass effects to irradiation are considered separately. It may well be that effects of irradiation on tumor mass differ from its influence on function.

RADIATION THERAPY TECHNIQUE

Techniques for conventional radiation therapy tend to be similar for all pituitary tumors; hence the technical aspects are reviewed separately from the considerations related to specific tumor types.

A few decades ago multiple small courses of radiation therapy, separated by periods ranging from several weeks to years, were commonly employed. Currently irradiation is given as a single course, usually consisting of four or five fractions per week, extending over about 5 weeks. At the University of California, San Francisco (UCSF), the present treatment policy utilizes five daily fractions per week. Generally each fraction is 180 rads with a total dose of 4,500 rads, calculated at the 95% isodose line. The total may be increased to 5,000 to 5,500 rads for unusually large or invasive tumors and for craniopharyngiomas. The size of treatment portals varies according to the tumor volume. The intent is to enclose the desired treatment volume within the 95% isodose line, with the dose throughout the tumor varying by $\pm 2.5\%$. In order to protect adjacent structures, treatment plans are designed so the dose outside the volume of interest decreases as rapidly as possible. Because of the sensitivity of the lens, and to a lesser extent the retina, care must be taken to avoid the eyes. With conventional irradiation it is impossible to protect the normal pituitary, and, especially with the larger tumors, the optic chiasm and hypothalamus are generally exposed.

Figures 1 and 2 illustrate treatment techniques for a radiocobalt teletherapy machine and a 4-MeV linear accelerator. These radiation sources are widely available and for this reason were chosen for illustration. Other suitable sources, however, are in use in many centers. In each illustration the tumor, represented by broken lines, was assumed to be quite large, i.e., 5 cm in diameter. The isodose curves were computer-generated and are appropriate for a radiation source-to-skin distance of 80 cm. Figure 1A is for a radiocobalt teletherapy machine using bilateral coaxial 6×6 cm fields. With this simple technique the absorbed dose is rather nonuniform and is appreciably greater in the temporal lobes than in the tumor. Figure 1B also utilizes bilateral opposed fields but is for a 4-MeV linear accelerator. Compared with ^{60}Co there is a modest improvement in tumor dose relative to that in the temporal lobes. Further improvement, not illustrated, could be obtained by adding a coronal field and introducing wedge filters on the lateral portals.

Figure 2A is for a 4-MeV linear accelerator with bilateral 110° coronal arcs and moving 30° wedge filters. Note that outside the 95% isodose line, which

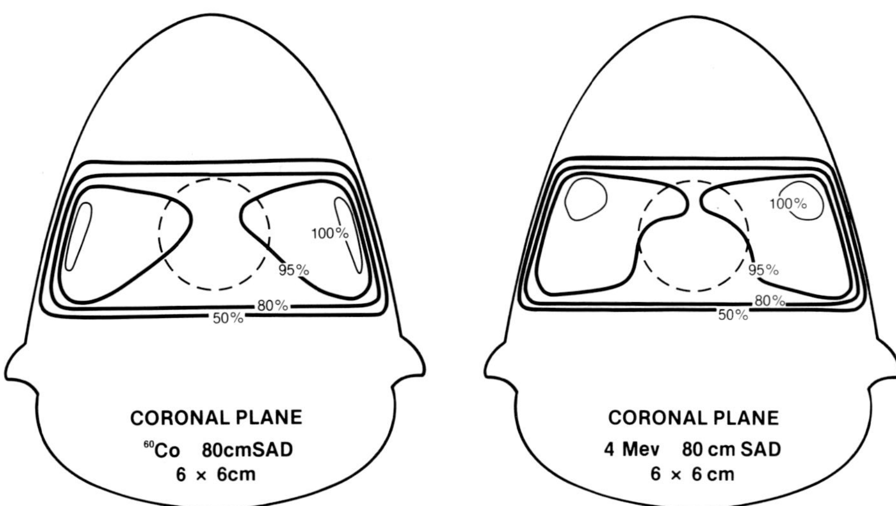

FIG. 1. A: Isodose curves for 5-cm diameter tumor volume (represented by dashed circle) centered in the sella, using a cobalt-60 teletherapy machine with bilateral coaxial 6 × 6 cm fields. **B:** Isodose curves for 5-cm diameter tumor volume (represented by dashed circle) centered in the sella, using a 4-MeV linear accelerator with bilateral coaxial 6 × 6 cm fields.

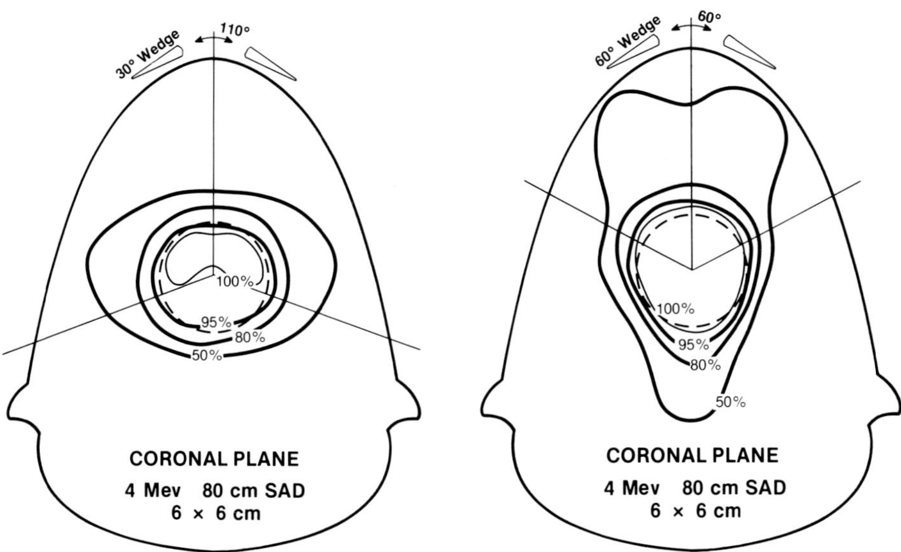

FIG. 2. A: Isodose curves for 5-cm diameter tumor volume (represented by the dashed circle) centered in the sella, using a 4-MeV linear accelerator, bilateral coronal arc (110°) fields with moving wedge (30°) filters. **B:** Isodose curves for 5-cm diameter tumor volume (represented by the dashed circle) centered in the sella, using a 4-MeV linear accelerator, bilateral coronal arc (60°) fields with moving wedge (60°) filters. This technique shifts the 50% isodose line away from the temporal lobes and toward the frontoparietal region.

encloses the hypothetical tumor volume, the dose decreases rapidly, with the temporal lobes receiving about one-half that delivered to the region of the sella. This is the basic technique currently used at UCSF. It must be emphasized that for a particular patient the technique must be tailored to the size and extension of the tumor. For a smaller tumor the field size and treatment volume would be correspondingly reduced. An asymmetrically extending tumor may require an asymmetrical treatment plan.

Figure 2B illustrates a variation designed to meet a special need. This treatment plan was developed for a patient with a large recurrent nonfunctioning adenoma. Over a period of 14 years he had had four surgical procedures and one course of radiation therapy to the pituitary. The latter had been given via bilateral opposed stationary fields using a teletherapy cobalt-60 machine with a 50-cm source-to-skin distance, a poor technique that resulted in a high dose to the temporal lobes. When retreating it was important to spare tissues lateral to the sella. To accomplish this goal the wedges were changed from 30° to 60° and the coronal arcs reduced from 110° to 60°. This technique shifted the extrasellar dose away from the temporal lobes into the previously nonirradiated frontoparietal area.

ACROMEGALY

Prior to the early 1960s radiation therapy was generally considered the treatment of choice for acromegaly. In the absence of major or progressing visual field deficits, radiation was given without biopsy or surgical decompression (41). Soon after the growth hormone assay became available, several studies suggested that conventional external radiation therapy was not effective for normalizing hGH levels. At about the same time, improved surgical techniques for the selective destruction or resection of pituitary tumors were coming into wide usage. Thus in many medical centers radiotherapy for acromegaly was virtually abandoned for the next several years. More recent data indicate that there is a role for conventional radiotherapy, and although in many instances it may not be the treatment of choice it is not time for its abandonment.

The second column of Table 1 summarizes results at UCSF for radiation therapy prior to 1959 (41). Forty-four percent of these patients had tumors sufficiently large to produce visual field deficits. Assay for hGH was not available at that time, and determination of control was based on adrenal, thyroid, and gonadal function; basal metabolic rate; blood chemistries; and the presence or absence of headaches, acral enlargement, and visual field deficits. Endocrine hyperactivity and pressure effects were controlled in 14 of 18 (78%) of these patients. As evidenced by a return to normal visual fields, mass or pressure effects were controlled indefinitely in 6 of the 8 patients with deficits present pretreatment. An additional 19 patients treated at UCSF (not included in Table 1) initially were given low-dose irradiation, i.e., $<3,500$ rads. In spite of repeated courses of radiotherapy, only a 63% control rate was achieved, indicating that doses higher than 3,500 rads were more effective.

TABLE 1. *Acromegaly: conventional radiation therapy*

Parameter	Sheline et al. (41)	Pistenma et al. (31)	Kramer (18)
Patients treated (No.)	18	19	29
Enlarged sella (No.)	14	18	—
Visual field defect(s) (No.)	8[a] (44%)	6 (32%)	—
Dose (rads)	4,400/5 wk (avg.)	5,800/6 wk (avg.)	4,500 ± 100/4.5 wk[b]
"Controlled" (No.)	14 (78%)	17 (90%)	25 (86%)
Acral improvement (No.)	—	7	—
Hypophysectomy for failure (No.)	1	2	4
Induced hypothyroidism (No.)	None	1/11	—

[a] Normalized in 6 patients (75%) postirradiation.
[b] Two patients received $<$ 4,000 rads and 7 received $>$ 5,000 rads.

Similar results have been reported from other institutions (Table 1). Pistenma et al. (31) described 19 acromegalic patients given radiation as primary therapy at Stanford. At least 18 had enlarged sellae and 6 had visual deficits. The control rate was 90%, with 2 patients requiring hypophysectomy for visual deterioration. Kramer (18) reported an 86% control rate, with 4 of 29 patients requiring hypophysectomy. Thus during the era before the hGH assay, conventional radiation therapy appeared to be an effective as well as a safe method for the treatment of acromegaly. This held true even for tumors large enough to cause a secondary visual field deficit.

In 1972, 24 patients irradiated at UCSF prior to the hGH assay were known to be alive (40). Seven had moved from the San Francisco Bay area and could not be fully re-evaluated. Of the remaining 17, 1 patient, who refused further therapy, had clinically active acromegaly and an hGH level of 200 ng/ml. The other 16 were clinically well and had fasting hGH levels equal to or less than 7.5 ng/ml. Thirteen of these 16 had received irradiation only; 3 had had transsphenoidal cryohypophysectomy because of persistently elevated hGH levels, but in 2 of the 3 the surgery had been performed within 1 year after irradiation. This interval is now known to be too short to evaluate results of radiation therapy. Excluding the two with early surgery, 13 of 15 (87%) had been controlled by irradiation alone.

The upper half of Table 2 presents results for 53 patients on whom postirradiation hGH determinations were done. These patients were treated before the hGH assay, and so their pretreatment hGH levels are unknown. The data were pooled from patients treated at UCSF, from reports of Lawrence et al. (20) and Kramer (18), and from information obtained by a poll of members of the Radiation Therapy Oncology Group (RTOG) (42). At the time of review 44 (83%) had normal hGH levels. Two had been operated on within 1 year after irradiation and hence were not evaluable. Seven still had active acromegaly. Obviously such a retrospective re-evaluation overlooks patients who were lost to follow-up or who died with uncontrolled disease and thus could yield a falsely high control rate.

TABLE 2. *Acromegaly: combined data*[a]

Parameter	No.	%
hGH measured only postirradiation		
Patients	53	
hGH normal	44	83
Surgery within 1 year	2	4
Clear failure	7	13
hGH $<$ 10 ng/ml measured pre- and postirradiation		
At 1 year	13/31	
At 2 year	24/32	
At 3 year	22/24	92

[a]Combined data from UCSF, Lawrence et al. (20), Kramer (18), and polled RTOG members (42).

TABLE 3. *Acromegaly: conventional irradiation*

No. of patients		47	
Dose		4,000–5,000 rads	
Mean decrease plasma hGH 5 years post-RT		77%	

Endocrine status	Before RT (%)	5 years (%)	10 years (%)
hGH < 10 ng/ml	13	73	81
hGH < 5 ng/ml	2	42	69
Hypothyroid	9	12	19
Hypoadrenal	6	30	38

Data from ref. 6.
RT = radiation therapy.

The lower half of Table 2 gives data for patients who had pre- and postradiotherapy hGH assays. These data also were pooled from reports by Lawrence et al. (20), Kramer (18), and Sheline and Wara (42). Although a total of 40 patients are represented, fasting hGH levels were not available for every patient at each posttreatment time; hence the numbers of patients indicated in Table 2 for each of the various intervals range from 24 to 32. Assuming that the upper limit of normal for hGH is 10 ng/ml, the control rate at 1 year was 42% (13 of 31 patients). By 3 years it had risen to 92%. The 3-year control rate was 100% when the pretreatment hGH was <45 ng/ml versus 71% for patients with pretreatment levels >50 ng/ml. This suggests that control is more likely if the hGH is <50 ng/ml. The number of patients, however, is small and the difference of questionable significance.

At the National Institute of Arthritis, Metabolism, and Digestive Disease, conventional irradiation has continued to be used as primary therapy for acromegalic patients with intact vision. Preliminary results were reported by Roth et al. in 1970 (34) and the data updated by Gorden and Roth (11) in 1973. A more definitive report is in preparation by Eastman et al. (6) from which selected data are presented in Table 3. Forty-seven previously untreated patients were irradiated using nonrotational techniques. The total doses were 4,000 to 5,000 rads, with daily fractions not exceeding 200 rads. Sixteen patients have been observed for at least 10 years. By 5 years there was a 77% decrease in mean plasma hGH, and 73% of patients had a hGH concentration <10 ng/ml. At 10 years 81% had a concentration of 10 ng/ml or less, and in 69% the level was <5 ng/ml. Throughout the observation period hGH concentrations continued to decrease. There was improvement in acral and facial changes and in metabolic effects that roughly paralleled the fall in plasma hGH concentration. There was no correlation between pretreatment hGH level and response to irradiation. After therapy no patient developed an extrasellar extension and headaches were said to have improved in the majority. Radiation complications, discussed later, were limited to hypothyroidism and hypoadrenalism.

Radiation therapy also is useful for treating acromegaly that persists after surgical resection, i.e., for treating surgical failures (Table 4). At UCSF 7 patients

TABLE 4. *Acromegaly: irradiation for surgical failure*

Author	Hypophysectomy	After irradiation	
		Interval (yr)	No. with normal hGH
Sheline	Cryohypophysectomy	1	2/7
		2	4/7
	Transfrontal	2	3/4
Williams et al. (47)	Transsphenoidal	—	4/6
Eastman et al. (6)	Transfrontal	2	4/5
Total			15/22

were irradiated 5 to 24 months following cryohypophysectomy. The postsurgical preirradiation hGH levels ranged from 17 to 48 ng/ml. Two years after irradiation (4,500 rads using conventional fractionation), 4 of the 7 had hGH concentrations <10 ng/ml. Four other patients with large incompletely resected suprasellar tumors and hGH levels of 54 to 200 ng/ml were treated by combined transfrontal hypophysectomy and postoperative radiation therapy. By 2 years the plasma hGH level was normal (1 to 8 ng/ml) in 3 of the 4 patients. In 4 of 6 patients irradiated after failure of transsphenoidal hypophysectomy by Williams et al. (47), the hGH levels returned to normal. Eastman et al. (6) irradiated 5 patients in whom the hGH concentration remained elevated (12 to 70 ng/ml) after transfrontal hypophysectomy. In 4 the hGH concentration decreased to 10 ng/ml or less by 2 years and was <6 ng/ml by 5 years. Of the total of 22 patients included in Table 4, 15 (68%) were controlled by radiotherapy within 2 years. It is expected that, as with primary irradiation for acromegaly, the control rate will continue to increase with time after irradiation.

In summary, there is no study which compares control rates for and complications of conventional megavoltage external radiation therapy with those for other therapeutic techniques, surgical or radiologic, for similar groups of acromegalic patients. The available data, however, suggest that, properly applied, all methods achieve similar control rates. Irradiation has the disadvantage of a slow response but produces relatively little morbidity and virtually no mortality, and eventually controls about 80% of patients. Irradiation is an appropriate and effective therapy for acromegaly if the disease is sufficiently mild that a slow response is of little concern. It is the treatment of choice for patients in whom surgery has failed to reduce adequately the hGH concentration or who for one reason or another are inoperable.

PROLACTIN-SECRETING TUMORS

When considering prolactin-secreting tumors, the small intrasellar adenomas that present with amenorrhea, hypogonadism, and/or galactorrhea but no mass effects must be distinguished from the large tumors with mass effects due to extrasellar extension. Hyperprolactinemia resulting from a microadenoma usually can be controlled quickly by transsphenoidal microdissection; with skilled surgery the control rate is high and the morbidity low, and to date reported recurrences are rare. Occasionally with microadenomas and frequently with large tumors control of excessive prolactin secretion is not achieved by surgery. Unfortunately, data on the effectiveness of irradiation in normalizing prolactin levels are limited.

Samaan et al. (38) reported 6 patients in whom basal serum prolactin levels were determined before pituitary surgery, after surgery but before irradiation, and after 4,900 to 5,400 rads to the pituitary. Only 2 of the 6 had elevated levels preirradiation; in one the concentration remained high 4 years after irradiation but was normal at 3 years in the other. In the 4 patients with normal preirradiation levels, the serum prolactin concentration was unchanged 6 months to 2.5 years after radiotherapy.

Kleinberg et al. (17) reported on 235 patients with galactorrhea from various causes (Table 5). (Interestingly, they had 5 patients with galactorrhea, an enlarged sella, but with an "empty sella" by pneumoencephalography.) Of 48 with pituitary tumors, 8 were irradiated. All 8 had enlarged sellae, several had abnormal visual fields, and 6 were amenorrheic. The mean prolactin level before therapy was 195 ng/ml with a range of 61 to 10,000 ng/ml. After irradiation the mean was reduced by about 75% and the range was 32 to 1,000 ng/ml. In 3 patients galactorrhea ceased and in the other 5 decreased to the point that it was no longer troublesome. Two of the 6 who presented with amenorrhea resumed menstruation. Results for patients treated by transsphenoidal resection were similar. The reasons for selecting surgery or irradiation, the radiation doses, and the intervals between irradiation and follow-up were not stated. Thus it is not possible to compare the efficacy of irradiation versus resection for their cases.

Gomez et al. (10) presented results for radiation therapy and/or microdissection in patients with a microadenoma, galactorrhea, and hyperprolactinemia (Table 5). Eight patients received conventional radiotherapy, and 11 underwent

TABLE 5. *Prolactin-secreting tumors*

Parameter	Kleinberg et al. (17)	Gomez et al. (10)	UCSF
Patients (No.)	8	8	4
Treatment	RT	RT	S & RT
Mean prolactin (ng/ml)			
Before treatment	195 (61–10,000)[a]	168 (38–480)	387 (37–1,300)
After treatment	50 (32–1,000)	64 (12–200)	192 (28–450)
Galactorrhea ceased (No.)	3/8	2/8	1/2
Menses resumed (No.)	2/6	4/?	0/3
Follow-up (months)	—	6–57	1–16

RT = radiation therapy. S = surgical resection (3 transsphenoidal, 1 transcranial).
[a] Range.

transsphenoidal surgery. Again, the basis for selection of therapy was not stated, and comparison of the two methods may be misleading. Prolactin levels were measured immediately following radiotherapy in 3 patients in each of whom there was a marked drop followed within a few months by a rebound to pretreatment levels. Six of the irradiated patients had been observed for at least 2 years at the time of reporting. Although the prolactin level had returned to normal in only 1 of the 6, menses had resumed in 4 and galactorrhea had ceased in 2.

At UCSF, although there has been no opportunity to give primary radiation therapy for a known prolactin-secreting tumor, in a number of patients irradiation after surgical resection failed to control excessive prolactin secretion. Four patients for whom postirradiation data are available are summarized in Table 5. A 50-year-old male with an initial prolactin of 1,300 ng/ml otherwise presented with panhypopituitarism. His tumor was thought to have been completely "shelled out," but postresection the prolactin level was 900 ng/ml. Sixteen months after irradiation the level had decreased to 250 ng/ml. There were 3 females, ranging in age from 27 to 36 years. All had amenorrhea, and 2 had galactorrhea. One, irradiated 6 months following transsphenoidal hypophysectomy for a 5-mm diameter tumor, has shown no decrease in prolactin level and remains amenorrheic 6 months postirradiation. Another, irradiated 1 month postsurgery, also has shown no change; this patient had a large tumor with suprasellar extension and bilateral visual field deficits. The third female had a 2-cm diameter hemorrhagic cystic tumor. Because of bleeding encountered at attempted transsphenoidal hypophysectomy, surgery was limited to biopsy. Three months postirradiation her prolactin level had decreased from 115 to 42 ng/ml, and galactorrhea had ceased. She is, however, still amenorrheic.

Recently Antunes et al. (2) (Table 6) presented data on 30 patients with prolactin-secreting pituitary adenomas for whom pre- and posttreatment prolactin concentrations were available. The adenomas were graded according to

TABLE 6. *Prolactin-secreting tumors reported by Antunes et al. (2)*

Parameter	T	T or C + RT	RT
Tumor grade (No. of patients)			
I	8	2	0
II	8	4	3
III	0	2	1
IV	0	0	2
Mean prolactin (ng/ml)			
Pretreatment	361 (27–900)	1,070 (21–3,600)	2,500 (110–10,000)
Posttreatment	80 (6–361)	144 (3–490)	165 (32–560)
Decrease of mean (%)	80	59	87
Prolactin normalized (No.)	7	2	0
Galactorrhea ceased (No.)	4/12	1/3	2/3
Menses resumed (No.)	3/13	0/3	1/3
Follow-up (months)	1–28	3–39	13–72

T = transsphenoidal resection. C = transcranial resection. RT = radiotherapy (4,500 rads/5 weeks).

Hardy's classification. Sixteen patients were treated by transsphenoidal resection alone, 8 by either transsphenoidal or transcranial resection plus irradiation, and 6 by irradiation alone. These authors tended to use radiation therapy in patients with high-grade tumors and high prolactin concentrations. Transsphenoidal resection alone was used for eight grade I and eight grade II tumors, whereas irradiation alone was used for three grade II, one grade III, and two grade IV tumors. Response, as indicated by a decrease in mean prolactin concentration, cessation of galactorrhea, and return of menses, was similar for the three treatment groups. However, normalization of prolactin levels occurred in 7 patients treated by transsphenoidal resection but in none of those treated by radiation alone. This may reflect either an actual difference in response, the fact that the larger tumors were irradiated and/or that response to irradiation is slow.

These data, although limited, suggest that irradiation, either as primary therapy or for surgical failure, controls amenorrhea and galactorrhea in about one-third of patients but only occasionally reduces serum prolactin to normal levels. For definitive conclusions a larger number of patients must be treated and observed for more extended periods of time. When assessing the efficacy of irradiation it must be kept in mind that suppression of prolactin secretion, like suppression of growth hormone, may be slow, and that observation periods of several years may be necessary.

NELSON'S SYNDROME

According to Moore et al. (26), if diagnosed and treated early the majority of patients with Nelson's syndrome have a favorable prognosis. Most authors, however, believe that the tumors associated with this syndrome are usually aggressive and often nonresponsive to therapy (23,35,44). Whatever the true nature of these rare tumors, radiation therapy of the pituitary has been advocated for prevention and treatment.

Orth and Liddle (29) (Table 7) found no instance of Nelson's syndrome in 43 patients who had pituitary irradiation for Cushing's disease even though

TABLE 7. *Nelson's syndrome in patients treated for Cushing's disease*

Author	Treatment for Cushing's	Mean observation (years)	Developed Nelson's
Orth and Liddle (29)	PRT	9	0/23
	PRT + A	8	0/20
Hopwood and Kenny (14)	A	3	>8/30
Jennings et al. (16)	PRT	8	0/11
	PRT + A	12	0/4
Wild et al. (46)	PRT + A	2	2/?
Moore et al. (26)	A	6	7/100
	PRT + A	12.5	2/20

A = adrenalectomy. PRT = pituitary irradiation.

20 also had bilateral adrenalectomies. In a nationwide survey Hopwood and Kenny (14) found that at least 8 of 30 patients (27%) who had had total adrenalectomy for childhood Cushing's disease developed sellar enlargement and hyperpigmentation. At least 10 others developed postadrenalectomy hyperpigmentation, but many did not have serial X-rays to document a possible change in the size of the sella. If their incidence of Nelson's syndrome—somewhere between 8 and 18 out of 30—is representative, it may be significant that Jennings et al. (16) failed to find a single case in 15 children who underwent pituitary irradiation for Cushing's disease. The absence of Nelson's syndrome in the patients of Orth and Liddle and of Jennings et al. has been advanced as presumptive evidence that pituitary irradiation prevents its development. Wild et al. (46), however, reported two cases of Nelson's syndrome in irradiated patients but did not indicate the total number of irradiated patients; hence the incidence in their material is unknown. Moore et al. (26) found about the same incidence of Nelson's syndrome in adrenalectomized patients regardless of whether they received pituitary radiotherapy. It may be that pituitary irradiation reduces the incidence but does not necessarily prevent Nelson's syndrome in all patients.

Available data on the effectiveness of irradiation for the treatment of Nelson's syndrome (Table 8) are also ambiguous. Moore et al. (26) used pituitary irradiation in 5 patients and irradiation plus partial excision in 2 others with Nelson's syndrome. The radiation doses ranged from 2,800 to 10,000 rads. Six patients were alive and "clinically stable" for an average of 9.4 years after discovery of the pituitary tumor. The seventh died from metastatic breast carcinoma 11 years after treatment of her pituitary tumor, which had remained controlled. McKenzie and McIntosh (25) reported "apparent benefit" from pituitary radiotherapy in 2 patients with Nelson's syndrome. Nelson et al. (27) had one patient in whom the ACTH level returned to normal within 1 month after partial excision plus a dose of 3,000 rads. In 2 patients treated with radiation only, the ACTH level was unchanged at 5 months. Our experience with irradiation is limited to 3 patients. One, who received 5,000 rads following unsuccessful hypophysectomy, was still uncontrolled 6 months after irradiation. The second, who had previously been unsuccessfully irradiated (4,400 rads), was treated by partial excision plus an additional 4,000 rads. This patient has been followed 5 years; although her ACTH concentration is unknown, her headaches have ceased and the abnormal pigmentation has cleared. The third patient, previously untreated, had a transsphenoidal subtotal hypophysectomy after which the ACTH was still 5,000 pg/ml. She then received 5,000 rads to the sella. Subsequently headaches ceased and pigmentation cleared. At 9, 18, and 26 months after irradiation the ACTH concentrations were 1,700, 500, and 240, respectively. This slow decrease of function is similar to that seen in patients irradiated for acromegaly.

Although these data are meager, they suggest that radiation alone controls some patients with Nelson's syndrome, and that it may be of value when pituitary surgery has not been completely effective. My present preference is excision

TABLE 8. *Nelson's syndrome: therapy*

Author	No. of patients	Therapy[a]	Follow-up	
			Interval	Status
Moore et al. (26)	5	2,800–10,000	9.4 years	6 Living and well
	2	S plus 3,000–5,000		1 DID[b]
McKenzie and McIntosh (25)	2	4,800	—	"Apparent benefit"
Nelson et al. (27)	1	S plus 3,000	1 month	Normal ACTH
	2	3,000–4,100	5 months	ACTH unchanged
Sheline	1	5,000	6 months	Uncontrolled
	1	S plus 4,000	5 years	Controlled
	1	S plus 5,000	2 years	Controlled

[a] Radiation dose in rads. S = surgical resection.
[b] DID = dead of intercurrent disease.

followed by irradiation if the excision is incomplete or the ACTH level remains elevated.

CUSHING'S DISEASE

Cushing's syndrome and the first patient with this syndrome to benefit from pituitary irradiation were described by Cushing in 1932 (4). Since that time many reports, usually concerning few cases, have appeared. Because of the small numbers, the changing surgical and radiotherapy techniques, and the widely differing criteria for success, the role of irradiation has only slowly emerged.

In 1957 Dohan et al. (5) (Table 9) reported on 12 patients irradiated at the University of Pennsylvania for Cushing's disease. Six patients who received pituitary doses of only 400 to 1,570 rads exhibited little or no response. Of the 6 who received larger doses (3,800 to 5,200 rads) 5 had an excellent response, with disappearance of the physical stigmata, improved glucose metabolism, lowered blood pressure, and resumption of menses in 4 of the 5 females. One patient with a dose of 4,550 rads failed to respond, but in this case therapy was given with unusually small individual fractions extended over a total of 85 days. As one example of an objective measure of improvement, among the 5 who responded to irradiation, diastolic blood pressure ranged from 100 to 120 mm Hg before treatment but after treatment was 78 to 92 mm Hg with a mean of 84 mm Hg. Depending on the indicator considered, the average interval between irradiation and evidence of marked improvement varied from 3 to 6 months. The patients with excellent results were observed 5.5 to over 7 years without evidence of relapse.

A decade later Heuschele and Lampe (13) (Table 10) reported 16 patients irradiated for Cushing's disease. The radiation dose to the pituitary was 4,000 rads within 4 to 4.5 weeks. Observation times ranged from 3 to 7 years after treatment. It was stated that complete and permanent remission was obtained in 10 of the 16 patients, but the criteria used to evaluate remission were not

TABLE 9. *Cushing's disease reported by Dohan et al. (5)*

Parameter	No. of patients
Pituitary dose: 400–1,570 rads	6
Little or no response	6
Pituitary dose: 3,800–5,200 rads	6
Excellent response	5
No response (treatment time 85 days)	1
Time to remission 3–6 months	
Complications	0
Recurrences	0
Follow-up	5.5–7 years

TABLE 10. *Cushing's disease reported by Heuschele and Lampe (13)*

No. of patients	16
Dose: 4,000 rads in 4–4.5 weeks	
Complete remission	10
Average to clinical remission	7.4 months
Average to biochemical remission	4.7 months
Mean age of patients	26 years
No improvement or recurred (No.)	6
Mean age of patients	45 years
Follow-up	3–7 years

given. The average time to clinical remission was 7 months and to biochemical remission 5 months. Six patients either failed to show improvement or developed a recurrence and were considered failures. The mean age for those with complete remission was 26 years, compared with 45 years for those who failed to respond, suggesting that younger patients are more responsive to radiotherapy.

Orth and Liddle (29) (Table 11) irradiated 51 patients with Cushing's disease. Radiation doses to the pituitary were 4,000 to 5,000 rads. Response was defined in terms of cortisol secretion. A patient was considered cured if the urinary 17-hydroxycorticosteroid excretion was <7 mg/g creatinine and the mean plasma cortisol concentration <10 μg/100 ml. If a normal diurnal rhythm was re-established, the low plasma cortisol value had to be <7 μg/100 ml. Of the 44 patients followed at least 1 year, 10 (23%) were cured and an additional 13 (30%) were improved to the extent that further therapy was unnecessary. Thus approximately 50% of their patients required only pituitary irradiation. When only adults were considered (16), 45% were improved (the cure rate decreased to 15%, but the "improved" rate remained 30%) to the point of needing no further treatment. The 21 patients not responding to irradiation were controlled by secondary bilateral adrenalectomy. There were no complications: specifically, no hypopituitarism and no visual or neurologic deficit. Finally, except for those adrenalectomized, no substitution therapy was required.

TABLE 11. *Cushing's disease reported by Orth and Liddle (29)*

Pituitary dose: 4,000–5,000 rads
Followed 1–14 years postirradiation: 44 patients
Needed no further therapy: 23 patients

No. of patients	24-hr 17-OHCS excretion (mg/g creatinine)	Mean plasma cortisol (μg/100 ml)
10 cured	< 7	< 10
13 improved	< 10	< 13

Adrenalectomy—for radiation failure (No.)	21
Complications	None
Follow-up (years)	1–14 (mean 9)

TABLE 12. *Cushing's disease: conventional pituitary radiotherapy reported by Edmonds et al. (7)*

Dose: 3,500 rads/3 weeks to 5,000 rads/5 weeks	
No. of patients	15
Complete biochemical remission	9
Biochemical improvement	1
Failure	5
Complications (No.)	0
Recurrences (1 transient) (No.)	0

Edmonds et al. (7) (Table 12) irradiated 15 patients with doses ranging from 3,500 rads in 3 weeks to 5,000 rads in 5 weeks. Postirradiation observation intervals were 5 months to more than 10 years. Biochemical remission was complete in 9 (60%) and partial in 1. The interval between radiation therapy and complete remission varied from less than 1 to over 6 months. There was one transient recurrence at 18 months that remitted spontaneously; this patient was observed an additional 10 years without further evidence of recurrence. Five patients (33%) failed to respond. There were no radiation complications.

Jennings et al. (16) recently reported results for pituitary irradiation of Cushing's disease in 15 patients less than 16 years of age at onset of symptoms and less than 19 years of age at time of treatment (Table 13). Some of these patients were included in the earlier report of Orth and Liddle (29). Cure was defined as a mean plasma cortisol <10 μg/dl with a 24-hr urinary 17-hydroxycorticosteroid excretion of <7 mg/g creatinine. Of the 15, 10 were cured within 9 months and 12 (80%) within 18 months. The three failures were controlled by bilateral adrenalectomy. Subsequent sexual development, including secondary sexual characteristics and sexual function, has been normal in all 15. Four have demonstrated fertility. Intellectual function has remained normal. Growth resumed in 12 patients. Although one patient had a subnormal hGH response to hypoglycemia, basal and stimulated hGH levels were normal in the other 11 tested. There was no complication attributable to irradiation.

It can be concluded that conventional pituitary irradiation controls Cushing's disease to the point where further therapy is unnecessary in 50 to 80% of patients. The control rate appears to be higher for childhood than for adult Cushing's disease. The average time to clinical or biochemical remission varies

TABLE 13. *Childhood Cushing's disease reported by Jennings et al. (16)*

No. of patients	15
Cures (dose 4,000–4,950) (No.)	12
Within 9 months	10
Within 18 months	12
Failures (dose 3,500–4,400) (No.)	3
Complications (No.)	0
Recurrences (No.)	0
Follow-up (years)	1–19 (mean 8)

from a few months to a year but is shorter than for hGH control in acromegaly. Complications are rare. With follow-up periods of 10 or more years, recurrence is virtually nonexistent.

LARGE INVASIVE PITUITARY TUMORS

Certain pituitary tumors, with or without endocrine hyperactivity, attain clinical significance because of their mass effects on surrounding structures. Most of these large, sometimes locally invasive tumors either cause hyperprolactinemia or are endocrinologically inactive. Occasionally, as noted earlier, they are associated with acromegaly or Nelson's syndrome. The endocrine aspects have been considered previously, and only mass effects are discussed at this point. These tumors usually present with some combination of headaches, hypopituitarism, an enlarged or eroded sella, and injury to optic nerves or chiasm. Depending on size and direction of growth, they may extend to involve oculomotor nerves or brain and grow inferiorly into the sphenoid sinus; they even may present as a tumor in the nasopharynx.

Growth tends to be slow, and identification of further growth or proof of permanent control requires many years of observation. For example, at UCSF the mean time to recurrence was 4 years (range 1 to 12 years) for patients who failed after surgery and 9 years (range 2 to 17 years) for those treated by surgery plus irradiation. Hence this discussion is based on tumors treated at least 10 years ago at UCSF. Although they were thought to be nonfunctional at the time of treatment, it is probable that many were in fact prolactin secretors.

Table 14 summarizes the initial findings in 140 consecutive patients treated prior to 1969 for large invasive pituitary tumors (39). Visual field deficits were present in 93%. Of the 11 (8%) patients with normal visual fields, 9 had suprasellar extension demonstrated radiographically and most had erosion into the sphenoid sinus. The 2 patients without suprasellar extension had tumors extending into the nasopharynx. Ninety-six percent had grossly enlarged sellae. Hypopituitarism was diagnosed in 53%. Many patients, however, were operated on with-

TABLE 14. *Adenomas presenting with mass effect: UCSF (1934–1968)*

	No. of patients by treatment			
Effect	RT	S	S + RT	Total
Visual defect	18	36	75	129
Enlarged sella	23	35	77	135
Hypopituitarism	16	17	41	74
Local invasion	1	7	6	14
Total patients	23	37	80	140

S = surgical resection (115 by craniotomy; 2 transsphenoidal). RT = radiation therapy.

TABLE 15. *Adenomas with mass effect: complications of therapy*

Complication	Surgery	Radiation therapy
Operative deaths		
1934–1944	4 (15%)	—
1945–1968	4 (4%)	—
Patients with increased visual defect		
Minor increase	10 (8%)	0
Major increase	7 (6%)	0
Wound infection	2	
CSF rhinorrhea	2 (transient)	1 (permanent)
Severe brain damage	1	0

out complete assessment of pituitary function, and the incidence of hypopituitarism was undoubtedly higher.

Twenty-three patients were treated with radiation therapy alone. Five of these had refused surgery. Seven elderly patients were considered poor surgical risks. Seven others had either minimal visual field deficits or were among those with normal visual fields. Thus of the irradiated-only group, approximately one-third had lesions of relatively modest size and another one-third consisted of elderly patients with short life expectancy. Among the group of 140, 117 patients had surgery with at least partial removal of the adenoma. Surgery was performed via craniotomy in 115 and by transsphenoidal resection in 2. Eighty patients were referred for and received postoperative radiation therapy. The reasons for referral of 80 but not the remaining 29 surviving surgical patients is unclear.

There were eight postoperative deaths, four of which occurred among the 90 patients undergoing craniotomy since 1945 (Table 15). Of the last four deaths, one was due to a cerebral infarct and the other three occurred in patients with extensive locally invasive adenomas. Surgery resulted in minor increases in visual deficits in 10 patients, with major loss of vision occurring in 7. There was one instance of late visual field deterioration associated with an empty sella syndrome in a patient who had been treated by surgery and irradiation. Cerebrospinal fluid (CSF) rhinorrhea occurred in 3 patients, each of whom had a tumor extending either through the floor of the sphenoid sinus or into the nasopharynx. Radiation-induced hypopituitarism was not recognized. It should be emphasized that these complications were primarily surgical and that most occurred in patients with locally invasive tumors. There were three operative deaths and two instances of epilepsy and severe mental deterioration among the 10 patients with tumors described at surgery as invasive. Other authors also have reported a poor experience with invasive adenomas (21,28,30,45).

Response to therapy was judged primarily on the basis of visual field deficit (Table 16). In the analysis each eye was considered separately, and it was assumed that if a patient underwent surgery the early response was due to the surgical procedure regardless of whether the patient was irradiated. Table 16 presents

TABLE 16. *Adenomas with mass effect: visual field response*

Pretherapy approximate field loss	Therapy	Fields posttherapy (%)			
		Normal	Improved	Unchanged	Worse
<1 Quadrant	RT (17)[a]	65	12	24	0
	S (42)	67	7	17	9
>1 to 2 Quadrants	RT (10)	0	60	40	0
	S (109)	32	28	29	11
>2 Quadrants	RT (0)	—	—	—	—
	S (17)	6	29	59	6

RT = radiation therapy. S = surgical resection.
[a]Number of eyes at risk.

response rates as a function of the extent of the pretreatment visual field deficit. Comparing eyes with equivalent visual deficits tends to reduce possible bias introduced by the manner in which patients were selected for irradiation. Of those eyes with a field deficit present but which involved one-fourth or less of a visual field, approximately two-thirds reverted to normal regardless of whether treatment was radiation therapy alone or began with a surgical decompression. After surgery 9% of visual fields deteriorated further. When the deficit involved more than one-fourth and up to one-half of a visual field, radiation therapy yielded a 60% improvement rate, but no deficit disappeared completely. Surgery produced the same overall improvement rate (i.e., 60%) but resulted in normalizing 32% of the visual fields, with 11% becoming worse. Thus although in patients with minimal visual deficits radiation therapy alone provided as good a response as surgical decompression, the surgical procedure produced more improvement for moderately advanced lesions.

Table 17 gives absolute recurrence-free survival rates as a function of time after treatment. Evaluation of recurrence or control was based primarily on repeated visual field examinations and roentgenograms of the sella. The number of patients at risk is indicated in parentheses. Those treated by radiation therapy

TABLE 17. *Adenomas with mass effect: recurrence-free (absolute) survival*

Interval (years)	% Recurrence-free survival		
	RT[a]	S	S + RT
2	86 (21)[b]	49 (37)[b]	96 (80)[b]
5	93 (15)	25 (36)	90 (72)
10	71 (7)	9 (32)	79 (47)
15	—	0 (25)	65 (31)
20	—	0 (23)	65 (17)

RT = radiation therapy. S = surgical resection.
[a]Excludes two treated with ≤ 1,900 rads.
[b]Number of patients at risk.

TABLE 18. *Adenomas with mass effect: recurrence-free (determinate) survival*

Interval (years)	% Recurrence-free survival		
	RT[a]	S	S + RT
2	100 (18)[b]	70 (26)[b]	98 (79)[b]
5	93 (15)	38 (24)	96 (68)
10	100 (5)	14 (21)	86 (43)
15	—	0 (16)	74 (27)
20	—	0 (14)	73 (15)

RT = radiation therapy. S = surgical resection.
[a]Excludes two treated with ≤ 1,900 rads.
[b]Number of patients at risk.

alone had recurrence-free survival rates similar to those treated by partial resection plus radiation therapy. Patients treated by surgery alone had markedly lower control rates at all times from 2 to 20 years following therapy than did those who underwent either irradiation alone or resection plus postoperative radiotherapy.

Table 18 shows determinate recurrence-free survival rates according to method of therapy. Excluded are 8 patients who died during the postoperative period, 23 dead of intercurrent disease, and 6 lost to follow-up. Exclusion of patients dead or lost to follow-up improves the surgical recurrence-free rates, whereas exclusion of those dead of intercurrent disease increases the radiation therapy rates. Those undergoing only irradiation experienced a determinate recurrence-free survival of 93% at 5 years and 100% at 10 years, but the number of patients is small. When recently reviewed, the 5 patients without recurrence at 10 years were still disease-free 15 years or more postirradiation. As with the absolute recurrence-free survival rates, the determinate control rates were superior for those who underwent postoperative radiation therapy compared with those who had surgery alone. The difference in favor of postoperative radiotherapy was progressively greater the longer the follow-up. Since 14 patients who underwent postoperative irradiation during the earlier part of the study period were given doses of <4,000 rads and the response is dose-dependent (42), 15- and 20-year control rates with current radiation therapy techniques are expected to be greater than the 73 to 74% indicated.

Others have reported similar experiences in the treatment of "chromophobic adenomas" (Table 19). Kramer (18) treated 16 patients by radiation therapy alone and observed them at least 5 years. These patients tended to be of advanced age and/or were poor surgical risks and hence had a short life expectancy. At the time of reporting, 6 were alive and well, 1 was lost to follow-up, 7 were dead of intercurrent disease, and 2 had had recurrences. The determinate 5-year relapse-free survival was 75%. For patients treated by surgery plus postoperative radiation therapy, Kramer's 5-year determinate recurrence-free survival rate was 83%. Emmanuel (8) had a 75% 4-year recurrence-free survival rate

TABLE 19. *"Chromophobic adenomas"*

Author	% Recurrence-free survival		
	RT	S	S+RT
Kramer (18) (5 yr)			
Absolute	38	—	75
Determinate	75	—	83
Emmanuel (8) (4 yr)			
Absolute	75	30	93
Pistenma et al. (30) (5 yr)			
Absolute	86	—	82

for radiotherapy alone, 30% for surgery alone, and 93% for surgery followed by radiotherapy. Pistenma et al. (30) reported an 86% 5-year control rate for irradiation versus 82% for surgery plus postoperative irradiation. Pistenma included 4 patients with invasive adenomas, 2 of whom were treated by radiotherapy and 2 by radiotherapy and resection; all died of problems related to the pituitary tumor.

Twenty-five patients initially treated at UCSF with either surgery or surgery plus irradiation have been retreated for recurrence of the adenoma (39). There were four serious complications, including two postoperative deaths and one patient who was incapacitated owing to brain damage. Fifteen of the 25 improved after retreatment, but 8 have already had recurrences again. Thus at UCSF the response rate to retreatment was 60%, but re-recurrence and complication rates were high. Kramer's (18) experience was similar. He irradiated 11 patients with recurrent "chromophobic adenomas." Six were alive and well 2 to 5.75 years after retreatment, 2 were lost to follow-up, and 3 expired within 1 year. As emphasized by Kramer, recurrence requires treatment carefully tailored to the previous therapy. If the earlier treatment included a full course of radiation therapy (e.g., a dose >4,500 rads), reliance must be primarily on surgery. Lesser doses may permit reirradiation with due consideration for the time interval and the initial treatment plan. Every effort must be made, however, to prevent recurrence and the problems of retreatment by the most effective initial therapy.

It is concluded that conventional radiation therapy is of value for controlling mass effects of large pituitary tumors. Although the evaluable experience is based on a mix of prolactin-secreting and nonfunctioning adenomas, this is probably true for each of these two tumor types. Radiotherapy alone may be effective, particularly with smaller tumors, but it is generally preferable to surgically debulk the tumor mass before administering the radiation. This permits confirmation of diagnosis and provides the most rapid means of decompressing the optic apparatus. The latter is especially important with extensive or progressive visual field deficits. Postoperative radiotherapy adds significantly to the recurrence-free survival rate, and complications are minimal. Since doses of <4,000 rads (180 to 200 rads per day) are associated with a high recurrence rate, and (as will be shown in the following section) at doses above 5,000 rads complications begin to appear, the radiation therapy must be carefully designed and delivered.

RADIATION COMPLICATIONS

Essentially the only side effect that appears during or shortly after radiation therapy is epilation. When treatment is given with a 4-MeV linear accelerator using the arc rotation–moving wedge filter technique described, epilation is minimal; it may not occur, and if it does it is generally transient.

Possible late complications include radiation-induced neoplasia, brain necrosis, damage to optic nerves or chiasm, and hypopituitarism. These may appear several months to years after completion of irradiation.

In 1966 Waltz and Brownell (43) reviewed the literature and found eight fibrosarcomas and one osteosarcoma reported in irradiated tissues following

TABLE 20. *Complications of irradiation for pituitary tumors*

Sarcomas reported[a]	14	
Fibrosarcoma	12	
Osteosarcoma	2	
Radiation therapy		
Dose unknown	4	
Multiple courses of therapy	7[b]	
Single course and dose ≤ 5,000	3	
Brain necrosis	Dose (rads)	Incidence
Sheline & Wara (42), Kramer (18), Pistenma et al. (30), Emmanuel (8)	4,000/4 wk to 5,800/6 wk	0/464
Martins et al. (22)	6,600 & 6,700	2/?
Almquist et al. (1)	5,000	1/?
Aristizabal et al. (3)	≤ 4,600	0/96
	> 4,600	1/26
Optic nerve/chiasm injury		
Aristizabal et al. (3)		
Total dose	≤ 4,600	0/96
Total dose	> 4,600	4/26
Daily dose	≤ 220	2/106
Daily dose	> 220	2/16
Harris & Levene (12)		
Daily dose	175 to < 250	0/27
Daily dose	≥ 250	5/28
Kramer (19)		
Acromegaly	5,000/5 wk	3/42
Chromophobe	4,500/4.5 wk	0/190
Sheline		
Total dose	4,500 ± 500	
Daily dose	≤ 200	0/180
Daily dose	225	1/1

[a] Data from refs. 32, 36, 43.
[b] Total dose usually very large.

radiotherapy for pituitary adenomas (Table 20). (They actually reported nine fibrosarcomas, but one was a duplication.) They presented two additional fibrosarcomas that followed radiation doses of 3,500 and 4,500 rads and one osteosarcoma after 6,000 rads. Subsequently Powell et al. (32) reported another fibrosarcoma. Their total dose was 5,000 rads, but neither the number of fractions nor the fraction size were specified. Rubinstein (36) added a twelfth fibrosarcoma but did not specify the dose. Of these 14 patients with presumably radiation-induced sarcomas, 7 had multiple courses of therapy, usually with an exceedingly high total dose. In 4 others the dose was not stated. Only 3 are known to have received a single course of treatment with a dose within the range currently advocated. Furthermore, sarcomas have been reported in unirradiated patients, and it is possible that some of these 14 were not radiation-induced. In view of the large number of patients who have been irradiated for pituitary adenomas, the incidence of radiation-induced malignant neoplasms must be small. It may be concluded that with modern fractionated radiotherapy, given as a single course with a dose <5,000 rads, radiation-induced neoplasia is rare and does not represent a major contraindication to radiotherapy.

The incidence of brain necrosis also is minimal. At UCSF (42) there was no instance of radiation necrosis in 115 pituitary patients irradiated 10 to 35 years earlier, even though most of these were treated by older techniques employing bilateral opposed fields, sometimes with multiple courses of therapy and often with orthovoltage radiation. Kramer (18), Pistenma et al. (30), and Emmanuel (8) found no necrosis in a combined total of 349 patients. Martins et al. (22) did report brain necrosis in 2 patients irradiated for pituitary adenomas, but these patients had received doses of 6,600 and 6,700 rads, which are well above those currently advocated. As far as I am aware, only two instances of necrosis have been reported with conventional doses. One of these followed 5,000 rads in 200-rad fractions (1) and the other 4,900 in 204-rad fractions (3).

Although rare, optic nerve and/or chiasmal injury may be more frequent than oncogenesis or necrosis. In 122 patients treated at Vanderbilt between 1952 and 1971, Aristizabal et al. (3) reported four optic nerve or chiasmal injuries attributable to irradiation. All four, however, occurred in the group of 26 patients who had received total doses >4,600 rads. In fact, no visual complication occurred with a dose <5,000 rads. Irrespective of total dose, when the daily increment was <220 rads, their complication rate was 2% (2/106) compared with 13% for daily fractions >220 rads. Harris and Levene (12) reported five radiation-induced optic nerve injuries among 55 patients treated at the Harvard Joint Center for Radiation Therapy. Each injury was associated with a daily fraction of 250 rads or more. With a total dose of 5,000 rads in 5 weeks, Kramer (19) had damage to optic nerves or chiasm in 3 of 42 acromegalic patients. He suggested that the patient with acromegaly may be unusually sensitive, probably because of abnormal vascularity. Since reducing the dose to 4,500 rads, he has had no further injury. Kramer has seen no optic injury among 190 "chromophobic" adenomas given 4,500 rads in 4.5 weeks. At UCSF we had one instance of radiation-induced blindness among 181 patients treated for pituitary adenomas between 1934 and 1975. Contrary to policy, this patient received daily increments of 225 rads, rather than the usual 180 rads. It is concluded that if the daily dose does not exceed 200 rads and the total is limited to 4,500 rads, at the 95% isodose line, radiation-induced optic nerve or chiasmal injury does not occur in more than a fraction of 1% of cases.

Only a few years ago it was believed that conventional radiation therapy would not influence the function of normal pituitary tissues. Richards et al. (33), however, reported 4 children irradiated at UCSF for nonpituitary nonhypothalamic brain tumors who subsequently were found to have hGH deficiencies (Table 21). One of the 4 also developed TSH, ACTH, and gonadotropin deficiencies. The pituitary doses were calculated to have been between 4,000 and 5,200 rads and were given in fractions of 160 to 180 rads per day. Similar findings appeared in the recent British literature. Samaan et al. (37) studied hypothalamic and pituitary function in 65 patients treated at the M.D. Anderson Hospital for cancer of the nasopharynx, paranasal sinuses, or orbit. These patients ranged from 14 to 76 years of age. In 60 (92%) the retrospectively calculated radiation dose to the hypothalamic–pituitary region was between 4,000 and 8,500 rads. At the time of the study, 3 to 20 years after irradiation, there was laboratory evidence of hypothalamic dysfunction in 54 and primary pituitary deficiency in 25 patients. Thirteen young adults showed growth failure and delayed bone age. An unspecified number of patients had signs and symptoms of Addisonian crisis which responded to cortisol administration. Unfortunately, neither the incidence of clinically significant hypothalamic–pituitary dysfunction nor the relationship between hypofunction and radiation dose was stated. It may be that clinical hypopituitarism was associated primarily with the higher end of their dose range.

With regard to patients with pituitary adenomas, it has been the impression of most radiation therapists that hypopituitarism is rarely if ever induced by conventional radiation therapy. Interpretation of the older data, however, pre-

TABLE 21. *Hypopituitarism after conventional radiotherapy*

Condition	Hypopituitarism (No. of patients)
Irradiated normal pituitary	
Richards et al. (33) (4,000–5,200 rads)	4/?
Samaan et al. (37) (4,000–8,500 rads)	
Hypothalamic	54/65
Primary pituitary	25/65
Irradiated pituitary adenomas (acromegaly)	
Goldfine and Lawrence (9)	3/12
Eastman et al. (6)	
Hypothyroid	9% → 19% (10 yr)
Hypoadrenal	6% → 38% (10 yr)

sents a number of problems: (a) Many of the patients for whom data have been reported were treated before the current sophisticated hormone assays became available. (b) Some degree of hypopituitarism was often present before therapy, especially with the "chromophobic" adenomas. (c) Many patients had resection and irradiation without a thorough, intervening endocrine evaluation. In 1972 Jenkins et al. (15) reported studies of endocrine function in 22 patients with various types of pituitary adenoma treated by external irradiation. One patient developed hypoadrenalism and hypothyroidism after radiation therapy, but this patient had had evidence of pituitary–adrenal dysfunction before treatment. Several of the 22 patients had increased pituitary function after irradiation. These authors concluded that in most cases irradiation of pituitary tumors has little impact on pituitary function. Goldfine and Lawrence (9) reported three instances of loss of trophic hormones following irradiation for acromegaly. Eastman et al. (6) studied hypothyroidism and hypoadrenalism in a group of 47 acromegalic patients treated by conventional supervoltage irradiation. The majority of their patients received between 4,000 and 5,000 rads to the pituitary with daily fractions not exceeding 200 rads. Sixteen were observed at least 10 years. Hypothyroidism, which increased from 9% before therapy to 19% at 10 years, is easily treatable and not of great concern. Hypoadrenalism was diagnosed in 6% before irradiation, 30% at 5 years, and 38% at 10 years. It was the policy of these authors that (a) if the onset of hypofunction was uncertain, it was attributed to the postirradiation period; and (b) if laboratory tests were equivocal, they were accepted as representing hypofunction. Thus the incidence of radiation-induced hypopituitarism probably is less than these data imply. Furthermore, of the 8 cases of hypoadrenalism Eastman et al. (6) allocated to the postirradiation period, only 4 required corticosteroid replacement therapy.

Although the relationship between radiation dose and incidence of clinical hypopituitarism is unknown, radiation-induced hypopituitarism can occur following conventional radiotherapy in patients with either normal pituitaries or pituitary tumors. It should be watched for and hormone replacement therapy instituted as necessary.

SUMMARY

Several illustrative techniques for conventional radiotherapy of pituitary tumors were presented. A good dose distribution may be obtained with megavoltage irradiation using bilateral coronal arcing fields and moving wedge filters. With modern treatment techniques irradiation complications (e.g., neoplasia, brain necrosis, or damage to optic chiasm or nerves) are exceedingly rare. Suppression of pituitary function may occur, but the incidence of clinically significant hypopituitarism—that requiring replacement therapy—is probably low.

Radiation therapy controls excessive hGH secretion in approximately 80% of acromegalic patients and ACTH production in 50 to 80% of patients with Cushing's disease. It appears to be more effective in childhood than adult Cushing's disease. Compared with surgery, the time to response is protracted. It requires one to several years to normalize the growth hormone level in acromegaly and a few months to a year or more to achieve remission in Cushing's disease. The role of irradiation in control of hyperprolactinemia is not well established.

Conventional radiation therapy is recommended for control of pituitary hypersecretion in patients where surgery fails. It is appropriate primary therapy when there is no urgency regarding normalizing circulatory hormone levels.

For large tumors with mass effects, postoperative radiation therapy is indicated to reduce the late recurrence rate. It may be used as primary therapy in patients medically inoperable and for invasive adenomas where the risks of attempted surgical excision are relatively high.

REFERENCES

1. Almquist, S., Dahlgren, S., Notter, G., and Sundbom, L. (1964): Brain necrosis after irradiation of the hypophysis in Cushing's disease: Report of a case. *Acta Radiol. [Diagn]*, 2:179–188.
2. Antunes, J. L., Housepian, E. M., Frantz, A. G., Holub, D. A., Hui, R. M., Carmel, P. N., and Quest, D. O. (1977): Prolactin secreting pituitary tumors. *Ann. Neurol.,* 2:148–153.
3. Aristizabal, S., Caldwell, W. L., and Avila, J. (1977): The relationship of time-dose fractionation factors to complications in the treatment of pituitary tumors by irradiation. *Int. J. Radiat. Oncol. Biol. Phys.,* 2:667–673.
4. Cushing, H. (1932): The basophilic adenomas of the pituitary body and their clinical manifestations. *Bull. Johns Hopkins Hosp.,* 50:137–195.
5. Dohan, F. C., Raventos, A., Boucot, N., and Rose, E. (1957): Roentgen therapy in Cushing's syndrome without adrenocortical tumor. *J. Clin. Endocrinol., Metab.,* 17:8–32.
6. Eastman, R. C., Gorden, P., and Roth, J.: *Personal communication.*
7. Edmonds, M. W., Simpson, W. J. K., and Meakin, J. W. (1972): External irradiation of the hypophysis for Cushing's disease. *Calif. Med. Assoc. J.,* 107:860–862.
8. Emmanuel, I. G. (1966): Symposium on pituitary tumours. 3. Historical aspects of radiotherapy, present treatment, techniques and results. *Clin. Radiol.,* 17:154–160.
9. Goldfine, I. D., and Lawrence, A. M. (1972): Hypopituitarism in acromegaly. *Arch. Intern. Med.,* 130:720–723.
10. Gomez, F., Reyes, F. I., and Faiman, C. (1977): Nonpuerperal galactorrhea and hyperprolactinemia: Clinical findings, endocrine features and therapeutic responses in 56 cases. *Am. J. Med.,* 62:648–660.
11. Gorden, P., and Roth, J. (1973): The treatment of acromegaly by conventional pituitary irradiation. In: *Diagnosis and Treatment of Pituitary Tumors,* edited by P. O. Kohler and G. T. Ross, pp. 230–233. Excerpta Medica/American Elsevier, New York.
12. Harris, J. R., and Levene, M. B. (1976): Visual complications following irradiation for pituitary adenomas and craniopharyngiomas. *Radiology,* 120:167–171.
13. Heuschele, R., and Lampe, I. (1967): Pituitary irradiation for Cushing's syndrome. *Radiol. Clin. Biol.,* 36:27–31.
14. Hopwood, N., and Kenny, F. (1975): Increased incidence of postadrenalectomy Nelson's syndrome in pediatric versus adult Cushing's disease: A nationwide study. *Pediatr. Res.,* 9:290.
15. Jenkins, J. S., Ash, S., and Bloom, H. J. G. (1972): Endocrine function after external pituitary irradiation in patients with secreting and nonsecreting pituitary tumours. *Q. J. Med.,* 41:57–69.
16. Jennings, A. S., Liddle, G. W., and Orth, D. (1977): Results of treating childhood Cushing's disease with pituitary irradiation. *N. Engl. J. Med.,* 297:957–962.
17. Kleinberg, D. L., Noel, G. L., and Frantz, A. G. (1977): Galactorrhea: A study of 235 cases, including 48 with pituitary tumors. *N. Engl. J. Med.,* 297:589–600.
18. Kramer, S. (1973): Indications for, and results of treatment of pituitary tumors by external

radiation. In: *Diagnosis and Treatment of Pituitary Tumors,* edited by P. O. Kohler and G. T. Ross, pp. 217–229. Excerpta Medica/American Elsevier, New York.
19. Kramer, S.: *Personal communication.*
20. Lawrence, A. M., Pinsky, S. M., and Goldfine, I. D. (1977): Conventional radiation therapy in acromegaly. *Arch. Intern. Med.,* 128:369–377.
21. Martins, A. N., Hayes, G. J., and Kempe, L. G. (1965): Invasive pituitary adenomas. *J. Neurosurg.,* 22:268–276.
22. Martins, A. N., Johnson, J. S., Henry, J. M., Stoffel, T. J., and DiChiro, G. (1977): Delayed radiation necrosis of the brain. *J. Neurosurg.,* 47:336–345.
23. Mason, A. S., and Greenbaum, D. (1962): Cushing's syndrome and skin pigmentation. *Br. Med. J.,* 2:445–448.
24. McCormick, W. F., and Halmi, N. S. (1971): Absence of chromophobe adenomas from a large series of pituitary tumors. *Arch. Pathol.,* 92:231–238.
25. McKenzie, A. D., and McIntosh, H. W. (1965): Hyperpigmentation and pituitary tumor as sequelae of the surgical treatment of Cushing's syndrome. *Am. J. Surg.,* 110:135–141.
26. Moore, T. J., Dluhy, R. G., Williams, G. H., and Cain, J. P. (1976): Nelson's syndrome: Frequency, prognosis, and effect of prior pituitary irradiation. *Ann. Intern. Med.,* 85:731–734.
27. Nelson, D. H., Meakin, J. W., and Thorn, G. W. (1960): ACTH-producing pituitary tumors following adrenalectomy for Cushing's syndrome. *Proc. R. Soc. Med.,* 52:560–569.
28. Ogilvy, K. M., and Jakubowski, J. (1973): Intracranial dissemination of pituitary adenomas. *J. Neurol. Neurosurg. Psychiatry,* 36:199–205.
29. Orth, D. N., and Liddle, G. W. (1971): Results of treatment in 108 patients with Cushing's syndrome. *N. Engl. J. Med.,* 285:243–247.
30. Pistenma, D. A., Goffinet, D. R., Bagshaw, M. A., Hanbery, J. W., and Eltringham, J. R. (1975): Treatment of chromophobe adenomas with megavoltage irradiation. *Cancer,* 35:1574–1582.
31. Pistenma, D. A., Goffinet, D. R., Bagshaw, M. A., Hanbery, J. W., and Eltringham, J. R. (1976): Treatment of acromegaly with megavoltage radiation therapy. *Int. J. Radiat. Oncol. Biol. Phys.,* 1:885–893.
32. Powell, H. C., Marshall, L. F., and Ignelzi, R. J. (1977): Postirradiation pituitary sarcoma. *Acta Neuropathol. (Berl),* 39:165–167.
33. Richards, G. E., Wara, W. M., Grumbach, M. M., Kaplan, S. L., Sheline, G. E., and Conte, F. A. (1976): Delayed onset of hypopituitarism: Sequelae of therapeutic irradiation of central nervous system, eye and middle ear tumors. *J. Pediatr.,* 89:553–559.
34. Roth, J., Gorden, P., and Brace, K. (1970): Efficacy of conventional pituitary irradiation in acromegaly. *N. Engl. J. Med.,* 282:1385–1391.
35. Rovit, R. L., and Duane, T. D. (1969): Cushing's syndrome and pituitary tumors. *Am. J. Med.,* 46:416–427.
36. Rubinstein, L. J. (1972): *Atlas of Tumor Pathology, Second Series, Fascicle 6: Tumors of the Central Nervous System,* p. 191. Armed Forces Institute of Pathology, Washington, D.C.
37. Samaan, N. A., Maor, M., Sampiere, V. A., Cangir, A., Jesse, R. H., Jr. (1978): Hypopituitarism after external irradiation of nasopharyngeal cancer. Presented at the International Symposium on Recent Advances in the Diagnosis and Treatment of Pituitary Tumors, San Francisco.
38. Samaan, N. A., Leavens, M. E., and Jesse, J. H., Jr. (1977): Serum prolactin in patients with "functionless" chromophobe adenomas before and after therapy. *Acta Endocrinol. (Kbh),* 84:449–460.
39. Sheline, G. E. (1974): Treatment of nonfunctioning chromophobe adenomas of the pituitary. *Am. J. Roentgenol. Radium Ther. Nucl. Med.,* 120:553–561.
40. Sheline, G. E. (1973): Treatment of chromophobe adenomas of the pituitary gland and acromegaly. In: *Diagnosis and Treatment of Pituitary Tumors,* edited by P. O. Kohler and G. T. Ross, pp. 201–216. Excerpta Medica, Amsterdam.
41. Sheline, G. E., Goldberg, M. B., and Feldman, R. (1961): Pituitary irradiation for acromegaly. *Radiology,* 76:70–75.
42. Sheline, G. E., and Wara, W. M. (1975): Radiation therapy of acromegaly and nonsecretory chromophobe adenomas of the pituitary. In: *Tumors of the Nervous System,* edited by H. G. Seydel, pp. 119–131. Wiley, New York.
43. Waltz, T. A., and Brownell, B. (1966): Sarcoma: a possible late result of effective radiation therapy for pituitary adenoma: Report of two cases. *J. Neurosurg.,* 24:901–907.
44. Welbourne, R. B. (1969): Cushing's syndrome. *Ann. R. Coll. Surg. Engl.,* 44:182–193.

45. Welbourne, R. B., Montgomery, D. A. D., and Kennedy, T. L. (1971): The natural history of treated Cushing's syndrome. *Br. J. Surg.,* 58:1–16.
46. Wild, W., Nicolis, G. L., and Gabrilove, J. L. (1973): Appearance of Nelson's syndrome despite pituitary irradiation prior to bilateral adrenalectomy for Cushing's syndrome. *Mt. Sinai Med. J.,* 40:68–71.
47. Williams, R. A., Jacobs, H. S., Kurtz, A. B., Miller, J. G. B., Oakley, N. W., Spathis, G. S., Sulway, M. J., and Nabarrow, J. D. N. (1975): The treatment of acromegaly with special reference to transsphenoidal hypophysectomy. *Q. J. Med.,* 44:79–98.

Clinical Management of Pituitary Disorders,
edited by G. T. Tindall and W. F. Collins.
Raven Press, New York © 1979.

17

Proton Radiosurgery for Functioning Pituitary Adenoma

Raymond N. Kjellberg and Bernard Kliman

Departments of Surgery and Medicine, Harvard Medical School and Massachusetts General Hospital, Boston, Massachusetts 02114

The detection and neurosurgical management of pituitary adenomas has made great progress during the past two decades, and it is anticipated that this progress will continue. Radioimmunoassay tests, as well as improving detection of acromegaly, have brought pituitary-dependent Cushing's disease and hyperprolactinemia firmly into the purview of neurosurgery. Microsurgical excision of adenomas and proton-beam therapy have provided unprecedented levels of effectiveness and safety in the therapy for these adenomas.

Patients with pituitary tumors face the most optimistic outlook of virtually any category of neoplasms below the skin. For the most part they should be able to look forward to 25 to 50 years free of the limitations of this disease. Further, it is timely in our present medical, social, and economic environment that our approach to the pituitary adenoma patient gives appropriate recognition to the roles of "informed consent" and "cost-effectiveness" of medical care, and this publication is written with these considerations in mind. To the extent that we have some further possibility of improving the care of pituitary adenoma patients, our existing deficiencies can be sought out. Two areas of deficiency are of major importance: (a) the epidemiology of pituitary tumors, and (b) long-term, lifetime follow-up of treated patients.

EPIDEMIOLOGY

Available information on the epidemiologic factors comes largely from two sources: Kurland's analysis (13) of the Rochester, Minnesota region from the 1960s in which the incidence of various cerebral neoplasms was computed, and federal government statistics from the U.S. National Center for Health Statistics (17). Kurland's figures give 1.5 pituitary tumor patients per 100,000 population per year, or about 3,000 per year in the United States. Government figures indicate about 10% of 8,000 to 10,000 brain tumors per year are adenomas, giving perhaps 1,000 pituitary tumors per year.

It is unlikely that these figures could have anticipated the role that radioimmunoassay has played in the detection of pituitary hyperfunction patients. This advance not only increases the detection rate but does so at an earlier age. Further, it is doubtful that the figures of Kurland or of the federal government include patients with pituitary-dependent Cushing's disease or the majority of patients with pituitary adenomas associated with hyperprolactinemia.

Because many of these patients appear to have the prospect of 25 to 50 years of productive life, from a socioeconomic viewpoint it should be cost-effective to invest our limited medical resources in such patients.

PATIENTS—INDICATIONS

Although proton hypophysectomy usually is preferred by the authors, there are specific indications for other methods. These indications can be considered in reference to the author's (RNK) total experience with surgical procedures on the pituitary (Table 1). There were 864 procedures for pituitary adenomas, of which 749 were performed by the proton-beam method. The figures may vary somewhat from those indicated elsewhere in this chapter, depending on the time at which the table was prepared. If a patient has suprasellar extension of an adenoma, particularly if visual field defects exist, open microsurgical transsphenoidal hypophysectomy is performed. Also, patients in whom a full course of radiation was already given usually are treated by transsphenoidal operation. Craniotomy is avoided because of the higher risks associated with this procedure. Transsphenoidal radiofrequency hypophysectomy has not been done by the author in recent years.

Two broad indications for therapy of pituitary adenomas exist: (a) hyperfunction and (b) mass effect. The majority of our adenoma patients were treated for hyperfunction as follows:

TABLE 1. *Surgical procedures on the pituitary*

	Open		Stereotactic		
	Frontal craniotomy	Transsphen.	Transsphen. radiofrequency	Bragg peak proton beam	Total
Functioning					
Acromegaly	3	32	—	431	466
Cushing's disease	3	4	—	113	120
Nelson's syndrome	—	2	—	23	25
Prolactinoma	—	17	—	64	81
Thyrotropinoma	—	1	—	1	2
Nonfunctioning	12	40	1	117	170
Total	18	96	1	749	864

1. A total of 466 procedures for acromegaly identified by characteristic clinical findings; nearly always elevated human growth hormone (hGH); hGH always refractive to glucose suppression; and usually, but not always, enlargement of the sella turcica.
2. Cushing's disease—120 procedures in patients with clinically active Cushing's disease; elevated urinary or, more currently, plasma steroids; and most frequently with a radiographically normal sella turcica.
3. Nelson's syndrome—25 procedures in totally adrenalectomized Cushing's disease patients; hyperpigmentation of the skin; elevated plasma ACTH; with or without sellar enlargement.
4. Hyperprolactinemia—81 procedures in patients with amenorrhea and galactorrhea; elevated prolactin; with or without evidence of enlargement of the sella turcica.
5. Hyperthyrotropinemia—a rare condition. We treated two such patients, previously thyroidectomized, with elevated TSH and irregular enlargement of the sella turcica.

Patients treated for nonfunctioning pituitary tumors often come to medical attention by virtue of a mass that produces visual field defects. Thus a relatively large number of our procedures in these patients are performed by the open microsurgical transsphenoidal method (40 procedures). Proton hypophysectomy may be performed following open excision hypophysectomy to control proved or suspected recurrence or residual tumor.

Fairly large nonfunctioning pituitary adenomas may be uncovered during the radiographic screening of patients with head injuries or troublesome headache, or for other reasons. Such patients may be simply followed periodically and reconsidered for therapy if the tumor progresses. Others are treated with proton therapy because either referring physicians or the patients themselves are reluctant to allow the harboring of an untreated proved tumor.

Proton hypophysectomy has been used in several patients with proved suprasellar extension, with or without visual field defects, considering the special circumstances of particular patients. Older, surgically unfit patients may be proton-treated to avoid the risks of a general anesthesia and a surgical convalescence. Younger patients, unwilling to risk hypopituitarism, particularly a compromise of fertility, may be proton-treated. In any case, the choice of alternative methods of treatment of pituitary adenoma patients is guided by consideration of the particular needs of the individual patient. We seek to minimize risk and maximize achievement of therapeutic goals at minimal cost, and thus have invoked proton hypophysectomy in 117 instances for nonfunctioning adenomas.

INFORMED CONSENT

An important factor influencing a patient's choice of a procedure is the risk, particularly the procedure-related mortality risk. Table 2 illustrates the reported

TABLE 2. *Operative mortality in pituitary tumors*

Series	Frontal craniotomy (%)	Transsphenoidal microsurgical (%)	Proton beam stereotactic (%)	"System" (%)
Present authors	5	0	0	0.12
Literature	1–13[a]	1.5–2.5[b]	—	—

Our mortality rate for the "system" reflects the fact that we try to elect the lowest risk procedure consistent with goals of "life time effective" therapy for pituitary adenoma, but that the over-all "system" shares the risk of employment of higher risk procedures when these are indicated as described in the text. The reported operative mortality of the several series cited from past publications probably does not reflect current mortality rates which are undoubtedly lower.

[a] From Ray, Mayo Clinic, Schwartz, and Lahey Clinic.

[b] From Hirsch, Guiot, and Hardy.

experience of several reputable series including our own. In general, craniotomy is associated with the highest mortality risk and currently is seldom used. Transsphenoidal hypophysectomy is quite safe, and experienced operators have mortality rates of 1% or less. In the process of securing "informed consent," patients are told that the risk of the transsphenoidal operation is in the range of 0.5 to 1.0%. Patients given a mortality risk of 1% versus 0% most often choose 0%, the mortality risk of proton hypophysectomy.

By selecting the treatment alternative with the lowest mortality risk and which is appropriate to the needs of the particular patient, our total experience reflects a "system" mortality risk of 0.12%. This represents a single death 16 years ago of a craniotomy patient, due to pulmonary embolus.

The other prominent feature of informed consent provided to adenoma patients is the prospect of recurrence. Interestingly, it is also important in cost-effective considerations. To appreciate an overview of recurrence rates, several series of treated patients were reviewed. Those shown in Table 3 were selected because the data allowed computation of annual recurrence rates; thus the variation in interval of follow-up did not seriously compromise comparison (3,6–8,14, 15,19).

In fact, several problems compromise the possibility of critical comparisons. In order to secure 25- or 50-year follow-up, one must deal with procedures performed 25 to 50 years ago. Only one series, that of Hirsch (8), falls within this range, a 37-year follow-up with an annual recurrence rate of 0.6%. Hirsch's method is not currently used. Beginning in 1910, he combined transsphenoidal evacuation of tumor with serial applications of a radium pellet. Nevertheless, the length of his follow-up and the low annual rate of recurrence of adenoma has been almost unequaled to this day.

Open excision by craniotomy with a 20-year follow-up is reported in two series of patients with recurrence rates of 7.5% per year and 1% per year, respectively (14,16). The supplementation of surgical excision by craniotomy

TABLE 3. *Pituitary adenoma: recurrence rates*

Procedure	Annual rate (%)	Cumulative (%)	
		25 Years	50 Years
Craniotomy	7.5	100.0	100.0
Craniotomy	1.0	25.0	50.0
Craniotomy and fract. X-ray ther.	1.2	30.0	60.0
Craniotomy and fract. X-ray ther.	2.0	50.0	100.0
Hirsch (TR-SP and radiation)	0.6	15.0	30.0
Transsphenoidal	1.5	38.0	75.0
Proton beam	0.15	3.8	7.5

The craniotomy alone and craniotomy plus fractionated X-ray therapy are present because they provided examples of series with sufficiently long intervals of follow-up (20 years) to justify the computations of annual recurrence rates and to justify the assumption that annual recurrence rates are relatively stable over such long intervals of time. Although Hirsch's interval of follow-up is the longest of any (37 years), it is uncertain as to the extent to which his transsphenoidal operation plus serial radium applications can be applied to contemporary surgical or radiation techniques. The transsphenoidal and proton beam recurrence rates are the authors' (see text).

with fractionated X-ray therapy improved the long-term prospects in one group and impaired it in the other (14,16). It is likely that selection of patients in both groups influenced the outcome.

It has been difficult to secure recurrence rates for microsurgical transsphenoidal hypophysectomy. We reviewed our own series of cases, which is admittedly a selected, nonrandom population. We defined recurrence as indicated in Table 4. Recurrence occurs when symptoms or abnormal laboratory values become abnormal following a remission. It differs from failure, wherein remission did not occur. The recurrence rate was 1.5% to 2% per year, depending on which of certain assumptions are made. The 2% rate, extrapolated to the 50-year interval, leads to recurrence in 100% of patients. The "effective" category includes cases not in remission but improved to the extent that no further therapy

TABLE 4. *Pituitary adenoma therapy: definitions*

Procedure mortality	Dead due to procedure
Failure	No better or worse
Effective	1. Cured or remission 2. Improved 3. Without symptoms
Ineffective	1. Procedure mortality 2. Failure
Recurrence	1. Endocrine remission followed by hyperfunction 2. Stable fields or findings followed by worsening, due to solid mass

TABLE 5. *Recurrent pituitary adenomas*

Adenoma	Open excision			Proton therapy		
	No. of pts.	No. of recur.	% Recur.	No. of pts.	No. of recur.	% Recur.
All adenomas	99	7	7	678	5	0.7
Nonfunctioning	45	5	11	114	1	0.9
Acromegaly	33	0	0	396	4	1.0
Cushing's disease	8	0	0	124	0	0
Prolactinoma	13	2	15	44	0	0

is immediately contemplated, especially when the prospect exists that remission may be forthcoming. We regard the concept and definition of recurrence to be of major importance in assessing "lifetime effectiveness."

In our proton-treated patients, recurrence occurred infrequently. Table 5 shows that one nonfunctioning adenoma recurred, but this patient was inadequately treated by a proton dose excessively low by our present standards. No patients with Cushing's disease or prolactinoma have had recurrence. Of four patients with recurrent acromegaly, three were operated by the author, and all three showed tissue culture features characteristic of "malignancy" (see below). Thus we are led to the impression that recurrence is very infrequent in proton-treated patients with typical benign adenomas.

This observation, if confirmed by longer detailed follow-up, is of paramount importance. Figure 1 shows the published and extrapolated cumulative recurrence prospects of therapy by various therapeutic alternatives. It becomes apparent that recurrence rates assume importance in assessing the prospects for lifetime cure or remission of the threat of pituitary adenomas. Recurrence rates following excision alone of 2% per year would indicate that a patient surviving 50 years probably will require further therapy. If the recurrence rate is reduced to 1% per year, a reasonable expectation from traditional excision plus conventional X-ray, only half the number of pituitary adenoma patients must undergo further therapy sometime in their lives.

If, however, informed consent leads a patient to choose the lowest procedure-related mortality rate and the greatest prospect of not requiring further therapy for pituitary adenoma, it appears that Bragg peak proton hypophysectomy best fulfills these prospects.

Additionally, informed consent, in our opinion, includes some other considerations added in the list in Table 6, which begins with the necessity of the procedure. We avoid "unnecessary" procedures. The necessity of therapy varies depending on the diagnosis and other factors.

The prospect of dying prematurely exists for acromegalic patients. Ninety percent of acromegalic patients are dead by age 60 (20). Before they die, they may become afflicted with hypertension, cardiomyopathy, diabetes mellitus, stroke, chronic pulmonary disease, carpal tunnel syndrome, and a broad spectrum of bone and joint complaints. The disfigurement of the disease is never

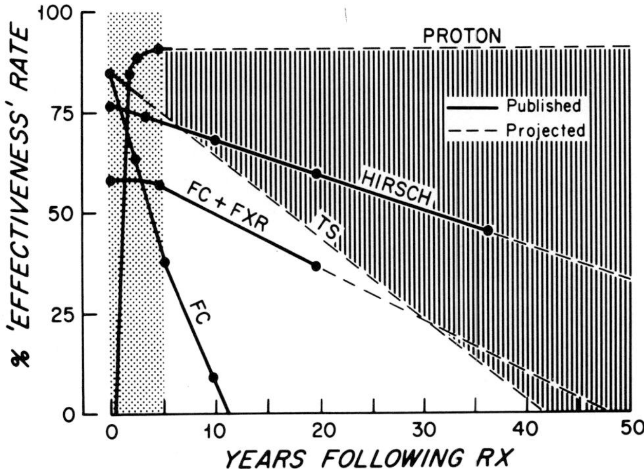

FIG. 1. This figure illustrates the importance of considering recurrence rates for judging the effectiveness of various forms of therapy when extrapolated to the anticipated lifetime of patients up to 50 years from the time of therapy. The vertical coordinate *(left)* represents the percent of patients "effectively" (remission and improved) treated at the time of hospitalization. The solid line for proton-treated cases is taken from Fig. 5. The stippled area on the left encompasses the first 5 years following therapy, during which the comparative effectiveness of various methods is rapidly changing. It is in the period beyond 5 years that the proton method appears to be increasingly effective, but long-term follow-up is required to document this anticipation more fully. (TS) transsphenoidal (author's). (FC) frontal craniotomy. (FXR) fractionated X-ray.

lethal and rarely disabling. Premature death and disability define the degree of "necessity" for therapy.

Untreated Cushing's disease is considered to lead to 50% mortality within 5 years. Hypertension, diabetes mellitus, osteoporosis, myopathy, obesity, and psychiatric disturbance contribute to disability; but disease-related mortality is often attributable to poor resistance to infection. This necessity for treatment is amply supported. However, alternate therapy exists, principally adrenalectomy. The risk of hypophysectomy seems to be less than adrenalectomy, and postoperative replacement therapy often is unnecessary. The development of Nelson's syndrome is avoided. The alternative of medical therapy is being evaluated.

Hyperprolactinemia due to prolactinoma stands in some contrast with acromegaly and Cushing's disease. Hyperprolactinemia per se is not understood to

TABLE 6. *"Informed consent"*

1. "Necessity" of therapy
2. Mortality risk
3. Disabling complications risk
4. Nondisabling complications risk
5. Alternative therapies
6. Late complications
7. Recurrence → further treatment

have lethal risks. Further, the principal disability, infertility, is eagerly sought after by a significant fraction of women of childbearing age. Hyperprolactinemia alone does not dictate necessity of therapy. The associated tumor may become threatening by virtue of growth. However, it is not entirely clear that all of these tumors grow progressively. In the original description of the amenorrhea–galactorrhea syndrome by Forbes et al. (4), 7 of their 15 patients had normal sellae up to 20 years following onset of symptoms.

Nonfunctioning adenomas develop necessity for therapy, usually by virtue of their mass. Mass effects are particularly threatening when the mass extends upward to affect the optic chiasm and the base of the brain. It is necessary to decompress these important neural structures promptly, and in these instances we recommend the open transsphenoidal method.

Nonfunctioning adenomas without suprasellar extension frequently do not produce disability. In the records of the Armed Forces Institute of Pathology (2) there are 1,000 pituitary adenomas, of which 51% were undetected prior to autopsy. We advise patients with asymptomatic nonfunctioning adenomas to be followed with annual radiographic, endocrine, and visual testing; then if the lesion shows evidence of progress, therapy is recommended. In some instances referring physicians and/or patients prefer that therapy be provided, in which case it is carried out.

COST-EFFECTIVENESS

Several determinants, or factors, contribute to cost-effectiveness. The emphasis may vary when different persons judge these determinants, and Table 7 was prepared with this in mind.

Hospital costs of proton-beam therapy are approximately half those of our transsphenoidal cases, a cost reduction due mainly to the short hospital stay, usually 6 or 7 days. The patients leave the hospital the day following the procedure. Further, proton-treated patients do not need time to convalesce but are free to resume work or activities immediately. Complications increase the cost of therapy by virtue of lengthening hospitalization and restricting a patient's life and work for variable periods of time. The prospect of recurrence also

TABLE 7. *Costs of therapy for pituitary adenoma*

1. Hospitalization
2. Not working during hospitalization
3. Not working during convalescence
4. Transient complications
5. Permanent complications
6. Late complications
7. Recurrent activity of disease

influences cost-effectiveness, and the prospect that further therapy will be required assures that the hospital and complication costs will be repeated. In general, proton treatment of adenomas is cost-effective on all of these counts.

METHOD

The stereotactic radiosurgical method is described elsewhere (10–12). In summary, patients are hospitalized 7 days or less for clinical evaluation, radiography, and therapy. General medical and special endocrine evaluations are done. Radiographic evaluation always includes pneumoencephalography for assessing suprasellar extension and the location of the optic nerves, cavernous sinography to determine the width of the pituitary, and calibrated "marker films." The proton-beam diameter and configuration are selected from these films, and heterodensity measurements are made to control the disposition of the Bragg peak of the proton beam. We always use the Bragg peak rather than intersecting portions of the plateau of the beam. There is no exit dose of beam passing beyond the sella. Also, the amount of radiation at the peak is two to three times greater than that along the entering plateau of the beam. Figure 2 illustrates that the

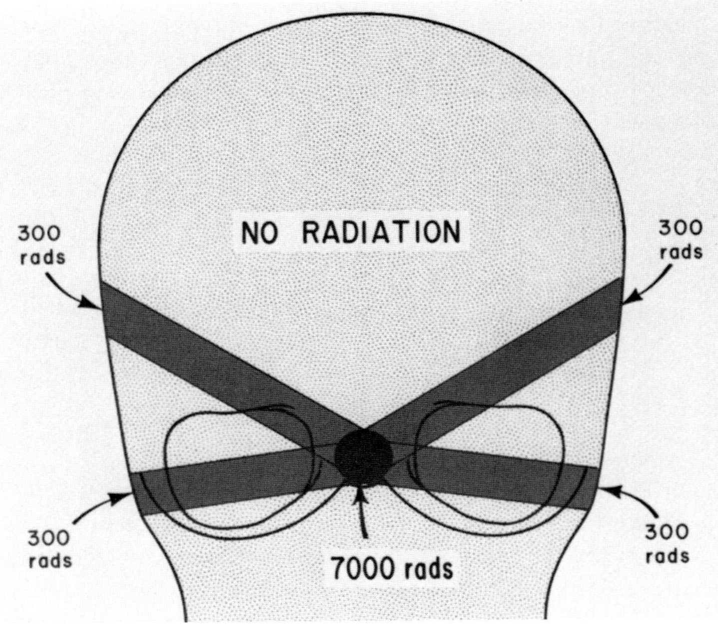

FIG. 2. Example of proton radiation dose and distribution in the coronal plane. By using multiple portals of beam entry that converge on the pituitary, the entrance dose and path dose through the brain can be kept at low levels while the pituitary target gets a high dose. Four paths are shown in the plane of the diagram; other paths (totaling 12) are in front of or behind the plane. The pituitary target dose (7,000 rads) is 23 times greater than the dose passing through skin and brain. 12 mm beam; 12 portals.

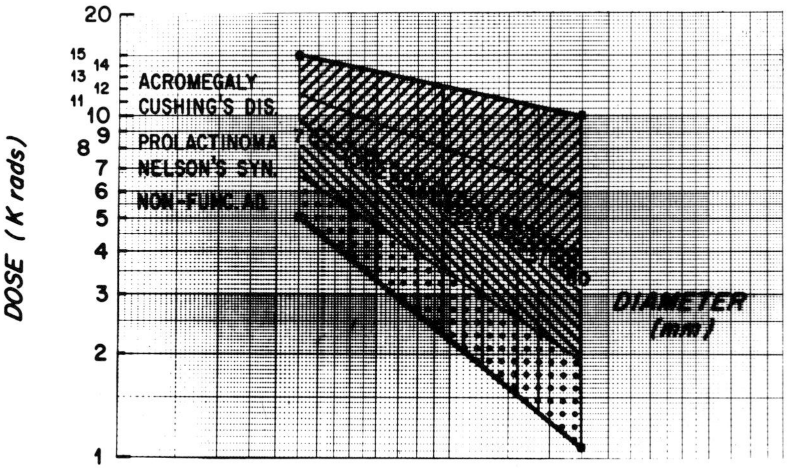

FIG. 3. Range of doses employed for various types of pituitary adenomas. Different dose ranges are used for different beam diameters, with smaller beams requiring larger doses.

pituitary target dose may be 20 to 25 times greater than the beam path dose. The dose required to induce an appropriate degree of radionecrosis is determined.

The dose required varies according to the beam diameter used and the therapeutic objective of the particular diagnostic category. Figure 3 illustrates our present schedule. Small beams (e.g., 7 mm) require much larger doses than large-diameter beams. The highest dose range is used for patients with acromegaly and Cushing's disease. Lower doses, still within the necrotizing range, are employed for hyperprolactinemia, Nelson's syndrome, and hyperthyrotropinemia. Subnecrotizing doses are sufficient for nonfunctioning adenomas where arrest of growth of the adenoma is the therapeutic objective. Higher doses are unnecessary, and the complication rates are higher.

PROCEDURE (RADIOSURGICAL)

The therapeutic radiosurgical procedure is performed at the 160 MeV Harvard Cyclotron. Figure 4 shows a patient in the stereotactic instrument. Local anesthesia is provided in the ear canals for stabilization of the stereotactic instrument. Local anesthesia is applied to the malar eminences and the nuchal line region where drill rods secure skeletal fixation of the instrument. Radiographs are performed to secure precise alignment of the Bragg peak of the proton beam to the pituitary tumor. Twelve portals (six to each side) are normally used for higher doses; six portals may be used for lower doses, but the skin dose is kept below 500 rads. Depilation rarely occurs. Within 1.5 to 2 hr the patient walks away from the procedure and returns to the hospital. Following overnight observation, the patient is discharged, fit for normal activities.

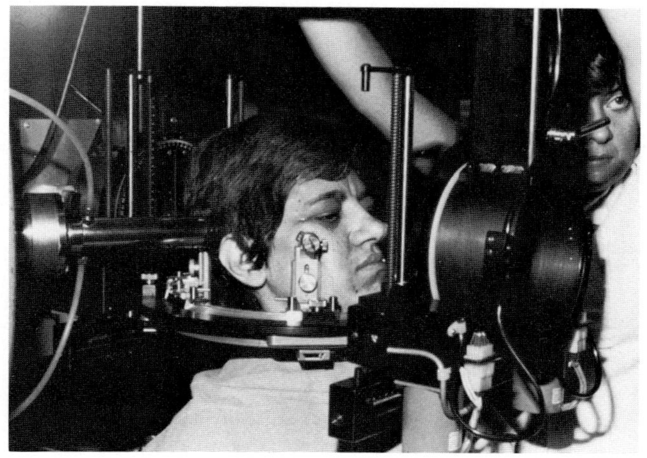

FIG. 4. Acromegalic patient in the stereotactic instrument undergoing proton radiosurgery.

PROCEDURE (MICROSURGICAL)

Our microsurgical procedure is similar to that used by others. A few technical details can be mentioned. We use a double-binocular microscope where access to the wound is equally facile to the assistant as to the operator. The patient is positioned supine, with head extended. The viewing axis through the microscope is straight down. Since the head is then about 10 cm below the spinal canal, the intracranial pressure is thought to be about 300 mm H_2O, which aids in expressing suprasellar tumor into the sella when the sellar contents have been removed. Normally the diaphragmatic dome of the tumor has reversed its curvature and balloons into the sella at the end of the procedure when the tumor has been evacuated.

Our method of closure differs slightly from that usually employed. The fascia lata is dried under an infrared lamp to a parchment-like appearance and consistency. The fascia is much easier to handle when it is stiff. A single piece is used and folded like two pages of a book. One leaf is applied to the diaphragmatic surface and the other against the anterior wall of the sella. We do not use muscle but, rather, use fat in the sellar cavity to back up the fascia. The low metabolism of fat permits it to survive as fat and not shrivel into a scar. Previously we frequently used folded gold foil to line the walls of the sellar cavity as a marker to permit early detection of recurrence by means of X-rays. This practice has been abandoned since radioimmunoassay of hormones functions as a marker of pituitary function, and CT scanning provides a basis for defining the mass.

RESULTS

Acromegaly

Most patients begin to exhibit a reversal of clinical features of acromegaly and a reduction of hGH 3 to 6 months following therapy; thereafter clinical

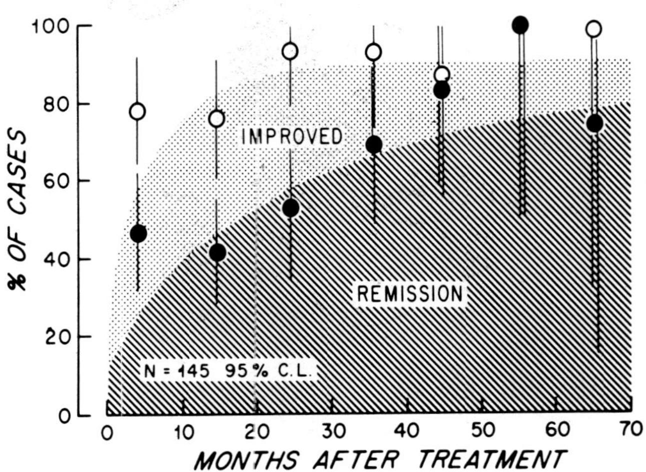

FIG. 5. Time course following proton treatment of acromegaly that patients enter into the categories of remission (hGH < 10 ng/ml) or improved (objective clinical change and hGH < 50% of the preoperative level). (●) remission. (○) remission plus improved.

change and hGH fall is progressive. Figure 5 shows the course of objective improvement and hormone fall which indicates that about 90% of patients are "improved" 24 months following treatment. At this interval, 60% of patients are in remission (hGH < 10 ng/ml); at the 4-year interval, the remission category has risen to 80%. About 10% of patients are failures, most of whom receive further therapy, usually open transsphenoidal hypophysectomy. We have not documented serious disabling complications in acromegalic patients. None has died as the result of therapy, and no patient is known to have been blinded, although a question of blindness was raised in two instances. Visual field defects did occur, but these were largely during our early experience. The incidence of transient extraocular movement disturbance has been reduced but not eliminated entirely. Diplopia and visual blurring continue to be reported in a few treated patients but frequently are not confirmed on ophthalmologic testing. About 10% of patients develop hypopituitarism and require replacement thyroid and/or steroid medication.

Cushing's Disease

In general, patients with Cushing's disease respond similarly to patients with acromegaly. Occasionally abrupt remission is seen within weeks of treatment. Figure 6 shows pre- and posttreatment values from a group of patients. Approximately 65% of treated patients undergo complete remission with restoration of normal clinical and laboratory findings. Another 20% are improved to the extent that no further therapy is considered desirable. Of the 10 to 15% failures, several were operated by either adrenalectomy or hypophysectomy prior to

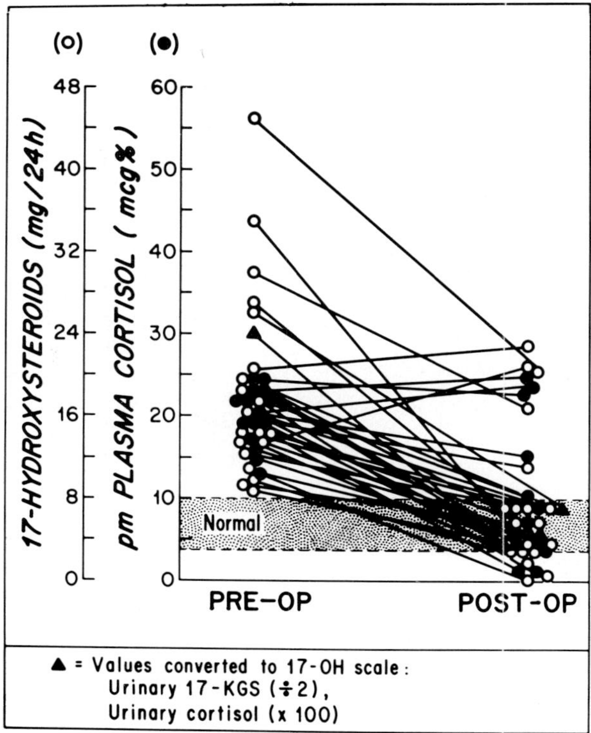

FIG. 6. Pre- and postoperative corticosteroid values in patients with Cushing's disease before and after proton beam therapy.

the 24-month interval we usually consider necessary to induce a completed radiosurgical result. Nevertheless, a patient is considered a failure if further ablative therapy is employed for any reason.

A histopathologic specimen (Fig. 7) was obtained from a patient with Cushing's disease who was proton-treated and who died 9 months later of a heart attack. Although the center of the tumor was amorphous owing to radionecrosis, a rim of remaining tumor was visible. The normal pituitary did not exhibit change. Prior to death, the patient exhibited clinical improvement and a reduction of steroid excess, but not to the normal range.

Complications have not been serious or disabling. One early patient developed a visual field defect. Temporary oculomotor disturbance continues to occur in 2 to 4% of treated patients. Thirteen percent of patients require replacement therapy, and a similar proportion develop impaired pituitary reserve.

Nelson's Syndrome

Patients with Nelson's syndrome are treated much like patients with Cushing's disease except that the dose is often lower, as shown in Fig. 3. Of 19 patients

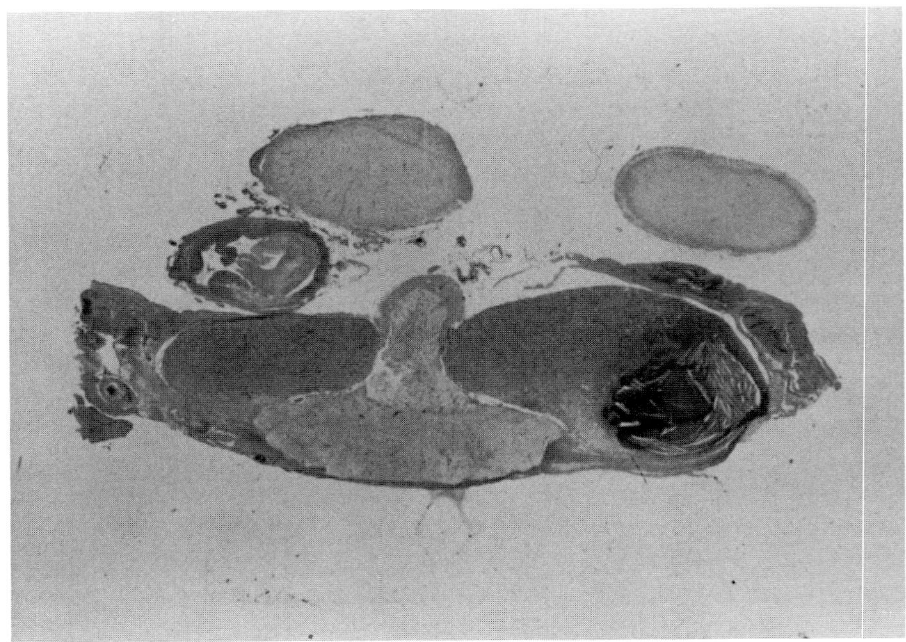

FIG. 7. Histologic specimen of the pituitary from a patient who died of a heart attack 9 months following proton therapy.

treated, follow-up was available on 14 (Table 8). Twelve of these experienced depigmentation following therapy. Headache was either reduced or eliminated in 8 of 11 patients with this complaint. One patient with residual headache was subsequently operated elsewhere twice by the transsphenoidal route to relieve the headache but without success. None of the patients had visual field defects prior to proton therapy, and none developed them afterward. The plasma ACTH

TABLE 8. *Nelson's syndrome in 19 patients: proton therapy*

Parameter	No.
Follow-up available	14/19
Depigmentation	12/14
Headache	11/14
Reduced headache	8/11
Headache relieved by 2° operation	0/1
Fields abnormal	0/19
Fields changed	0/14
ACTH fell	4/4
ACTH normalized	1/4
Deaths	0/14
Transient EOM	0/14
2° Operation for mass (invasive)	1/14
Other complications	0/12

fell in 4 patients on whom data was available but became normal in only 1 patient. One patient with a tumor widely invading the base of the skull was subsequently operated on and died from cancer of the liver. There have been no other deaths or complications.

Prolactinemia

We have treated patients with amenorrhea/galactorrhea and pituitary adenoma for a decade or more. Prior to the advent of radioimmunoassay of plasma prolactin, they were treated according to the low-dose schedule indicated in Fig. 3 for nonfunctioning adenomas. Currently we treat hyperprolactinemic patients with substantially larger doses. We are satisfied from our inflow of data (Fig. 8) that satisfactory responses are being obtained, but there has been no systematic follow-up of these cases.

Nonfunctioning Adenomas

As indicated above, patients with nonfunctioning adenomas are a nonhomogeneous group and are less subject to analysis by uniform criteria that objectively

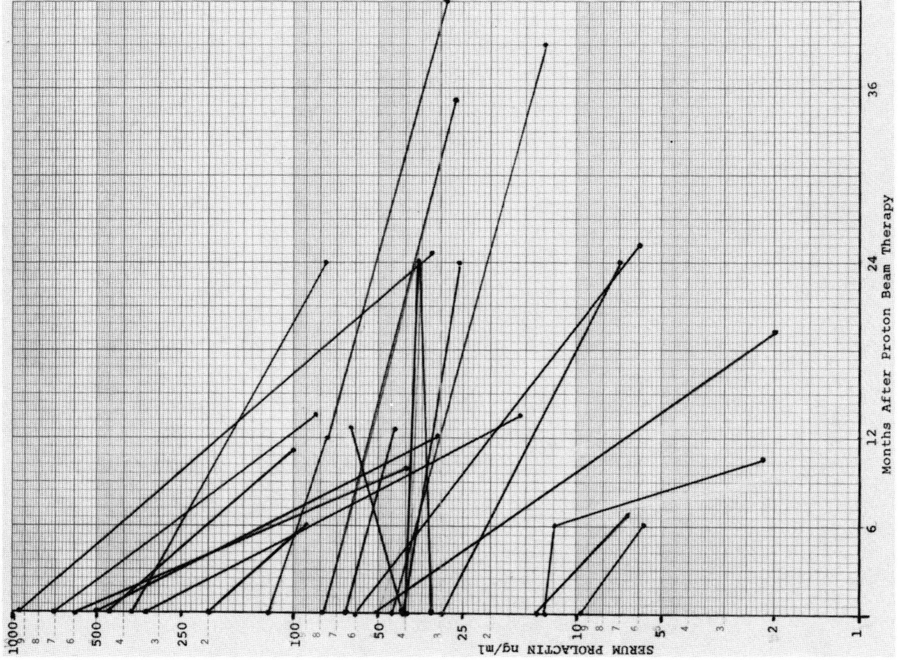

FIG. 8. Prolactin responses in prolactinoma patients. Note the log scale of prolactin levels and the time in months on the horizontal scale. A pretreatment value of 14 is in error; it should be 140. The two other pretreatment values of prolactin below 25 ng/ml were in women with amenorrhea, galactorrhea, and sella enlargement by tumor. The symptoms subsided about 6 months after proton therapy.

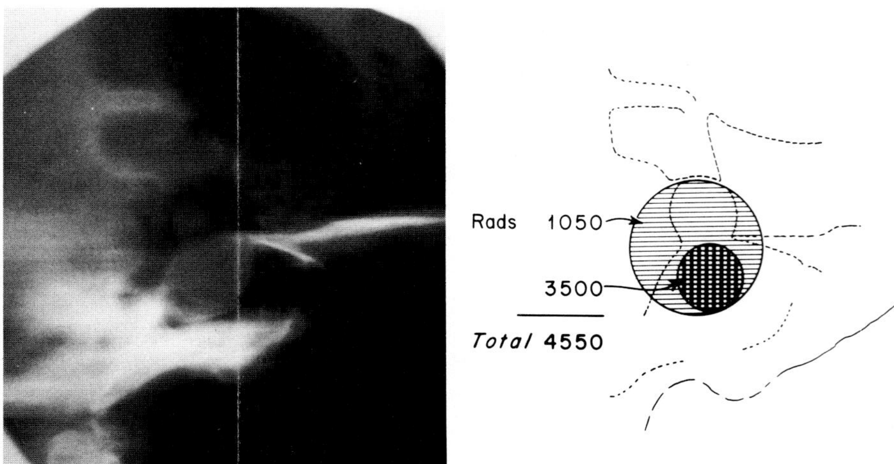

FIG. 9. "Double beam technique." The larger volume that is proton-treated is directed to inducing growth arrest of adenoma without risk to visual or other neural structures. The larger infraclinoid dose can be expected to induce radionecrosis.

document response to therapy. In any case, recurrence or the need for further treatment following proton therapy in adequately treated patients has been negligible to date.

Complications have been few since we initiated a policy of avoiding irradiation of patients with suprasellar extension with generous doses of radiation. During the first 2 years of our therapeutic trials with proton therapy, three patients experienced complication outcomes in which we were concerned that proton treatment may have contributed to an untoward result. More recently we treated selected patients with a "double-beam technique," an example of which is shown in Fig. 9. The larger-diameter beam delivers a dose which our data indicate is safe from injury to neural structures but is capable of arresting the growth of the adenoma. The smaller beam, confined to subclinoid adenoma, can be anticipated to induce radionecrosis within the adenoma. With our present dose schedule, there have been no deaths, blindness, visual field defects, extraocular motor disturbance, or hypopituitarism. One elderly patient with many surgical procedures has a memory disturbance, but we doubt that it is related to proton therapy.

RADIOGRAPHIC CLASSIFICATION

In the categorization of patients, details of radiographic features are receiving increasing attention, especially as they may guide the selection of patients for one means of treatment or another. In general, selection by means of radiographic features is the consequence of analysis of prior therapeutic results according to such criteria.

Adenomas certainly exist in normal sellae, particularly in patients with Cushing's disease and prolactinoma. In the absence of deformity, the difficulties of locating the microadenoma are increased. The size should be computed from polytomograms using DiChiro's formula (1). The presence or absence of suprasellar extension is relevant to sellae of any size and is established by either pneumoencephalography or CT scan. A deformed sella of normal volume typically houses a microadenoma, and the deformity leads to detection of the location, particularly the laterality. The size of an enlarged sella is important. The prospects for cure or remission by any single procedure when the sella is modestly enlarged is different than one which is massive. If parasellar extension exists, prospects for cure are much modified. We avoid using the term "invasive" for bony change in plain X-rays because this implies a biological variant of uncertain relevance to a radiographic observation. Erosion of bone does occur, and this term is adequately descriptive without implications of biological character. Extension into the sphenoid sinus can be demonstrated on polytomograms of the sella. Invasion into the cavernous sinus can be seen on CT scan and sometimes with cavernous sinography. Cavernous sinus invasion is particularly prejudicial to a good outcome for patients treated by either transsphenoid or proton techniques. The use of the term "invasion" is justified in the cavernous sinus because the adenoma must clearly pass through its dural envelope to enter the sinus.

The term "invasive" above may imply some biologic quality similar to "malignant," but the latter term is virtually never confirmed by changes recognized by light microscopy or the presence of metastases. This consideration is to be discussed further below.

MALIGNANCY

The optimistic outlook faced by pituitary adenoma patients is attributable to the fact that most of these tumors are benign. Nevertheless, malignant tumors do occur in the pituitary, although we have not encountered any patient with a proved carcinoma.

Another risk of irradiation is the production of sarcoma in brain following "effective" radiation therapy (18). In the report cited, two cases of sarcoma developed in 65 patients treated by fractionated X-ray. These and other cases reviewed were treated with 3,500 rads or more. The sarcomas developed at intervals of 5 and 15 years, respectively. We also had a single instance of sarcoma in an acromegalic patient in whom the symptoms began 7 years following proton treatment. Fractionated X-ray therapy was given without benefit. The patient died, and an autopsy revealed sarcoma.

That some seemingly benign pituitary adenomas have a more aggressive growth character than others was recognized by Hirsch (8) and Gordon et al. (5). These tumors are not malignant in the sense of having distinguishing malignant features by light microscopy, nor do they metastasize. They have a greater

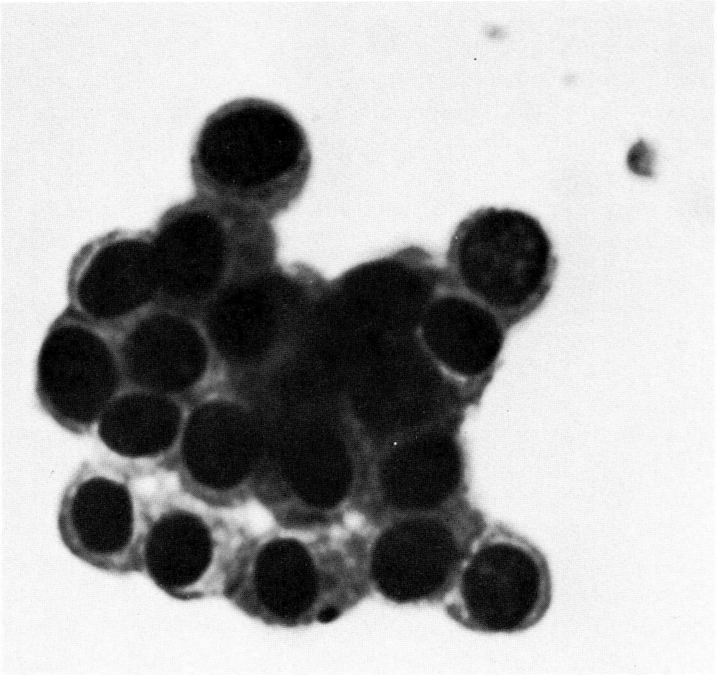

FIG. 10. Photomicrograph of typical benign pituitary cells growing in tissue culture. They float in the medium and are fairly uniform in size and staining characteristics.

tendency to recur and may transdurally invade the cavernous sinus and base of the skull (9).

For a period of time, all excised pituitary tumors in our series were grown in tissue culture. Figure 10 represents the usual appearance of a typically benign tumor. Small clusters of uniform cells float about in the culture medium. Infrequently the cells grow in a different manner (Fig. 11): they grow more rapidly, tend to adhere to container walls, and are less uniform in size and staining, features frequently associated with malignancy in other tumors. The three acromegalic patients who underwent operation for recurrent tumor had these features. Although the term "malignant" was used to describe their growth character, it is probably inappropriate to call them malignant cells for the reasons given above; i.e., they were light microscopically indistinguishable from benign tumors and nonmetastasizing. However, there does appear to be a small percentage of such cases that have a more biologically aggressive growth character, are not as readily brought into remission, and invade surrounding structures. We agree with Gordon et al. (5), who estimate on incidence of 1 to 3% of such tumors in acromegalic patients.

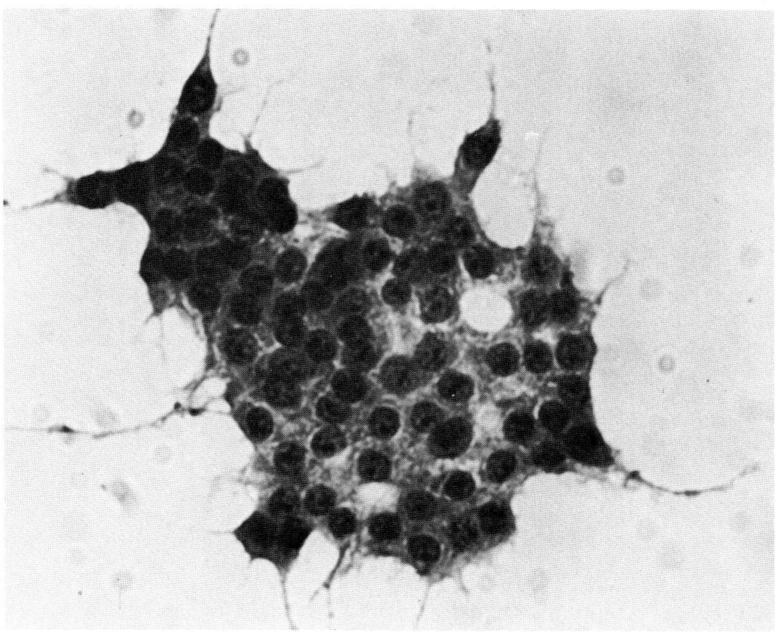

FIG. 11. This photomicrograph can be compared with that in Fig. 10. The specimens from recurrent acromegalic patients showed features of adherence to the walls of the container and more variation in size and staining characteristics of the cells.

SUMMARY

Bragg peak proton beam hypophysectomy widely employed for over a decade is safe, clinically efficacious, and cost-effective. The absence of procedure-related mortality and very low recurrence rates are major advantages of the procedure. Cyclotrons providing particle beam therapy serve as area-wide resources for the provision of special therapeutic capability for specific situations.

REFERENCES

1. Di Chiro, G., and Nelson, K. B. (1962): The volume of the sella turcica. *Am. J. Roentgenol. Radium Ther. Nucl. Med.,* 87:989–1008.
2. Earle, K. M., and Dillard, S. H., Jr. (1973): Pathology of adenomas of the pituitary gland. In: *Diagnosis and Treatment of Pituitary Tumors,* edited by P. O. Kohler and G. T. Ross, pp. 3–16. Excerpta Medica, Amsterdam.
3. Fager, C. A., Poppen, J. L., and Takaoka, Y. (1973): Indications for and results of surgical treatment of pituitary tumors by the intracranial approach. In: *Diagnosis and Treatment of Pituitary Tumors,* edited by P. O. Kohler and G. T. Ross, pp. 146–155. Excerpta Medica, Amsterdam.
4. Forbes, A. P., Henneman, P. H., Griswold, G. C., and Albright, F. (1954): Syndrome characterized by galactorrhea, amenorrhea and low urinary FSH: Comparison with acromegaly and normal lactation. *J. Clin. Endocrinol. Metab.,* 14:265–271.

5. Gordon, D. A., Hill, F. M., and Ezrin, C. (1962): Acromegaly: A review of 100 cases. *Can. Med. Assoc. J.*, 87:1106–1109.
6. Guiot, C. (1973): Transsphenoidal approach in surgical treatment of pituitary adenomas: general principles and indications in non-functioning adenomas. In: *Diagnosis and Treatment of Pituitary Tumors*, edited by P. O. Kohler and G. T. Ross, pp. 159–178. Excerpta Medica, Amsterdam.
7. Hardy, J. (1973): Transsphenoidal surgery of hypersecreting pituitary tumors. In: *Diagnosis and Treatment of Pituitary Tumors*, edited by P. O. Kohler and G. T. Ross, pp. 179–194. Excerpta Medica, Amsterdam.
8. Hirsch, O. (1959): Life-long cures and improvements after transsphenoidal operation of pituitary tumors (thirty-three patients, followed-up for 20–37 years). *Acta Ophthalmol.* [*Suppl*] *(Kbh)*, 56:5–60.
9. Kernohan, J. W., and Sayre, G. P., editor (1956): *Tumors of the Pituitary Gland and Infundibulum.* Armed Forces Institute of Pathology, Washington, D.C.
10. Kjellberg, R. N., Shintani, A., Frantz, A. G., and Kliman, B. (1968): Proton beam therapy in acromegaly. *N. Engl. J. Med.*, 278:689–695.
11. Kjellberg, R. N., and Kliman, B. (1973): A system for therapy of pituitary tumors. In: *Diagnosis and Treatment of Pituitary Tumors*, edited by P. O. Kohler and G. T. Ross, pp. 234–252. Excerpta Medica, Amsterdam.
12. Kjellberg, R. N., and Kliman, B. (1976): Treatment of acromegaly by proton hypophysectomy. In: *Current Controversies in Neurosurgery*, edited by T. P. Morley, pp. 392–405. Saunders, Toronto.
13. Kurland, L. T. (1968): Geography of neural tumors. In: *Pathology of the Nervous System*, edited by J. Minckler, pp. 2803–2808. McGraw-Hill, New York.
14. MacCarty, C. S., Hanson, E. J., Jr., Randall, R. V., and Scanlon, P. W. (1973): Indications for and results of surgical treatment of pituitary tumors by the transfrontal approach. In: *Diagnosis and Treatment of Pituitary Tumors*, edited by P. O. Kohler and G. T. Ross, pp. 139–145. Excerpta Medica, Amsterdam.
15. Ray, B. S., and Patterson, R. H., Jr. (1971): Surgical experience with chromophobe adenomas of the pituitary gland. *J. Neurosurg.*, 34:726–729.
16. Sheline, G. E. (1973): Treatment of chromophobe adenomas of the pituitary gland and acromegaly. In: *Diagnosis and Treatment of Pituitary Tumors*, edited by P. O. Kohler and G. T. Ross, pp. 201–216. Excerpta Medica, Amsterdam.
17. U.S. National Center for Health Statistics, International Classification of Diseases, Adapted for Indexing Hospital Records by Diseases and Operations. U.S. Dept. of Health, Education, and Welfare, Public Health Service, Washington, D.C.
18. Waltz, T. A., and Brownell, M. B. (1966): Sarcoma: a possible later result of effective radiation therapy for pituitary adenoma: Report of two cases. *J. Neurosurg.*, 24:901–907.
19. Wirth, F. P., Schwartz, H. G. and Schwetschenau, P. R. (1974): Pituitary adenomas: factors in treatment. In: *Clinical Neurosurgery. Proceedings of the Congress of Neurological Surgeons, Honolulu, Hawaii, 1973*, edited by R. H. Wilkins, pp. 8–25. Williams & Wilkins, Baltimore.
20. Wright, A. D., Hill, D. M., Lowy, C., and Fraser, T. R. (1970): Mortality in acromegaly. *Q. J. Med.*, 39:1–16.

Clinical Management of Pituitary Disorders,
edited by G. T. Tindall and W. F. Collins.
Raven Press, New York © 1979.

18

Neurosurgical Management of Large and Invasive Pituitary Tumors

Charles B. Wilson

Department of Neurological Surgery, University of California San Francisco, San Francisco, California 94143

The present task concerns the formulation of neurosurgical approaches to pituitary adenomas based on the tumor's size and manner of growth, irrespective of its endocrinological characteristics. In order to characterize a particular tumor according to its intrasellar and extrasellar components, I modified slightly the excellent classification system proposed by Hardy (1,2). Further, it seems useful to clarify terms—such as "malignant adenoma"—that have been applied to adenomas extending beyond the sella. Others may disagree with the terminology used, but until a standard system of classification finds universal approval ambiguous terms should be defined.

My primary reliance on the transsphenoidal approach will become apparent. Large tumor size, by itself, does not preclude this approach, and unless stated otherwise all varieties of pituitary tumors are considered suitable for transsphenoidal removal.

TERMINOLOGY AND CLASSIFICATION

In his 1940 address to the Royal Society of Medicine, Jefferson introduced the terms "massive," "malignant," and "extension" to describe the extrasellar growth of pituitary adenomas (3). Slightly more than a decade later, when he defined a small group of malignant tumors that invade the cavernous sinus (4), he changed his earlier terminology to avoid ambiguity when describing the local extension of an adenoma through its capsule. In fact, pituitary adenomas are not encapsulated in the customary sense, but the use of "capsule" to indicate the generally smooth and convex surface of most adenomas is descriptive of the stretched and thinned mesodermal tissues that encase the extrasellar extensions of large adenomas.

A slight modification of Hardy's classification permits inclusion of the "locally malignant" variants described by Jefferson. Tumors that penetrate into the cavernous sinus deserve a separate category. Although they are rare, clinically they represent an entity that Jefferson described with characteristic clarity. Anatomically their location precludes complete operative removal.

The classification to which subsequent descriptions refer is depicted in Table 1. Hardy's grade I tumor, the entirely intrasellar (enclosed) adenoma having a diameter of less than 10 mm, excluded from the main subject of this chapter because of its size, is included in the classification scheme for completeness. Arbitrarily, any tumor of greater dimensions is considered "large." Hardy's grade III and IV categories contain adenomas that have perforated the dural membrane and cortical bone of the anterior wall and floor of the sella. Extension into the air-containing sphenoid sinus or into the nonpneumatized sphenoid bone can be either localized (grade III) or diffuse (grade IV). Adenomas that perforate the dura covering the dorsum sellae must be rare, if they exist at all.

Hardy placed suprasellar extensions into three categories: type A, those expanding into the suprasellar cistern without causing deformity of the third ventricle; type B, those obliterating the anterior recesses of the third ventricle; and type C, those deforming and elevating the floor of the third ventricle. He added a fourth type (D) for expansions into temporal or frontal fossa.

The majority of pituitary adenomas retain a globular configuration, regardless of their size, although the interclinoid aperture often imposes a waist-like indentation between the intrasellar and suprasellar components of larger tumors. Jeffer-

TABLE 1. *Anatomic (radiographic and operative) classification of pituitary adenomas*

Extension
Suprasellar extension
0: None
A: Occupies cistern
B: Recesses of 3rd ventricle obliterated
C: 3rd Ventricle grossly displaced
Parasellar extension
D[a]: Intracranial (intradural)
E: Into or beneath cavernous sinus (extradural)
Site of adenoma
Floor of sella intact
I: Sella normal or focally expanded; tumor < 10 mm
II: Sella enlarged; tumor ≥ 10 mm
Sphenoid
III: Localized perforation of sellar floor
IV: Diffuse destruction of sellar floor
Distant spread
V: Spread via CSF or blood-borne

[a]Designate anterior (1), middle (2), or posterior (3) fossa.

son originally applied the term "malignant" to those tumors that deviate from a globular configuration because of relative overgrowth from one or more surfaces of the adenoma, much as a bud perforates the skin of a potato. He imagined that a relatively more rapid growth of one part of an adenoma resulted in a focal "bursting" through the capsule; and although he referred to any extrasellar growth of this nature, he was concerned primarily with suprasellar extensions since he was using a transfrontal approach as his frame of reference. Jefferson considered this asymmetrical outgrowth a reflection of locally malignant behavior, although he pointed out that the process was benign in a biological sense. His later decision to discard the term "malignant" when describing this manner of growth avoided further misunderstanding of the term. Still, those tumors that extend into the anterior, middle, and posterior fossas as asymmetrical outgrowths belong in a separate class. I have chosen to place this group of tumors in Hardy's scheme as *parasellar extensions* under (D). The same focal overgrowth can involve the uppermost surface of a suprasellar tumor, but for convenience this variant is included with the symmetrical suprasellar expansions into the third ventricle under categories A through C.

I have added a separate category (E) for those adenomas that invade the cavernous sinus through the lateral dural envelope of the sella. Typically, tumors that invade the cavernous sinus cause trigeminal anesthesia and ophthalmoplegia, often accompanied by severe trigeminal pain. Jefferson referred to these tumors as "invasive," a term that is no longer unambiguous since Hardy used "invasive" to describe perforation into the sphenoid.

Pituitary adenomas have certain features in common with meningiomas: absence of capsule derived from the tumor; a usually globular configuration and expansive growth; asymmetrical extension of nodules produced by focal overgrowth; and the capacity to perforate dura, erode bone, occupy dural venous sinuses, and extend into extracranial cavities (paranasal sinus and orbit). The term "malignant" has been imprecise as applied to pituitary adenomas and meningiomas. In both, distant spread, either through the cerebrospinal fluid (CSF) or blood-borne metastases, is rare. Without engaging in a discussion of the histological distinction between benign and malignant, I propose a separate grade (V) for those rare pituitary adenomas that exhibit distant spread.

Finally, Jefferson's use of the term "massive" requires brief comment. He applied the term to a tumor, "which is merely a very large tumor, the diameters of which are equal" (3). These tumors retain their globular shape, and in the majority the massive size of the tumor reflects three factors: "the innate urge of the adenoma to enlarge" (3), an optic chiasm that is either prefixed or postfixed, and characteristics of the sellar diaphragm and the bone constituting the sellar floor. The massive adenomas should not be classified separately, and most occupy grade II-C and II-D categories. However, the use of this term has precedent, and for any huge tumor regardless of its location "massive" can be added to the anatomical classification.

In the proposed classification, the categories introduced by Hardy are maintained. Additional designations (0, E, and V) were added after reviewing the radiological studies and operative findings in our series of patients (5). The preoperative classification of all tumors necessarily was based on radiographic studies: polytomograms of the sella and pneumoencephalograms in 99%; carotid angiography in tumors of grades II through IV; and, rarely, cavernous venography. At the time of operation the preoperative anatomical diagnosis is changed by any of the following findings:

1. A small tumor nodule, not evident by pneumoencephalography, extending into the suprasellar cistern through an incomplete sellar diaphragm.
2. Extension of tumor into the cavernous sinus or through the dura at the junction of the floor and cavernous sinus.
3. Small perforations of dura and cortical bone of the sellar floor, with tumor occupying the sphenoid body. Polytomograms permit detection of defects in the cortical bone facing the sphenoid sinus but fail to do so in some cases where the body of the sphenoid is invaded.

Category 0 was added to indicate that the tumor has no extension above the level of the diaphragm. This designation applies to all grades of tumor. Grade I–0 designates the classic microadenoma contained entirely within the sella. If a microadenoma extends through the floor of the sella—and our series contains several small tumors with such focal perforations—the tumor is classified III–0. When reviewing the prolactinomas, extension into or beneath the cavernous sinus was documented unequivocally at operation in association with grade I and II tumors. This operative finding implied a poor chance for endocrinological cure. Typically, the tumor extended over the lateral edge of the sella, and retrospectively subtle erosion of bone was evident on polytomograms in most cases. The tumor produces lateral displacement of the cavernous sinus and, after perforating the dura, extends for varying distances in an extradural position between the cavernous sinus and sphenoid bone. Frank but asymptomatic perforation of the lateral dura and extension into the cavernous sinus has been documented in two grade I tumors. In the proposed classification these invasive tumors would be separated from the favorable grade I–0 tumors by the designation I–E.

Category D contains those suprasellar tumors, otherwise assigned to grade II–B or II–C in most cases, which exhibit significant asymmetrical growth into the anterior, middle, or posterior fossa. Because the classification is used primarily by surgeons who prefer the transsphenoidal approach, this additional category is important: A signficant proportion of tumors in the grade II–C and III–C categories can be removed completely, or nearly so, by the transsphenoidal route, but significant extensions away from a direct suprasellar location preclude total removal by any route—or at the least render it unlikely. For this reason, the latter tumors should be placed in a separate category, although their number is small.

TRANSSPHENOIDAL APPROACH FOR SUPRASELLAR EXTENSION

Our preoperative preparation and transsphenoidal approach to the sella, which were described in an earlier paper (5), differ in no significant details from the procedures originally described by Hardy (1). After the induction of general anesthesia, air is injected through a lumbar catheter to outline the suprasellar mass; demarcation of the mass is sometimes poor, but it is a worthwhile maneuver. As tumor is removed and air fills the excavated cavity, the thickness of remaining tumor is defined between the air overlying it and air that has entered the excavated tumor. The anesthesiologist can inject saline or withdraw CSF to control intracranial pressure and thereby the relation of the "capsule" to the sella.

The usual adenoma is soft and relatively avascular. As the intrasellar component of the tumor is removed, the suprasellar component moves down into the operative field; if the suprasellar component does not descend, saline is injected through the lumbar catheter. Perhaps one-third of patients develop intracranial hypotension as a consequence of the lumbar puncture used for pneumoencephalography 1 or 2 days earlier, and without a ready means of reversing this unfavorable differential pressure (negative relative to atmospheric pressure) in the semisitting position the suprasellar component remains above the sella, literally being drawn upward by the negative intracranial pressure.

The surgeon should visualize the entire surface of the suprasellar "capsule." This is a simple matter if the extension is not large, but it is difficult with large suprasellar masses, particularly if large nodules of tumor have formed irregular extensions from the major globular mass. When the suprasellar component is large, the redundant and inverted "capsule" falls to the bottom of the excavated sella, obscuring the tumor's posterior extension above and behind the dorsum sellae. In this instance withdrawal of CSF elevates the capsule to allow visualization of tumor remaining in a posterior–superior direction. A dental mirror can be used for inspecting all surfaces of larger tumors, and with practice one can obtain an excellent view of otherwise inaccessible areas by using it.

One or more silver clips are attached to the midportion of the suprasellar capsule for two purposes: first, they serve as a guide to avoid excessive packing of the sella; and second, they provide a marker to follow during the postoperative period—early on for hematoma, and later for regrowth of tumor.

Postoperative retraction of the optic nerves and chiasm into an emptied sella is uncommon, but the possibility exists. I have had a single case. If the sella is unusually large and the chiasm markedly elevated by the tumor's dome, I take the precaution of either packing much of the sella with fat or elevating the dura from the sellar floor by placing bone and cartilage beneath the dura.

I now pack the sella to reduce the possibility of an unexpected postoperative CSF leak, although this is an uncommon complication unless CSF is encountered during the course of the procedure. A sudden increase in intracranial pressure (e.g., because of coughing or vomiting) may tear the redundant capsule suspended within an emptied sella. If the arachnoid has been exposed, fascia lata should be placed over it before packing the sella with fat. Obtaining a fascia lata graft causes minimal postoperative discomfort, in contrast to the pain caused by excising muscle. Packing fat is simplified by holding it in place with strips of Surgicel. The sellar opening is closed using cartilage slipped inside the dural edges; if the cartilage is insecure, it can be held in place with a few drops of biologic adhesive.

A few tumors, perhaps as many as 5%, contain an inordinate amount of connective tissue that often produces a woody consistency. These tumors do not collapse into the operative field, and I have been unable to achieve a radical or near-complete removal of any large tumor possessing this characteristic.

The preceding approach is suitable for tumors in categories A through C. If a substantial part of the tumor has extended out of the suprasellar space (e.g., into the middle fossa), craniotomy may be indicated, primarily if the mass is very large or in rare cases secondarily after a delay of 2 to 3 weeks following transsphenoidal decompression of the optic nerves. In the latter situation the sella should be packed with particular care at the end of the transsphenoidal operation.

TRANSSPHENOIDAL APPROACH FOR SPHENOID EXTENSION

Grade III tumors present no particular problem unless the sphenoid sinus has been filled with tumor escaping from a limited perforation in the sella. By contrast, removal of tumor that has eroded through dura into sphenoid bone can be difficult. The tumor cannot be removed with assurance unless the excavated bone is directly visualized by drilling away the bone separating the bony concavity and the sphenoid sinus. The bone immediately surrounding the tumor should be drilled away because tumor cells can permeate the interstices of cancellous bone in this situation. I hesitate to depend solely on the cytocidal action of alcohol. The floor of the sella can be reconstituted as indicated in the preceding section.

Grade IV tumors present a special problem. One of the worst nonfatal complications I have encountered occurred after the radical removal of a tumor of this kind; two reoperations were required, one for a postoperative hematoma and the other for a persistent CSF leak. First, the sphenoid sinus is often packed with tumor and the rostral sphenoid may be thinned or eroded. More importantly, with neither intact dura nor intact bone to maintain a cartilage graft, closure of the sella will be tenuous. Consequently, I am conservative in approaching these tumors and have as my objectives decompression of the chiasm (if involved), removal of the intrasphenoid mass and some of the intrasellar and suprasellar (if present) tumor, and absolutely avoiding entry into the subarachnoid space. With rare exceptions, grade IV tumors are not cured by operation, and the preceding objectives can be met without the risk of a postoperative CSF fistula.

INVASION INTO AND BENEATH THE CAVERNOUS SINUS

When perforation of the dura is recognized and invasion of the cavernous sinus can be identified without question, pursuit of the tumor inside the sinus is ill-advised. Complete removal of tumor is improbable, and injury to the carotid artery and the nerves to the extraocular muscles—the oculomotor nerve in particular—is likely. Whenever involvement of the cavernous sinus is recognized during the course of the operation, the remainder of the procedure should be conducted with the knowledge that surgical cure is precluded.

More frequent, although still uncommon, is perforation of the dura beneath the cavernous sinus with tumor extending into a lateral extradural position. I have followed such tumors to the junction of dorsum sellae and petrous apex. Any tumor that has gained an extradural location by this means can be considered incurable by operation. I have used currettes and copious volumes of alcohol in an effort to eradicate extradural extensions, most particularly when the remainder of the tumor was removed cleanly, but I doubt that permanent "cure" has been achieved in any case.

ABSOLUTE INDICATIONS FOR CRANIOTOMY

Although rarely, and probably because of a weak or incomplete diaphragma sella, a massive suprasellar extension can arise out of a moderately enlarged sella, creating a narrow interclinoid aperture bridging the intrasellar and suprasellar components. If the tumor is shown to be cystic by computerized tomographic scanning, the problem is not serious; but without assurance of a cyst, craniotomy is preferred over a transsphenoidal approach—even though, at times, unpredictably fortunate circumstances permit removal of the suprasellar mass through the narrow opening into the sella.

Craniotomy for major extension into the anterior, middle, or posterior fossa was discussed earlier. Using the rule of performing a craniotomy in cases of doubt, in my experience with 480 adenomas only nine cases (< 2%) were unsuited to the transsphenoidal approach.

SUMMARY

Large (≥ 10 mm) and invasive pituitary adenomas exhibit variable anatomical patterns of growth. For comparability of different therapeutic approaches and to predict the outcome of treatment for a specific category, the excellent grading system introduced by Hardy is used with slight modification.

Using the transsphenoidal approach, the majority of pituitary tumors can be removed totally, or nearly so. Adenomas that destroy the sellar floor (grade IV), extend into parasellar locations [intradural (D) or extradural (E)], or spread to distant sites (grade V) cannot be cured by operation regardless of size, but incomplete removal can relieve chiasmal compression and enhance the effect of irradiation by reducing the volume of remaining tumor.

The author has followed the transsphenoidal techniques described by Hardy with only slight variation. In a series of 480 pituitary adenomas, only 9 cases (< 2%) were treated initially by craniotomy because of contraindications to a primary approach.

REFERENCES

1. Hardy, J. (1973): Transsphenoidal surgery of hypersecreting pituitary tumors. In: *Diagnosis and Treatment of Pituitary Tumors,* edited by P. O. Kohler and G. T. Ross, pp. 179–194. Excerpta Medica/American Elsevier, New York.
2. Hardy, J., and Vezina, J. L. (1976): Transsphenoidal neurosurgery of intracranial neoplasm. In: *Advances in Neurology, Vol. 15: Neoplasia in the Central Nervous System,* edited by R. A. Thompson and R. Green, pp. 261–274. Raven Press, New York.
3. Jefferson, G. (1960): *Selected Papers of Sir Geoffrey Jefferson.* Thomas, Springfield, Ill.
4. Jefferson, G. (1955): *The Invasive Adenomas of the Anterior Pituitary* (The Sherrington Lectures III). Thomas, Springfield, Ill.
5. Wilson, C. B., and Dempsey, L. C. (1978): Transsphenoidal microsurgical removal of 250 pituitary adenomas. *J. Neurosurg.,* 48:13–22.

Clinical Management of Pituitary Disorders,
edited by G. T. Tindall and W. F. Collins.
Raven Press, New York © 1979.

19

Management of Recurrent Pituitary Tumors

William F. Collins

Department of Neurological Surgery, Yale University School of Medicine, New Haven, Connecticut 06510

The management of recurrent pituitary tumors is one of the more arduous tasks encountered by physicians in general and practicing neurosurgeons in particular. As there is no solitary cause for the symptoms, no sole response to therapy, or even a single indication for treatment, management of these lesions can best be accomplished if three concepts are considered. First, it is important to recognize that persistent pituitary tumor with recurrent symptoms, in contrast with recurrent tumor or *de novo* development of a second pituitary tumor, usually is the problem. Second, depending on either proliferative or secretory aspects of the tumor, the recurrent symptoms can be categorized into those caused by mass effects relating to progressive growth of the tumor, endocrinopathy due to hypersecretion or impairment of pituitary function, or a combination of mass effects and endocrinopathy; as a general rule, the recurrent symptoms are similar to the initial symptoms caused by the tumor. Finally, treatment goals should be realistic, tempered by the therapy used initially in the treatment of the tumor, and take into account whether the clinical situation threatens life, central nervous system activity, and/or pituitary function.

Diagnostic assessment and the rationale for therapy of symptomatic recurrent pituitary tumors associated with mass effect are more easily recognized and explicable because of the resulting serious morbidity and significant mortality. In contrast, the recurrent symptoms of the endocrinopathy caused by pituitary tumors vary from slowly progressive hypopituitarism to the overt endocrinopathies of a hypersecreting adenoma. The various endocrinopathies differ in their effects and need for treatment. The endocrinopathy of Cushing's disease (i.e., hypercortisolism) has severe morbidity and a high mortality within a few years (13) and therefore justifies aggressive and often radical therapy for control. The systemic effects of acromegaly not only cause frequent complications and morbidity but the disease is known to shorten life expectancy (19), thus justifying aggressive therapy to control excessive secretion of growth hormone (hGH). Hyperprolactinemia has not been demonstrated to affect life expectancy or to cause significant mortality or morbidity unless the tumor causes mass effect. It is not clear that the presence of a prolactin-secreting adenoma even justifies the institution of treatment (e.g., surgery) that may be associated with some risks to the patient. This is true especially in women whose principal symptom is infertility since medical therapy with bromocriptine is effective. Thus the clinical findings and the effects of the tumor (i.e., visual loss, progressive hypopituitarism, and debilitating endocrinopathy) rather than the demonstrated presence of recurrent or persistent tumor (i.e., an asymptomatic patient with progressive, serial rises in serum prolactin) should dictate the need for therapy regardless of which therapeutic option is chosen. When there is the potential for serious morbidity and/or shortening of life, a full evaluation and consideration of therapy is mandatory. The evaluation and management of recurrent pituitary tumors is discussed in this chapter with the therapeutic goal of alleviating the morbidity and mortality that can be caused by recurrent symptoms of pituitary tumor after failure of initial treatment.

TREATMENT OF MASS EFFECT

The most immediate and threatening symptoms of persistent pituitary tumors are those caused by mass effects. Treatment modalities to control mass effects include surgical decompression, removal of the pituitary and tumor by hypophysectomy, drug therapy, and/or cerebrospinal fluid (CSF) shunting. The use of pharmacological agents to reduce tumor mass has not undergone significant clinical trials, although steroids may provide a positive temporary effect by reducing edema of adjacent tissues; further, thyroid replacement, particularly in the hypothyroid child, has been shown to have significant mass reducing action on pituitary tumors (9). Dopamine agonists (e.g., bromocriptine) although altering secretory aspects of pituitary tumor, have not been demonstrated to alter proliferative growth of these lesions even though isolated reports of a decrease in mass effects with improvement in vision have been reported (3,18) and is encouraging. The factors to be considered when using the different treatment modalities for the care of the patient with recurrent pituitary tumor include age and general condition of the patient, rate and growth of the tumor, size and position of the tumor, and the previous treatment given including what, how much, and when it was applied.

Clinical experience over the past 70 years has demonstrated that mass effects of pituitary tumors are best controlled by radiation therapy (8). Irradiation of persistent pituitary tumors with recurrent mass effects that have not been treated previously is a good therapeutic option (15) and, in the author's opinion, the treatment of choice. Since radiation therapy is most effective when tumor size is reduced as much as possible, surgical decompression of the recurrent mass should be done when feasible before irradiation is started. The method for decompression (i.e., transcranially or transsphenoidally) is dependent on the position and extent of the mass. Tumors confined by either the diaphragma sella or a reconstituted fibrous diaphragma, and which are large enough to encroach on the third ventricle and/or the prepontine cisterns, can often be handled transsphenoidally, whereas a smaller tumor with lateral extension into the middle fossa or without an enlarged sella turcica are probably best approached transcranially. Tumors invading the base of the skull are usually more easily decompressed with the transsphenoidal approach, whereas those with a sheet-like extension or multiple small tumor extensions into the subarachnoid space may best be handled by irradiation alone or by shunting without decompression since removal of such multiple small masses is hazardous and ineffectual. Surgical cure of recurrent mass effect symptoms is at best difficult and usually can be accomplished only by removing all intrasellar tissue, a procedure which obviously involves hypophysectomy. The decision for the latter approach is determined by the physical characteristics of the tumor, surgical accessibility, extent of encapsulation, and the ability to sterilize the capsule chemically. The capsule of large pituitary tumors is not a tumor capsule per se but rather a blend of structures including the dura of the clivus, cavernous sinus, and sella turcica; the diaphragma sella or its reconstitution by fibrous connective tissue, arachnoid, or glia connected to cranial nerves, and the pituitary stalk. Almost always some (and frequently all) of these tissues contain islands of tumor (20), and therefore chemical sterilization of these islands is indicated if a cure is to be accomplished. Because of the types of tissue involved, careful preoperative definition of the tumor and its relation to intracranial structures, as well as experience at recognizing the various tissue that can constitute the pseudocapsule, are necessary before deciding to attempt hypophysectomy and chemical sterilization of the tumor bed. For such sterilization, I prefer Zenker's solution, a carryover from my experience using Bronson Ray's hypophysectomy technique. Other considerations to weigh in the decision for hypophysectomy, although perhaps less applicable in persistent pituitary tumors with recurrent mass effects, include the patient's age and whether the patient is mentally capable of handling replacement therapy. The latter consideration enters the evaluation since there is a continuing mortality with the passage of time relating to the need for steroid replacement for illness and injury that can result in significant mortality. The incidence of such mortality is difficult to determine; in our hypophysectomy cases done mostly for breast carcinoma and diabetic retinopathy, we estimated it at 1.5 to 2.5% per year. This is a significant mortality rate for the benign disease of pituitary tumor that can encompass decades, but it seems to take on less significance if repetitive surgical treatment and/or recurrent mass effects are the alternatives.

If the patient previously received an adequate amount of radiation therapy, the control of mass effect symptoms usually are more difficult. Although hypophysectomy may seem to be an appropriate option, it should be realized that it will probably control only a small percentage of cases. In fact, there is no series in the literature using hypophysectomy for recurrent mass effects. I have used it in three cases, and only one patient survived more than 5 years without further recurrence. The principle reason for failure of the operation to eradicate the tumor probably relates to the biological aggressiveness of the tumor that has already failed to be controlled by decompression and radiation. Not infrequently, repetitive surgical decompression and/or shunting of CSF to control hydrocephalus are the only practical options. Reevaluation of previous X-ray therapy, including the interval since it was administered and the dosage, helps determine whether more radiation can be used. The dangers of exceeding 5,000 to 5,500 rads, even in divided doses, for the initial therapy of pituitary tumor, or in the course of giving repetitive doses of therapy for control of recurrent symptoms over extended periods, is well documented (2,10,12) and must enter into the decision.

It is difficult to know the true incidence of complications of radiation therapy when treating pituitary tumors since most studies are either case reports or combined in series of patients that include treatment of malignant brain tumors with short life expectancy. In a series of 85 patients reported from our institution (17), 8 patients received either large fractional doses or over 6,500 rads in repetitive treatment sequence. Three of the eight patients showed evidence of chiasmatic, optic nerve, or hypothalamic damage within the next 18 months, and one showed sudden loss of optic nerve function about 4 years after treatment. Further problems may be encountered in these patients, for although radiation necrosis usually occurs within 4 to 18 months it has been reported as late as 12 years following treatment (7). Four patients in my series with surgical decompression and radiation as either the initial therapy or the treatment of the first recurrence underwent radical excision of the tumor for symptoms of recurrent mass effects. As already mentioned, three of these patients had hypophysectomy. The four patients had an average remission of 23 months, a discouragingly short period of palliation, although one of the four has been free of symptoms for more than 5 years since the operation. Although I have had no experience with heavy-particle radiation in these recurrent cases, it may be that with modern stereotactic control of this modality perhaps it should be considered. CSF shunting is indicated in patients with signs and symptoms of hydrocephalus when the condition cannot be controlled by surgical decompression of the tumor and/or irradiation. Hydrocephalus should always be considered in patients with persistent pituitary tumors with recurrent mass effects as it is a common complication. Not infrequently shunting has provided long periods of palliation.

TREATMENT OF ENDOCRINOPATHIES

Persistent or recurrent symptoms of endocrinopathy also can be difficult to control but fortunately are usually less life-threatening than mass effects, and often there is an alternative method for controlling the symptoms. With the availability of radioimmunoassays for detecting pituitary hormones, either failure to control by treatment or recurrence usually is diagnosed in the laboratory rather than from the patient's symptoms. Symptoms of hypersecretion of pituitary tumors can cause no serious symptoms as in prolactin-secreting adenomas, or can be quite grave and disabling as in Cushing's disease. Separation of the complication of secretory and mass effects, at least for considerable periods of time, is common; hence increasing levels of circulating hormone, while indicating persistent tumor, often do not signify that symptoms from mass effect are imminent. The opposite circumstance is probably also true, although I have no example in our series of over 300 pituitary tumors, i.e., mass effects occurring in a patient with a formerly endocrine-active adenoma who now has evidence only of mass effect and decreasing pituitary function. When this was suspected in our series (i.e., the latter sequence of decreasing pituitary function being a sign of mass effect), it was, as far as our work-up can determine, the result of radiation therapy, either alone or after surgical therapy. Although persistent elevation of circulating pituitary hormone indicates, with the possible exception of a moderate elevation of prolactin, persistent tumor, it does not indicate increasing mass but suggests a need for careful definition of the sellar and parasellar areas. Computerized axial tomography (CT) can demonstrate large extensions of tumor, and although the results of CT scanning of the parasellar regions have improved with technical improvements in the scanners and the use of water-soluble contrast material, pneumoencephalography with laminography is necessary to determine accurately the extrasellar extent of tumor during the initial work-up of patients suspected of having a pituitary tumor and for evaluating recurrent symptoms in patients with known pituitary tumors if surgical or radiation therapy is being considered.

The treatment of endocrinopathy resulting from persistent endocrine-active pituitary tumors is determined by the effects of the endocrinopathy and is tempered by the morbidity and mortality of the treatment. Certainly hypercortisolism must be controlled, and excess hGH should be controlled since both cause significant morbidity and a shortened life expectancy. The mortality and morbidity of the effects of hyperprolactinemia are not as clear, although it can relate to hypoestrogenism with osteoporosis and vaginal tissue atrophy or can cause impotence, situations with considerable distress. On the other hand, hyperprolactinemia may be a welcome cause of infertility in many women. Recurrent symptoms of the endocrinopathy of pituitary tumors usually relate directly to changes in the levels of the circulating hormone produced by the tumor, in contrast to the poor correlation of the hormone levels with recurrent mass symptoms.

Since previous pituitary tumor literature recounts mainly data relative to mass effect (e.g., morbidity and mortality), and since the ability to measure accurately the circulating pituitary hormones has been available for only a few years, it is difficult to discuss recurrent endocrinopathies of pituitary tumors because an adequate and significant data base is unavailable. In our series of endocrine-active tumors, the major cause of recurrent symptoms has been the failure to control the endocrinopathy with the initial treatment as measured by laboratory studies even though following such treatment the symptoms of the endocrinopathy may have been controlled temporarily. The gradual increase in the level of circulating hormones with passage of time has forecast the return of the symptoms. Thus the situation is rarely cure followed by recurrence of disease; rather, it is treatment followed by improvement but not complete control, followed by progressive loss of control and return of symptoms of endocrinopathy. Part of the problem, particularly when evaluating the treatment of pituitary endocrinopathies in more recent series, is to determine the criteria for cure, control, and failure. In acromegaly, for instance, a common criterion for measuring cure of the disease is to restore resting hGH to a value below 10 ng/ml following treatment (4). Applying this criteria to our series with a 4- to 8-year follow-up, 13 of 16 patients (81%) would be cured. If the resting hGH level is set at less than 5 ng/ml, a more acceptable level, only 9 of 16 (56%) would be controlled. If the criteria are to reverse all metabolic dysfunction of hGH, however, (i.e., resting levels below 5 ng/ml), depression of circulating levels with a glucose load, correction of any paradoxical rise with glucose intake, no response to TRH (see Chapters 9 and 10), and no suppression with dopamine agonists, then only 5 of 16 (31%) are controlled. The latter criterion can be justified if few or no late recurrences of the symptoms of acromegaly occur in these patients compared to the others; however, long, careful follow-up is required to determine if such strict criteria are necessary. Certainly only a few years has been necessary to show in our series that many patients with resting hGH levels of 6 to 10 ng/ml have a rise in hGH with the passage of time if no further treatment is given. It is clear, therefore, that as a criterion of control of acromegaly, resting hGH levels of 6 to 10 ng/ml are inadequate.

If a major consideration in the treatment of recurrent symptoms of the endocrinopathy of pituitary tumors is balancing the morbidity of the endocrinopathy against the morbidity of the treatment, then treatment of progressive hypopituitarism is obvious since the difficulty of controlling the symptoms by adequate replacement therapy is negligible whereas the morbidity of hypopituitarism is considerable. As alluded to above, whether progressive mass effects of pituitary tumor are causing the hypopituitarism should always be determined.

Other treatment modalities to control the symptoms of recurrent endocrinopathy of hypersecreting pituitary tumors include: (a) further surgical removal of the tumor; (b) hypophysectomy; (c) irradiation; (d) removal of the target endocrine gland; and (e) medical therapy. Surgical excision of the tumor is certainly the most desirable therapy for controlling the symptoms; however, often in those patients in whom the disease recurred following the first surgical attempt, aggressive growth characteristics of the tumor and invasion of the remaining pituitary gland and/or surrounding structures at the first attempt frequently were the causes of the failure and make a second attempt fruitless unless hypophysectomy and chemical sterilization of the surrounding tissues is done. Hypophysectomy and its morbidity and life-shortening effects must be compared to the morbidity of the endocrinopathy. Hypercortisolism and excessive hGH merit such radical treatment but hyperprolactinemia does not (16). Radiation has been used to control the symptoms of endocrinopathy; but in contrast to its documented effects on the proliferative characteristics of pituitary tumor and the resulting mass effect, its action on the secretory aspects is neither as well documented nor as clear. Series of cases that show an improvement reflected in a 40 to 50% reduction in circulating levels of hormone (5,14) are scarcely worth commenting on, for it is clear that reducing prolactin from 1,000 to 500 ng/ml or hGH from 80 to 40 ng/ml does not affect the morbidity of the endocrinopathy even though the percentage drop in circulating hormone levels is impressive mathematically. In our series, irradiation has had a differential effect on the hormone levels of the various endocrine-active tumors. Early in our series I believed that all pituitary tumors should be irradiated, and so any patient with an endocrine-active tumor who postoperatively did not have completely normal levels of hormone underwent irradiation. Of nine patients with hGH-producing adenomas who received 5,000 rads in fractionated doses from a linear accelerator over a 5-week period, seven had levels of hormone gradually reduced below 5 ng/ml over an 18- to 24-month period. In one patient the hGH level gradually increased, and in another it remained the same. None of the patients fulfilled all the criteria for control of hGH-producing tumors mentioned earlier. By way of contrast, 15 prolactin-secreting adenomas received X-ray therapy, and in none of these patients were the elevated prolactin values reduced to normal levels. This failure might be explained by damage to the stalk or hypothalamus from the radiation but also might be explained by a difference in sensitivity of the tumor. Of six patients with ACTH-producing pituitary tumors, in none was the hypercortisolism controlled by radiation therapy.

The problems, therefore, of radiation therapy for endocrine-active tumors include: (a) an apparent difference in sensitivity of the different tumors and therefore differential ability of the radiation to control the endocrinopathy; (b) a long delay in the effectiveness of the control of the endocrinopathy; and (c) the small but definite risk of receiving radiation therapy in the usual therapeutic doses and the increased risk when these levels are exceeded or when repetitive courses of therapy are given (6).

When the hypercortisolism of Cushing's disease cannot be controlled by pituitary surgery, it can be treated with adrenalectomy. Orth and Liddle suggested that radiation be given at the time of adrenalectomy, and their results indicate that this approach controls the growth potential of most of the tumors (11). However, no data are available concerning the proportion of ACTH-producing tumors of the pituitary that have marked growth potential. Unfortunately, circulating levels of ACTH remain difficult to interpret. Metyrapone has been used to control hypercortisolism while awaiting the effect of either proton-beam or conventional radiation therapy, but no other medication appears to have a significant effect on hypercortisolism. In contrast, bromocriptine is effective in small doses for controlling hyperprolactinemia and in larger doses for controlling the excess production of hGH (1,5).

Keeping in mind the treatment options available, the morbidity and mortality of the mass effects, and the endocrinopathies of recurrent or persistent pituitary tumors, the type of follow-up necessary to prevent mortality and morbidity becomes clear. Although the need to be certain that recurrent symptoms from persistent pituitary tumors are treated before the patient sustains functional damage is obvious, the rarity of recurrent symptoms, particularly from mass effects during the first few years after treatment, causes many physicians to have a false sense of security. The treatment of pituitary tumors in the early series was confined mainly to the treatment of mass effects or the acromegaly, the evaluation of which did not include hGH assays. The classic follow-up for pituitary tumors, therefore, was to (a) watch for symptoms and signs of encroachment on the parasellar structures, particularly the optic nerves and chiasm, at yearly or biyearly intervals; (b) evaluate the bony sella with skull X-rays; and (c) evaluate pituitary function, particularly hypothyroidism, so it could be treated when diagnosed.

During more recent years corticosteroid replacement was added to the treatment of hypopituitarism; and with the advent of radioimmunoassays, recurrent evaluation of pituitary function is done in many clinics. This recurrent endocrine evaluation, however, can be disconcerting unless the differential between the diagnosis of mass effect and endocrinopathy is considered.

For instance, over a period of 10 years I followed an asymptomatic man who had been treated for a large chromophobe adenoma. He had mentioned many times that he was impotent and was placed on testosterone with little effect. No symptoms of mass effect appeared in his work-up, but when prolactin assays became available his blood level of prolactin was found to be 600 ng/ml, or approximately 30 times the normal level. He was one of the first patients who suggested to me the separation of mass effects and endocrinopathy in recurrent or persistent pituitary tumors. The marked elevation of prolactin led to a complete re-evaluation of his tumor, including pneumoencephalography and re-exploration of his sella. The latter showed small islands of fibrous connective tissue, normal pituitary, and tumor whose removal barely changed his hyperprolactinemia. He had received approximately 5,000 rads of radiation therapy following his surgery, which had obviously controlled the proliferative aspects but not the secretory aspects of the tumor. Bromocriptine restored his potency and normal levels of prolactin.

The follow-up of the treatment of pituitary tumors must be prolonged to at least two decades and preferably for the life of the patient. The patient should be instructed at the time of initial treatment that the recurrence of the tumor is always possible and that continued follow-up is necessary. Follow-up evaluation should include appropriate periodic studies to rule out mass effects and to determine if any changes occur in the function of the parasellar structures, adjacent brain, and bones of the skull as a result of mass effect. Studies should also include reappraisal of pituitary function, particularly evaluation of any abnormal levels of pituitary hormones produced by endocrine-active tumors, and assessment of levels of circulating hormones to diagnose progressive hypopituitarism. How frequently these studies should be done is not a settled issue, but perhaps within a decade or so information will be available that defines the need accurately. At our institution the protocol is to evaluate the patient 6 months after treatment is complete and then at yearly intervals. No time limit for deciding that further evaluation is no longer necessary has been made, and each patient is instructed that any untoward symptoms should be used as an indication for more frequent evaluation. It is hoped that with this protocol we can better evaluate therapy and, hopefully, protect the patients from unnecessary morbidity. Thorough, careful, periodic evaluation of the treatment of pituitary tumors may ultimately lead to better treatment techniques, and thus the problems of recurrent symptoms will become less frequent and the need to concern ourselves with the management of recurrent pituitary tumors will diminish with the passage of time.

REFERENCES

1. Besser, G. M., and Thorner, M. O. (1976): Bromocryptine in the treatment of the hyperprolactinameia-hypogonadism syndromes. *Postgrad. Med. J. (Suppl 1),* 52:64–70.
2. DiLorenzo, N., Nolletti, A., and Palma, L. (1978): Late cerebral radionecrosis. *Surg. Neurol.,* 10:281–290.
3. Eskildsen, P. C., Svendsen, P. A., Vang, L., and Nerup, J. (1978): Long-term treatment of acromegaly with bromocriptine. *Acta Endocrinol. (Kbh),* 87:687–700.
4. Giovanelli, M. A., Motti, E. D. F., Paracchi, A., et al. (1976): Treatment of acromegaly by transsphenoidal microsurgery. *J. Neurosurg.,* 44:677–686.
5. Holdaway, I. M., Frengley, P. A., Scott, D. J., and Ibbertson, K. (1978): Bromoergocryptine treatment of acromegaly persisting following conventional therapy. *Clin. Endocrinol.,* 8:45–54.
6. Jenkins, J. S., Ash, S., and Bloom, H. J. G. (1972): Endocrine function after external pituitary irradiation in patients with secreting and non-secreting pituitary tumors. *Q. J. Med.,* 41:57–69.
7. Kindt, P. H. (1953): Rontgenshaden nach bestrahlung medianer hirngewachse. *Arch. Psychiatry,* 191:55–72.
8. Kohler, P. O., and Ross, G. T., editors (1973): *Diagnosis and Treatment of Pituitary Tumors.* Excerpta Medica/American Elsevier, New York.
9. Lawrence, A. M., and Hagen, T. C. (1973): Alternatives to ablative therapy for pituitary tumor. In: *Diagnosis and Treatment of Pituitary Tumor,* edited by P. O. Kohler and G. T. Ross, pp. 297–312. Exerpta Medica, Amsterdam.
10. Martins, A. N., Johnston, J. S., Henry, J. M., et al. (1977): Delayed radiation necrosis of the brain. *J. Neurosurg.,* 47:336–345.
11. Orth, D. N., and Liddle, G. W. (1971): Results of treatment in 108 patients with Cushing's syndrome. *N. Engl. J. Med.,* 285:243–247.
12. Peck, F. C., and McGovern, E. R. (1966): Radiation necrosis of the brain in acromegaly. *J. Neurosurg.,* 25:536–542.
13. Plotz, C. M., Knowlton, A. I., and Ragan, C. (1952): The natural history of Cushing's syndrome. *Am. J. Med.,* 13:597–614.
14. Roth, J., Gorden, P., and Brace, K. (1970): Efficacy of conventional pituitary irradiation in acromegaly. *N. Engl. J. Med.,* 282:1385–1391.
15. Sheline, G. E. (1971): Untreated and recurrent chromophobe adenomas of the pituitary. *Am. J. Roentgenol. Radium Ther. Nucl. Med.,* 112:768–773.
16. Tyrrell, J. B., Brooks, R. M., Fitzgerald, P. A., et al. (1978): Cushing's disease: Selective transsphenoidal resection of pituitary microadenomas. *N. Engl. J. Med.,* 298:753–758.
17. Urdaneta, N., Chessin, H., and Fischer, J. J. (1976): Pituitary adenomas and craniopharyngiomas: Analysis of 99 cases treated with radiation therapy. *Int. J. Radiat. Oncol. Biol. Phys.,* 1:895–902.

18. Wass, J. A. H., Thorner, M. O., Morris, D. V., et al. (1977): Long-term treatment of acromegaly with bromocriptine. *Br. Med. J.,* 1:875–878.
19. Wright, A. D., Hill, D. M., Lowy, C., and Fraser, T. R. (1970): Mortality in acromegaly. *Q. J. Med.,* 39:1–16.
20. Wrightson, P. (1978): Conservative removal of small pituitary tumors: Is it justified by pathological findings? *J. Neurol. Neurosurg. Psychiatry,* 41:283–289.

Clinical Management of Pituitary Disorders,
edited by G. T. Tindall and W. F. Collins.
Raven Press, New York © 1979.

20

Transcranial Microsurgical Approaches to the Sellar Region

Albert L. Rhoton Jr.

Department of Neurological Surgery, Health Center, University of Florida, Gainesville, Florida 32610

Microsurgery is defined as surgery using the 3× to 40× magnification provided by the surgical microscope. A recent study of surgical services in the United States by the American College of Surgeons and the American Surgical Association ranked the application of microsurgical techniques to the treatment of tumors of the nervous system as one of the most significant advances in surgery during the period 1945–1970 (5). Microsurgery, in addition to permitting new dimensions in transsphenoidal surgery, has improved the technical performance of the older standard transfrontal-intracranial approaches to the sellar region (8–12) (Fig. 1). This chapter reviews the different transcranial microsurgical approaches to the sellar region and the selection and use of microinstruments for these approaches. Valuable adjuncts to the use of the surgical microscope include bipolar coagulation, improved devices for immobilizing the head, and self-retaining brain retractors.

INSTRUMENT SELECTION

Conventional microsurgical instruments are designed with working tips as small as 2 to 3 mm. Most microinstruments are modifications of these well-known surgical instruments, e.g., bayonet forceps and dissectors with miniature tips. One should try to obtain microsurgical instruments with handles and designs similar to those which one uses for surgery with the naked eye. The instruments should have a dull finish because the brilliant light from highly polished instruments reflected back through the surgical microscope can interfere with the surgeon's vision and detract from the quality of photographs taken through the surgical microscope. Sharpness and sterilization are not affected by the dull finish.

The separation between the instruments' tips should be only great enough

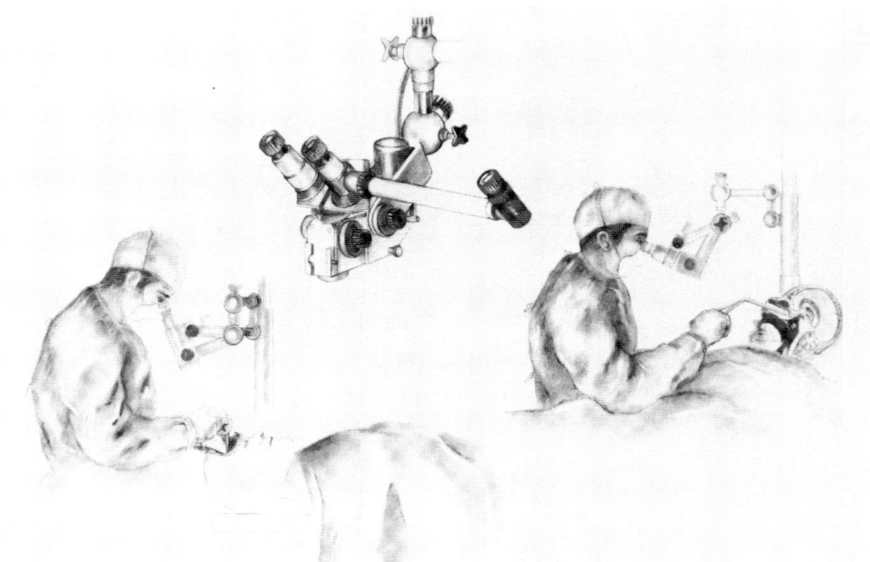

FIG. 1. Surgical microscope. Observer tube projecting to right for surgical assistant **(center)**, use of microscope for transfrontal craniotomy **(left)**, and use of microscope for transsphenoidal approach to sella **(right)**. (From ref. 8.)

to allow them to straddle, cut, or grasp the tissue accurately. Excessive opening and closing movements necessitated by wide-tip separation reduces the functional accuracy of the instrument during delicate manipulation under high magnification. The finger pressure required to bring widely separated tips together against firm spring tension often initiates a fine tremor and inaccurate movement.

The length of the instruments should be adequate for the particular microsurgical task being contemplated (Fig. 2). Standard jewelers' forceps (11 cm in length) are barely long enough for use on the cerebral surfaces. Straight forceps, needle holders, and scissors approximately 18 cm in length are a more satisfactory length for use on the scalp and near (but not below) the surface of the brain. Bayonetted instruments (forceps, needle holders, and scissors) having 8-cm shafts (the length between the handles and tips) may be used near or just below the cortical surface, but a 10-cm length is needed for the sellar region or near the circle of Willis. For transsphenoidal operations instruments having shafts 9.5 to 12 cm are needed.

Bipolar Coagulation

Bipolar coagulation is required because it allows accurate, fine coagulation of small vessels, minimizing dangerous spread of current to the optic nerves and other structures (3) (Fig. 3). Surgeons with experience in conventional coagulation are conditioned to acquire maximal dryness at the surface of application,

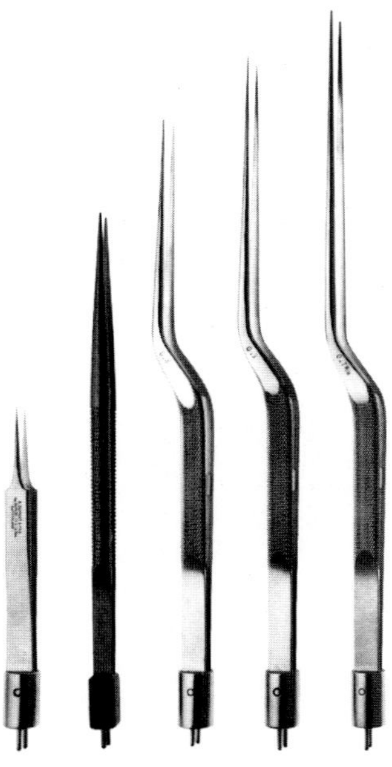

FIG. 2. Bipolar coagulation forceps of different lengths. **From left to right**: Modified jeweler's forceps for use on surface tissues (11 cm). Straight forceps for work at and just below the surface (18 cm). Short bayonet forceps for use 3 to 5 cm below the surface (21 cm). Long bayonet forceps for work in deeper areas, such as the sellar region and cerebellopontine angle (23 cm). Longest bayonet forceps for use in long narrow transsphenoidal exposures (25 cm). (From ref. 12.)

but with bipolar coagulation some moistness is preferable. Coagulation takes place even if the tips are immersed in saline, and indeed keeping the tissue moist with local cerebrospinal fluid (CSF) or saline irrigation during coagulation reduces heating and minimizes drying and sticking of tissue to the forceps. The points of the forceps should be cleaned after each application to the tissue to avoid sticking after coagulation. If charred blood coats the tips, it should be removed with a damp cloth rather than by scraping with a scalpel blade because the blade may scratch the tips and make them more adherent to tissue during coagulation. The tips of the forceps should be polished if they become pitted and rough after long use.

The bipolar unit allows coagulation in areas where unipolar coagulation would be hazardous, e.g., near the optic and other cranial nerves, within the ventricles, and around the brainstem. It is important to remember that when the electrode tips touch each other, the current is short-circuited and no coagulation occurs. There should be enough tension in the handle of the forceps to allow the surgeon to control the distance between the tips. Some forceps, so attractive for their delicacy, compress with so little pressure that even with a delicate grasp one cannot avoid closing them during coagulation. It is preferable to test forceps for tension and tactile qualities by holding them in the gloved rather than the naked hand. Forceps which are perceived to have adequate resistance to closure in the naked hand may become almost imperceptible in the gloved hand. The forceps may be used to develop tissue planes by inserting the partially closed forceps between the structures to be separated and releasing the tension so that the blades open and separate the structures. This form of dissection requires greater tension in the handles than is found in some delicate forceps. The bayonet

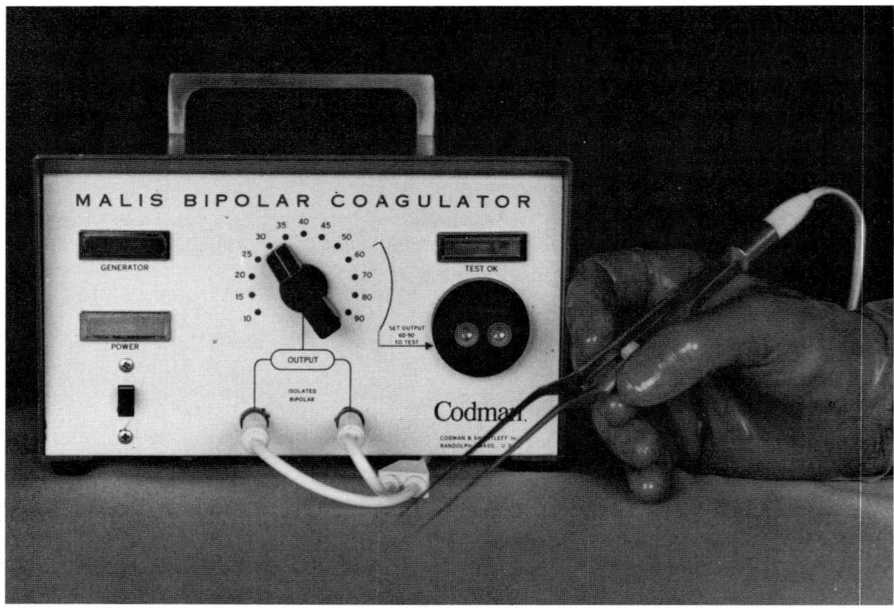

FIG. 3. Bipolar coagulation unit with round handle bayonet forceps attached. (From ref. 10.)

forceps should be properly balanced so that, when its handle rests across the radial side of the middle finger and the web between the thumb and index finger, it remains there without falling forward when the grasp of the index finger and thumb is released. Poor balance prevents the delicate grasp needed for microsurgery. Some surgeons prefer round-handled bayonet forceps because the handles make it possible to rotate the instrument between the thumb and forefinger rather than having to rotate the entire wrist.

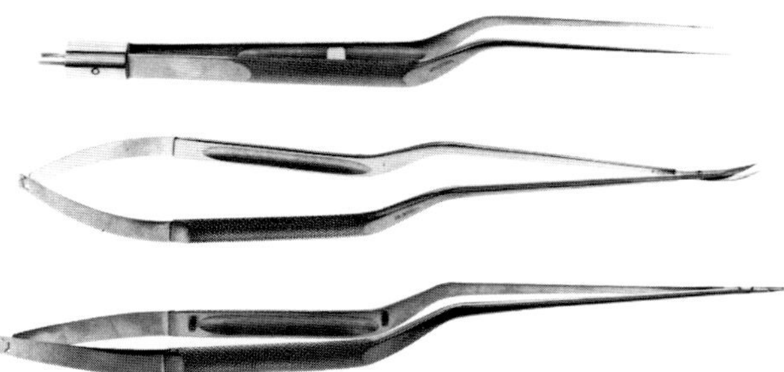

FIG. 4. Bayonet bipolar coagulation forceps **(top)**, scissors **(center)**, and needle holder **(bottom)** with round handles. The working distance from handle to tip is 8 cm, suitable for most neurosurgical operations. For deeper work, similar instruments, but with 10-cm shafts, are used. For surface work, straight, not bayonetted, instruments as shown in Fig. 5 are used. (From ref. 12.)

Standard bayonet forceps have blades 8 cm in length (Fig. 4); however, for transfrontal approaches to the sellar region, 10-cm blades are needed. Bayonet bipolar coagulation forceps with the same length of blades are also required. A series of bipolar forceps having tips of 0.3 to 1.5 mm allow coagulation of almost any size vessel. Tips of 0.3 mm are like those found on jewelers' forceps and are suitable for the finest work.

Brain Retraction

Self-retaining brain retraction is used for the transfrontal approach because it allows the surgeon to work in the relatively confined space of the subfrontal area unhindered by the assistant's hand and because it is more dependable in maintaining constant gentle retraction of the brain than the surgeon's or assistant's hand (Fig. 5). Removal of a pituitary tumor commonly requires several

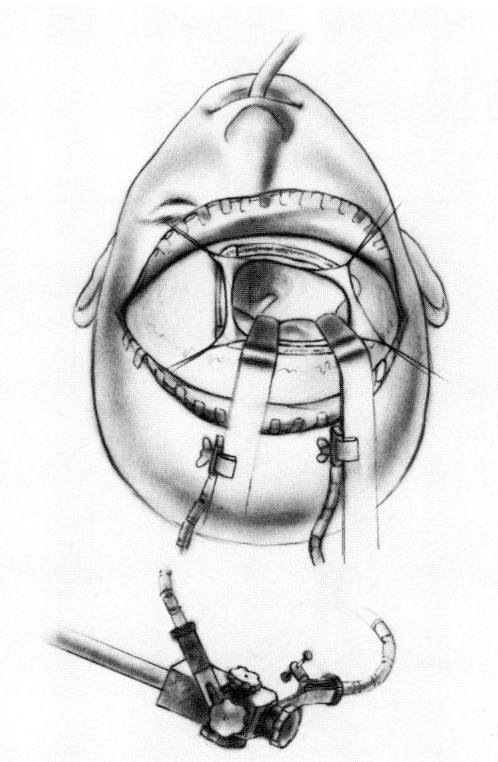

FIG. 5. Self-retaining brain retractor as used for transfrontal operative approach to the sella. Leyla self-retaining brain retractor designed by Yasargil (Aesculap, Tuttlingen, Germany). The retractor arm shown here is locked to a bar which attaches to the operating table rather than directly to the bone margin. Attachments are available for locking the arm of the retractor to the craniotomy margin. (From ref. 11.)

hours of retraction, which can lead to severe edema and irreversible damage to the frontal lobe. When utilizing self-retaining retractors, normal-appearing frontal lobe is often found after removing a retractor that has been in position for hours. The surgeon should learn to manipulate the retractor while looking through the microscope. The retractor should not be applied so firmly that it blanches the cortical vessels and causes infarction of the underlying brain. This occurs infrequently if blood pressure is normal; however, if hypotension is used,

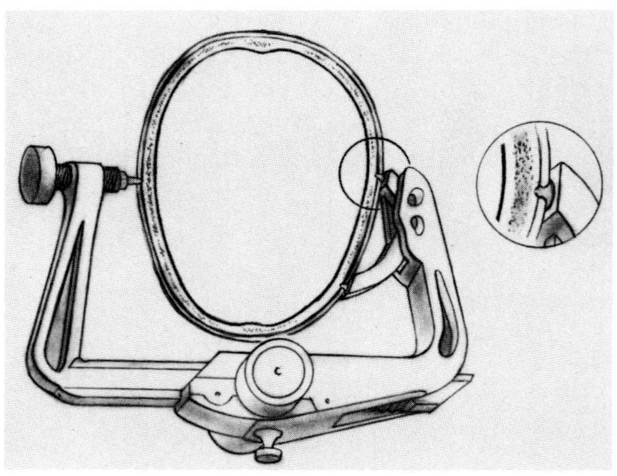

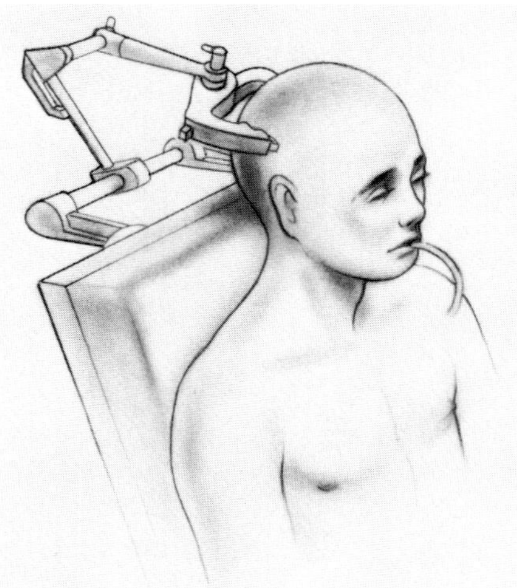

FIG. 6. Pinion head holder used to immobilize head during microsurgical operations. **A:** Pins penetrate scalp and are firmly fixed to the outer table of the skull. **B:** Pinion head holder as used for craniotomy in prone position or for transsphenoidal operations. For the latter, the head holder should be placed high enough on the head so that it does not obscure the sellar region on intraoperative fluoroscopy. (From ref. 11.)

inadequate perfusion under the retractor may cause infarction with subsequent hemorrhage after the retractor is removed. The most frequently used self-retaining brain retractors are the Yasargil (Aesculap, Tuttlingen, Germany) and the Greenberg type (Codman, Randolph, Massachusetts). Each consists of a series of ball-and-socket units resembling a chain of pearls with an internal cable which, when tightened, holds in the desired position. For some procedures the retractor may be attached directly to the craniectomy margin, but the small craniotomy openings often used for the transfrontal approach to the sella makes this impractical. The author prefers to attach the retractor arm to a bar fixed to the operating table and not to the craniectomy margin.

Cranial Fixation

Firm cranial fixation is essential for the transcranial and transsphenoidal approaches and is best achieved by a pinion head holder consisting of a clamp with three pins that penetrate the scalp and are firmly fixed to the outer table of the skull (Fig. 6). During transsphenoidal surgery it is important that the pinion head rest be placed above the sellar region so it does not obscure the sella during intraoperative fluoroscopy.

Suction

The most commonly used suction tubes, the No. 9 and 10 French sizes of the Frazier and Adson types, are too large for many microsurgical procedures; stretched nerve fascicles or small vessels can easily become entrapped in such large tubes. Suction tubes of No. 3, 5, and 7 French size of the type one customarily uses are needed for microsurgery (Fig. 7). The French designation applies

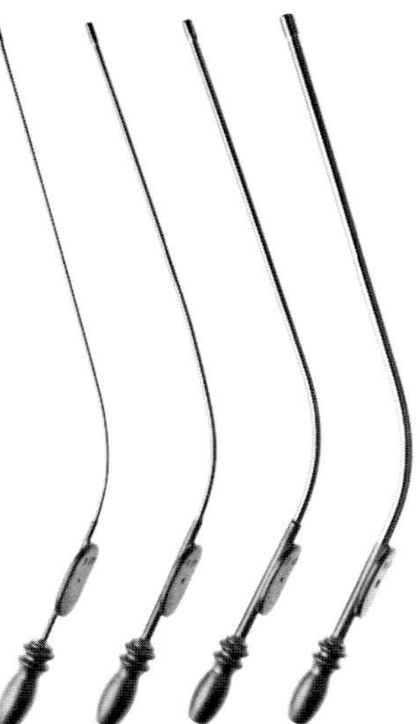

FIG. 7. Rhoton-type suction tubes from left to right are the 3, 5, 7, and 9 French size. Tips are thicker than tubes to prevent tissue damage when they are used for retraction. (From ref. 12.)

to the outer diameter of the instrument; No. 3 French is equivalent to 1 mm outer diameter; thus No. 15 French has an outer diameter of 5 mm, and so forth. A No. 3 French tube is preferred when the most delicate suction is needed.

A suction system with a mechanism to control the negative pressures to very low levels is needed. The suction should be finely adjusted so as to eliminate the hazard of fine neural and vascular structures being entrapped and damaged. Many neurosurgical suction tubes are constructed to allow regulation of suction strength by adjusting the degree to which the thumb occludes an air hole. If one relies on this technique, the hole should be large enough that removal of one's thumb will reduce suction to near zero. In place of wall suction, some surgeons prefer an electric suction pump easily regulated by adjusting the dials on the pump (1; M. G. Yasargil, *personal communication,* 1975).

Cup Forceps

A cup forceps, as used for intervertebral disc removal, is commonly used for removing tumor within the capsule of sellar tumors (Fig. 8). The most frequently used forceps or punch has a tip 3 mm wide. For removal of smaller tumors or small fragments of tumor around optic nerves, we prefer cup forceps having a smaller diameter. For grasping small bits of tumor directly on or near nerves, the 1.0-mm cup forceps is used. The 2-mm tip is suitable for the intercapsular removal of some small tumors. Angle microcup forceps enable one to reach behind the nerves within the tumor capsule for removal of tumor.

Dissectors

Another important consideration is the selection of appropriate dissectors for defining the cleavage plane between the tumor capsule and neural tissue.

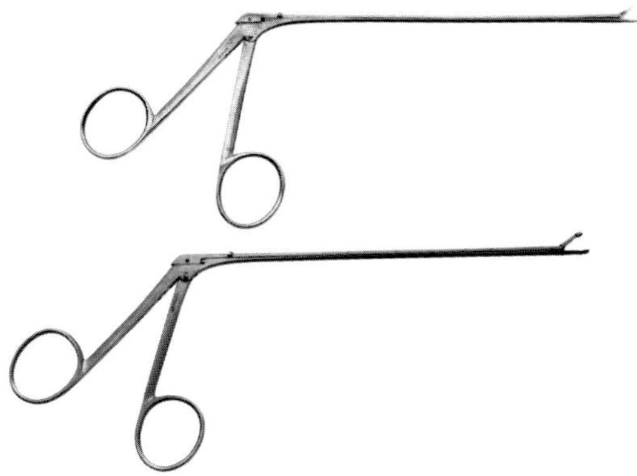

FIG. 8. Alligator-type scissors **(top)** and cup forceps **(bottom)** suitable for cutting or grasping in deep narrow openings. Cup forceps with cups 1 to 3 mm in diameter are needed for transsphenoidal surgery. (From ref. 12.)

If the pia–arachnoid membrane is adherent to tumor capsule, or if there is a mass of tumor within the capsule preventing collapse of the capsule away from the chiasm, there is a tendency to apply traction to both layers and to tear neural vessels running on the pial surface. Prior to separating the pia–arachnoid from the capsule, it is important to have all of the tumor removed so the capsule is so thin it is almost transparent. If one is uncertain about the margin between the capsule and pia–arachnoid membrane, several sweeps of a small dissector through the area help clarify the appropriate plane for dissection.

The most widely used neurosurgical dissectors are of the Penfield or Freer type; however, the size and weight of these instruments make them unsuitable for dissection between the optic nerves and chiasm and tumor. The smallest Penfield dissector (No. 4) has a width of 3 mm. For microsurgery, dissectors with working tips of 1 and 2 mm are needed. Roundtipped dissectors resembling the Sheehy canal knives used by otolaryngologists but with longer handles are suitable for separation of tumor from nerve (Figs. 9 through 13). An alternative method of fine dissection is to use straight-pointed instruments we call needles (Figs. 9 and 10, below). It may be difficult to grasp the margin of the tumor with forceps, and in some situations a small, pointed needle introduced into the margin of the tumor may be helpful for retracting the tumor in the desired direction. This type of pointed instrument can also be used to develop a cleavage plane between tumor and arachnoid membrane, nerves, and brain.

Cutting

A fresh No. 11 or 15 blade on a suitable handle is adequate for most microsurgical procedures on the sella requiring a knife (Fig. 10A, below). For more delicate cutting a razor blade fragment or diamond knife is recommended. Blades that crack cleanly without bending are being manufactured especially for use in preparing razor knives, and some manufacturers offer precut razor blade fragments. Diamond knives have the sharpest cutting edge, but their use is limited by the cost.

Scissors having fine blades on bayonetted handles are frequently used during transfrontal pituitary surgery. Cutting should be done by the distal half of the blade (Figs. 4, 10 through 12, below). If the scissors open too widely, cutting ability and accuracy suffer. Scissors on an alligator-type shank having a long shaft may be needed for cutting in deep and narrow openings, e.g., in transsphenoidal operations (Fig. 8).

Drilling

A drill is frequently used during microsurgical operations for removing the sphenoid ridge, clinoid process, tuberculum sellae, or other protrusions of the cranial base (Fig. 12, below). A drill that can reverse its direction is preferred to one that cuts in only one direction. The operation should be planned so

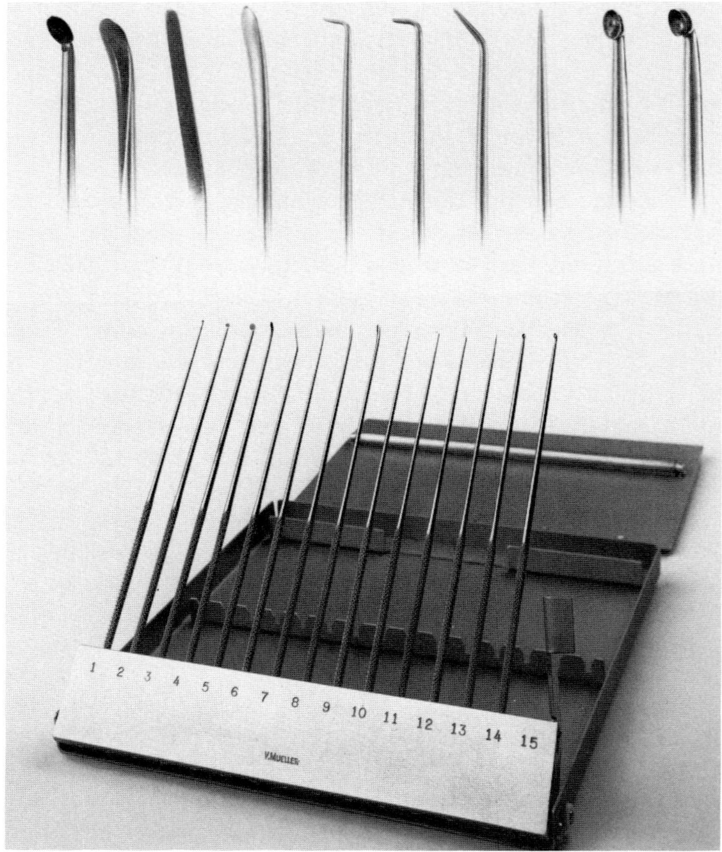

FIG. 9. Microsurgical dissectors for neurosurgery. Beginning on left **(top)** are four types of dissectors: round, spatula, flat, and micro-Penfield dissectors in that order. The next two instruments are sharp and blunt microhooks, and the next two are angled and straight needle dissectors. The two instruments on the right are straight and angled microcurettes. **(Bottom):** Storage case of type shown permits easy access to instruments and yet protects the delicate tips between uses. (From ref. 11.)

that the burr rotates away from critical structures; thus if skidding occurs it will be away from them. Diamond burrs are used near important structures. One should become acquainted with and skilled in the application of the drill in the laboratory prior to using it in a neurosurgical operation.

Drills are available which function at speeds of 6,000 to nearly 100,000 rpm. At speeds greater than 25,000 rpm the bone melts away so easily the drill poorly transmits the tactile details of bony structure to the surgeon's hand. Speeds less than 25,000 rpm should be used for delicate surgery in which tactile control of the drill is important. A diamond bit used at speeds below 8,000 rpm is preferable for the most delicate bone removal.

The drill should be held like a pen, and cutting should be done with the side rather than the end of the burr. The most accurate and controlled use of the drill is obtained at higher speeds if a light brush action is used to remove the bone. Dangerous skidding may ensue at the lower speeds because greater pressure is needed to cut the bone. Avoid running the burr across bone by using light, intermittent pressure rather than constant pressure of the burr on one spot. A constant suction irrigation with physiologic saline reduces heat transmission to nearby neural structures. The teeth of the burr should be clean of bone dust. A coarse burr clogs less easily but is harder to control because it runs across bone more easily; irrigation reduces this skidding. Rather than use a burr blindly to make a long, deep hole, the field should be beveled and as wide open as possible. A small curette rather than a drill should be used to follow a small track. Bone dust should be meticulously removed.

Curettes

Small curettes are sometimes used for removing the last shell of bone between the drill surface and the optic canal or for removing a clinoid process (Figs. 9 and 12, below). A straight curette is satisfactory for this, although 45° angled curettes may be needed for special purposes, e.g., curetting a tumor from the sphenoid ridge or other areas on the cranial base. Curettes having a tip as small as 1.5 mm are available (Fig. 9). The curette should be held so the cutting edge is in full view, and cutting should be done with the side rather than the tip. Pressure is applied parallel to or away from important structures rather than toward them. Properly sharpened curettes cut with less pressure and are safer than dull ones. Try to use the largest curette that will do the job.

SURGICAL APPROACHES

Some surgeons still prefer the intracranial approach for all tumors with suprasellar extension. Magnification permits the procedure to be done through a smaller cranial opening and with less brain retraction than is required for conventional macrosurgical techniques. Although we prefer to use the transsphenoidal approach for most suprasellar tumors, those associated with a small sella or asymmetrical upward extension require a transfrontal intracranial approach. The intracranial approaches include: (a) the subchiasmatic approach between the optic nerves and below the chiasm; (b) the opticocarotid approach, between the carotid artery and the optic nerve; (c) the transfrontal–transsphenoidal approach; and (d) the lamina terminalis approach posterior to the optic chiasm medial to the optic tracts, anterior to the anterior cerebral arteries through the thin anterior lamina of the third ventricle.

In completing the transfrontal skin incision, a small four-hole bone flap is placed just above the eyebrow (Fig. 5). The frontal sinus is not avoided if entering it allows lower placement of the flap and reduces the need for brain

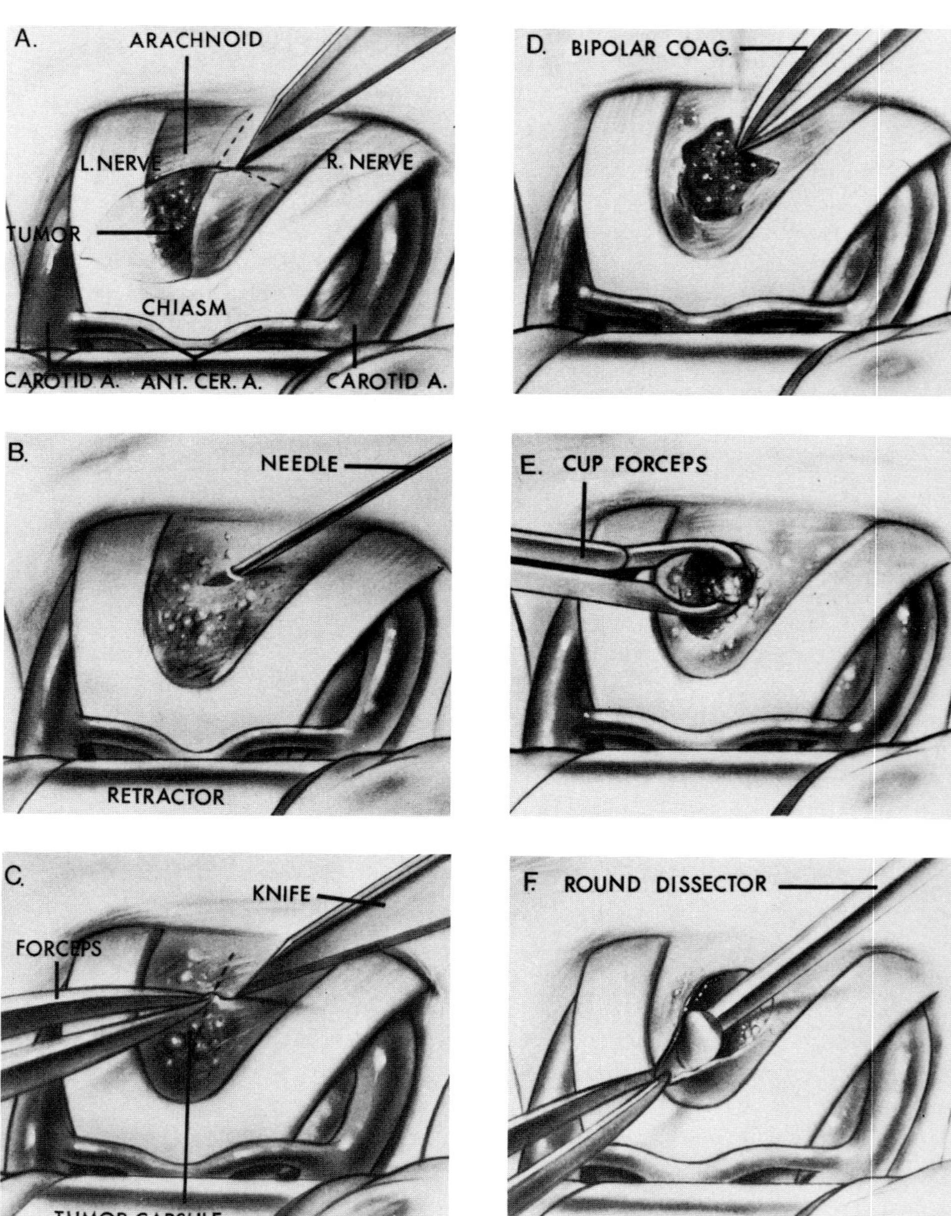

FIG. 10.A–F. Subchiasmatic approach to a suprasellar tumor. (Orientation and exposure as in Fig. 5.) **A:** Arachnoid incised so that it is not removed but is left over the optic nerves as a protective layer. **B:** Tumor aspirated for cyst prior to starting removal. **C:** Tumor capsule incised. **D:** Bipolar coagulation used on bleeding points on capsule. **E:** Microcup forceps used to remove tumor within capsule. **F:** Small, round dissector used to push tumor inferiorly for removal. (From ref. 10.)

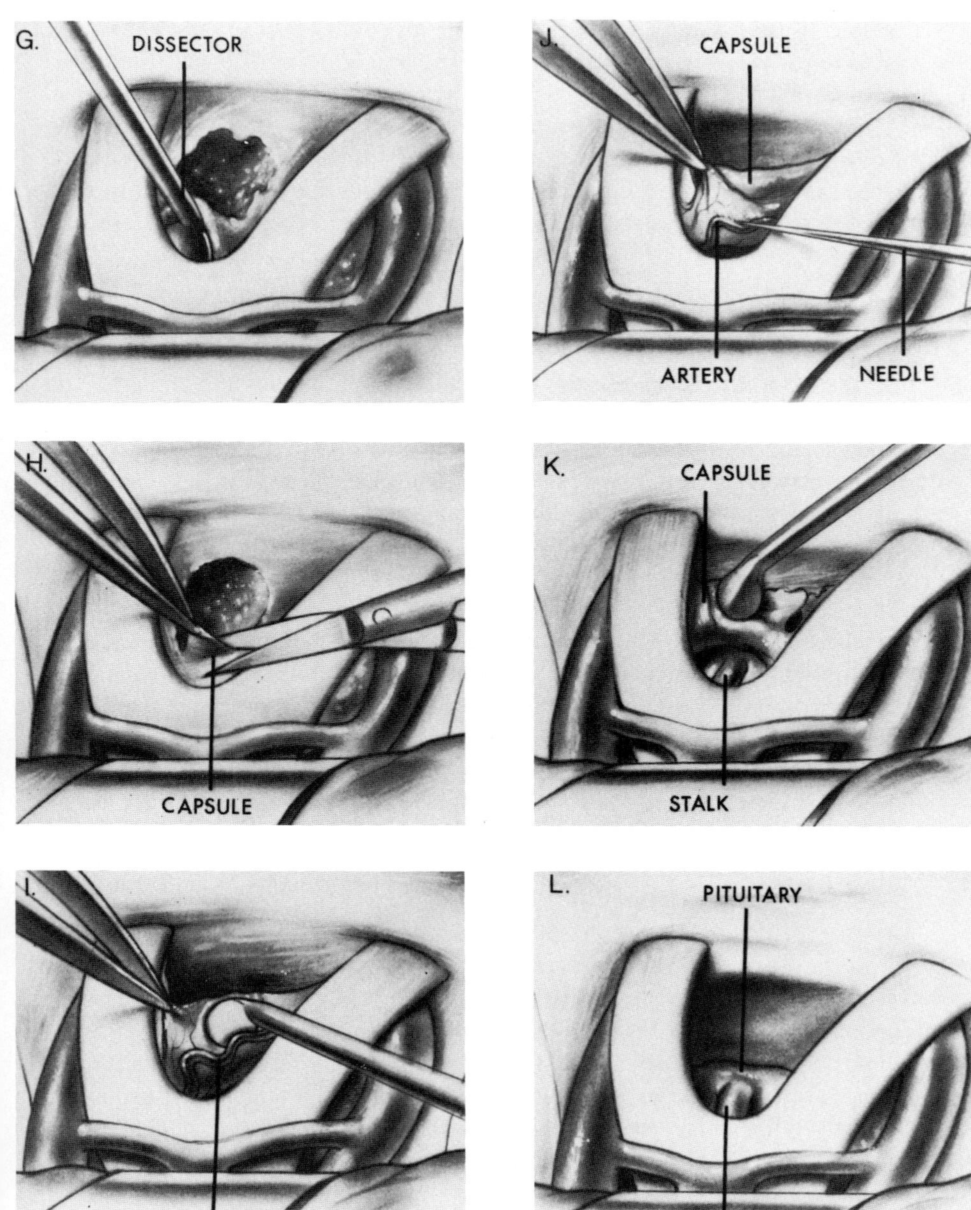

FIG. 10G–L. Subchiasmatic approach to a suprasellar tumor. **G:** Capsule pushed inferiorly away from chiasm rather than chiasm being retracted to expose capsule. **H:** Portion of capsule being excised. **I:** Perforating artery being dissected away from tumor capsule using a round dissector. **J:** Perforating vessel being removed from capsule using a needle dissector. **K:** Capsule depressed inferiorly and pituitary stalk exposed. **L:** Removal complete. (From ref. 10.)

retraction. If the frontal sinus is entered, the mucosa is pushed downward and a thin layer of soft acrylic is applied over the opening and allowed to harden. A pericranium flap is then reflected over the sinus and sutured to the dura. The head is extended slightly so the frontal lobes tend to fall away from the floor of the anterior cranial fossa, thereby reducing the need for brain retraction. This need is further reduced by draining CSF through a lumbar puncture and administering intravenous dehydrating agents (e.g., mannitol) as the scalp flap is elevated.

Subchiasmatic Approach

For the approach between the optic nerves and below the chiasm, the arachnoid of the anterior wall of the chiasmatic cistern is incised so that it falls downward over the nerves and chiasm and provides a protective layer during surgery (Fig. 10). The optic nerves and chiasm are not retracted. The tumor is aspirated with a small lumbar puncture needle prior to incision of the capsule (Fig. 10B). Tumor is removed within the capsule until tumor and capsule collapse away from the nerves and chiasm. This is preferable to retracting the optic nerves and chiasm to expose the tumor (Fig. 10K). Gentle retraction of stretched nerves with a compromised blood supply may increase visual loss. No attempt should be made to see the dome of a suprasellar tumor when the frontal lobe is initially elevated. To achieve satisfactory removal, one need only see the inferior 5 mm of the tumor. Attempts at further exposure of the tumor initially can lead to frontal lobe and chiasmal injury. An initial intercapsular removal of tumor, working through a small opening in the inferior part of the tumor, allows the tumor mass to shrink. Some advocate frontal lobe resection early in the procedure to expose large tumors; however, this is only rarely required even with the largest tumors.

The most common cause of tumor appearing to be "tightly adherent" to the hypothalamus and optic nerves and chiasm is not a result of adhesions between the capsule and nerve tissue but of residual tumor within the capsule wedging the tumor into position. As the intercapsular contents are removed, the tumor collapses; further removal causes a further inferior shift of the tumor, thus making it possible to remove more tumor through the small exposure. Only rarely is the tumor so densely adherent to the nerves that it defies easy removal after the intercapsular contents are removed. If the tumor does not collapse after the intercapsular contents have been removed, a brief wait allows the pulsation of the brain to dislodge the tumor further inferiorly, and more tumor can be removed. No attempt should be made to remove the capsule from the chiasm and optic nerves until the capsule has collapsed.

Special attention is given to preserving the perforating arteries that pass over the capsule to supply the optic nerves, chiasm, and hypothalamus (Fig. 10 I–J). Any vessel that stands above the surface of the capsule should be dealt with initially as if it were a vessel supplying the brain. These vessels can frequently be preserved with accurate dissection. One should try to displace the vessel off the tumor capsule using a small dissector after the tumor has been removed from within the capsule. The branches arising from the anterior choroidal, internal carotid, posterior communicating, and posterior cerebral arteries and the basilar apex pass over the tumor and are important because they supply the optic nerves, chiasm, and tracts; the hypothalamus; and the upper diencephalon. Injury of the pericapsular arteries can lead to visual loss, diabetes insipidus, autonomic disturbances, limb paresis, loss of consciousness, and even loss of life.

Structures that must be dissected free of tumor include the optic nerves, optic chiasm, oculomotor nerves, pituitary stalk, hypothalamus, cerebral peduncles, anterior third ventricle, and the internal carotid, posterior communicating, posterior cerebral, basilar, anterior choroidal, and anterior cerebral arteries (Fig. 10K,L). Under magnification, individual adhesions between these structures and the tumor can be divided with microinstruments. The technique has been especially helpful in removing craniopharyngiomas because they are more densely adherent to surrounding structures than are chromophobe adenomas.

It is frequently possible to remove the capsule of craniopharyngiomas but not of chromophobe adenomas. The capsule of the chromophobe adenoma is the dura of the diaphragma sella, which has been stretched upward over the tumor. The stretched dura over the dome of the tumor may be removed, as shown in Fig. 10G–K, but an attempt to pull this capsule from its attachment to the cranial base may cause severe bleeding and cranial nerve injury.

Opticocarotid Approach

The approach between the optic nerve and carotid artery is referred to as the opticocarotid approach (Fig. 11A–F). It is used if there is asymmetrical extension of tumor that widens the interval between the carotid artery and optic nerve; if there are no major perforating branches of the carotid artery passing across this area to the optic nerve, chiasm, and hypothalamus; and if the visual fields indicate that the lateral portion of the nerve, adjacent to the carotid artery, is damaged by the tumor. Injury to the lateral part of the nerve with a resulting nasal field defect is more disabling than injury to the medial portion, with a resulting temporal defect. The lateral portion of the nerve is the last part to be compressed by most tumors. The same general principles of tumor removal reviewed for the subchiasmatic approach apply to removal by this route. Tumor is removed within the capsule until it collapses away from the optic nerve and carotid artery. An attempt is made to save all perforating arteries.

Transfrontal–Transsphenoidal Approach

An example of how magnification has led to the refinement and improvement of the conventional transfrontal approach is the transfrontal–transsphenoidal

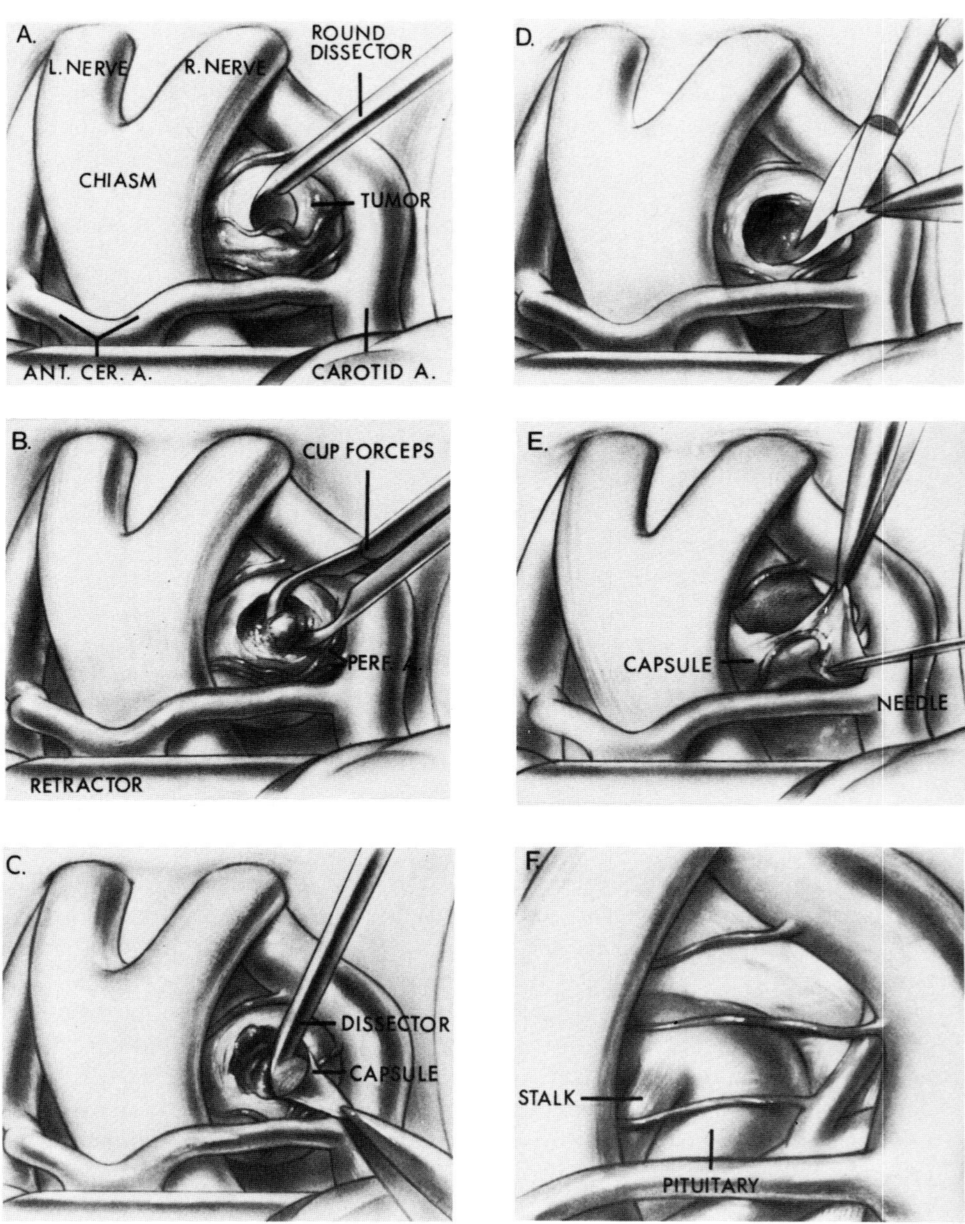

FIG. 11. Opticocarotid approach to suprasellar tumor. (Orientation and exposure as in Fig. 5.) The approach is through the triangle between the optic nerve, carotid artery, and anterior cerebral artery. **A:** Tumor exposed and perforating arteries moved off tumor capsule to expose an area for incision of the capsule. **B:** Cup forceps used to remove tumor. **C:** Round dissector pushes tumor down into area of exposure away from the arteries and nerves. **D:** Tumor capsule being excised. **E:** Perforating arteries being dissected from the tumor capsule. **F:** Tumor removed. Pituitary gland and stalk intact. (From ref. 10.)

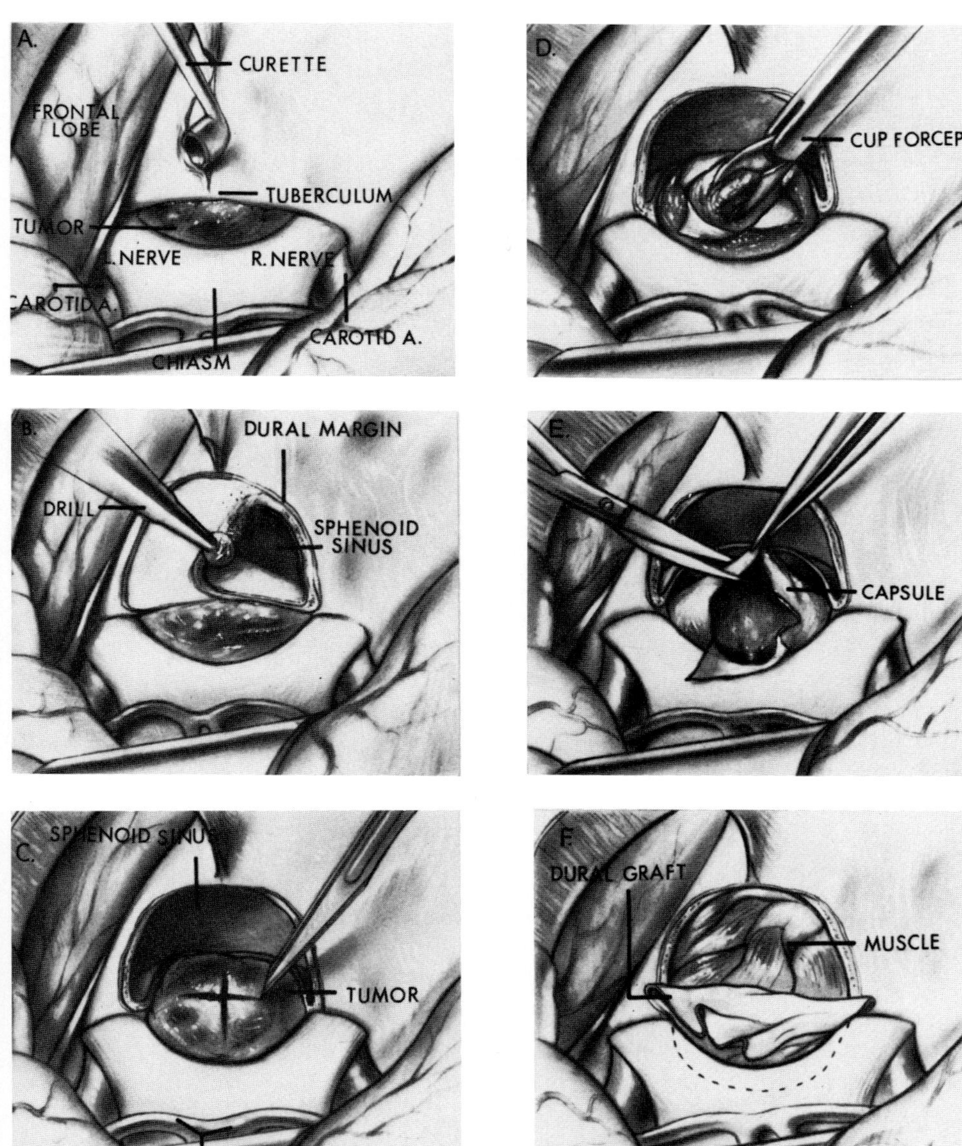

FIG. 12. Transfrontal-transsphenoidal approach. (Orientation and exposure as in Fig. 5.) **A:** Prefixed chiasm blocks the approach to a tumor with suprasellar extension. Dura is removed from the tuberculum with a microcurette. **B:** Dental drill used to remove planum sphenoidale and tuberculum in area between nerves. Sphenoid sinus opened and mucosa pushed inferiorly. **C:** Tumor capsule incised with No. 11 knife blade. **D:** Cup forceps used to remove tumor. **E:** Upper portion of capsule being removed. **F:** Sphenoid sinus and sella packed with muscle. Dural graft laid over the area of bone removal for closure. (From ref. 10.)

approach developed by Rand (6) (Fig. 12A–F). This technique is used when the transfrontal exposure is limited by a prefixed position of the optic nerves and chiasm; these anatomic obstacles are overcome by a transsphenoidal approach through the transfrontal cranial opening. The sphenoid sinus is exposed by resection of the planum sphenoidale, tuberculum sellae, and anterior wall of the sella (Fig. 12A,B). The sinus mucosa is depressed inferiorly. The greater exposure of tumor without trauma to the chiasm allows free access to the sellar portion of the tumor and a more extensive removal (Fig. 12C,D). In this approach the capsule is allowed to collapse away from the neural structures rather than the neural structures being retracted to expose the capsule (Fig. 12E). The sphenoid sinus and cranial base is closed by packing the area with muscle and a dural graft (Fig. 12F).

A preoperative radiographic assessment of the anatomic relationships between the sphenoid sinus and sella turcica is helpful in planning the transfrontal–transsphenoidal exposure and is indispensable to the transnasal–transsphenoidal exposure. Hamberger and associates (2) classified these relations into three types—the conchal, presellar, and sellar—depending on the extent to which the sphenoid bone is pneumatized. The sellar type of sphenoidal sinus is completely pneumatized and extends under the sella to the anterior aspect of the clivus. The presellar type is pneumatized only in the portion of the sinus anterior to the sella. The conchal type is not pneumatized, and the sphenoid below the sella consists of dense bone up to 2 cm in thickness. Fortunately, the sellar type, which occurs in 80% of adults, has a thin sellar floor that bulges into the sphenoid sinus and is easily removed (7). The conchal type occurs in only 3% of the cases.

Lamina Terminalis Approach

The lamina terminalis approach is used if the tumor cannot be seen in the subchiasmatic space, does not occupy the sella, and stretches and distends the thin anterior lamina of the third ventricle (Fig. 13A–F). Craniopharyngiomas are the tumors most frequently removed by this approach. Special attention is required to see that the operative approach is sufficiently posterior to the optic chiasm and medial to the optic tract to prevent injury to these structures. Tumors qualifying for this approach have usually thinned the lamina terminalis so the tumor is visible through this lamina. After opening through the lamina, one is working within the third ventricle. Meticulous attention is given to separating the tumor from the walls of the third ventricle in order to prevent injury to the pillars of the fornices and other structures in the walls of the third ventricle.

Radiation Therapy

Radiation therapy should be given following removal of large chromophobe tumors of the type that were frequently submitted to transfrontal surgery in the past. The frequency of recurrence when radiation therapy is given after surgery is less than with either treatment used alone. Radiation therapy is used

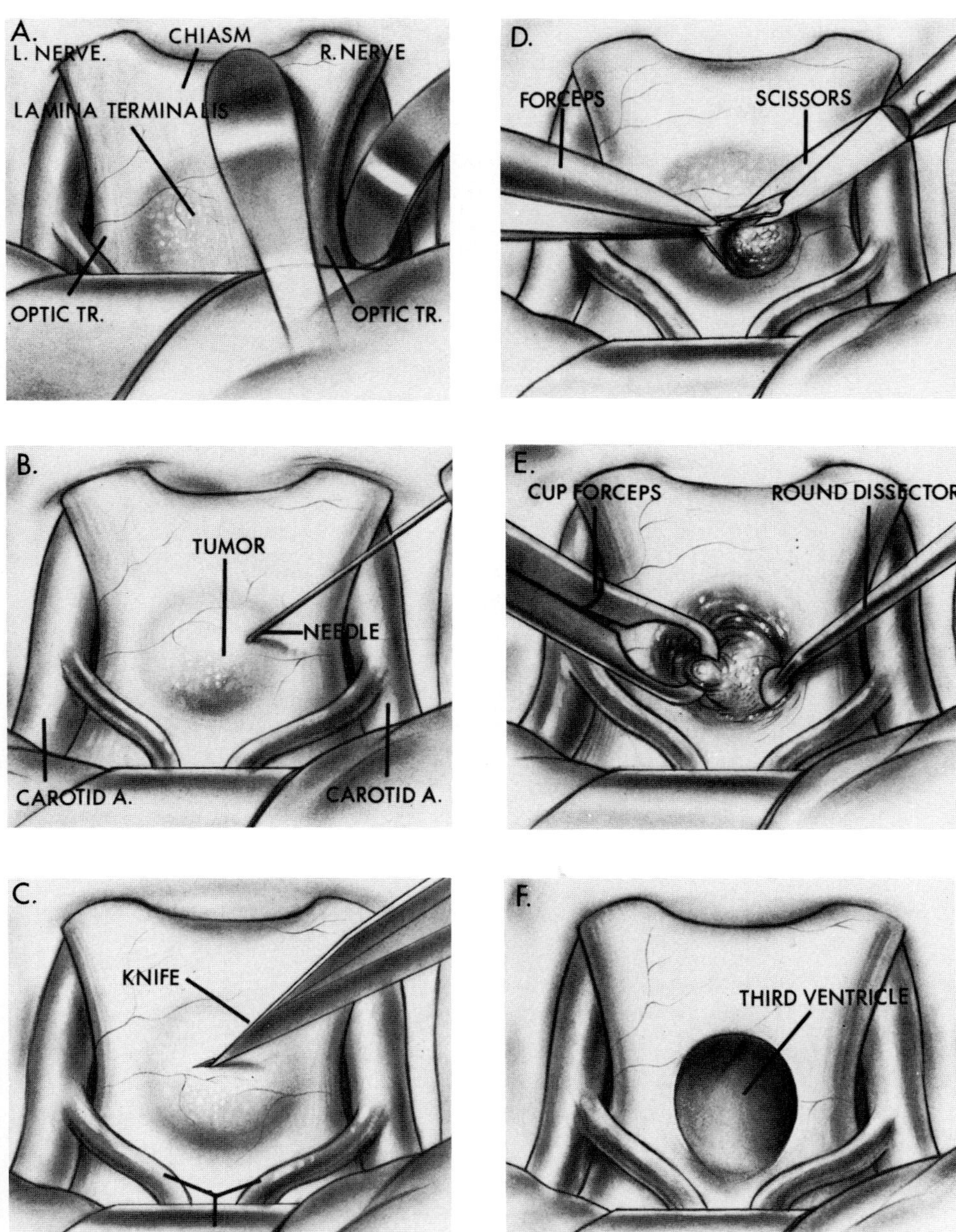

FIG. 13. Lamina terminalis approach to a suprasellar tumor (Orientation and exposure as in Fig. 5.) **A:** Prefixed chiasm blocks the approach to a tumor with suprasellar extension. Finely calcified particles can be seen through the lamina terminalis. Tumor cannot be exposed by the opticocarotid approach. **B:** Tumor aspirated for cyst prior to starting removal. **C:** Thin lamina terminalis and tumor capsule incised with No. 11 knife blade. **D:** Tumor capsule being delivered through small opening and being excised with scissors. **E:** Cup forceps and round dissector being used to remove tumor. **F:** Tumor removal complete, exposing interior of third ventricle. Optic chiasm, optic tracts, and anterior cerebral arteries preserved. (From ref. 9.)

for all tumors including craniopharyngiomas if the tumor cannot be completely removed or if it has produced extensive sellar destruction. With small tumors, especially the microadenomas, the indications for radiation therapy are less well defined. It is not used following removal of an hypersecreting intrasellar microadenoma if the level of elevated hormone returns to normal after surgery. If the abnormal hypersecretion recurs at any later time, the sella is re-explored and the tumor removed. Radiation would be given if the abnormal hypersecretion persists or if there has been extensive destruction of the sellar floor.

Pituitary Ablation

Pituitary ablation, although frequently performed by the transcranial route in the past, is currently regarded as a procedure that should be done by the transsphenoidal route. A recent review of 1,642 cases treated by hypophysectomy gave an average remission rate of 56% (46 to 81%) (4). However, pain was relieved more often. The presence of estrogen-binding sites in breast cancer tissue gives strong predictive evidence that hypophysectomy will prove beneficial. Hypophysectomy often relieves pain caused by bone metastasis from prostatic carcinoma, but it is doubtful that it prolongs life. Although the palliative effect results from ablation of the anterior lobe, the total gland is usually removed because the anterior lobe occasionally surrounds the superior aspect of the posterior lobe, and in these cases total pituitary removal is the only method of removing the anterior lobe completely. A low stalk section helps prevent diabetes insipidus.

REFERENCES

1. Bader, D. C. H. (1975): Microtechnical nursing in neurosurgery. *J. Neurosurg. Nursing,* 7:22–24.
2. Hamberger, C. A., et al. (1961): Transanterosphenoidal hypophysectomy. *Arch. Otolaryngol.,* 74:2–8.
3. Malis, L. I. (1969): Bipolar coagulation in microsurgery. In: *Microsurgery Applied to Neurosurgery,* edited by M. C. Yasargil, pp. 42–45. Academic Press, New York.
4. Morrison, G. (1976): Transsphenoidal hypophysectomy in metastatic breast cancer. *J. Fla. Med. Assoc.,* 63:844–846.
5. Potter, R. A., editor (1975): *Surgery in the United States,* Vol. 1, pp. 155.
6. Rand, R. W. (1969): Transfrontal transsphenoidal craniotomy in pituitary and related tumors using microsurgical techniques. In: *Microneurosurgery,* edited by R. W. Rand, pp. 74–86. Mosby, St. Louis.
7. Renn, W. H., and Rhoton, A. L., Jr. (1976): Microsurgical anatomy of the sellar region. *J. Neurosurg.,* 43:288–298.
8. Rhoton, A. L. (1972): Microneurosurgery of the pituitary gland. *Med. Clin. North Am.,* 56:915–930.
9. Rhoton, A. L., Jr., Hardy, D. G., and Chambers, S. M. (1979): Microsurgical anatomy and dissection of the sphenoid bone cavernous sinus and sellar region. *Surg. Neurol.,* 12:63–104.
10. Rhoton, A. L., Jr., and Maniscalco, J. E. (1977): Microsurgery of the sellar region. *Neuroophthalmology,* 9:106–127.
11. Rhoton, A. L., Jr. (1978): Micro-operative techniques. In: *Neurological Surgery,* 2nd ed, edited by J. R. Youmans. Saunders, Philadelphia *(in press).*
12. Rhoton, A. L., Jr. (1978): *Microsurgical Instrumentation for World Microsurgery Congress II Proceedings.* Houghton Mifflin, Pacific Palisades, California *(in press).*

Clinical Management of Pituitary Disorders,
edited by G. T. Tindall and W. F. Collins.
Raven Press, New York © 1979.

21

Craniopharyngiomas

Raymond N. Kjellberg

Department of Surgery, Harvard Medical School and Massachusetts General Hospital, Boston, Massachusetts 02114

"These cases offer the most baffling problems which confront the neurosurgeon" (11). That these words of Cushing begin so many essays on the subject is testimony to the difficulty of developing a systematic, effective means for managing patients with craniopharyngiomas. The author, preparing this communication, appreciated that the problems are not yet solved. However, the technical and conceptual developments of the past decade present exciting prospects.

It is the author's intention to draw attention to the "state of the art" by a selected review of the principal treatment methods currently used, i.e., (a) total excision by craniotomy; (b) cyst aspiration, biopsy, limited excision, plus fractionated X-ray therapy; (c) transsphenoidal excision; and (d) radiosurgery—stereotactic radioisotopes in cysts and focal beam therapy.

The author has further taken the liberty of redefining the following terms: method-related mortality, function capability, and recurrence. The redefinition of terms is imposed on reports of various methods with the intention of making the treatment methods more comparable. Reports that include patients treated prior to 1950 were excluded because since that time steroids have been available for substitution therapy and as antiedema agents in "pharmacologic" doses, and this resource has influenced significantly the therapeutic outcome. The advent of microsurgical technique is equally important, although the microscope is of comparatively recent application. Few reports distinguish this technical capability. This chapter is confined to published information, and anecdotal or expectant reports are not included. The author personally communicated with most of the authors to invite their current estimate of the role of their advocated methods.

Published accounts of many methods suffer from the inherent liability that long periods of follow-up, 10 to 25 years, inevitably include methods and capability now regarded as outdated. Evaluation of the frequency of recurrence inevitably suffers in this regard. However, because the frequency of recurrence of craniopharyngioma is such an important aspect when appraising the effectiveness of particular therapy methods, we cannot ignore this consideration and so seek balance by evaluating each method as equally as the available published accounts allow. The author appreciates that recurrence rate data depend heavily on the interval of follow-up in each report. As a rule, it is preferable to compute recurrence rate on a yearly basis than to compare total recurrence rates between reports with widely different intervals of follow-up. The author believes that annual recurrence rates are more similar than different for both short and long intervals.

In the selected review which follows, the following aspects of craniopharyngiomas are considered: epidemiology; presentation; anatomy; therapy—methods and results; and considerations and conclusions.

EPIDEMIOLOGY

The rate of appearance of craniopharyngiomas may have some influence on the judgment of neurosurgeons as they seek to formulate policy regarding the care of patients harboring the tumor. Table 1 shows that in Olivecrona's series (10) of pituitary region tumors, adenomas comprised two-thirds of the total number whereas craniopharyngiomas occurred one-fifth as frequently. Meningiomas were seen slightly less frequently than craniopharyngiomas. The other five lesions identified appeared individually at one-tenth the frequency of the craniopharyngiomas, or about 1% for each.

United States government figures (21) for the frequency of all brain tumors indicate that currently over 8,000 are diagnosed each year and that the number is expected to rise to 10,000 per year during the next few years (Table 2). Table 3 shows the proportion of craniopharyngiomas in several large series of brain tumors (10). The average incidence of craniopharyngioma among all brain tumors is just under 2.5%. If we apply this rate to the estimated 10,000 brain tumors per year in the United States, the number of craniopharyngiomas in the United States annually approaches 250 cases.

TABLE 1. *Olivecrona's series of pituitary region tumors (up to 12/31/58)*

Tumor	No.	%
Hypophyseal adenomas	517	68.20
Craniopharyngiomas	108	14.25
Suprasellar meningiomas	83	10.95
Hypothalamus gliomas	9	1.18
Optic chiasm gliomas	12	1.58
Suprasellar cholesteatomas	14	1.85
Retrosellar chordomas	9	1.18
Suprasellar teratomas	6	0.81
Total	758	100

Modified from ref. 10.

TABLE 2. *Selected estimated frequencies of craniopharyngioma in the U.S.*

1. Intracranial tumors in United States	≅ 10,000/year
Percent of intracranial tumors	≅ 2.5%
No. of craniopharyngiomas in United States	≅ 250/year
2. No. of neurosurgeons in United States	≅ 2,500
No. of neurosurgeons per craniopharyngioma	≅ 10/year
3. No. of major medical centers	≅ 50
No. of craniopharyngiomas per center	≅ 5/year

TABLE 3. *Proportion of craniopharyngiomas in series of brain tumors*

Authors	Intracranial tumors	Craniopharyngiomas No.	Craniopharyngiomas %
Cushing	2,004	92	4.59
Grant	1,001	30	2.99
Droguet (Vincent's series)	5,000 ?	100 ?	2.00
Horrax	1,814	48	2.65
	9,819	270	2.74
Olivecrona	6,135	108	1.76
	15,954	378	2.37

Modified from ref. 10.

Thus for any one of the 2,500 neurosurgeons in the United States, the calculated relation allows 10 neurosurgeons for each case per year, or one case for each neurosurgeon in 10 years, or 3 or 4 cases in the lifetime of an average neurosurgeon. Many of these patients tend to find their way to "major medical centers." No list of "major centers" is available, but if we assume there are 50 such centers, each might expect to see approximately five craniopharyngiomas each year. Interestingly, this figure is not significantly different from the average annual rates of patients seen in several of the large reported series (Table 4).

TABLE 4. *Craniopharyngioma case frequency*

Author	Cases	Years	Cases/year
Sweet	42	22	1.9
Matson & Crigler	58	18	3.3
Hoffman et al. (Toronto)	48	25	1.9
Kramer et al.	43	20	2.3
Bloom (London)	99	20	5.0
Hardy	32	16	2.0
Backlund	34	10	3.4
Total	348	133	2.6

The largest number of patients are treated during the second decade of life (10). The median age, however, is the third decade of life. There is a slight preponderance in males.

CLINICAL PRESENTATION

A constellation of clinical features induce patients to seek medical attention. The clinical presentation varies significantly between children and adults. Radiographic features most often lead to a fairly confident diagnosis or at least a high suspicion of the diagnosis. Additionally, radiography furnishes important anatomic information for the surgeon planning an operation. Histologic examination provides ultimate confirmation of diagnosis.

Children develop a multitude of clinical findings (6). Headache, vomiting, papilledema, and hydrocephalus collectively are expressions of intracranial hypertension. Preliminary routine examination often reveals field defects and intracranial calcification, findings which direct attention to the sellar region. Endocrine disturbance is less prominent. On the other hand, adults more often have visual problems and seek relief of headache (7). Mental, endocrine, and altered consciousness are comparatively infrequent.

Radiologic examination traditionally begins with plain skull X-rays. In approximately 80% of children, calcification is present in the tumor (7). This frequency decreases during young adulthood until it stabilizes in the mid-thirties, after which 80% of patients show no roentgenologic evidence of calcification.

Currently the trend is toward computerized tomography (CT scan) as the initial radiographic procedure, as this important diagnostic instrument distinguishes solid tumors, cysts, and calcification, as well as indicating ventricular size (19). Computer-reconstructed CT scans improve resolution to 2-mm cubes and also display the image in horizontal, coronal, and/or sagittal planes.

Ventriculography with either air or metrizamide provides further anatomic detail when desired. Metrizamide in the ventricles or basal cisterns can provide dramatic contrast imaging for CT scanning. Arteriography contributes relatively little additional information. Postoperative, periodic CT scans are valuable for evaluating residual or recurrent tumor and should be done on a routine basis.

ANATOMY

Several anatomic features of craniopharyngioma deserve the attention of neurosurgeons. These tumors are believed to arise from epithelial rests of Rathke's pouch. The cell rests are distributed along the pituitary stalk from the pars distalis to the floor of the third ventricle, with most of the cells concentrated in the middle portion of the stalk (10). Those rests situated in the upper portion of the stalk may give rise to tumors that extend into the third ventricle. Tumors confined to the third ventricle may be excised by craniotomy via either the lamina terminalis or the foramen of Monro. Either approach is technically very demanding. Tumors in the middle third of the stalk may be infrachiasmatic and supraclinoid. This most common site is traditionally approached via subfrontal craniotomy. Tumors arising from the lower third of the stalk or pars distalis may extend into the sella turcica, in which case the transsphenoidal route offers a low-risk route of excision. Cysts, which may be single or multiple, occur in 70% of craniopharyngiomas (3). Largely cystic lesions may be aspirated by stereotactic or open craniotomy methods. Excision or radiation may be directed to the cyst walls.

The boundary between craniopharyngioma and hypothalamus may be difficult to discern (20). Additionally, diverticulae of tumor into brain have been observed. The prospect of preserving an effective cleavage plane under these circumstances should not be anticipated by surgeons performing excisions.

THERAPY—METHODS

The various treatment modalities include: (a) radical or total excision by craniotomy (RadEx); limited excision by craniotomy plus fractionated X-ray therapy (LimEx + FXR); transsphenoidal excision (TrsphenEx); and radiosurgery (Radiosg). As already mentioned, the series of patients evaluated here were treated after 1950 when corticosteroids came into general use.

A general method may include more than a single technique, e.g., limited excision plus X-ray therapy. We believed it appropriate to group the techniques that are interdependent. Further, we considered it important that when two techniques were used together, the mortality risk, disability, and recurrence frequency should be shared by the techniques.

Radical (Total) Excision

Sweet (20) and Matson and Crigler (18) used essentially similar methods. Using general anesthesia, an adequate frontal craniotomy flap was turned. After aspirating cystic lesions the cyst wall was dissected from surrounding structures. Solid tumors were gutted and, when possible, the margins dissected free and excised. Frequently these surgeons believed that they had determined that total excision had been achieved, an assessment that did not always prove correct, even though the procedures were performed carefully and meticulously, and were often quite lengthy. The operating microscope was not used by either surgeon in the majority of cases. The intervals of follow-up were of long duration for the early cases.

The Toronto series (13) differs somewhat. A number of operators were involved, and a variety of techniques, surgical and radiological, were employed in various combinations. One group of 17 of the total 48 patients are categorized as "total excision;" 9 of these were operated on with the aid of the microscope. Other groups of the Toronto series were 16 cases in which the tumors were aspirated, biopsied, or partially removed, and 15 cases in which they were subtotally removed. These groups are not comparable with the series of Sweet and Matson but are discussed under *Results,* below.

Limited Excision by Craniotomy Plus Fractionated X-Ray Therapy

Prominent advocates of the (LimEx + FXR) method are Kramer (15–17) and Bloom (8,9), both radiotherapists. Kramer used 2-MeV X-rays and cobalt-60 sources to deliver 7,000 rads within 7 weeks to adults and 5,500 rads within 6 weeks to children. Bloom used 2-MeV X-rays to deliver 5,000 rads within 6 to 7 weeks. Kramer reported on mortality attributed to the limited surgical excisions whereas Bloom did not. Thus Bloom's report does not provide adequate data to allow comparisons between this multimodel technique and other methods. The report is included, however, because of the author's extensive experience.

Transsphenoidal Excision

Currently Hardy *(personal communication, 1978)* has treated 32 cases using transsphenoidal microsurgery, 15 of whom were included in a previous report (12). This method deserves particular attention because there was no procedure-related mortality in a significant number of cases. Hardy advocates total excision as the preferred initial therapy in patients in whom the sella turcica is enlarged. Usually X-ray therapy is not used unless patients are known to have residual tumor. In view of the evident importance of the method, it would be illuminating if Hardy would indicate the percentage of craniopharyngioma patients that qualify for the transsphenoidal route, compared with those who require other approaches.

Radiosurgery

Radiosurgery applies stereotactic neurosurgical technique to biopsy tumors, it injects isotopes into cysts, and it delivers focal radiation—gamma or proton—to defined intracranial target neoplasms. The principal method described is that of Backlund (1–5; and *personal communication* with W. H. Sweet, 1975). This method may not be widely known, but the results with the technique are sufficiently encouraging for it to be considered in a general review of the treatment of craniopharyngiomas. Using special equipment, suspected craniopharyngiomas are biopsied stereotactically. CT scans may be used to indicate the presence of cysts that can be aspirated. Examination of the fluid can support the diagnosis of craniopharyngioma. Some craniopharyngiomas are purely cystic, whereas others are a combination of cystic and solid components. Cystic portions may be aspirated stereotactically, and solid components may be biopsied. Cysts can be aspirated and refilled with a colloidal suspension of yttrium-90 carefully computed to provide a dose of 20,000 rads of pure beta radiation to the cyst walls. Solid components of mixed cystic/solid tumors and purely solid (histologically confirmed) are treated by the "gamma unit." The latter (4) consists of sharply collimated, multiple (several hundred) sources of cobalt-60 that precisely deliver high-dose radiation (focal radiosurgery) in a single session. The surrounding uninvolved brain receives negligible radiation. The results of this technique as well as similar procedures are discussed below. The author has treated two patients with tumor residuals following craniotomy with the Bragg peak proton method. One patient had a calcific component impacted below the optic chiasm, and the other had a tumor which on two occasions developed cysts that filled the third ventricle. The latter case also had a mixed cyst/solid component below the optic chiasm. On the basis of X-ray, polytomography, air encephalography, CT scan, and reconstructed CT scans, beam dimensions and isodose plots are prepared so that it is possible to necrose the center and cause arrest of growth in the margins of the tumor.

THERAPY—RESULTS

Results of therapy of the methods reviewed above were compared according to method-related mortality, function capability, and recurrence.

Method-Related Mortality

The term "method-related mortality" is preferred to "operative mortality" as the latter does not invariably include all deaths which occur as a result of the therapeutic procedure. For instance, in the present discussion, Matson's "operative mortality" and "later deaths due to hypothalamic or hypophyseal dysfunction" are grouped under "method-related mortality." Also, death due to radiation necrosis of the brain would not appropriately be termed "operative mortality" but can be considered "method-related mortality." "Method-related mortality" includes treated patients who died because the therapy failed regardless of the type of treatment. In each of the above categories, ranks have been assigned.

We divided the function capability category into two groups of patients—those who are functioning appropriate to their station and those who are not. Further detailed categories are not possible as the source material would not support further gradations. An individual is considered to be functioning appropriate to one's station if: a male adult is working at any level, a female adult is working or caring for a household, a child or young adult is attending a normal school, not a school for the disabled.

"Recurrence" refers to the situation when the condition of a treated patient seemed to be improved or arrested but the patient later developed clinical findings related to the tumor. When patients died for this reason, the "recurrent" category was divided between "recurrence—dead" and "recurrence—alive." Whether a patient with recurrence is dead or alive may depend on the interval after the procedure or if further therapy was employed. The intervals of recurrence are

TABLE 5. *Method-related mortality*

Method	Mortality (%)	Rank
Radical excision—craniotomy		2
Sweet ($N = 30$)	9	
Matson ($N = 34$)	7	
Toronto ($N = 17$)	6	
Limited excision, biopsy—craniotomy + FXR		3
Kramer ($N = 43$)	16	
Bloom ($N = 99, 43$)	16+	
Excision—transsphenoidal		1
Hardy ($N = 15$)	0	
Radiosurgery		1
Backlund/Leksell ($N = 34$)	0	
Kjellberg ($N = 2$)	0	

difficult to compare in the source material available. The results of therapy for recurrence generally were poor.

Radical Excision (Primary Operation)

The mortality of the Sweet (20) and Matson (18) series (Table 5) treated after 1950 are similar: 7% and 9%, respectively. Matson's mortality included late deaths attributed to hypophyseal and hypothalamic disturbance attributable to the surgical procedure.

The Toronto series (13) cannot be compared directly with the series of Sweet and Matson because a wider range of procedure was employed by several operators with possibly differing therapeutic goals. Of the 48 cases in the Toronto series, 17 were "totally excised" with a mortality of 6%.

Limited Excision by Craniotomy Plus Fractionated X-Ray Therapy

The two helpful accounts for the multimodel method of LimEx + FXR are those of Kramer (15–17) and Bloom (8,9). When evaluating this treatment modality, it is appropriate that the mortality risk includes that attributable to the craniotomy as well as to X-ray. Kramer (Table 6) described three deaths attributable to the limited excision craniotomy. In addition, 3 patients died because X-ray was ineffective, two died of radiation necrosis of the brain, and two died of endocrine problems presumably related to either the surgical or the radiotherapeutic procedure. Thus the procedure-related mortality of this combined method is 16%, approximately twice that of total excision by craniotomy. Bloom's report included no acknowledgment of the risks of the limited excision craniotomy; no deaths or other details are reported. Bloom mentioned experience with 99 cases but limited his reports to 43 cases. The basis for exclu-

TABLE 6. *Limited excisions by craniotomy plus fractionated X-ray therapy*

Author	No. dead				No. alive		
	Total	2°FXT	2°LimEx	2°Unrel.	Total	Known recur.	No known recur.
Kramer ($N = 43$)	13 (30%)	4 (9%) 2 necr. 2 fail.	3 (7%)	6 (14%)	30 (70%)	8 (19%)	22 (51%)
Bloom (Total $N = 99$; reported $N = 46$)	7 (16%)	7 (16%) 3 fail. 2 necr. 2 endo.	N.A.	N.A.	34 (74%)	1 (2%)	33 (72%)

sion of the remainder is not clear. A summary of these reports is shown in Table 4.

Transsphenoidal Excision

Hardy operated on 32 patients (12) by the transsphenoidal route without mortality. Although this method can be assumed to have low risk, it suffers from the limitation that it is applicable only to some unknown fraction of the total population of craniopharyngioma patients. Further, the report is not clear in regard to the use of radiation and to the recurrence rate.

Radiosurgery

Backlund has had extensive experience with radiosurgery (1–5, and *personal communication*). In 34 patients treated during a 10-year interval, there was no procedure-related mortality. Two late deaths—one due to status epilepticus and the other to acute infection—are not considered procedure-related. A third

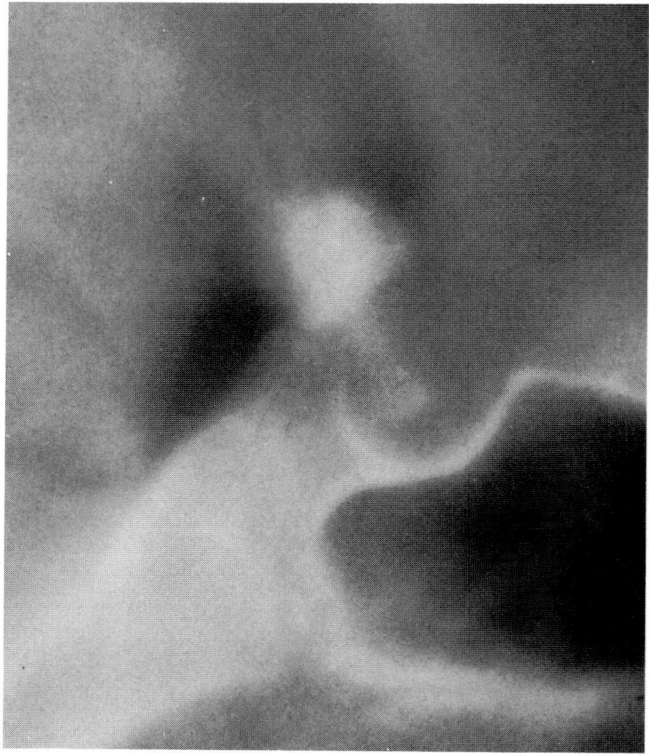

FIG. 1. Lateral polytome of sella turcica showing calcification in a craniopharyngioma just above the dorsum sella.

death occurred in a patient in whom a cyst had been aspirated and who subsequently underwent craniotomy and died. The latter case is complicated, but the death does not appear to be directly related to the radiosurgical procedure. Stereotactic radiosurgery alone was the treatment in 25 cases, and 12 had various other forms of treatment in addition to stereotactic radiosurgery.

The author has treated two cases of craniopharyngioma with radiosurgery, both of whom had previously had craniotomy. One, a 16-year-old boy had a calcific tumor mass (Fig. 1) below the optic tracts that could not be extracted via the translamina terminalis route. The calcific mass was stereotactically irradiated with Bragg peak proton beam, and the patient remains asymptomatic and is attending school (with prior field defect) 18 months after treatment. A second patient had undergone two previous operations, and each time a cystic mass filling the third ventricle was incompletely excised. CT scan and pneumoencephalogram showed residual tumor in the floor of the third ventricle (Fig. 2). An isodose pattern was calculated that would produce radionecrosis in the center and posterior wall of the tumor and growth arrest in the margin of tumor while keeping the optic nerve and chiasm dose sufficiently low as to not preclude further radiation therapy (either proton or X-ray). Six months following proton treatment, a CT scan showed disappearance of most of the infrachiasmatic

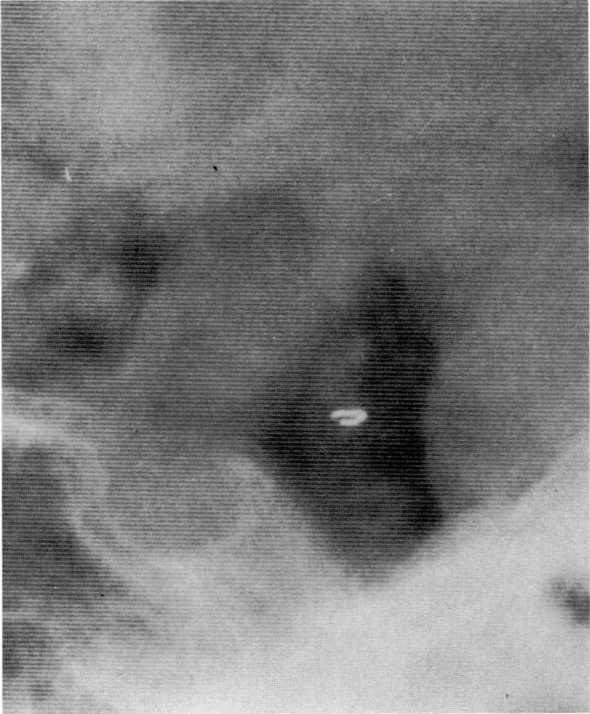

FIG. 2. Lateral pneumoencephalogram showing residual tumor in floor of third ventricle.

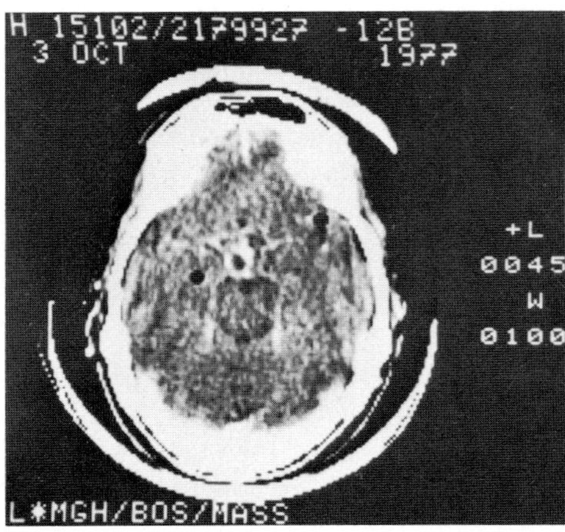

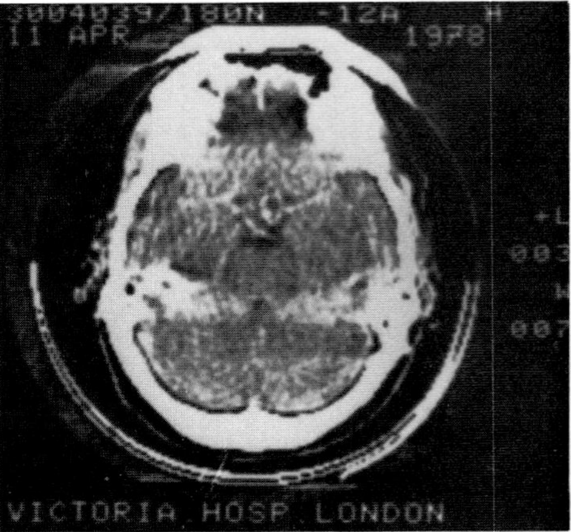

FIG. 3. CT scan on left shows residual tumor in third ventricle floor (same case as in Fig. 2). Six months following proton treatment, CT scan on right shows disappearance of most of the infrachiasmatic craniopharyngioma.

craniopharyngioma (Fig. 3), with a small amount of residual tumor in the retrochiasmatic floor of the third ventricle. Radiosurgical methods reported here have no associated procedure-related mortality.

The ranks of these methods are shown in Table 7.

Functional Capability

Radical Excision

Sweet (20) compared his series to that of Katz (Matson's series) (14) in regard to "primary total excision" according to "quality." He used the term "functional" and further divided the categories. Patients classified as "dependent" or "nonfunctional" are those not functioning appropriate to their station. The figures for those treated by "primary total" excision by Matson and by Sweet are 68% and 95%, respectively (Table 8). As can be anticipated, those operated for recurrence or which were partially excised did not equal the "primary total" group. The Toronto report (13) provides limited information regarding the functional capability of the 17 patients included in their "total excision" group.

TABLE 7. *Results of therapy: method-related mortality (primary procedure)*

Procedure	%	Rank
Radical excision	7–9	2
Limited excision + FXR	16	3
Transsphenoidal excision	0	1
Radiosurgery	0	1

TABLE 8. *Function capability (primary procedure)*

Procedure	Working (%)	Rank
Radical excision	68–95	2
Limited excision + FXR	85	3
Transsphenoidal excision	—	—
Radiosurgery	87–100	1

Although anecdotal visual and endocrine data are provided, there is no mention of school or work function.

Limited Excision Plus Fractionated X-Ray Therapy

Kramer's report of the functional status of his cases is difficult to adapt to our format. The term "alive and well" was applied to 18 of 26 cases (69%). If we deduct his method-related mortality (16%) from the 31% remaining, 15% of survivors are nonfunctional. From Bloom's data one is unable to establish the number of patients who were attending school or working; thus his experience cannot be ranked in this category.

Transsphenoidal Excision

Hardy's data includes ophthalmologic and endocrine status but does not include school or work function capacity. Thus no comment can be made regarding these aspects.

Radiosurgery

As already mentioned, 2 of 34 cases in Backlund's series (1–5, and *personal communication*) died of circumstances not related to the therapy. Of the remaining 32 cases, 2 were preschool children. He reported 2 patients "partially disabled"—one with craniotomy developed epilepsy and the other was "not working—under treatment." Thus 30 of 32 patients (94%) were without functional impairment.

Of the author's two proton radiosurgical cases, one, a schoolboy, is performing at his previous capacity, and the other, a male physician, is practicing medicine without difficulty. Both are categorized as "functioning." The ranking of function capability for the methods described is shown in Table 8.

Recurrence

Radical Excision

The recurrence rates for Sweet's and Matson's radical primary excision are 19% and 29%, respectively, for procedure survivors (Table 9). Katz (14) deter-

TABLE 9. *Recurrence (primary procedure)*

Procedure	%	Rank
Radical excision	19–29	3
Limited excision + FXR	14	2
Transsphenoidal excision	—	
Radiosurgery	0	1

mined that all three of the deaths reported by Matson were in patients considered to have "total" removal of tumor who went on to die of hypothalamic/hypophyseal dysfunction. None of 25 believed to have "total" removals developed recurrence. Thus total removal in fact occurred in 65% of survivors of the original 34 patients in Matson's series.

Limited Excision Plus X-Ray Therapy

Kramer (17) reported recurrence in 17% of 43 patients and Bloom (9) in 13% of 46 patients (of the 99 he treated). Of Kramer's recurrent cases, 2 were dead and 6 living. Of Bloom's 6 recurrent cases, 5 were dead.

Transsphenoidal Excision

There is inadequate case material available currently to compute either recurrence rates or ranking.

Radiosurgery

This author did not identify in Backlund's publications (1–5, and *personal communication*) any cases of recurrence following radiosurgery. As noted, 12 patients had various therapies, and possibly some of these were recurrent, but this possibility was not apparent.

It is evident that recurrence rates are significantly influenced by the total or average intervals of follow-up. Further, occasional patients may survive long intervals with known residual or recurrent tumor. No attempt has been made to account for these intervals in the assessment. The ranking of recurrence rates for the various methods is shown in Table 9.

CONSIDERATIONS AND CONCLUSIONS

The results of therapy are summarized in Table 10, in which mortality, function, and recurrence rates are ranked. The best (lowest) mortality is given the rank "1." When percent rates are similar or nearly so, the same rank is given to each method. Thus transsphenoidal excision and radiosurgery, each with zero mortality, are given the rank 1.

TABLE 10. *Comparison of ranks*

Procedure	Mortality	Function	Recurrence
Radical excision	2	2	3
Limited excision + FXR	2	3	2
Transsphenoidal excision	1		
Radiosurgery	1	1	1

On each account—mortality, function, and recurrence—radiosurgery as described by Backlund (1–5, and *personal communication*) achieves a rank of 1. Unfortunately, this method of treatment is not available in the United States.

There are several features of the current state of the art that call for optimism. Dramatic technical and conceptual advances are regularly emerging. Steroid replacement, dating from 1950, began an epoch in endocrinologic capability which we have not yet seen consummated. The risk of general anesthesia has become less, and is further reduced when general anesthesia is omitted in favor of local anesthesia, which is usually the case in stereotactic procedures.

It is obvious that the operating microscope is having a substantial favorable impact on technical neurosurgery. As in many other areas of neurosurgery, the use of the operating microscope by a skilled neurosurgeon offers the distinct potential for safer, more complete removal of craniopharyngiomas.

The route of excision needs to be more fully evaluated. Although transsphenoidal microsurgery has demonstrated exceptional promise, there are certain limitations of the procedure. Additional data are needed to appreciate the role of adjuvant therapies, irradiation, and long-term outcome.

Considering the role of limited excision by craniotomy plus X-ray therapy, the data of its advocates indicate it to be less satisfactory than other principal alternatives. On the basis of Backlund's data, it appears that radiosurgery offers considerable promise as a mode of treatment. Certainly efforts should be made to provide similar treatment facilities so that this treatment method can be investigated further.

REFERENCES

1. Backlund, E. O. (1972): Studies on craniopharyngiomas. I. Treatment: past and present. *Acta Chir. Scand.,* 138:743–747.
2. Backlund, E. O., Johansson, L., and Sorby, B. (1972): Studies on craniopharyngiomas. II. Treatment by stereotaxis and radiosurgery. *Acta Chir. Scand.,* 138:749–759.
3. Backlund, E. O. (1973): Studies on craniopharyngiomas. III. Stereotaxic treatment with intracystic yttrium-90. *Acta Chir. Scand.,* 139:237–247.
4. Backlund, E. O. (1973): Studies on craniopharyngiomas. IV. Stereotaxic treatment with radiosurgery. *Acta Chir. Scand.,* 139:344–351.
5. Backlund, E. O. (1971): A new instrument for stereotaxic brain tumour biopsy. *Acta Chir. Scand.,* 137:825–827.
6. Banna, M., Hoare, R. D., Stanley, P., and Till, K. (1973): Craniopharyngioma in children. *J. Pediatr.,* 83:781–785.
7. Banna, M. (1973): Craniopharyngioma in adults. *Surg. Neurol.,* 1:202–204.

8. Bloom, H. J. G. (1975): Combined modality therapy for intracranial tumors. *Cancer,* 35:111–120.
9. Bloom, H. J. G., and Harmer, C. L. (1976): Craniopharyngioma: general aspects and treatment. In: *I Tumori Infantili,* edited by P. Bucalossi, U. Veronesi, H. Emanuelli, and F. Fossati Bellani, pp. 119–128. Casa Editrice Ambrosiana, Milan.
10. Carmichael, H. T. (1931): Squamous epithelial rests in the hypophysis cerebri. *Arch. Neurol. Psychiatry,* 26:966–975.
11. Cushing, H. (1932): *Intracranial Tumors. Notes upon a Series of Two Thousand Verified Cases with Surgical Mortality Percentages Pertaining Thereto.* Thomas, Springfield, Illinois.
12. Hardy, J., and Vezina, J. L. (1976): Transsphenoidal neurosurgery of intracranial neoplasm. *Adv. Neurol.,* 15:261–274.
13. Hoffman, H. J., Hendrick, E. B., Humphreys, R. P., Buncic, J. R., Armstrong, D. L., and Jenkin, R. D. T. (1977): Management of craniopharyngioma in children. *J. Neurosurg.,* 47:218–227.
14. Katz, E. L. (1975): Late results of radical excision of craniopharyngiomas in children. *J. Neurosurg.,* 42:86–90.
15. Kramer, S., Southard, M., and Mansfield, C. M. (1968): Radiotherapy in the management of craniopharyngiomas—further experiences and late results. *Am. J. Roentgenol. Radium Ther. Nucl. Med.,* 103:44–52.
16. Kramer, S. (1974): Radiation therapy in the management of craniopharyngiomas. In: *Central Nervous System Tumours,* edited by T. J. Deeley, pp. 204–223. Butterworths, London.
17. Kramer, S. (1976): Craniopharyngioma: the best treatment is conservative surgery and postoperative radiation therapy. In: *Current Controversies in Neurosurgery,* edited by T. P. Morley, pp. 336–343. Saunders, Toronto.
18. Matson, D. D., and Crigler, J. F., Jr. (1969): Management of craniopharyngioma in childhood. *J. Neurosurg.,* 30:377–390.
19. New, P. F. J., and Davis, K. R. (1978): Intrasellar and perisellar lesions. In: *Central Nervous System,* edited by S. M. Wolpert, Grune & Stratton, New York *(in press).*
20. Sweet, W. H. (1977): Radical surgical treatment of craniopharyngioma. In: *Current Techniques in Operative Neurosurgery,* edited by H. H. Schmidek and W. H. Sweet, pp. 199–221. Grune & Stratton, New York.
21. U.S. National Center for Health Statistics: *International Classification of Diseases, Adapted for Indexing Hospital Records by Diseases and Operations.* U.S. Department of Health, Education, and Welfare, Public Health Service, Washington, D.C.

Clinical Management of Pituitary Disorders,
edited by G. T. Tindall and W. F. Collins.
Raven Press, New York © 1979.

22

Hypophysectomy—Current Status

George T. Tindall and Suzie C. Tindall

Division of Neurosurgery, Department of Surgery, Emory University School of Medicine, Atlanta, Georgia 30322

The beneficial influence of endocrine manipulation on certain breast cancers has been known since 1896, when Beatson (3) showed that some patients with disseminated disease achieved regression following oophorectomy. Subsequently, adrenalectomy, hypophysectomy, and additive hormonal therapy were shown to induce tumor regression (21). Hypophysectomy, as a method for achieving palliation of malignant disease, was first reported during the early 1950s by Perrault et al. (47) in a case of breast cancer with pulmonary metastases and by Shimkin et al. (56) in a man with malignant melanoma. In 1962 Scott and Schirmer (55) related that hypophysectomy was actually first performed in September 1948 in a patient with disseminated prostatic cancer. The procedure proved unsuccessful, and the patient died 11 days after surgery. In 1953 Luft and Olivecrona (34) cited their experiences with hypophysectomy in 26 cases for a variety of conditions including Cushing's syndrome, diabetes mellitus, hypertension, and malignant tumors. In the latter category were nine breast cancers and one prostatic cancer, all in an advanced stage. These workers, who performed hypophysectomy via a transcranial approach, concluded that the procedure was well tolerated by patients, and that when total pituitary ablation was accomplished cancer regression was possible. Subsequently several others showed that hypophysectomy is a worthwhile palliative operation in metastatic breast (4,5,9,20,25,27,46,51–53,58,61,64) and prostate gland (12, 36,42,55,57,59–61,65) cancer.

In 1953 Poulsen (48) described a patient who later experienced a 15-year regression (49) of diabetic retinopathy following the development of Sheehan's syndrome in 1945. This report along with the pioneering work by Luft and Olivecrona (33,34) stimulated interest in treating diabetic retinopathy with hypophysectomy; and by 1972 over 1,000 patients had been treated by pituitary ablation for this condition (68). Although results were generally favorable in certain patients, the interest in pituitary ablation has decreased significantly with the advent of photocoagulation.

Originally hypophysectomy required craniotomy. Although beneficial effects resulted, many physicians considered this operative approach too extensive and risky for many patients with diabetes mellitus and advanced breast and prostatic cancer, particularly elderly patients with prostatic cancer. Fortunately, easier and safer methods for accomplishing hypophysectomy (e.g., cryohypophysectomy, radiofrequency coagulation, and transsphenoidal microsurgical removal of the pituitary gland) have been developed; as a result, hypophysectomy currently can be recommended to patients who are not good candidates for craniotomy.

In this chapter the indications and contraindications for hypophysectomy in breast cancer, prostatic cancer, other malignancies, and diabetic retinopathy are discussed. Additionally, factors influencing responsiveness in breast and prostate cancer pre- and posthypophysectomy evaluation and management, techniques available for performing hypophysectomy, and results of this procedure in patients with breast and prostate cancer in achieving pain relief and tumor regression are stressed.

RATIONALE FOR HYPOPHYSECTOMY IN DISSEMINATED BREAST AND PROSTATE GLAND CANCER

Since the metabolism of certain breast cancers is significantly influenced by estrogenic hormones, the major effect of hypophysectomy is probably the suppression of estrogen production by the gonads and adrenal glands because of the removal of gonadotropin and ACTH, respectively. Although estrogenic substances appear to be the chief hormones influencing breast cancer, others (e.g., growth hormone and prolactin) conceivably could exert a direct or indirect role in tumor growth.

Huggins and Hodges (22) contended that androgens stimulate growth of prostatic cancer and thus reasoned that eliminating testicular androgens by castration or countering the effects of androgen by estrogen administration frequently would retard the growth of prostatic cancer. In patients with prostatic cancer who relapse after castration, it is likely that the adrenals have begun to elaborate a significant amount of extragonadal androgen. Thus in this situation hypophysectomy removes the source of ACTH, thereby abolishing androgen production by the adrenal gland. The circumstances surrounding the effectiveness of hypophysectomy in prostatic cancer may be more complex than simply removing the stimulus for androgen production. For instance, prolactin and growth hormone may synergize the action of testosterone and therefore could have a stimulating effect on this tumor. Thus as with breast cancer, the possible effects of hormones other than those elaborated by the gonads on tumor growth remain unknown.

FACTORS INFLUENCING REMISSION FOLLOWING HYPOPHYSECTOMY IN BREAST AND PROSTATE CANCER

Breast Cancer

In patients with breast cancer the following factors may be helpful in predicting whether a patient will achieve an objective remission following hypophysectomy:

1. *Previous response to castration.* Authorities agree that the most reliable index for predicting a satisfactory remission from hypophysectomy is a previous, favorable response to oophorectomy in the premenopausal patient. Pearson and Ray (45,46) contend that approximately 90% of the patients who have shown remission after oophorectomy obtain objective improvement from hypophysectomy. Conway and Collins (5) noted similar results in their series of 100 cases, obtaining remission in 86%. However, not all investigators have obtained response rates comparable to those just cited. For instance, Kennedy and French (27) obtained a favorable response following hypophysectomy in only 19 (49%) of 39 patients who had obtained a previously positive response from oophorectomy.

2. *Previous response to hormone therapy.* The response to androgen and/or estrogen therapy is useful for predicting the result following hypophysectomy. Kennedy and French (27) found that 14 of 20 (70%) postmenopausal women who had exhibited a salutary response following hormonal therapy had an improvement after hypophysectomy. Similar data were reported by Conway and Collins (5). However, in our opinion the selection of patients for hypophysectomy should not be restricted to those who have shown a previous remission after oophorectomy and/or hormonal therapy. Not infrequently patients who fail to achieve a remission from either of these measures respond favorably to hypophysectomy. As shown by the data of Conway and Collins (5), in a series of 100 patients 25% of women who did not obtain benefits following oophorectomy subsequently experienced remission after hypophysectomy. Similarly, 24% of women who failed to respond to androgen/estrogen therapy later obtained a remission from hypophysectomy. These workers also found that pain relief follows hypophysectomy despite failure to achieve an objective remission. Thus these data appear to justify recommending hypophysectomy in some patients who have not shown a previous favorable response to castration and/or hormonal therapy.

3. *Presence of estrogen and progesterone receptors.* The presence of specific estrogen-binding protein (i.e., estrogen receptors), which can be demonstrated from excised malignant tissue in a significant number of patients with breast cancer, may be helpful in selecting those for endocrine therapy and/or hypophysectomy (30,37,45). In a summary (37) of the results of an international workshop held in 1974 to correlate data on estrogen receptors and responsiveness of breast cancer to endocrine therapy, it was reported that only 8 (8.5%) of 94 patients

with negative tumor estrogen receptor values experienced a positive response following endocrine ablative therapy (i.e., castration, adrenalectomy, and/or hypophysectomy). This compares with 59 (55%) of 107 patients with positive tumor estrogen receptor values in whom the treatment succeeded. Patients with borderline tumor estrogen receptor values had a 30% response rate. These data indicate that when there are no demonstrable estrogen receptors there is little chance (<10%) of obtaining objective remission from hypophysectomy. On the other hand, the presence of estrogen receptors forecasts a good chance, but no guarantee, that an objective response will result.

McGuire et al. (37) found progesterone receptors in approximately 60% of breast cancer specimens that also contained estrogen receptors. These workers found that the response rate following endocrine therapy was significantly higher if the tumor contained estrogen and progesterone receptors, as opposed to containing only estrogen receptors, implying that prediction of response may be enhanced by determining estrogen and progesterone receptors in biopsied tissue.

An interesting observation was recently reported by Lippman et al. (31) relative to estrogen receptors and response to chemotherapy. These workers found that 34 (76%) of 45 patients with low or absent estrogen-receptor values had objective responses to chemotherapy, whereas only 3 (12%) of 25 with higher estrogen-receptor values responded. These findings, which were not affected by different types of chemotherapy, indicate that estrogen receptor values might well become an important predictor of response to cytotoxic chemotherapy in metastatic breast cancer.

4. *Duration of free interval.* The free interval is defined as the period of time between original treatment of breast cancer and discovery of the first metastasis. Most authors believe that a comparatively long (i.e., >3 years) free interval is a relatively good prognostic sign in terms of response to hypophysectomy. In 45 patients in whom the interval was greater than 2 years Edelstyn et al. (9) found that the remission rate was 65%, whereas in 24 patients in whom the interval was less than 2 years the remission rate was 43%.

5. *Age.* The incidence of remission in premenopausal women, particularly those under 40 years of age, appears to be slightly lower than the general average. In older women (i.e., those 60 to 75 years of age) the remission rate is higher.

6. *Site of metastases.* Although most authorities agree that the best response is obtained in patients with bony metastases, patients with visceral metastases also can be considered for hypophysectomy. Contrary to popular belief, the presence of liver metastases does not prognosticate a poor response to hypophysectomy. Indeed, in Conway and Collins' series (5), 37% of 30 patients with liver metastases had remission after pituitary ablation.

7. *Predictive value of L-DOPA.* Therapeutic doses of L-DOPA alleviate bone pain in a significant number of patients with metastatic breast cancer. Encouraged by the results in a relatively small number of patients, Minton et al. (38,39) concluded that the responsiveness of the tumor to ablative therapy could be predicted on the basis of the response to this drug; i.e., patients showing relief

of bone pain would be expected to respond objectively and subjectively to either hypophysectomy or adrenalectomy. However, this study was not definitive in that 20 of the 30 who did not respond to L-DOPA were never subjected to any type of ablative procedure. Consequently, the value of L-DOPA in predicting objective remission remains unproved. As the majority of patients with severe bone pain are relieved by transsphenoidal hypophysectomy (perhaps 85 to 90%), the results of a predictive test to determine the effects of an endocrine ablative procedure on pain appear academic. For these reasons the present authors do not recommend the use of L-DOPA test for predicting response of breast cancer patients to hypophysectomy.

Prostate Cancer

Unfortunately factors that predict hypophysectomy responses are not as clear-cut in disseminated prostatic cancer as in breast cancer, and in general the clinical results following orchiectomy and/or estrogen therapy bear no consistent relationship to the outcome following hypophysectomy. However, there are differences of opinion in this regard. Based on their small but well-studied group, Scott and Schirmer (55) decided that a good response to castration–estrogen therapy is usually followed by a good response to hypophysectomy. Their results led them to state further, however, that failure to respond to castration–estrogen therapy does not preclude a response to hypophysectomy. Silverberg (57) found that patients with liver involvement and hematocrit values less than 30% usually did not achieve a good response. His conclusions were based on relatively small numbers of patients (i.e., 17); more importantly, the absence of liver involvement and/or hematocrit values above 30% do not imply that the patient will achieve a good response. Thompson et al. (60) found that patients who had pain relief more than 3 months following estrogen therapy or castration had a 64% chance of responding to hypophysectomy for at least 6 months. However, Thompson et al. (60) used pain relief rather than objective remission as evidence of a positive response.

As is well known from more recent work, pain relief which represents subjective remission occurs even in cases that do not get an objective remission. Based on their experiences with 100 cases, Fergusson and Hendry (11) concluded that the results of previous orchiectomy and estrogen therapy did not have definite predictive value in patients undergoing hypophysectomy for prostatic cancer. These workers did note, however, that a long history of the disease prior to hypophysectomy was likely to be associated with a good result.

REMISSION CRITERIA FOR DISSEMINATED BREAST AND PROSTATE CANCER FOLLOWING HYPOPHYSECTOMY

Subjective remission is assessed by relief of pain, correction or improvement of anemia, gain in weight, and improvement in appetite. An objective remission is measured by a decrease in lesion size following hypophysectomy without advance of other lesions or development of new lesions, disappearance of a neurologic deficit, increase in function of an obstructed organ (e.g., ureter), and/or a significant decrease in serum acid and/or alkaline phosphatase activity. Most authorities believe that the objective remission should last a minimum of 3 months to be considered a positive response.

INCIDENCE OF OBJECTIVE REMISSION

Breast Cancer

Although a comprehensive survey of hypophysectomy results for breast cancer is beyond the scope of this chapter, a summary (Table 1) of several selected large series (4,5,25,27,51,58) indicates that remissions occur in nearly one-half of women who have hypophysectomy; further, the period of survival in those who respond to hypophysectomy is significantly increased. Conway and Collins (5) obtained remission in 40% of 100 patients undergoing cryohypophysectomy. Of this number, 13 patients were alive and in remission 14 to 30 months (mean 18.6 months) after hypophysectomy; 2 were alive who had had remissions of 9 and 12 months, respectively; and 25 patients were dead after remissions of 3 to 28 months (mean 11.3 months). The latter group survived for periods ranging from 5 to 40 months (mean survival 20.3 months). Ray (51,52) obtained objective remission in 42% of 630 patients. For those having a remission longer than 6 months, the average duration was more than 17 months. In this same group the average survival after hypophysectomy was more than 24.5 months, with some still living after 3 to 5 years. In those patients who failed to obtain a remission, the average survival was only 5.6 months.

The remission statistics from many reports in the literature represent data from unselected series of cases; consequently it is not surprising that the overall incidence of objective remission is just under 50%. The importance of selection is emphasized in a report by Collins (4) summarizing his personal experience

TABLE 1. *Results of hypophysectomy in patients with disseminated cancer of the breast*

Series	No. of patients	Patients achieving remission		Average survival after hypophysectomy (months)	
		No.	%	Patients with remission	Patients without remission
Kennedy & French (27)	71	39	55	28	6.2
Stevens (58)	50	29	58	20	5.0
Kapur & Dalton (25)	63	29	46	—	—
Conway & Collins (5)	100	40	40	20.3	4.4
Collins (4)	394	184	47	—	—
Ray (51)	630	264	42	24.5	5.6

with hypophysectomy for breast cancer. He obtained a 27% response rate in 156 unselected women compared to a 57% response in 238 selected cases. Thus a higher response rate can be expected in those patients who have met one or more of the previously discussed criteria predisposing to a positive response.

Prostate Cancer

The incidence of beneficial results in patients with prostatic cancer following hypophysectomy varies widely, with favorable response rates ranging from as low as 19% to as high as 80% among the reported series (11,12,36,42,55,59–61,65). The principal reasons for this wide variation among reports are: (a) differentiation between objective and subjective types of remission are not made clear in many reports; (b) a variety of surgical techniques (e.g., craniotomy, yttrium implants) rather than a single standard method have been used to accomplish hypophysectomy; and importantly (c) most authors are reporting relatively small numbers of cases. Among reports that specifically identify patients with objective remission, the incidence of this type of remission ranges from 19 to 37%. The lowest reported incidence (19%) of objective remission occurred in the series of 47 cases reported by Thompson et al. (60), who performed hypophysectomy via the transcranial, or craniotomy, approach. Maddy et al. (36) obtained objective remission in 7 (35%) of 20 patients following cryohypophysectomy. The mean durations of remission and survival were 7 and 11.5 months, respectively. Using the transsphenoidal microsurgical technique, objective remission occurred in 5 (29%) of 17 patients in Silverberg's series (57) and in 18 (36%) of 53 patients treated at our institution.

Following yttrium hypophysectomy in 100 cases of prostatic cancer, Fergusson and Hendry (11) obtained a "good" response in 39 and no response in 29; 32 cases were listed simply as having responded. In their series a "good" response meant that pain or the symptom complex resulting from some major complication such as paraplegia or bladder neck obstruction was relieved completely, and the relief continued until death or only shortly before. Patients in the "responded" category achieved either partial but worthwhile relief of symptoms or complete relief followed by subsequent relapse. These authors made no attempt to identify specifically those patients showing an objective remission.

INCIDENCE OF PAIN RELIEF IN BREAST AND PROSTATE CANCER

Breast Cancer

After hypophysectomy approximately 75% (61) of patients with severe pain due to metastatic breast cancer obtain gratifying relief of pain, particularly osseous pain. Relief occurs within 24 to 36 hr, and often within 2 to 4 hr, of the operative procedure; moreover, as already mentioned, even patients who fail to gain an objective remission after hypophysectomy are relieved of their pain.

Prostate Cancer

The incidence of pain relief for prostatic cancer varies among the reported series but usually is significantly higher than the incidence of objective remission. As with breast cancer, pain relief occurs in many patients who fail to achieve an objective remission. In the series of 53 patients treated at our hospital, the remarkably high incidence (91%) of pain relief probably reflects the completeness of pituitary ablation accomplished via the transsphenoidal microsurgical method.

The striking relief of pain following hypophysectomy is intriguing from the standpoint of possible mechanisms. Several explanations that might be offered include structural or regressive alterations in the tumor, placebo effect, nonspecific steroid effect, and removal of one or more pituitary trophic hormones and/or related substances. Although the constraint of space does not permit extensive discussion of every possible mechanism, certain points can be made either for or against some explanations.

Temporal aspects of the relief argue against placebo effect, steroids, and regressive changes in the tumor. Also, many patients achieve relief despite failure to obtain an objective remission. Conceivably, certain pituitary trophic hormones (i.e., gonadotropins, growth hormone, and prolactin) may influence pain associated with cancer. Certain clinical observations in patients undergoing pituitary surgery are inconsistent with either growth hormone or prolactin having a direct relationship with pain relief following hypophysectomy. For instance, the removal of prolactin-inhibiting factor (PIF) by pituitary stalk section normally is associated with postoperative blood levels of prolactin that are significantly above normal (63); yet despite hyperprolactinemia, many patients undergoing stalk section for palliation of breast cancer obtain relief of pain (7,10). As another example, levodopa stimulates the release of growth hormone (8), but in a significant number of patients the administration of L-DOPA alleviates pain associated with breast cancer and, in fact, has been tried on occasion as a screening test to identify possible responders to hypophysectomy (38,39).

Recently peptides having significant pain-relieving properties have been discovered in the brain and pituitary gland of several mammals (16–18,32). These peptides, which include enkephalins and alpha- and beta-endorphins, were shown in animal studies to have considerably greater analgesic properties than morphine. The mechanism of action and circumstances of potential release of these substances into brain substance, cerebrospinal fluid (CSF), and/or ventricular fluid, or the peripheral circulation remain to be determined. However, it is interesting to speculate that pituitary ablation in humans may stimulate an inappropriate release of these peptides, which act in some as yet unknown manner to alleviate pain. Since the structures of alpha- and beta-endorphins are known, it will probably be possible ultimately to develop an appropriate radioimmunoassay, thereby allowing pre- and postoperative blood and/or CSF assays in hypophysectomized patients. It is possible that some insight into the potential role of these peptides in relieving cancer pain may be gained through this approach.

INDICATIONS FOR HYPOPHYSECTOMY IN BREAST AND PROSTATE CANCER

Breast Cancer

Hypophysectomy can be recommended for most patients with widespread and advancing cancer of the breast whose recurrent disease is not suitable for local excision or radiation therapy. In premenopausal patients oophorectomy should be considered as the initial palliative procedure. An oophorectomy failure does not necessarily contraindicate hypophysectomy, however. In postmenopausal patients the effects of androgen/estrogen therapy should be evaluated before performing hypophysectomy. It is still uncertain whether a trial of chemotherapy should precede or follow hypophysectomy in patients who have failed previous endocrine therapy. Hypophysectomy should be considered relatively early in the course of metastatic breast cancer because when this procedure is performed either as a last resort or after extensive chemotherapy, radiation therapy, and/or adrenalectomy, relatively poor results in terms of a useful remission can be expected.

The results of hypophysectomy for alleviating pain in patients with disseminated breast cancer have been so consistently gratifying that the presence of severe pain, particularly osseous pain, constitutes one of the principal indications for hypophysectomy in disseminated breast cnacer.

Prostate Cancer

Hypophysectomy can be recommended in all patients with proved progressive prostatic cancer who have previously undergone orchiectomy and estrogen therapy regardless of the response to these two methods of treatment. However, bearing in mind that many patients are elderly, that the majority have been through several treatment programs, and that a few are in marginal general health, one could reasonably question if hypophysectomy is an appropriate palliative operative procedure in patients with disseminated carcinoma (stage IV) of the prostate. For instance, considering the relatively low incidence (35%) of objective remissions, which last only approximately 1 year, the frequent occurrence of postoperative diabetes insipidus, and the potential risk of operating on elderly individuals with metastatic disease, one could reasonably question if hypophysectomy has an undisputed role in patients with this disease. In regard to the high complication rate of diabetes insipidus, it is appropriate to point out that the disorder is partial and in the majority can be satisfactorily controlled by the regular oral adminstration of clofibrate-S (Atromid-S) (41). In the authors' experience this complication has been an annoying but not a disabling problem. Hypophysectomy can be performed on elderly individuals without significant risk provided the patients are in reasonably good general health and do not have extensive, widespread metastatic disease. Although an objective remission rate of 35% is not comparable with the higher remission rate that is usually achieved in certain patients with disseminated carcinoma of the breast, some patients may choose to proceed with the operation knowing that their chances of obtaining an objective remission are relatively low. The most significant benefit of hypophysectomy and one that does appear to justify the operation is the dramatic pain relief that follows the procedure in the great majority of patients. For this reason the authors believe that hypophysectomy is an appropriate procedure especially in patients with severe osseous pain who are in reasonably good health.

CONTRAINDICATIONS

The contraindications for hypophysectomy in patients with prostate cancer are the same as in those with breast cancer who are being considered for the procedure. They include the following:

1. Debilitation
2. Poor general health
3. Significant hematologic disorders (e.g., deficient platelets)
4. Widespread, extensive metastatic disease
5. Brain metastases (relatively rare in prostatic cancer)
6. Unreliability from the standpoint of taking replacement medications

Although patients with prostatic cancer are usually elderly, advanced age alone is not a contraindication to hypophysectomy. As an example, Fergusson and Phillips (12) obtained remission in 14 of 21 patients over age 70 following hypophysectomy.

HYPOPHYSECTOMY VERSUS ADRENALECTOMY

Hypophysectomy and adrenalectomy are effective endocrine ablative procedures for disseminated carcinoma of the breast and prostate gland when the procedure is performed by a competent and experienced operator. Judging from reports in the literature, there does not appear to be a clear advantage of either operative procedure over the other in terms of objective remission rate for breast cancer (1,13,66). In our opinion, adequate data are not available on the use of the two operative procedures for prostatic cancer to make a comparative analysis. When craniotomy was the method for performing hypophysectomy, the risks and magnitude of the two operative approaches for achieving endocrine ablation were approximately equal. However, present-day techniques for performing hypophysectomy—e.g., the transsphenoidal microsurgical approach (19)—are considerably simpler and less troublesome to patients than bilateral adrenalectomy. Currently an experienced neurosurgeon can perform transsphenoidal hypophysectomy within a relatively short period of time with extremely low mortality. In premenopausal women bilateral oophorectomy is also necessary when adrenalectomy is performed. Perhaps the major advantage of hypophysectomy over adrenalectomy other than simplicity is the high incidence of significant pain relief. In patients having adrenalectomy pain relief occurs only when the patient acquires an objective remission, whereas with hypophysectomy patients obtain pain relief even when an objective remission fails to occur.

HYPOPHYSECTOMY FOR PAIN RELIEF IN METASTATIC CANCER OTHER THAN IN BREAST AND PROSTATE GLAND

Pain due to disseminated breast and prostate gland cancer is usually relieved shortly after hypophysectomy even in patients who do not attain objective regression of the disease, as noted. This observation, implying that endocrine alterations following hypophysectomy which result in tumor regression may be different from those responsible for pain relief, led to the development of the hypothesis that the relief of pain induced by hypophysectomy may not be limited to patients with potentially endocrine-sensitive tumors (i.e., breast and prostate gland) but may occur in patients with other neoplasms. A modicum of support for this hypothesis comes from the clinical studies of Moricca (40), Katz and Levin (26), and Corrsen et al. (6) in which pain relief from a wide variety of metastatic cancers was achieved by injecting absolute alcohol into the sella turcica. In many of the cases reported by these workers, it was necessary to reinject alcohol into the pituitary to sustain the pain relief.

Stimulated somewhat by these observations, we undertook a pilot study in a small group of patients to determine whether hypophysectomy would relieve severe pain in metastatic cancer other than breast and prostate gland (62). Transsphenoidal microsurgical hypophysectomy was performed in six patients with advanced and disseminated carcinoma (pancreas 2; testicle 2; adrenal 1; and urethra 1 case). Interestingly, two patients received significant and lasting relief of pain; one achieved relief but died from progression of disease 5 weeks after surgery; one patient, initially relieved, had recurrence of pain 3 months later; one had about 50% relief; and one received no benefit. Although these observations are intriguing and raise many interesting questions about the mechanisms for pain relief in patients with metastatic cancer, they are not to be interpreted as an endorsement for hypophysectomy for all metastatic cancers.

HYPOPHYSECTOMY FOR DIABETIC RETINOPATHY

Sufficient data have accumulated to indicate that hypophysectomy has a beneficial effect in certain cases of diabetic retinopathy. The mechanism by which hypophysectomy brings about an arrest of the angiopathy and visual improvement is unknown. The role of growth hormone in aggravating diabetes makes it reasonable to suspect that elimination of this hormone or some other unidentified diabetogenic pituitary substance underlies the explanation for these results (2). Although growth hormone appears to be the major diabetogenic factor, other trophic hormones that have diabetogenic action (e.g., ACTH and thyrotropin) also should be considered when discussing the possible mechanisms of the beneficial effects of hypophysectomy.

The selection of candidates for hypophysectomy should adhere to strict criteria. Diabetic patients who present with only background retinopathy (microaneurysms, hard and soft exudates, irregularities in retinal vessels, and small capillary hemorrhages in the deeper retina that appear as dot and blot hemorrhages) are not considered for pituitary ablation because such retinopathy poses relatively little threat to vision (54). Candidates for hypophysectomy include patients who have progressive proliferative retinopathy with impending blindness, at least one clinically healthy macula with corrected vision not worse than 20/60 to 20/80, and no serious cardiovascular and renal disease.

The results of hypophysectomy in properly chosen candidates are good, and reports indicate that the procedure arrests the progression of proliferative retinopathy in more than 60% of diabetic patients (54). Objective changes include clearing of vitreous opacities, improvement in vision, involution and disappearance of new vessels with decrease and cessation of leakage and hemorrhage, resorption of retinal edema, and reduction of venous caliber. Two well-controlled reports (23,24,35,44) concluded that pituitary ablation provides substantial benefit in highly selected cases, and that for maximal benefit all pituitary tissue within the sella should either be removed or destroyed. Thus the modern transsphenoidal microsurgical technique, which not only accomplishes total removal of the gland but also carries relatively little risk, probably is the procedure of choice in diabetic retinopathy. At least one form of diabetic retinopathy (i.e., florid retinopathy) has been shown to respond considerably better to hypophysectomy than photocoagulation (28).

The advent of photocoagulation has considerably decreased the number of diabetic patients being referred for hypophysectomy. Although hypophysectomy may not be the ultimate answer to the problem of diabetic retinopathy, it has been shown to reverse ocular changes and to prolong the retention of useful vision in many diabetic patients. When considering therapeutic options for diabetic retinopathy, photocoagulation and hypophysectomy should be given thoughtful consideration.

HYPOPHYSECTOMY TECHNIQUES

Craniotomy, which was the original approach, is probably too major a procedure for most patients and currently is not recommended as the method for achieving hypophysectomy. Because of the relative resistance of the normal pituitary gland to irradiation, X-ray therapy directed at the sella turcica for purposes of pituitary destruction is neither practical nor effective and should not be used. Transsphenoidal stereotactic insertion of either yttrium or other radioactive substance is not recommended because of the high complication rate that usually develops several weeks or months following instillation of the radioactive material (14).

Procedures that are effective and relatively safe include stereotactic cryohypophysectomy (50), stereotactic radiofrequency lesioning (67), and open transsphenoidal microsurgical removal (19) of the gland. In experienced hands any one of these three procedures yields good results in properly chosen patients.

Stereotactic radiofrequency hypophysectomy (67) induces prompt and effective cessation of pituitary function, and the procedure can be performed with minimal risk and little discomfort to the patient. Likewise, stereotactic cryohypophysectomy (50) has been used with success by several neurosurgeons. A large series with disseminated breast cancer treated with cryohypophysectomy by Conway and Collins (5) typifies the results (40% objective remission rate in 100 cases) that can be accomplished with this operative technique.

Although safe and well tolerated by patients, neither cryohypophysectomy nor radiofrequency coagulation accomplishes complete pituitary destruction, or at least complete ablation of all intrasellar pituitary tissue. The study of Norrell et al. (43) is germane to this issue. These investigators evaluated residual pituitary tissue following cryohypophysectomy in 18 autopsied cases and found, significantly, that in 7 of the 18 cases more than 10% of the anterior lobe remained viable. However, whether it is necessary to produce total destruction of all intrasellar pituitary tissue in order to achieve remission in a significant number of patients is a controversial issue (29,59,65). For instance, Norrell et al. (43) believe that a remission in patients with advanced cancer can still occur despite failure to destroy the entire gland. Edelstyn et al. (9) challenge this viewpoint, and as support for their opinion cite the finding of Ganong and Hume (15) that as little as 5% of the anterior pituitary can stimulate the adrenal cortex.

Currently the open transsphenoidal microsurgical operation described by Hardy (19) probably is the most commonly used procedure for performing hypophysectomy. It is an operation that is safe and associated with relatively little patient discomfort. The open transsphenoidal operation is the only one that consistently accomplishes complete removal of the pituitary gland, and this feature represents the principal advantage of this procedure over the stereotactic methods. The results with the open transsphenoidal microsurgical technique are comparable with any other method for performing hypophysectomy in terms of achieving objective remission, and are probably superior to other methods in alleviating pain, a feature most likely related to the completeness of pituitary ablation.

There are no special anesthetic techniques required for patients undergoing hypophysectomy. It is necessary to administer hydrocortisone 100 mg i.v. immediately before and during the operative procedure. The question of prophylactic antibiotics during operation (particularly via the transsphenoidal approach) and during the postoperative course is not a settled issue. The authors prefer to use ampicillin (1 g every 6 hr) for a period of 24 hr, beginning the antibiotic immediately prior to starting the operation. Some authorities believe that the prolonged use of antibiotics encourages the overgrowth of opportunistic organisms.

PRE- AND POSTOPERATIVE MANAGEMENT OF HYPOPHYSECTOMY PATIENTS

Preoperative Management

Appropriate preoperative studies in patients who are to undergo hypophysectomy include a history and complete physical examination, complete blood count and platelet count, either a metastatic X-ray survey or bone scan to assess the extent of disease, a lateral skull X-ray to visualize the sella turcica and sphenoid sinus, and, if possible, determination of either fasting growth hormone or prolactin. Pre- and 10-day postoperative comparison of the growth hormone or prolactin values may provide some index to the completeness of the pituitary ablation.

Postoperative Management

During the immediate postoperative period the primary concerns are adequate corticosteroid coverage and fluid balance. Hydrocortisone is administered in a dosage of 50 mg i.m. every 8 hr for the first 2 days and every 12 hr for the third day following surgery. For the remainder of the patient's hospital stay, hydrocortisone is administered orally in a dosage of 20 mg every 12 hr. Fluid balance is followed by strict attention to the hourly fluid intake and output and the specific gravity of the urine. Incomplete diabetes insipidus is present in the majority of patients postoperatively, and the surgeon performing hypophysectomy should be prepared to recognize and manage this complication (see below).

By the time of discharge from the hospital, the patient is on a maintenance dose of hydrocortisone, 20 mg in the morning and 10 mg in the late afternoon. The patient and family must be instructed to increase the steroids by two to three times the usual dose in the event of severe physical or traumatic stress (fever, respiratory infection, accident, etc.) and to notify the physician of the problem. Thyroid replacement therapy is started only when it is ascertained that the patient has become hypothyroid clinically and chemically, usually 4 to 6 weeks after surgery. Thereafter corticosteroids and thyroid replacement therapy are maintained indefinitely.

COMPLICATIONS OF HYPOPHYSECTOMY AND THEIR MANAGEMENT

Diabetes insipidus is the most common complication following hypophysectomy in the majority (perhaps more than 75%) of patients. Diagnostic criteria for diabetes insipidus is as follows:

1. Urine specific gravity <1.005 for two consecutive hours
2. Urine output > total intake by 250 ml during any 1-hr period (or by 1,000 ml during any 4-hr period)
3. Serum osmolality >300 mOsm/kg
4. Urine osmolality <200 mOsm/kg
5. Serum Na >150 mEq/liter and urine specific gravity <1.005

Fortunately, the complication is transitory and in many patients terminates by the time of discharge. In others the diabetes may be so mild as to be managed by the patient by simply controlling fluid intake despite moderate thirst. Frequently the condition can be managed effectively with clofibrate in a dosage of 500 mg q.i.d. administered orally (41). It is unusual for posthypophysectomy diabetes insipidus not to respond to clofibrate, but in cases refractory to this medication it is necessary to use vasopressin (Pitressin Tannate) in oil administered intramuscularly.

CSF rhinorrhea is the most serious complication following hypophysectomy, particularly when the transsphenoidal approach is used. The frequency of this complication after transsphenoidal operations for pituitary removal varies, but in general the incidence in experienced hands is probably less than 5%. This complication should be corrected promptly because of the potential threat of meningitis. The diagnosis of CSF rhinorrhea is confirmed by testing the fluid with a Dextristik and demonstrating the presence of glucose. In our opinion the condition should be managed initially by performing a lumbar puncture and slowly removing CSF to as low a pressure as the patient's headache will tolerate. If the CSF leak persists, an indwelling spinal subarachnoid catheter should be inserted percutaneously and left in place for 3 days, during which time the patient remains in bed with the head elevated to 40°. The catheter is connected to a sterile reservoir, which is placed no higher than the lumbar puncture site. Should the fluid continue to leak following removal of the catheter, the surgeon should reopen the transsphenoidal wound and pack the sella and sphenoid sinus with adipose tissue. Reopening the wound after a transsphenoidal operation is relatively easy. Whenever persistent CSF rhinorrhea follows cryohypophysectomy or stereotactic radiofrequency hypophysectomy, then transnasal, transsphenoidal exposure of the sella is performed as described by Hardy (19).

Other complications that occur infrequently include sinusitis and adrenal insufficiency. Sinusitis is uncomfortable, but usually clears spontaneously. Adrenal insufficiency requires either readjustment of the replacement medication or reemphasizing to a patient the importance of taking the medication regularly.

SUMMARY AND CONCLUSIONS

Hypophysectomy is a useful, gratifying palliative operative procedure in patients with disseminated breast and prostatic cancer. Objective remission occurs in nearly 50% of patients with breast cancer and approximately 35% of patients with prostatic cancer. In women with breast cancer who have shown a positive response to previous oophorectomy, the remission rate following hypophysectomy may be as high as 80 to 85%. In a significant number of patients with breast and prostatic cancer a remission follows hypophysectomy despite the fact that a previous castration procedure and/or endocrine manipulation did not effect regression of the tumor. The relief of pain, particularly osseous pain, is one of the principal benefits of hypophysectomy and occurs in the majority of patients with breast and prostatic cancer, irrespective of whether there is other evidence of remission of the lesion. Hypophysectomy has also been shown to be a beneficial surgical procedure in selected cases of diabetic retinopathy.

The procedures of choice for performing hypophysectomy include stereotactic cryohypophysectomy, stereotactic radiofrequency lesioning, and the open transsphenoidal microsurgical technique. All three operations yield comparable results in terms of objective remission of disease, and all are considerably safer and less troublesome to the patient than craniotomy. The open transsphenoidal technique appears to provide pain relief in a higher percentage of patients than the stereotactic methods. Most likely this is because the majority of patients achieve complete pituitary ablation that does not invariably occur with stereotactic methods.

As a result of many advances in pituitary surgery in recent years, all of which have resulted in safer procedures, the authors conclude that hypophysectomy should be given early and serious consideration in patients with disseminated breast and prostatic cancer. When this operation is delayed until after extensive chemotherapy, irradiation treatment, and other methods have been exhausted, hypophysectomy becomes a "last resort" procedure, and in this situation it is likely that unsatisfactory results will be obtained in most of the patients.

REFERENCES

1. Atkins, H., Falconer, M. A., Hayward, J. L., MacLean, K. S., and Schurr, P. H. (1966): The timing of adrenalectomy and of hypophysectomy in the treatment of advanced breast cancer. *Lancet,* 1:827–830.
2. Balodimos, M. C. (1971): Treatment of diabetic retinopathy: Pituitary ablation and retinal photocoagulation. *Med. Clin. North Am.,* 56:989–999.
3. Beatson, G. T. (1896): On the treatment of inoperable cases of carcinoma of the mamma: Suggestions for a new method of treatment, with illustrative cases. *Lancet,* 2:104–107, 162–165.
4. Collins, W. F. (1974): Hypophysectomy: Historical and personal perspective. *Clin. Neurosurg.,* 21:68–78.
5. Conway, L. W., and Collins, W. F. (1969): Results of transsphenoidal cryohypophysectomy for carcinoma of the breast. *N. Engl. J. Med.,* 281:1–7.
6. Corssen, G., Holcomb, M. C., Moustapha, I., Langford, R., Vitek, J. J., and Ceballos, R.

(1977): Alcohol-induced adenolysis of the pituitary gland: A new approach to control of intractable cancer pain. *Anesth. Analg.,* 56:414–421.
7. Dugger, G. S., Van Wyke, J., and Newsome, J. F. (1958): Transection of the hypophyseal stalk in the management of metastatic mammary carcinoma. *Am. Surg.,* 24:603–608.
8. Eddy, R. L., Gilliland, P. F., and Ibarra, J. D. (1974): Human growth hormone release: Comparison of provocative test procedures. *Am. J. Med.,* 56:179–185.
9. Edelstyn, G., Gleadhill, C., and Lyons, A. (1968): Total hypophysectomy for advanced breast cancer. *Clin. Radiol.,* 19:426–432.
10. Ehni, G., and Eckles, N. E. (1959): Interruption of the pituitary stalk in the patient with mammary cancer. *J. Neurosurg.,* 16:628–652.
11. Fergusson, J. D., and Hendry, W. F. (1971): Pituitary irradiation in advanced carcinoma of the prostate: Analysis of 100 cases. *Br. J. Urol.,* 43:514–519.
12. Fergusson, J. D., and Phillips, D. E. H. (1962): A clinical evaluation of radioactive pituitary implantation in the treatment of advanced carcinoma of the prostate. *Br. J. Urol.,* 34:485–492.
13. Fracchia, A. A., Farrow, J. H., Miller, T. R., Tollefsen, R. H., Greenberg, E. J., and Knapper, W. H. (1971): Hypophysectomy as compared with adrenalectomy in the treatment of advanced carcinoma of the breast. *Surg. Gynecol. Obstet.,* 241–246.
14. Fraser, R., Joplin, G. F., and Laws, J. W. (1959): Needle implantation of yttrium seeds for pituitary ablation in cases of secondary carcinoma. *Lancet,* 1:382–386.
15. Ganong, W. F., and Hume, D. M. (1956): The effect of graded hypophysectomy on thyroid, gonadal, and adrenocortical function in the dog. *Endocrinology,* 59:293–301.
16. Goldstein, A. (1976): Opioid peptides (endorphins) in pituitary and brain. *Science,* 193:1081–1086.
17. Goldstein, A., Lowney, L. I., and Pal, B. K. (1971): Stereospecific and nonspecific interactions of the morphine congener levorphanol in subcellular fractions of mouse brain. *Proc. Natl. Acad. Sci. USA,* 68:1742–1747.
18. Guillemin, R., Ling, N., Burgus, R., and Fontaine, M. (1976): Endorphines, peptides, d'origine hypothalamique et neurohypophysaire a activite morphinomimetique: Isolment et structure moleculaire de l'a-endorphone. *C R Acad. Sci. Paris,* 282:783–785.
19. Hardy, J. (1971): Transsphenoidal hypophysectomy. *J. Neurosurg.,* 34:581–594.
20. Harrold, B. P., Cates, J. E., and James, J. A. (1968): Treatment of advanced breast cancer by trans-sphenoidal hypophysectomy. *Br. J. Cancer,* 22:19–31.
21. Heusen, J. C. (1974): Hormones by administration. In: *Treatment of Breast Cancer,* edited by H. Atkins, pp. 113–164. University Park Press, Baltimore.
22. Huggins, C., and Hodges, C. V. (1941): Studies on prostatic cancer. I. The effect of castration, of estrogen and of androgen injection on serum phosphatases in metastatic carcinomia of the prostate. *Cancer Res.,* 1:293–297.
23. Joplin, G. F., Fraser, R., Hill, D. W., Oakley, N. W., Scott, D. J., and Doyle, F. H. (1965): Pituitary ablation for diabetic retinopathy. *Q. J. Med.,* 34:443–462.
24. Joplin, G. F., Oakley, N. W., Hill, D. W., Kohner, E. M., and Fraser, T. R. (1967): Diabetic retinopathy. II. Comparison of disease remission induced by various degrees of pituitary ablation by Y^{90}. *Diabetologia,* 3:406–412.
25. Kapur, T. R., and Dalton, G. A. (1969): Trans-sphenoidal hypophysectomy for metastatic carcinoma of the breast. *Br. J. Surg.,* 56:332–337.
26. Katz, J., and Levin, A. B. (1977): Treatment of diffuse metastatic cancer pain by instillation of alcohol into the sella turcica. *Anesthesiology,* 46:115–121.
27. Kennedy, B. J., and French, L. (1965): Hypophysectomy in advanced breast cancer. *Am. J. Surg.,* 110:411–415.
28. Kohner, E. M., Hamilton, A. M., Joplin, G. F., Fraser, T. R. (1976): Florid diabetic retinopathy and its response to treatment by photocoagulation or pituitary ablation. *Diabetes,* 25:104–110.
29. LaRosa, J. T., Strong, M. S., and Milby, J. C. (1978): Endocrinologically incomplete transethmoidal, trans-sphenoidal hypophysectomy with relief of bone pain in breast cancer. *N. Engl. J. Med.,* 298:1332–1335.
30. Leung, B. S., Fletcher, W. E., and Krippachne, W. W. (1973): Estrogen receptors: A valid test for selection of breast cancer patients for endocrine ablation. *Surg. Forum,* 24:125–127.
31. Lippman, M. E., Allegra, J. C., Thompson, E. B., and Simon, R. (1978): The relation between estrogen receptors and response rate to cytotoxic chemotherapy in metastatic breast cancer. *N. Engl. J. Med.,* 298:1223–1228.

32. Loh, H. H., Tseng, L. F., Wei, E., and Li, C. H. (1976): Beta-endorphin is a potent analgesic agent. *Proc. Natl. Acad. Sci. USA,* 73:2895–2898.
33. Luft, R., Olivecrona, H., and Sjögren, B. (1955): Hypophysectomy in man: Experiences in severe diabetes mellitus. *J. Clin. Endocrinol. Metab.,* 15:391–408.
34. Luft, R., and Olivecrona, H. (1953): Experience with hypophysectomy in man. *J. Neurosurg.,* 10:301–316.
35. Lundback, K., Malmros, R., Anderson, H. C., Rasmussen, J. H. (1969): Hypophysectomy for diabetic angiopathy: a controlled clinical trial. In: *The Treatment of Diabetic Retinopathy,* edited by M. Goldberg and S. Fine, p. 291. U.S. Public Health Service, Washington, D.C.
36. Maddy, J. A., Winternitz, W. W., and Norrell, H. (1971): Cryohypophysectomy in the management of advanced prostatic cancer. *Cancer,* 28:322–328.
37. McGuire, W. L., Horwitz, K. B., Pearson, O. H., and Segaloff, A. (1977): Current status of estrogen and progesterone receptors in breast cancer. *Cancer,* 39:2934–2947.
38. Minton, J. P. (1974): The response of breast cancer patients with bone pain L-DOPA. *Cancer,* 33:358–363.
39. Minton, J. P., Bronn, D. G., and Kibbey, W. E. (1976): L-DOPA effect in painful bony metastases. *N. Engl. J. Med.,* 294:3210.
40. Morrica, G. (1974): Chemical hypophysectomy for cancer pain. In: *Advances in Neurology, Vol. 4, Pain,* edited by J. J. Bonica. Raven Press, New York.
41. Moses, A. M., Howanitz, J., and van Bimert, M. (1973): Clofibrate-induced antidiuresis. *J. Clin. Invest.,* 52:535–542.
42. Murphy, G. P., Boctor, Z. N., Gailani, S., and Belmusto, L. (1969): Hypophysectomy for disseminated prostatic carcinoma. *J. Surg. Oncol.,* 1:81–95.
43. Norrell, H., Alves, A. M., Winternitz, W. W., and Maddy, J. (1970): A clinicopathologic analysis in cryohypophysectomy in patients with advanced cancer. *Cancer,* 25:1050–1060.
44. Oakley, N. W., Joplin, G. F., Kohner, F. M., and Blach, R. K. (1969): The treatment of diabetic retinopathy by pituitary implantation of radioactive yttrium. In: *The Treatment of Diabetic Retinopathy,* edited by M. Goldberg and S. Fine, p. 315. U.S. Public Health Service, Washington, D.C.
45. Pearson, O. (1976): Endocrine treatment of breast cancer. *CA,* 26:165–173.
46. Pearson, O. H., and Ray, B. S. (1960): Hypophysectomy in the treatment of metastatic mammary cancer. *Am. J. Surg.,* 99:544–552.
47. Perrault, M., Lebeau, J., and Klotz, B. (1952): L'hypophysectomie totale dans le traitement du cancer sein: Premier cas francais: avenir de la method. *Therapie,* 7:290–300.
48. Poulsen, J. E. (1953): Recovery from retinopathy in a case of diabetes with Simond's disease. *Diabetes,* 2:7–12.
49. Poulsen, J. E. (1966): Diabetes and anterior pituitary insufficiency: Final course and postmortem study of a diabetic patient with Sheehan's syndrome. *Diabetes,* 15:73–77.
50. Rand, R. W., Daske, A. M., Paglia, D. E., Conway, L. W., and Solomon, D. H. (1964): Stereotactic cryohypophysectomy. *JAMA,* 189:255–259.
51. Ray, B. S. (1967): Hypophysectomy as palliative treatment. *JAMA,* 200:974–975.
52. Ray, B. S. (1973): Hypophysectomy by craniotomy. In: *Neurological Surgery,* Vol. 3, edited by J. R. Youmans, pp. 1915–1927. Saunders, Philadelphia.
53. Robin, P. E., Powell, D. J., Waterhouse, J. A. H., and Dalton, G. A. (1975): Transsphenoidal hypophysectomy in disseminated carcinoma of the breast. *Br. J. Surg.,* 62:85–91.
54. Saglam, S., Wilson, C. B., and Seymour, R. J. (1970): Indications for hypophysectomy in diabetic retinopathy and cancer of the breast and prostate. *Calif. Med.,* 113:1–6.
55. Scott, W. W., and Schirmer, H. K. A. (1962): Hypophysectomy for disseminated prostatic cancer. In: *On Cancer and Hormones: Essays on Experimental Biology,* pp. 175–204. University of Chicago Press, Chicago.
56. Shimkin, M. B., Boldrey, E. B., Kelly, K. H., Bierman, H. R., Ortega, P., and Naffziger, H. C. (1952): Effects of surgical hypophysectomy in a man with malignant melanoma. *J. Clin. Endocrinol. Metab.,* 12:439–453.
57. Silverberg, G. D. (1977): Hypophysectomy in the treatment of disseminated prostate carcinoma. *Cancer,* 39:1727–1731.
58. Stevens, D. (1968): Hypophysectomy: A report on 50 operations for metastasizing breast cancer. *Laryngoscope,* 82:73–77.
59. Straffon, R. A., Kiser, W. S., Robitaille, M., and Dohn, D. (1968): Yttrium hypophysectomy

in the management of metastatic carcinoma of the prostate gland in 13 patients. *J. Urol.,* 99:102–105.
60. Thompson, J. B., Greenberg, E., Pazianos, A., and Pearson, O. H. (1974): Hypophysectomy in metastatic cancer. *NY State J. Med.,* 74:1006–1008.
61. Tindall, G. T., Ambrose, S. S., Christy, J. H., and Patton, J. (1976): Hypophysectomy in the treatment of disseminated carcinoma of the breast and prostate gland. *South. Med. J.,* 69:579–587.
62. Tindall, G. T., Nixon, D. W., Christy, J. H., and Neill, J. D. (1977): Pain relief in metastatic cancer other than breast and prostate gland following transsphenoidal hypophysectomy. *J. Neurosurg.,* 47:659–662.
63. Turkington, R. W., Underwood, L. E., and Van Wyck, J. J. (1971): Elevated serum prolactin levels after pituitary-stalk section in man. *N. Engl. J. Med.,* 285:707–710.
64. VanGilder, J. C., and Goldenberg, I. S. (1975): Hypophysectomy in metastatic breast cancer. *Arch. Surg.,* 110:293–295.
65. West, C. R., and Murphy, G. P. (1973): Pituitary ablation and disseminated prostatic carcinoma. *JAMA,* 225:253–256.
66. Wilson, R. E., Piro, A. J., Aliapoulios, M. A., and Moore, F. D. (1969): Evaluation of adrenalectomy and hypophysectomy in the treatment of metastatic cancer of the breast. *Cancer,* 24:1322–1330.
67. Zervas, N. T. (1969): Stereotaxic radiofrequency surgery of the normal and the abnormal pituitary gland. *N. Engl. J. Med.,* 280:429–437.
68. Zimmerman, B. R., and Molnar, G. D. (1977): Prolonged follow-up in diabetic retinopathy treated by sectioning the pituitary stalk. *Mayo Clin. Proc.,* 52:233–237.

Clinical Management of Pituitary Disorders,
edited by G. T. Tindall and W. F. Collins.
Raven Press, New York © 1979.

23

Transsphenoidal Hypophysectomy: Pathophysiology and Results

Jules Hardy

Service of Neurosurgery, Notre-Dame Hospital and University of Montreal, School of Medicine, Montreal H2L 4K8, Quebec, Canada

Functional hypophysectomy is essentially removal of the normal pituitary gland. It is not concerned with the treatment of hypersecreting disorders (e.g., acromegaly, Cushing's disease, and galactorrhea–amenorrhea syndrome). Our experience over the last several years with transsphenoidal microsurgical exploration of the sella turcica has shown that, even if the size of the sella appears normal radiologically, there is always an intrapituitary circumscribed nodule—a "microadenoma"—responsible for the clinical syndrome (9,11,13). For this reason the treatment of oversecreting pituitary disorders should be dealt with under the subject of pathology of pituitary adenomas (3–5,9).

Historically the first hypophysectomy was performed in France in 1934 by Puech (2) in a patient with severe juvenile diabetes; the decision to try this treatment was based on the Houssay phenomenon (15), which demonstrated the diabetogenic role of pituitary hormones. Following the extensive works of Huggins (16), who demonstrated the hormonal dependency of certain cancers of the breast and prostate, hypophysectomy was attempted in humans during the early 1950s (17,18,21). After several years of empiricism, there remain only two clinical indications for hypophysectomy: (a) advanced metastatic cancer of the breast and prostate, and (b) the prevention of blindness in diabetic retinopathy.

PATHOPHYSIOLOGY

The clinical results are obvious but the pathophysiological mechanism of the effects produced by hypophysectomy is not yet completely understood. Recent progress in endocrinology and experimental biological correlations, however, has suggested certain explanations.

In hormone-dependent cancer of the breast, patients submitted to hypophysectomy have experienced a sudden arrest of the rapid flare-up of the generalized cancerous process, regression of metastases, and improvement of general condition. It is probable that these long-term objective results may be dependent on the suppression of gonadotropins and especially of prolactin (23), which has been shown to induce breast cancer in mice (19,20). Similarly, growth hormone (hGH), which is responsible for skeletal growth until adulthood, could be involved in the process of cellular growth in young neoplastic tissues. It appears that the relief of osseous pain may be related to the sudden suppression of hGH since it has been shown that infusion of this hormone into hypophysectomized patients temporarily reproduces the bone pain (21). Further support for this supposition is seen in acromegalic patients with severe arthritic pain, which is suppressed immediately following removal of the hGH-oversecreting adenoma.

In diabetes mellitus accompanied by retinopathy, improvement of visual function associated with retinal changes following hypophysectomy may also depend on suppression of the diabetic hormone, a biochemical substance closely related to hGH although not necessarily with the same molecular structure. The effect on diabetes mellitus is constant in that following hypophysectomy hyperglycemia is normalized and in all cases the insulin requirement is markedly reduced, even completely suppressed in some patients. The lipotropic hormone, although not yet isolated in humans, may be involved also since the normalization of hypertriglyceridemia is observed in diabetic patients following hypophysectomy (8).

INDICATIONS AND RESULTS

In advanced metastatic cancer of the breast the various results with different metastatic lesions better clarify the indications for hypophysectomy. The best results are obtained in patients suffering from uncontrollable skeletal metastases. In premenopausal women ovariectomy should precede hypophysectomy since this estrogenic suppression allows a period of remission which is further extended by hypophysectomy. In postmenopausal women hypophysectomy should be the method of choice. Complete suppression of pain occurs in 92% of cases following total transsphenoidal hypophysectomy (14). Partial suppression has been obtained in patients in whom technical difficulties did not allow a complete hypophysectomy.

In the presence of visceral metastases, pulmonary or liver metastases without bone pain is a doubtful indication since objective remission is obtained in only 30% of cases and it is unnecessary to produce panhypopituitarism in a patient who is already bedridden with a prognosis of markedly reduced life expectancy. On the other hand, the presence of visceral metastases in a patient suffering from uncontrollable bone pain is not a contraindication provided the patient can tolerate general anesthesia. In these cases "hypophysiolysis" with needle introduction of radioactive material (24,25), heating (27), or cold (22) performed under local anesthesia is a less traumatic procedure although the statistical results are less consistent.

The indication for hypophysectomy for patients with prostatic cancer is similar to that for breast cancer, i.e., diffuse metastatic bone pain at the stage of the second flare-up following orchidectomy. Clinical results have corroborated the validity of relying on this indication (26).

There are reports of surprising results after hypophysectomy in patients with various other conditions associated with diffuse metastatic lesions. For instance, patients who presented with pathological fractures of long bone and treated simultaneously with orthopedic osteosynthesis and hypophysectomy experience immediate pain relief, thus permiting early ambulation (14). Moreover, patients presenting with paraplegia due to metastases verified by myelography experience improvement in motor function following hypophysectomy to the point that they become partially ambulant. Finally, patients with peritoneal carcinomatosis and bowel obstruction recover normal function after hypophysectomy (14).

In patients with diabetic retinopathy, steady deterioration of vision can progress to blindness within 5 years (1). In these cases hypophysectomy produces regression of diabetic retinopathy and particularly neovascularization (7,8): 65% of these patients retained a normal visual index after 5 years. However, at the stage of fibrotic retinopathy, hypophysectomy is not indicated as it has no effect on scar tissue. At the present time, hypophysectomy is indicated in patients under age 40 who have severe retinopathy and in whom photocoagulation does not allow the treatment of neovessels from the papilla or in whom neovascularization is diffuse over the retina (10).

Patients who undergo pituitary ablation should be given hydrocortisone 300 mg i.v. on the day of surgery. The corticotherapy is reduced progressively over the following days until a physiological dose of 37.5 mg cortisone acetate is administered daily. Patients should also receive thyroid replacement therapy (L-thyroxine 0.2 mg daily).

Following hypophysectomy approximately 40% of patients develop transitory diabetes insipidus which is well controlled with injections of vasopressin (Pitressin Tannate in Oil). In 10% of these patients the diabetes will be permanent but can be controlled with oral clofibrate (Atromid-S).

REFERENCES

1. Caird, F. I. (1968): Diabetic retinopathy as a cause of visual impairment. In: *Symposium on the Treatment of Diabetic Retinopathy,* pp. 41–46. U.S. Department of Health, Education, and Welfare, Public Health Service, Washington, D.C.
2. Chabanier, H., Puech, P., Lobo-Onell, C., and Lélu, E. (1936): Hypophyse et diabète (à propos de l'ablation d'une hypophyse normale dans un cas de diabète grave). *Presse Med.,* 44:986–989.
3. Guiot G., et al. (1958): *Adènomes Hypophysaires.* Masson et Cie, Paris.
4. Guiot, G., Rougerie, J., and Hertzog, E. (1958): L'utilisation de l'amplificateur de brillance en neurochirurgie. *Ann. Chir.,* 12:689–695.
5. Hardy, J., and Wigser, S. M. (1965): Transsphenoidal surgery of pituitary fossa tumors with televised radiofluoroscopic control. *J. Neurosurg.,* 23:612–620.

6. Hardy, J. (1967): La chirurgie de l'hypophyse par voie transsphénoidale ouverte: Etude comparative de deux modalités techniques. *Ann. Chir.,* 21:1011–1022.
7. Hardy, J., and Ciric, I. S. (1968): Selective anterior hypophysectomy in the treatment of diabetic retinopathy: A transsphenoidal microsurgical technique. *JAMA,* 203:73–78.
8. Hardy, J., Panisset, A., Marchildon, A., and Lanthier, A. (1969): Microsurgical selective anterior pituitary ablation for diabetic retinopathy. *Can. Med. Assoc. J.,* 100:785–792.
9. Hardy, J. (1969): Transsphenoidal microsurgery of the normal and pathological pituitary. *Clin. Neurosurg.,* 16:185–217.
10. Hardy, J. (1970): Hypophysectomie et diabète. *Med. Hyg.,* 916:743–744.
11. Hardy, J. (1971): Microchirurgie des adènomes hypophysaires hypersécrétants. In: *Les Adènomes Hypophysaires Sécrétants,* pp. 195–196. Masson et Cie, Paris.
12. Hardy, J. (1971): Transsphenoidal hypophysectomy. *J. Neurosurg.,* 34:582–594.
13. Hardy, J. (1973): Transsphenoidal surgery of hypersecreting pituitary tumors. In: *International Conference on Diagnosis and Treatment of Pituitary Tumors,* pp. 179–194. Excerpta Medica, Amsterdam.
14. Hardy, J., Grisoli, F., Leclercq, T. A., and Somma, M. (1975): Le traitement du cancer du sein métastatique par l'hypophysectomie transsphènoidale. *Un. Med. Can.,* 104:1557–1562.
15. Houssay, B. A., and Brasotti, A. (1930): La diabetes pancréatica de los perros hipofisoprivos. *Rev. Soc. Argent. Biol.,* 6:251–296.
16. Huggins, C. (1942): Effect of orchiectomy and irradiation on cancer of prostate. *Ann Surg.,* 115:1192–1200.
17. Le Beau, J. (1958): *L'hypophysectomie dans le Traitement du Cancer.* Doin, Paris.
18. Luft, R., and Olivecrona, H. (1953): Experiences with hypophysectomy in man. *J. Neurosurg.,* 10:301–316.
19. McGuire, W. L., Chamness, G. C., Costlow, M. E., et al. (1974): Hormone dependence in breast cancer. *Metabolism,* 23:75–100.
20. Mühlbock, O., and Boot, L. M. (1959): Induction of mammary cancer in mice without the mammary tumor agent by isografts of hypophyses. *Cancer Res.,* 19:402–412.
21. Pearson, O. H., Ray, B. S., Lipsett, M. B., Hood, H., and Greenberg, E. (1958): Hypophysectomy in man. *Arch. Surg.,* 77:144–152.
22. Rand, R. W., Dashe, A. M., Paglia, D. E., et al. (1964): Stereotactic cryohypophysectomy. *JAMA,* 189:255–259.
23. Smithline, F., Sherman, L., and Kolodny, D. (1975): Prolactin and breast carcinoma. *N. Engl. J. Med.,* 292:784–792.
24. Talairach, J., Aboulker, J., David, M., and Tournoux, P. (1954): Utilisation de la mèthode radio-stéreotaxique pour l'abord de l'hypophyse par voie nasale. *Rev. Neurol. (Paris),* 90:658.
25. Talairach, J., and Sedam, R., with Szikla, G., Bonis, A., Schaub, C., and Harter, M. (1966): La chirurgie stéréotaxique de l'hypophyse non tumorale par les radio-isotopes. *Neurochirurgie,*
26. Tindall, G. T., Payne, N. S., and Nixon, D. W. (1979): Transsphenoidal hypophysectomy for disseminated carcinoma of the prostate gland. *J. Neurosurg.* 50:275–282.
27. Zervas, N. T. (1969): Stereotaxic radiofrequency surgery of the normal and the abnormal pituitary gland. *N. Engl. J. Med.,* 280:429–437.

Clinical Management of Pituitary Disorders,
edited by G. T. Tindall and W. F. Collins.
Raven Press, New York © 1979.

24

Anesthetic Considerations for Patients Undergoing Transsphenoidal Surgery

Yung-Fong Sung

Department of Anesthesiology, Division of Neurosurgical Anesthesia, Emory University Hospital, Atlanta, Georgia 30322

When Harvey Cushing was a third-year medical student he was called down from the seats, sent into a side room with a patient and an orderly, and told to put the patient to sleep, as the attending surgeon was preparing to operate for the class. He knew nothing about the patient, merely that a nurse came in and gave the patient a hypodermic injection. He proceeded as best he could under the orderly's directions, and in view of the repeated urgent call for the patient from the amphitheater it seemed to him an interminable time for the old man, who kept gagging, to go to sleep. The operation was started, and at this juncture there was a sudden gush of fluid from the patient's mouth, most of which was inhaled, and he died.

Cushing stood aside, burning with chagrin and remorse. No one paid the slightest attention to him though he supposed that he had killed the patient. The operation was completed in spite of the episode, as a demonstration to the class. Cushing slunk out of the hospital, walked the streets of north Boston the rest of the afternoon, and in the evening went to the surgeon's house to ask if there was any possible way he could atone for the calamity to the man's family before he left the medical school and went into some other business. To his amazement he was told that he had had nothing to do with the man's death—the man had had a strangulated hernia and had been vomiting all night. Further, that sort of thing happened frequently, and Cushing had better forget about it and go on with medical school. Harvey Cushing continued with medical school but never forgot the incident (3). It led to his developing a continuous record of blood pressure, heart rate, respiratory rate, and body temperature for patients undergoing anesthesia—records that continue to be a baseline for all modern monitoring of anesthetized patients.

Cushing was aware of the importance of anesthesia and control of vital functions in surgical patients early in his medical training. Although endotracheal anesthesia was used as early as 1880 by William MacEwen (28), during World War I Cushing adopted the use of local anesthesia to treat war wounds, a measure that subsequently became popular for intracranial surgery. From 1917 to 1932 local anesthesia was used almost universally in neurosurgical clinics (47) despite the deficiencies of local anesthesia for major neurosurgical operative procedures. During the early 1930s neurosurgeons began using general anesthesia with endotracheal intubation, thus allowing more complicated and longer operative procedures to be performed safely (13).

Impressive and significant progress in anesthesia over the years has allowed and stimulated the development of surgical techniques. During the last few decades subspecialties within anesthesia—e.g., neurosurgical anesthesia (4,10,19,40,44,51)—have emerged to meet the requirements for better care of patients, and specialized techniques have been developed to accomplish this.

Initially pituitary surgery was indicated primarily to relieve mass effects (23), i.e., optic chiasm compression. A further indication for pituitary surgery (i.e., hypophysectomy) is palliation, and the procedure is now used in the treatment of metastatic cancer of the breast (27,32) and prostate (49); diabetic retinopathy (20,48,58); and uncontrolled exophthalmus associated with hyperthyroidism (31,34). The transsphenoidal approach to pituitary tumors, which was first done by Schloffer in 1907 (7,8), was used prior to the introduction of transcranial approaches to these lesions.

PREOPERATIVE EVALUATION AND ASSESSMENT

The preoperative visit is important in pituitary surgery for the patient and the anesthesiologist. The patient can be relieved of unnecessary anxiety, and the anesthesiologist can better understand how to handle problems related to the patient's disease process that may arise later.

1. General status is determined. The preoperative visit provides the anesthesiologist a chance to evaluate the status of the different systems, e.g., respiration, circulation, kidney, liver function, homeostatic function, endocrine status, allergy problems (9).
2. The anesthetic agent of choice and the monitoring necessity is determined largely by the preoperative visit. The patient should be asked about any previous anesthetic problems. If he has had previous troubles (e.g., nausea and vomiting after surgery, a hereditary disorder, reaction to muscle relaxants), the anesthesiologist can take appropriate steps to prevent a recurrence.

The existence of specific problems must be reviewed for each patient undergoing transsphenoidal microsurgery. Potential problems include the following:

1. The tumor produces excessive hormone secretions (59).
   A. The tumor associated with elevated prolactin level is usually found in young, healthy, adult women. The symptoms (amenorrhea, galactorrhea)

presented by these women do not pose significant anesthetic difficulties. Occasionally the patients complain of headache but otherwise are young, healthy adults. Little preoperative management is necessary except to alleviate their anxiety.

B. hGH-secreting tumor usually presents in patients as giantism or acromegaly. Not infrequently these patients have concomitant diseases and thus may present several major problems with respect to anesthesia. Some of these problems can be summarized as follows:

a. Cardiovascular system (2,22,24,36,43,56). The patient may have heart muscle disease such as cardiomyopathy, congestive heart failure, and/or arrhythmias. He may also have coronary artery disease and hypertension. For these patients a cardiology consultation should be provided to bring the patient to the most optimal condition before surgery (15) so he tolerates anesthesia and surgery much better and has a smoother postoperative recovery.

b. Airway difficulty (21,29). The acromegalic patient often has a large nose, prognathism, spread teeth, and a large tongue. These may make airway management difficult. He may also have a decreased width of the cricoid cartilage and an increased anterior–posterior diameter of the larynx. Some even have paralysis of one vocal cord, which should warn of possible postoperative airway difficulty. Some acromegalic patients have arthralgia and hypertropic osteoarthritis with limited neck mobility, or "frozen neck." This condition may also affect airway management.

c. Other endocrine dysfunction (14,16) may coexist in acromegalic patients, including diabetes mellitus, hyper- or hypothyroidism, or adrenal cortical or pituitary insufficiency. These should be evaluated preoperatively.

2. Tumor-produced symptoms of local compression, e.g., impairment in visual fields and/or acuity. This may be the first complaint of the patient. These patients are likely to be in relatively good health.
3. Tumor-produced hormone deficiency or recurrent tumor. These patients have varying degrees of hypopituitarism, and their history of previous medications is very important.
4. Ablative hypophysectomy for metastatic cancer. Pituitary surgery in this case is usually a final measure, done after all other treatment regimens are exhausted. Often these patients are in marginal health. Various medical problems including anemia; low platelet count; lung metastases with associated localizing pneumonitis, pleuritis, and pleural effusion with decreased lung compliance; bronchial obstruction due to metastases may also be present and complicate anesthetic management. The presence of metastatic bone disease, particularly in the cervical spine, emphasizes the need for caution during induction of anesthesia and positioning for surgery. Anemia and/or low platelet counts may require the appropriate blood replacement either

before or during surgery. Chest X-ray and pulmonary function tests must be evaluated preoperatively. Breast cancer patients may have had chemotherapy with adriamycin, which is a cardiac toxin and may cause cardiomyopathy (12,46). It is especially important to obtain an accurate history from these patients so they can be treated correctly. During the preoperative visit it is important to ascertain if patients are taking antidepressant drugs such as tricyclic compounds (5). These drugs may cause arrhythmias, and if hypotension occurs during anesthesia vasopressor agents must be used with extreme caution.

5. Hypophysectomy for diabetic retinopathy. These patients may be in marginal health as a consequence of decompensation of vascular, renal, and myocardial function secondary to long-standing diabetes mellitus. These patients should be completely evaluated and brought to their most optimal condition before surgery.

Preoperative medications include hypnotic drugs, narcotics, and anticholinergic agents. As mentioned previously, the preoperative visit is very important for alleviating the patients' anxiety. In healthy patients hypnotic drugs or narcotics may be combined, although narcotics are not used routinely in healthy patients.

Cancer patients may have been taking narcotics regularly; therefore preoperative medications must be adjusted accordingly to prevent an additive effect of the preoperative medications. This combination could result in serious respiratory depression prior to the patient's arrival in the operating room.

During the preoperative visit, the nature of the anesthetic and operative procedures should be explained to the patient. It is also necessary to explain that upon recovery from anesthesia soft rubber airway tubes will be in place in each nostril to facilitate nose breathing and serve as a pack to reattach the nasal mucosa.

INDUCTION, POSITIONING, AND EMERGENCE

Induction

Increased intracranial pressure is rare in transsphenoidal pituitary surgery patients. Infrequently, however, a large tumor may extend sufficiently above the sella turcica to block the third cerebral ventricle with resulting hydrocephalus. In this unusual situation the same precautions should be taken as for induction for patients with increased intracranial pressure, described elsewhere (35, 40,50).

1. *Pituitary tumor:* Induction for pituitary tumor is not substantially different from other general anesthesia and is usually accomplished using thiopental in incremental dosage, succinylcholine 1.5 mg/kg, and pretreatment with either *d*-tubocurarine 3 mg or gallamine 10 to 20 mg (6).

2. *Metastatic cancer:* A slow induction is required primarily because of the debilitation of the chronically ill patient. Small increments of thiopental and narcotics (i.e., fentanyl) should be given to avoid hypotension. If the patient has metastatic cervical spine lesions, the neck should be handled with care during intubation and positioning. In these cases the neck should probably be braced before the patient is taken to the operating room for surgery. A fiberoptic laryngoscope should be utilized. These patients must be handled with extreme care to avoid pathological fractures of the involved cervical vertebrae.

3. *Acromegaly:* This usually requires two anesthetists present for induction. The induction may present difficulties because of the large facial structure and tongue, and so a large mask, large laryngoscopes, and long endotracheal tubes should be available. These patients usually should be preoxygenated before induction because there may be prolonged apnea if the intubation is difficult. The patient's blood pressure and heart rate must be monitored carefully during induction to avoid increased or decreased blood pressure and heart rate since most of these patients have increased sensitivity of the vasculature to stimuli. In this group of patients hypertension may not respond to increased depth of anesthesia. In this situation a vasodilating agent such as a nitroglycerin drip (100 μg/ml) should be administered intravenously (26) at a rate that maintains blood pressure at the desired level during induction and thus avoids hypertension and increased myocardial oxygen consumption. This drug has minimal effect on heart rate, and no toxic side effects have been seen.

4. *Cerebrospinal fluid rhinorrhea:* These patients require a "crash induction" to avoid aspiration of cerebrospinal fluid (CSF) and positive pressure that could introduce bacterial intracranially.

5. *Diabetic retinopathy:* These patients, who are usually in marginal health, require a slow induction with small incremental dosages of medication to avoid hypotension.

Positioning

After intubation the patient's tube should be securely taped at the left corner of the mouth with the esophageal stethoscope and temperature probe in place (Fig. 1). No oral airway should be used in this case. The tube should be well secured to avoid accidental extubation during the surgical procedure. After induction the patient's eyes are examined for pupil size and reaction, and are then taped shut to avoid accidental corneal abrasion during surgery. The patient's head is placed in three-point skeletal fixation using a Mayfield skull clamp and table attachment. The position of the patient is arranged such that the skull is extended slightly and tilted to the patient's left, the face toward the right side, and the head elevated 10° to 15° from the operating table. The surgeon stands on the patient's right side (Fig. 2).

After the patient's head is fixed and before draping, the endotracheal tube is reevaluated for its security. Breath sounds over both lungs should be obtained again to be sure the endotracheal tube is above the carina (Fig. 3).

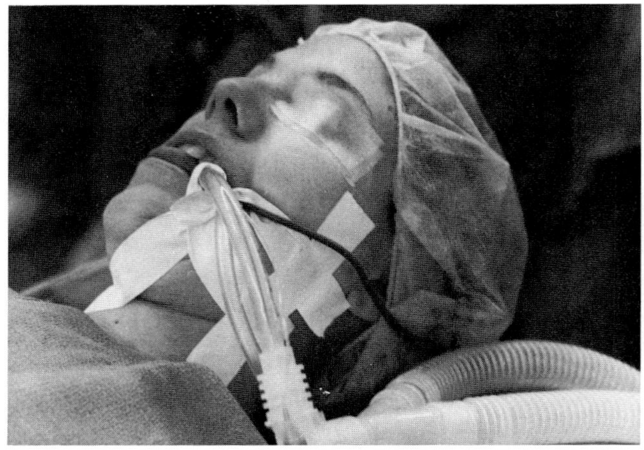

FIG. 1. After induction and intubation the patient's tube should be well taped at the left corner of the mouth with the esophageal stethoscope and temperature probe in place.

Emergence

After undraping the patient the pharyngeal area is suctioned for blood and secretions. Extubation is preferably done as soon as the patient's cough and gag reflexes have returned in order to avoid aspirating blood or blood clots. However, vigorous coughing should be avoided in order to avoid acute rises

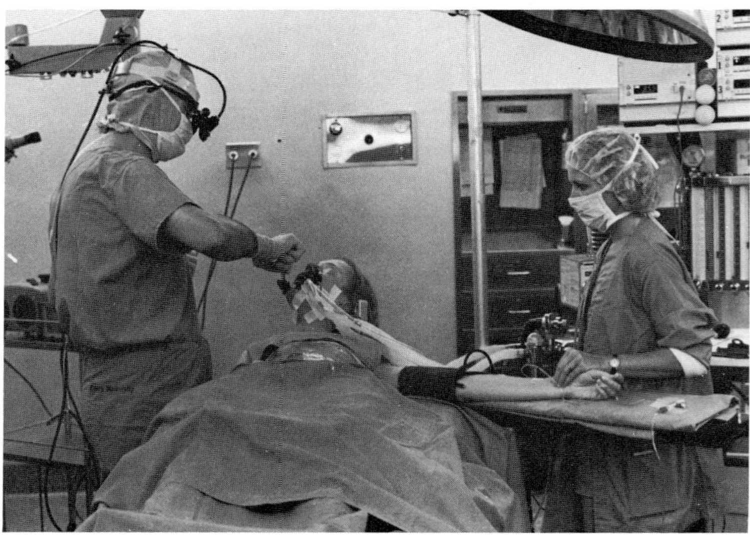

FIG. 2. The patient is positioned as such: the skull is extended slightly and tilted over to the patient's left, the face toward the right side with the head elevated 10° to 15° from the operating table as though he/she was looking at the surgeon's face.

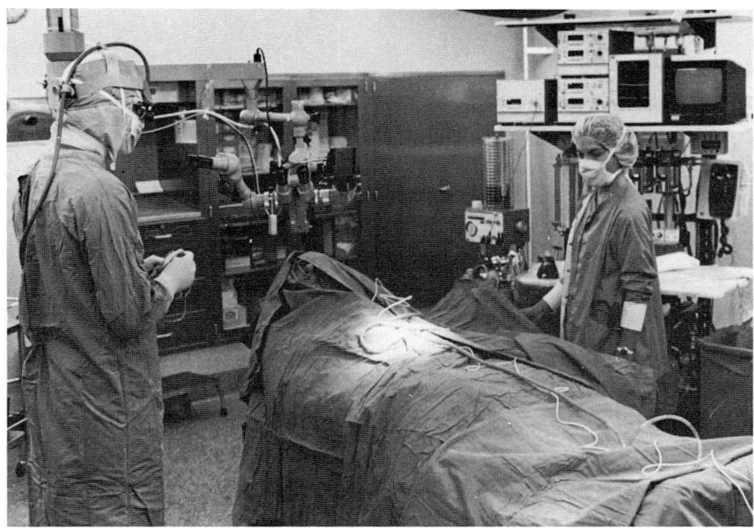

FIG. 3. Positions of surgeon, microscope, anesthesiologist, and anesthesia equipment in relation to the patient.

in intracranial pressure, which might result in detachment of the adipose tissue graft in the sella and sphenoid sinus thus predisposing to a CSF leak.

ANESTHETIC AGENTS OF CHOICE

Because of the uncomfortable positioning for the patient and length of the procedure (operating time varies from 2 to 4 hr), general anesthesia with endotracheal intubation is used in our institution for transsphenoidal pituitary surgery. Selection of the anesthetic agents was based primarily on the personal preference of the particular anesthesiologist who made preoperative rounds. These agents include halothane–N_2O–O_2, enflurane–N_2O–O_2, or balanced anesthesia (N_2O–narcotic–relaxants). The author's preference is enflurane–N_2O–O_2 anesthesia, as our experience indicates that the incidence of cardiac arrhythmias intraoperatively is approximately one-third as great with this anesthetic mixture as with halothane–N_2O–O_2.

MONITORING AND SPECIAL TECHNIQUE

Monitoring is important in any type of anesthetic management including neurosurgery (37). In transsphenoidal hypophysectomy patients the following parameters are monitored routinely:

1. Heart rate using the precordial stethoscope, which is changed to an esophageal stethoscope (55) after intubation

2. Indirect arterial blood pressure with the cuff on the patient's left arm
3. Temperature with temperature probe placed in the esophagus and taped at the left corner of the mouth with the esophageal stethoscope and endotracheal tube
4. Urinary output via Foley catheter
5. Respiration either assisted or controlled
6. Electrocardiograph, which permits recognition of arrhythmias, electrolyte imbalance, or myocardial ischemia in anesthetized patients (61)

In addition, in some patients a direct intra-arterial line is inserted for continuous blood pressure monitoring during intravenous infusion of peripheral vasodilators and for the determination of blood sugar, blood gases, or electrolytes. In patients who have diabetes insipidus (52), serum electrolytes and serum and urinary osmolarity should be monitored throughout the procedure. In patients who have severe heart disease, central venous line, pulmonary arterial pressure, and pulmonary wedge pressure (57) are also monitored.

Certain special monitoring such as intraoperative recording of visual evoked responses (62) was not performed in our series of approximately 350 cases. Although lumbar CSF drainage is not needed in transsphenoidal hypophysectomy, it may apply to the transcranial procedure for hypophysectomy (18,33, 39,41).

After emergence from anesthesia the first neurological examination usually takes place in the operating room. Pupillary size and reaction are checked as soon as the drapes are removed. Movement of all extremities is also briefly checked before transfer to the recovery room. After the patient is fully awake in the recovery room, further neurological examination is performed (38). Special techniques such as controlled hypotension (30) or hypothermia anesthesia (17,41) were not utilized in this group of patients.

FLUID, BLOOD, AND STEROID REPLACEMENT

Fluids

Balanced salt solution or 5% dextrose in balanced salt solution (5% dextrose in normal saline, 5% dextrose in Ringer's lactate solution) (40) is used for maintenance intravenous fluid throughout the procedure. Five percent dextrose in water is not used because it can increase CSF pressure to about twice that following administration of an equal volume of the salt solutions mentioned above (11). Diabetes insipidus occurs very rarely during surgery unless the condition existed prior to surgery as a consequence of the disease (e.g., craniopharyngioma), or it may become manifest 2 hr to a few days postoperatively. Fluid replacement in these cases is controversial. Shucart and Jackson (52) suggest that a dextrose in water solution should be used as the sole intravenous infusion, whereas Messick et al. (39) believe that a glucose infusion is contraindicated because it may induce osmotic diuresis in the diabetes insipidus patient.

Over the past 5 years we have used Ringer's lactate and 5% dextrose in 0.2 or 0.5 N saline solution to replace urine loss, insensible fluid loss, and mild blood loss. Serum electrolytes and osmolarity and urine osmolarity are closely monitored during surgery even though changes in serum electrolyte levels were reported not to occur (45). In severe cases vasopressin (Pitressin) may be used in small dosages.

Blood

Blood loss is minimal during surgery in these cases. For the anemic patient we usually transfuse one or two units of blood prior to surgery. Most patients do not require transfusion during surgery. For patients with normal hemoglobin and/or hematocrit the blood loss is usually less than 200 ml. Approximately 15% of patients require one unit of blood, and less than 3% require more.

Steroids

Steroid replacement and its importance are discussed elsewhere (1,25,42, 54,60). Patients with either hypopituitarism or hypoadrenal function have already been receiving steroids prior to surgery and generally require a large dose of steroid replacement during operation. In patients with normal pituitary function we follow a prescribed protocol for steroid replacement. A total of 100 mg hydrocortisone is administered intramuscularly as part of the preoperative medication. During surgery an additional 50 mg hydrocortisone is added to each liter of intravenous fluid. Beginning in the recovery room the patients receive 50 mg intramuscularly or intravenously every 8 hr throughout the second postoperative day. Thereafter steroid dosage depends on the operative procedure performed, e.g., hypophysectomy or pituitary tumor removal with sparing of pituitary gland.

COMPLICATIONS

1. Endotracheal tube kinking or cuff leakage: To date, we have had only one patient who had cuff leakage intraoperatively, and he developed pneumonia postoperatively due to CSF and blood aspiration. Five patients developed significant kinking of the endotracheal tube. Two were discovered before the surgery started, and so we were able to straighten the tube and redrape before surgery. Three were discovered during surgery, requiring that we hold the endotracheal tube throughout the rest of the procedure.
2. Cardiac arrhythmias: This was discussed above.

CONCLUSIONS

Transsphenoidal pituitary microsurgery is a relatively benign procedure with a low mortality and morbidity rate. The anesthetic management of this procedure is relatively simple. The success of this procedure is reliant on a group of physicians' teamwork, one of whom is the anesthesiologist. A good result comes from following certain practices: (a) carefully selecting the patients; (b) accurately identifying potential problems preoperatively; (c) maintaining good communication between the surgeon and the anesthesiologist pre-, intra-, and postoperatively; (d) adequately monitoring the patient during and after anesthesia; (e) having thorough familiarity with the anesthetic technique; and (f) providing sufficient blood, steroid, and fluid replacement pre-, intra-, and postoperatively.

REFERENCES

1. Ballantine, R. I. W. (1960): *General Anesthesia for Neurosurgery,* pp. 94–95. Little Brown, Boston.
2. Balzer, R., and McCullagh, E. P. (1959): Hypertension in acromegaly. *Am. J. Med. Sci.,* 237:449–452.
3. Beecher, H. K. (1940): The first anesthesia records (Codman, Cushing). *Surg. Gynecol. Obstet.,* 71:689–693.
4. Brunelle, J. P., and Lepage, C. (1964): Anæsthesia for transsphenoidal hypophysectomy. *Can. Anaesth. Soc. J.,* 11:101–103.
5. Byck, R. (1975): Drugs and the treatment of psychiatric disorders. In: *The Pharmacological Basis of Therapeutics,* ed. 5, edited by L. S. Goodman and A. Gilman, pp. 174–179. MacMillan, New York.
6. Cullen, D. J. (1971): The effect of pretreatment with nondepolarizing muscle relaxants on the neuromuscular blocking action of succinylcholine. *Anesthesiology,* 35:572–578.
7. Cushing, H. (1909): Partial hypophysectomy for acromegaly. *Ann. Surg.,* 50:1002–1017.
8. Cushing, H. (1914): Surgical experiences with pituitary disorders. *JAMA,* 63:1515–1525.
9. Dripps, R. D., Eckenhoff, J. E., and Vandam, L. D. (1977): *Introduction to Anesthesia. The Principles of Safe Practice,* pp. 11–21, 36–48. Saunders, Philadelphia.
10. Durshordwe, C. J. (1942): Anesthesia in neurosurgery. *Anesth. Analg.,* 21:61–74.
11. Fishman, R. A. (1953): Effects of isotonic intravenous solutions on normal and increased intracranial pressure. *Arch. Neurol. Psychiatry,* 70:350–360.
12. Friedman, M. A., Bozdech, M. D., Billingham, M. E., and Rider, A. K. (1978): Doxorubicin cardiotoxicity. *JAMA,* 240:1603–1606.
13. Gillespie, N. A. (1950): *Endotracheal Anesthesia,* ed. 2, p. 8. University of Wisconsin Press, Madison, Wisc.
14. Goldfine, I. D., and Lawrence, A. M. (1972): Hypopituitarism in acromegaly. *Arch. Intern. Med.,* 130:720–723.
15. Goldman, L., Caldera, D. L., Nussbaum, S. R., et al. (1977): Multifactorial index of cardiac risk in noncardiac surgical procedures. *N. Engl. J. Med.,* 297:845–850.
16. Gordon, D. A., Hill, F. M., and Ezrin, C. (1962): Acromegaly: A review of 100 cases. *Can. Med. Assoc. J.,* 87:1106–1109.
17. Gordon, E. (1975): Induced hypotension and hypothermia. *Monogr. Anesthesiol.* 2:219–238.
18. Gordon, E. (1975): The technique of reduction of the intracranial pressure. *Monogr. Anesthesiol.,* 2:209–218.
19. Hadfield, C. F. (1933): Discussion on anaesthesia in intracranial surgery. *Proc. R. Soc. Med.,* 26:953–958.
20. Hardy, J., and Ciric, I. S. (1968): Selective anterior hypophysectomy in the treatment of diabetic retinopathy. *JAMA,* 203:95–100.
21. Hassan, S. Z., Matz, G. J., Lawrence, A. M., and Collins, P. A. (1976): Laryngeal stenosis in acromegaly: A possible cause of airway difficulties associated with anesthesia. *Anesth. Analg.,* 55:57–60.
22. Hejtmancik, M. R., Bradfield, J. Y., Jr., and Herrmann, G. R. (1951): Acromegaly and the heart: A clinical and pathologic study. *Ann. Intern. Med.,* 34:1445–1456.
23. Henderson, W. R. (1939): The pituitary adenomata: A follow-up study of the surgical results in 338 cases (Dr. Harvey Cushing's series). *Br. J. Surg.,* 26:811–921.

24. Hirsch, E. Z., Sloman, J. G., and Martin, F. I. R. (1969): Cardiac function in acromegaly. *Am. J. Med. Sci.,* 257:1–8.
25. James, M. L. (1970): Endocrine disease and anaesthesia. *Anaesthesia,* 25:232–252.
26. Kaplan, J. A., Dunbar, R. W., and Jones, E. L. (1976): Nitroglycerin infusion during coronary-artery surgery. *Anesthesiology,* 45:14–21.
27. Kennedy, B. J., French, L. A., and Peyton, W. T. (1956): Hypophysectomy in advanced breast cancer. *N. Engl. J. Med.,* 255:1165–1172.
28. Keys, T. E. (1945): *The History of Surgical Anesthesia,* pp. 63–69. Schuman, New York.
29. Kitahata, L. M. (1971): Airway difficulties associated with anaesthesia in acromegaly. *Br. J. Anaesth.,* 43:1187–1190.
30. Larson, A. G. (1964): Deliberate hypotension. *Anesthesiology,* 25:682–706.
31. Luft, R., Olivecrona, H., Ikkos, D., et al. (1955): Hypophysectomy in man: Further experiences in severe diabetes mellitus. *Br. Med. J.,* 2:752–756.
32. Luft, R., Olivecrona, H., Ikkos, D., et al. (1958): Hypophysectomy in the management of metastatic cancer of the breast. In: *Endocrine Aspects of Breast Cancer,* edited by A. R. Currie, pp. 27–35. Livingstone, Edinburgh.
33. McComish, P. B., and Bodley, P. O. (1971): *Anesthesia for Neurological Surgery,* pp. 200–217. Year Book Medical Publishers, Chicago.
34. McCullagh, E. P., Clamen, M., and Gardener, W. J. (1957): Clinical progress in the treatment of exophthalmos of Graves' disease, with particular reference to the effect of pituitary surgery. *J. Clin. Endocrinol. Metab.,* 17:1277–1292.
35. McDowall, D. G. (1975): The influence of anaesthetic drugs and techniques on intracranial pressure. *Monogr. Anesthesiol.,* 2:135–170.
36. McGuffin, W. L. Jr., Sherman, B. M., Roth, J., et al. (1974): Acromegaly and cardiovascular disorders: A prospective study. *Ann. Intern. Med.,* 81:11–18.
37. Martin, J. T. (1973): Neurosurgery. *Clin. Anesth.,* 9:261–282.
38. Mayo Clinic and Mayo Foundation (1976): *Clinical Examinations in Neurology,* ed. 4. Saunders, Philadelphia.
39. Messick, J. M., Laws, E. R., and Abboud, C. F. (1978): Anesthesia for pituitary surgery. *Anesth. Analg.,* 57:206–215.
40. Michenfelder, J. D., Gronert, G. A., and Rehder, K. (1969): Neuroanesthesia. *Anesthesiology,* 30:65–100.
41. Michenfelder, J. D., Gronert, G. A., and Rehder, K. (1969): Anesthesia for neurosurgical procedures. *Clin. Anesth.,* 3:383–414.
42. Mushin, W. W. (1957): The adrenals and the anaesthetist. *Anaesthesia,* 12:15–29.
43. Pepine, C. J., and Aloia, J. (1970): Heart muscle disease in acromegaly. *Am. J. Med.,* 48:530–534.
44. Poznak, A. V. (1968): Anesthesia for surgery of the pituitary gland. In: *Clinical Anesthesia. Anesthesia for Patients with Endocrine Disease,* Vol. 3, edited by Jenkins, pp. 118–125. Davis, Philadelphia.
45. Randall, R. V., Clark, E. C., Dodge, H. W., Jr., and Love, J. G. (1960): Polyuria after operation for tumors in the region of the hypophysis and hypothalamus. *J. Clin. Endocrinol. Metab.,* 20:1614–1621.
46. Rinehart, J. J., Lewis, R. P., and Balcerzak, S. P. (1974): Adriamycin cardiotoxicity in man. *Ann. Intern. Med.,* 81:475–478.
47. Sachs, E. (1952): *The History and Development of Neurological Surgery,* 1st ed., p. 85. Hoeber, New York.
48. Schimek, R. A. (1956): Hypophysectomy for diabetic retinopathy: A preliminary report. *Arch. Ophthalmol.,* 56:416–425.
49. Scott, W. W. (1954): Role of pituitary in normal and abnormal prostatic growth. *Trans. Am. Assoc. Genitourin. Surg.,* 46:33–39.
50. Shapiro, H. M. (1975): Intracranial hypertension: Therapeutic and anesthetic considerations. *Anesthesiology,* 43:445–471.
51. Shapiro, H. M., and Aidinis, S. J. (1975): Neurosurgical anesthesia. *Surg. Clin. North Am.,* 55:913–928.
52. Shucart, W. A., and Jackson, I. (1976): Management of diabetes insipidus in neurosurgical patients. *J. Neurosurg.,* 44:65–71.
53. Silinková-Málková, E., and Kölbel, F. (1970): Relationship between symptoms of acromegaly and its complications, principally cardiovascular in 86 patients. *Acta Univ. Carol. [Med] (Praha),* 16:553–569.

54. Slaney, G., and Brooke, B. N. (1957): Postoperative collapse due to adrenal insufficiency following cortisone therapy. *Lancet,* 1:1167–1170.
55. Smith, C. (1954): An endo-oesophageal stethoscope. *Anesthesiology,* 15:566.
56. Souadjian, J. V., and Schirger, A. (1967): Hypertension in acromegaly. *Am. J. Med. Sci.,* 254:629–633.
57. Swan, H. J. C., Ganz, W., Forrester, J., et al. (1970): Catheterization of the heart in man with use of a flow-directed balloon-tipped catheter. *N. Engl. J. Med.,* 283:447–451.
58. Teuscher, A., Escher, F., Knoig, H., and Zahnd, G. (1970): Long-term effects of transsphenoidal hypophysectomy on growth hormone, renal function and eyeground in patients with diabetic retinopathy. *Diabetes,* 19:502–518.
59. Tindall, G. T., McLanahan, C. S., and Christy, J. H. (1977): Transsphenoidal microsurgery for pituitary tumors. *J. Med. Assoc. Ga.,* 66:951–957.
60. Tung, P. P., Randall, H. T., and Howland, W. S. (1956): The anesthetic management of hypophysectomized patients. *Anesthesiology,* 17:739–744.
61. VanderArk, G. D. (1974): Cardiovascular monitoring in neurosurgery. *Clin. Neurosurg.,* 22:462–475.
62. Wilson, W. B., Kirsch, W. M., Neville, H., et al. (1976): Monitoring of visual function during parasellar surgery. *Surg. Neurol.,* 5:323–329.

Clinical Management of Pituitary Disorders,
edited by G. T. Tindall and W. F. Collins.
Raven Press, New York © 1979.

25

Postoperative Management Following Pituitary Surgery

Earl A. Zimmerman

Department of Neurology, College of Physicians & Surgeons, Columbia University, New York, New York 10032

Fortunately the great majority of patients undergoing transsphenoidal surgery (e.g., those with prolactin-secreting microadenomas) do not have significant endocrine deficiency before or after surgery. Even among the otherwise healthy patients in this group, however, and especially in those with more advanced disease, there are important exceptions; these are the patients with abnormal thyroid and/or adrenal function. An adequate preoperative endocrine work-up such as outlined by Christy (Chapter 7) is necessary for planning postoperative management. If thyroid and adrenal function are significantly impaired before surgery, or if total hypophysectomy is performed, these hormones often require chronic replacement.

The intent of this chapter is to outline common problems encountered after pituitary surgery. They include transient and in some cases chronic diabetes insipidus, hypoadrenalism, hypothroidism, and in some cases persistent hypogonadism with or without hyperprolactinemia.

DIABETES INSIPIDUS

Diabetes insipidus is the most common endocrine abnormality following transsphenoidal pituitary surgery. In my experience with 50 patients with small prolactin-secreting adenomas, transient diabetes insipidus that lasted 1 to 5 days was found in about 25% undergoing surgery. It persisted for several weeks in 8%, and in 3 cases (6%) it lasted for months. In 1 patient, it lasted 1.5 years and then disappeared a few months after delivery of a spontaneous pregnancy. All 3 patients with prolonged vasopressin deficiency had normal anterior pituitary function, including return of menses and reduction of elevated serum prolactin levels to normal. A possible pathogenesis of this problem is discussed later. Tindall (16) reported an incidence of diabetes insipidus in 59% after transsphenoidal surgery which lasted long enough to require treatment with clofibrate in 27%; in 5% it was more persistent. Wilson and Dempsey (17) found a lower total number of patients with diabetes insipidus (9.2%); of these, 3.6% had partial and 2.0% had total persistent diabetes insipidus. Hardy reports elsewhere in this volume that 37% of patients undergoing total hypophysectomy developed diabetes insipidus.

Diabetes insipidus is generally a disorder of the hypothalamus and upper pituitary stalk. These areas should be spared by intrapituitary microsurgery. It has long been known that experimental diabetes insipidus requires a lesion of the supraoptic and paraventricular nuclei or their pathways in the median eminence or upper pituitary stalk. Nerve terminals on blood vessels in this area (15), recently confirmed by immunocytochemistry (8,18), can probably maintain adequate vasopressin secretion to the peripheral circulation. What then is the mechanism by which diabetes insipidus is produced by transsphenoidal surgery below the diaphragma sella (Table 1)? One can envision that the common occurrence of several days of transient diabetes insipidus may be caused by inadvertent gentle traction on the pituitary stalk and/or temporary disruption of its blood supply with transient functional loss of vasopressin secretion may occur. This transient functional diabetes insipidus may well be potentiated by high doses of glucocorticoids and relieved by their withdrawal after a few days since glucocorticoids inhibit vasopressin secretion. The late recovery after weeks or months may be due to regeneration of nerve terminals in the stalk, which is known to occur after damage in this region (15). One must postulate more than a functional lesion of the infundibulum in the persistent cases of diabetes insipidus. The problem with this postulated lesion in the infundibulum is the normality of the endocrine functions of the anterior pituitary observed in these patients which are regulated by releasing factor hormones of the (parvocellular) tuberoinfundibular system secreted into the hypophyseal portal system at this site. How could gonadotropin and therefore luteinizing hormone releasing hormone be intact in the three patients I described? In these patients there must have been a selective disturbance of the (magnocellular) supraoptic–paraventricular neurosecretory system. At present it is suspected, but not proved, that the accepted practice of absolute alcohol instillation into the tumor bed at surgery, presumed to destroy residual tumor cells, may cause a selective disturbance of the magnocellular system. These neurons are normally sensitive to alcohol,

TABLE 1. *Operative causes of diabetes insipidus*

1. Destruction or trauma to upper stalk or supraoptic nuclei
2. Usually recovers
   Days—"stalk shock"
   Weeks—regeneration
   Months to years—?regeneration
3. Potentiation by steroid therapy
4. Possible role of instilled alcohol in tumor bed?

which inhibits vasopressin secretion, and inadvertent dissection of the drug upward (12) might selectively destroy them. Alternatively, instilled alcohol reaching magnocellular nerve fiber terminals in the posterior pituitary might destroy these neurons. These considerations are at present speculative, but the clinical paradox and the annoyance of diabetes insipidus demands further observation and experimentation. Closer evaluation of patients after pituitary surgery for functional diabetes insipidus (14) is likely to reveal an even higher incidence than is currently appreciated.

MANAGEMENT OF POSTOPERATIVE DIABETES INSIPIDUS

Frank diabetes insipidus is usually easy to recognize (4,13). There is a sudden increase in urinary volume (Table 2), greater than 150 ml/hr, with a low accompanying osmolality of the urine. Although it may be noted during the intraoperative period, its appearance is most often delayed for 12 to 24 hr after pituitary surgery. Other causes of polyuria (e.g., excessive hydration or severe glycosuria) are easily recognized. The urine volume is determined hourly and insensible loss replaced; short-acting aqueous vasopressin (Pitressin) is generally used at this time. Urine specific gravity or osmolality and plasma electrolytes and osmolality are checked at appropriate intervals. It is best to let patients who are not very ill and can take oral fluids regulate their own intake and water balance. As soon as possible, remove their intravenous fluids and taper the glucocorticoids. By the second or third postoperative day, the polyuria and polydipsia have usually attenuated to several liters a day and do not require treatment. As a general principle, it is best not to overuse vasopressin if the patient can regulate his own fluids. In this situation the diabetes insipidus is more of an annoyance.

In those in whom major diabetes insipidus persists, Pitressin Tannate in Oil (2.5 to 5.0 IU) can provide relief for 24 to 36 hr. Clofibrate or chlorpropamide are oral agents that can be used to ameliorate significant persistent partial diabetes insipidus (Table 3). The patient must have some of his own secretion of vasopressin to be further stimulated by these drugs. Chlorpropamide may cause hypoglycemia, and this should be watched for if the drug is used. Intranasal prepara-

TABLE 2. *Postoperative diabetes insipidus*

1. Polyuria (3–15 liters/24 hr; 150 ml/hr); other causes = usually less output
2. Low urine osmolality; 1.001–1.005 specific gravity ($<$200 mOsm/kg); (1.008–1.014 = 300–400 mOsm; 1.020 = $>$800 mOsm)
   Increased plasma osmolality (NL 286–294); Na increased; to calculate osmolality: 2 × Na + (G/18) + (BUN/2.5)
3. Appears 12–24 hr; rule out overhydration, glycosuria
4. Replace last hourly output and insensible loss (25 ml/hr)
5. Aqueous vasopressin 5 IU i.m. q 4–6 hr
6. Encourage patient to regulate own fluids

Na = sodium. G = glucose. BUN = blood urea nitrogen. NL = normal range.

TABLE 3. *Postoperative diabetes insipidus*

1. Common a few days after transsphenoidal surgery, occasionally weeks, rarely months or years
2. Treatment of choice: DDAVP 10–20 μg/day or b.i.d.
3. Lysine vasopressin (LVP) nasal spray—often rhinitis
4. Pitressin Tannate in Oil 0.5 ml (5 units/ml) q 2 days
5. Chlorpropamide 250 mg/day or b.i.d.; carbamazepine, clofibrate

tions of vasopressin, of course, should be avoided immediately after transsphenoidal surgery. We have found, however, that gentle instillation of 1-desamino-8-D-arginine vasopressin (DDAVP) (7) can be used safely after the first week with great benefit. Unlike lysine vasopressin nasal spray, DDAVP has no smooth-muscle-constricting effects, obviating the usual complaints of nasal irritation and dryness with lysine vasopressin.

TRIPHASIC DIABETES INSIPIDUS

Triphasic diabetes insipidus is an unusual pattern of postoperative diabetes insipidus that may occur after operations in the region of the pituitary stalk (2,13). After several days of diabetes insipidus, it suddenly disappears to be replaced by the syndrome of inappropriate secretion of antidiuretic hormone (SIADH) (12) originating from degenerating transected nerve terminals to the posterior gland (Table 4). Polydipsia disappears, and the urine output falls with a concomitant increase in urine osmolality usually greater than 700 mOsm. If unanticipated, the patient may rapidly become water-intoxicated and severely hyponatremic on parenteral fluids (10).

The condition may be expected after pituitary stalk transection or operations in that region, e.g., removal of a craniopharyngioma or some other suprasellar lesion. We have not yet seen it after microadenoma surgery, but in some instances it might be expected to occur with drugs such as chlorpropamide (2).

If severe water intoxication occurs with mental changes or seizures, fluid restriction alone is inadequate as therapy, and furosemide diuresis with electrolyte replacement (3% NaCl) should be instituted (5). Several days of inappropri-

TABLE 4. *Triphasic diabetes insipidus*

1. Follows several days after postoperative diabetes insipidus
2. Excess of AVP from degenerating nerve terminals (form of SIADH)
3. Anticipate especially after operating around the pituitary stalk—prevent by avoiding excess intake
4. Hyponatremia (plasma hyposmolality), inappropriately increased urinary osmolality (>700 mOsm)
5. Treatment of SIADH: for a mild case, fluid restricted to 1 liter/day; for a severe case, furosemide and 3% NaCl
6. Disappears within days; may be replaced with total, partial, or no diabetes insipidus

ate vasopressin secretion is usually followed by reappearance of diabetes insipidus, which may be transient or permanent.

POSTOPERATIVE GLUCOCORTICOIDS

If the pituitary–adrenal axis is normal before microadenoma surgery, in most cases it is normal afterward. Tindall et al. (16) reported 2 of 37 patients in whom it was abnormal. It is our practice to taper rapidly the high-dose dexamethasone (16 mg/day) commonly employed in these patients during and right after surgery to maintenance levels (0.75 mg) (Table 5) by the third or fourth day; in this way we can observe the patients for clinical evidence of adrenal insufficiency for several days prior to discharge. This schedule also reduces the incidence of glucose intolerance and the potentiating effects of the steroid on diabetes insipidus (Table 6). Furthermore, treatment with glucocorticoids for less than a week is usually not associated with adrenal suppression. The tapering schedule is delayed if the patient is not doing well for a variety of reasons and must be tailored to the particular patient. At some centers patients are routinely discharged on replacement glucocorticoids (25 mg cortisone per day) until postoperative evaluation is carried out a month or so later (17). The peripheral thyroid hormone level a week after surgery can provide some indication of the state of the anterior pituitary gland (Tables 6 and 7). This can be obtained just before discharge, and if it is in the normal range we do not usually discharge the patient on replacement medication. Patients operated on for Cushing's disease usually require larger than normal replacement steroid doses for several months (6). An ACTH stimulation test or a 24-hr urinary collection for adrenal steroids can be done at this time or later as a guide to the need for therapy if there is any doubt. The possibility of a need for steroids and the symptoms of insufficiency are discussed with the patient and family when leaving the hospital; the patient is given cortisone tablets and the physician's telephone number in case of an emergency.

Patients with preoperative pituitary–adrenal insufficiency usually have more advanced disease, often have thyroid insufficiency, and require replacement ste-

TABLE 5. *Adrenal steroid preparations*

Steroid	Potency relative to cortisol: Glucocorticoid	Potency relative to cortisol: Mineralocorticoid	Replacement dose (approximate) (mg)
Cortisol	1	1	20
Cortisone	0.7	0.7	25
Prednisone	4	0.7	5
Dexamethasone	30	2	0.75
Fluorocortisone[a]	10	400	—

[a]No need to replace in pituitary failure.

TABLE 6. *Postoperative glucocorticoids*

1. Glucose intolerance on high-dose steroids
2. Aggravation of diabetes insipidus
3. Treatment for a week or less does not require tapering
4. Ambulatory and off steroids a day or two before discharge
5. Anticipate glucocorticoid replacement if thyroid requires replacement

TABLE 7. *Postoperative thyroid function*

1. Half-time of T_4 is 6.7 days
   A. Often a fall in T_3 and T_4 within a week
   B. Often rises again a week or two later; may wait for this prior to committing to thyroid (and adrenal) replacement
2. Dilantin lowers T_4 (not more than 1 μg/ml)
3. Desiccated thyroid 1–2 grains; L-thyroxine 0.1–0.2 mg

roids after surgery. There are occasional exceptions to this rule among patients with small tumors (16). In these patients and those subjected to total hypophysectomy, the high-dose steroids are tapered to replacement levels, which are adjusted when the patient is fully ambulant prior to discharge. Thyroid replacement is never given without full assessment of adrenal reserve, as institution of thyroid therapy increases the need for adrenal hormone and may precipitate an adrenal crisis. When thyroid replacement is needed, adrenal replacement is usually required as well. Patients receiving adrenal replacement should always be appraised of the probable need for additional hormones in times of stress.

THYROID HORMONE

Like adrenal replacement, thyroid hormone therapy is usually not needed after microadenoma surgery. A slight fall of the peripheral T_3 and T_4 to the borderline low normal range is often noted in these patients a week postoperatively (Table 7). It usually rises to normal a week later. This probably reflects a transient disturbance in pituitary thyroid-stimulating hormone (TSH) function around the time of surgery since the half-time of T_4 is about a week. If thyroid values remain low, and the T_4 is not falsely low due to the use of phenytoin, for example, thyroid and adrenal function should be fully reassessed for the possible need for replacement therapy. Patients requiring thyroid medication before surgery or those who had a total hypophysectomy are usually started on replacement thyroid as soon as they can take oral medications. As in the case of pituitary ACTH deficiency, an occasional patient with a small pituitary adenoma may have return of TSH function after microsurgery (16).

LONGER-RANGE FOLLOW-UP

Samples for one or more of the hypersecreted hormones (prolactin, growth hormone, ACTH), when appropriate, are obtained prior to discharge, and the hormone levels are followed at regular intervals afterward. Reduction of the blood level to normal is a good indication of total removal. Consistent and progressive evidence of hypersecretion can be a useful warning of persistent or recurrent tumor. However, one should be aware that a single high value may reflect a laboratory error or simply a variation of its concentration in blood at that particular instant. For example, prolactin values occasionally vary from normal to several times normal in patients with or without tumor obtained on the same or consecutive days. Elevated basal growth hormone values should be tested with glucose suppression in the acromegalic patient. A return of the diurnal rhythm of cortisol is a good indication that Cushing's disease has been cured (6).

The patient is usually seen about a week or 10 days after discharge from the hospital. Visual fields and acuities are retested and their clinical status reassessed. Headaches are usually not a problem, although there may be minor nasal congestion or fullness, which soon disappears. Galactorrhea or some acromegalic features previously present may have improved. General well-being and water intake are reassessed. Blood samples are obtained to test for anemia, and thyroid hormones are measured to reassess the need for, or the amount of, replacement needed. The amount and timing of cortisone administration is assessed clinically. Cortisone acetate 12.5 mg twice a day is appropriate for most adults, although larger individuals may need a total dose of 37.5 mg/day. There is a danger of producing Cushing's syndrome with larger doses of cortisone. Mineralocorticoid replacement is not needed in ACTH deficiency.

The patient is usually seen again about a month later, at which time endocrine function is retested (this is about 6 weeks after surgery) (17). By this time, menses might have returned, although they may not appear for another several months if at all. If thyroid function has been borderline without therapy, it and adrenal function are retested. The adrenal response to ACTH stimulation is a useful test in this situation. Gonadotropins, prolactin level, and testosterone assay in males may also be useful guides at this time if clinically warranted. The sperm count is the most sensitive test of fertility in the male, and menstrual cycles with evidence of ovulation in the female (temperature rise at midcycle or progesterone elevation at late cycle). Gonadotropin (luteinizing hormone, follicle-stimulating hormone) concentrations are frequently in the normal range in pituitary hypogonadism. The appearance of infertility in men who desire children should be actively sought because, once established, it is much more difficult to treat than in women. It often requires gonadotropin administration. Testosterone propionate, about 200 mg i.m. once a week for 3 weeks and then every 2 to 3 weeks, may improve libido and sexual performance.

If menses do not return by 6 months after microadenoma removal and a pregnancy is desired, the present trend is to employ bromergocriptine (3) 2.5 mg two or three times a day. In this situation there is usually persistent hyperprolactinemia and probably residual tumor. The drug is a dopamine agonist and thereby acts as a prolactin-inhibiting factor, which is probably dopamine. Inhibition of prolactin permits return of fertility in a majority of women. The decision to induce fertility with drugs (e.g., parenteral gonadotropins) is best made in concert with an obstetrician–gynecologist expert. Some neurosurgeons elect to reoperate for residual tumor if hyperprolactinemia persists. The neurosurgeon or neurologist should continue to follow the pregnant patient with a probable pituitary tumor as there is some risk of reversible swelling of the pituitary during the pregnancy (3,9,11). Headache and visual field disturbances due to pressure upward from the sella are the usual problem, although lateral pressure occasionally causes cranial nerve deficits, e.g., extraocular muscle palsies. The true incidence of such complications of pregnancy in patients with a pituitary adenoma is not yet fully known; a reasonable estimate from the literature is 3 to 5%, although it may be greater (3). If these problems occur, they can be treated by high-dose steroids (11), transsphenoidal surgery (9), or possibly bromergocriptine (3). The problem may disappear a few days after delivery probably owing to reduction of circulating estrogens, which cause the pituitary to enlarge in pregnancy (11).

Most patients are seen at 3-month intervals the first year after surgery and, if stable, every 6 or 12 months thereafter. Evaluation of visual fields, thyroid function, and measurement of the previous hypersecreted hormone comprise the minimal work-up. In some patients visual problems or hypopituitarism may appear months or years after treatment, which may not be appreciated in the early stages. Tomography of the sella is not usually a useful routine follow-up tool. In my opinion lateral coned-down X-ray views of the sella about every 2 years are just as useful in most instances.

COMMENT

What I outlined in this chapter is one approach to the patient after pituitary surgery. The management of pituitary tumor is in a state of evolution. What therapy we chose as the best today may differ a year or more from now. Which microadenomas to remove and when, or whether to reoperate for persistent prolactin-secreting tumor or even to irradiate are not settled issues. We do not know the natural history of the prolactinomas, which radioimmunoassay and polytomography have allowed us to discover in recent years (1). Are these early forms of the same tumors associated with visual disturbance and hypopituitarism? How many untreated or partially removed microadenomas will become troublesome to the patient in later years? In retrospect, we know that some of these have been present in patients for 25 years or more without much effect. Some of these women even had children without treatment, whereas others developed visual and further endocrine problems. The lack of information about the natural history and pathogenesis of prolactinomas has led to a "wait and see" attitude in many medical centers concerning treatment. The availability of bromergocriptine recently provided a more-simple, inexpensive means of establishing fertility in hyperprolactinemic individuals. Some of these patients who have not had surgery or radiation therapy will have trouble during pregnancy, but how many and how severe the problem will be remains to be seen. This approach must be balanced against the small complication rate of surgery and the recurrence rate, which is not yet known. In any case, we will probably have a group of untreated microadenomas to follow but will not have the answers for many years to come.

ACKNOWLEDGMENTS

The author thanks his colleagues at Columbia University, Drs. Peter Carmel and Edgar Housepian (neurosurgery), Donald Holub and Andrew Frantz (endocrinology), and Rapheal Jewelewicz and Raymond VandeWiele (obstetrics and gynecology); our patients for the experience provided in this chapter; and Cindy Topping for assistance with the manuscript.

REFERENCES

1. Antunes J. L., Housepian, E. M., Frantz, A. G., Holub, D. A., Hui, R. M., Carmel, P. W., and Quest, D. O. (1977): Prolactin-secreting pituitary tumors. *Ann. Neurol.,* 2:148–153.
2. Bartter, F. C. (1973): The syndrome of inappropriate secretion of antidiuretic hormone (SIADH). *Disease-A-Month,* November, pp. 1–47.
3. Bergh, T., Nillius, S. J., and Wide, L. (1978): Clinical course and outcome of pregnancies in amenorrheic women with hyperprolactinaemia and pituitary tumors. *Br. Med. J.,* 1:875–880.
4. Berl, T., Anderson, R. J., McDonald, K. M., and Schrier, R. W. (1976): Clinical disorders of water metabolism. *Kidney Int.,* 10:117–132.
5. Beroniade, V., Leblanc, P., and Beaupre, A. (1977): Oral furosemide and NaCl supplements in chronic treatment of inappropriate secretion of antidiuretic hormone (SIADH). *Kidney Int.,* 12:462.
6. Carmalt, M. H. B., Dalton, G. A., Fletcher, R. G., and Smith, W. J. (1977): The treatment of Cushing's disease by transsphenoidal hypophysectomy. *Q. J. Med.,* 46:119–134.
7. Cobb, W. E., Spare, S., and Reichlin, S. (1978): Neurogenic diabetes insipidus: Management with dDAVP (1-desamino-8-D arginine vasopressin). *Ann. Intern. Med.,* 88:183–188.
8. Defendini, R., and Zimmerman, E. A. (1978): The magnocellular system of the mammalian hypothalamus. In: *The Hypothalamus,* edited by S. Reichlin, R. J. Baldessarini, and J. B. Martin, pp. 137–154. Raven Press, New York.
9. Falconer, M. A., and Stafford-Bell, M. A. (1975): Visual failure from pituitary and parasellar tumors occurring with favorable outcome in pregnant women. *J. Neurol. Neurosurg. Psychiatry,* 38:919–930.
10. Hantman, D., Rossier, B., Zohlman, R., and Schrier, R. (1973): Rapid correction of hyponatremia in the syndrome of inappropriate secretion of antidiuretic hormone. *Ann. Intern. Med.,* 78:870–875.
11. Jewelewicz, R., Zimmerman, E. A., and Carmel, P. W. (1977): Conservative management of a pituitary tumor during pregnancy following induction of ovulation with gonadotropins. *Fertil. Steril.,* 28:35–40.
12. Lipton, S., Miles, J., Williams, N., and Jones, N. B. (1978): Pituitary injection of alcohol for widespread cancer pain. *Pain,* 5:73–82.
13. Martin, J. B., Reichlin, S., and Brown, G. M. (1977): Neural regulation of water and salt metabolism: Physiologic function and disease. In: *Clinical Neuroendocrinology,* pp. 63–92. Davis, Philadelphia.
14. Miller, M., Dalakos, T., Moses, A. M., Fellerman, H., and Streeten, D. H. P. (1970): Recognition of partial defects in antidiuretic hormone secretion. *Ann. Intern. Med.,* 73:721–729.
15. Rothballer, A. B., and Skoryna, S. C. (1960): Morphological effects of pituitary stalk section in the dog with particular reference to neurosecretory material. *Anat. Rec.,* 136:5–25.

16. Tindall, G. T., McLanahan, C. S., and Christy, J. M. (1978): Transsphenoidal microsurgery for pituitary tumors associated with hyperprolactinemia. *J. Neurosurg.,* 48:849–860.
17. Wilson, C. B., and Dempsey, L. C. (1978): Transsphenoidal microsurgical removal of 250 pituitary adenomas. *J. Neurosurg.,* 48:13–22.
18. Zimmerman, E. A., and Robinson, A. G. (1976): Hypothalamic neurons secreting vasopressin and neurophysin. *Kidney Int.,* 10:12–24.

Clinical Management of Pituitary Disorders,
edited by G. T. Tindall and W. F. Collins.
Raven Press, New York © 1979.

26

Complications of Transsphenoidal Surgery

Edward R. Laws Jr. and Eugene B. Kern

Departments of Neurologic Surgery and Otorhinolaryngology, Mayo Clinic, Mayo Medical School, Rochester, Minnesota 55901

In 1910 Halstead reported two patients operated on for pituitary tumor via the transsphenoidal approach (6). One of these patients died shortly after surgery with symptoms suggestive of hypothalamic damage; this constitutes the first known complication of transsphenoidal surgery. It is noteworthy that several large series of pituitary tumors treated by transsphenoidal surgery began during the first two decades of the twentieth century when neither antibiotic therapy nor cortisol replacement were available to document the efficacy of this operative approach in terms of results, complications, and mortality rates.

Cushing used the transsphenoidal approach between 1909 and 1928 with a 5.4% mortality rate in some 242 cases (8). Hirsch had a career of performing transsphenoidal surgery that extended from 1910 through 1962, with an overall mortality rate less than 5% in 425 cases (9). Dott used the transsphenoidal approach throughout his neurosurgical career, and it was from Dott that Guiot learned the technique. Guiot (3) and Hardy (7) currently have series of over 1,000 patients operated on transsphenoidally, and each has a mortality rate close to 1%.

CATEGORIES OF COMPLICATIONS

Intracranial Complications

The hypothalamus may be injured by direct trauma or secondary vascular effects. The characteristic clinical course of coma and high fever is usually irreversible. Intracranial hemorrhage, in the form of an organized hematoma or subarachnoid bleeding, may occur, causing varying degrees of neurologic dysfunction or fatality. Branches of the circle of Willis may be injured, and symptomatic cerebral vasospasm may develop. Meningitis may develop if the subarachnoid space is contaminated by oronasal flora during surgery or later if a cerebrospinal fluid (CSF) leak is present. A large tumor extension into

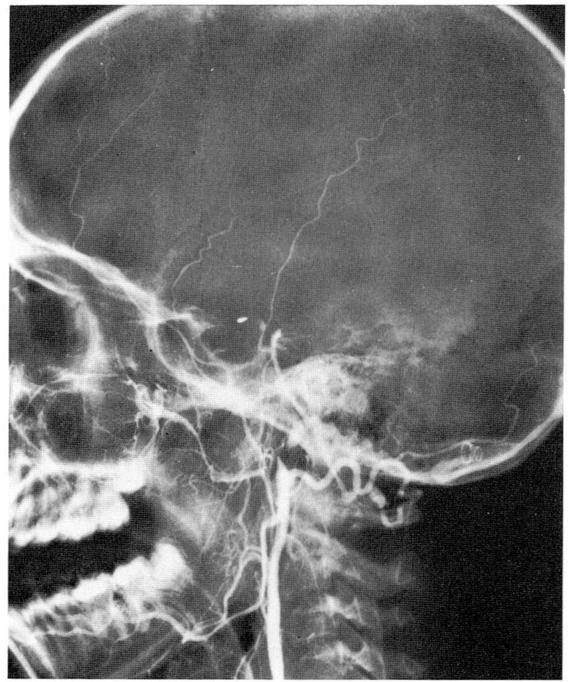

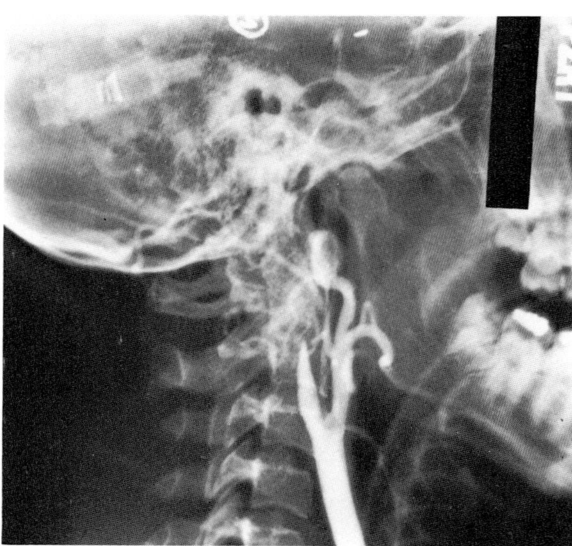

FIG. 1. Craniopharyngioma. Postoperative fatal vascular occlusion. Note obstruction of both internal carotid arteries and filling of the basilar artery via the occipital artery.

the anterior or middle cranial fossa is a relative contraindication to the transsphenoidal route, and complications may develop from tumor nodules that are inaccessible from this approach.

Carotid Artery Complications

Laceration, avulsion, and/or perforation of the cavernous carotid artery is a potential cause of either serious complications or death. Arterial hemorrhage from the carotid may be difficult to control without interfering with distal flow. Dissection against the walls of the cavernous sinus may provoke immediate or delayed vascular occlusion, thrombosis, spasm, and/or embolus formation (Figs. 1 and 2). Tortuous carotid arteries which course within the sella are occasionally present and if unrecognized may be injured. Likewise, a carotid aneurysm may simulate, or coexist with, a pituitary tumor (10,12,16), and this is why preoperative cerebral angiography is recommended for many patients. Delayed carotid artery complications in the form of carotid-cavernous fistula or false aneurysm may occur and may be difficult to correct.

Visual Complications

The optic nerves and chiasm may be injured directly (Fig. 3) or secondarily through vascular effects. Compression of these structures may develop as a

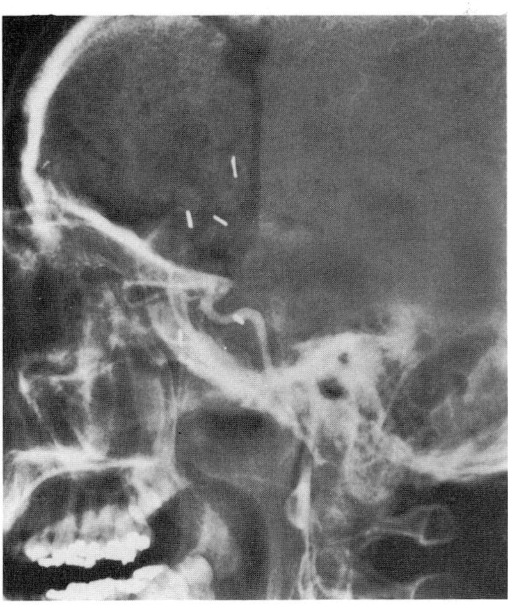

FIG. 2. Nonfunctioning pituitary adenoma. Postoperative vascular occlusion of the supraclinoidal left internal carotid artery.

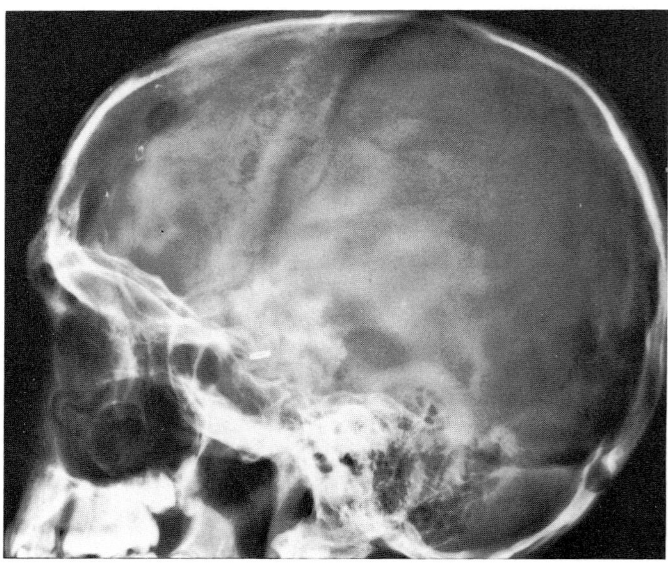

FIG. 3. Craniopharyngioma. Visual loss followed an unsuccessful attempt at removal of this large calcified tumor.

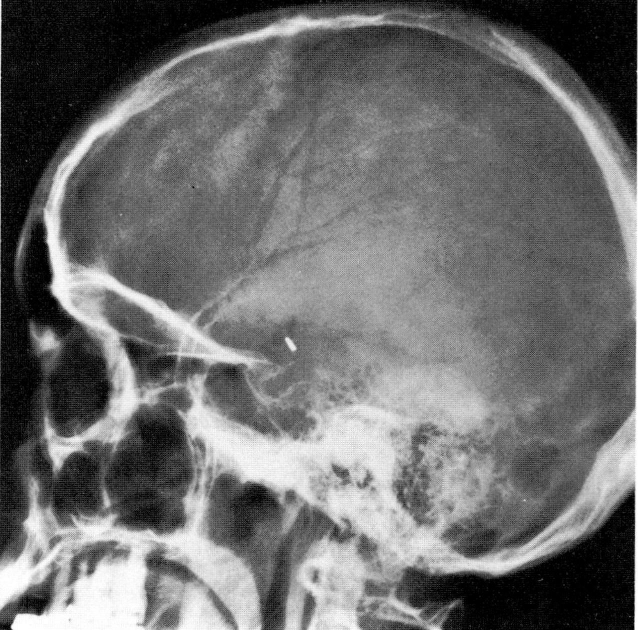

FIG. 4. Nonfunctioning pituitary adenoma. Transient visual loss was caused by the muscle graft used to fill the tumor cavity. The clip is on the muscle.

result of postoperative hematoma extending to the suprasellar space as well as by inadvertent suprasellar extension of the muscle or fat graft used to pack the sella following tumor removal (Fig. 4). If the empty sella is not adequately filled with muscle or fat, the chiasm may prolapse into the sella with resulting visual impairment. Aggressive use of the transsphenoidal speculum and spreader may result in fracture of the base of the skull through the optic foramen, resulting in blindness.

Cavernous Sinus Complications

Venous hemorrhage may occur as a result of violation of the walls of the cavernous sinus or from injury to the connections between the two cavernous sinuses. If the operating position calls for the patient's head to be elevated, venous air embolism may occur (13). The 3rd, 4th, 5th, and 6th cranial nerves traverse the cavernous sinus, and any of these may be injured during intrasellar dissection, with the most common injuries affecting the 3rd and 6th nerves. Fortunately, the resultant palsies are usually transient.

Sellar Complications

The most common problems related to the sella are CSF rhinorrhea related to either violation or incompetency of the diaphragma sellae. A poorly pneumatized sphenoid sinus can pose a major problem in exposure (Figs. 5 and 6), requiring the use of a drill and the image intensifier (1). Excessive enlargement

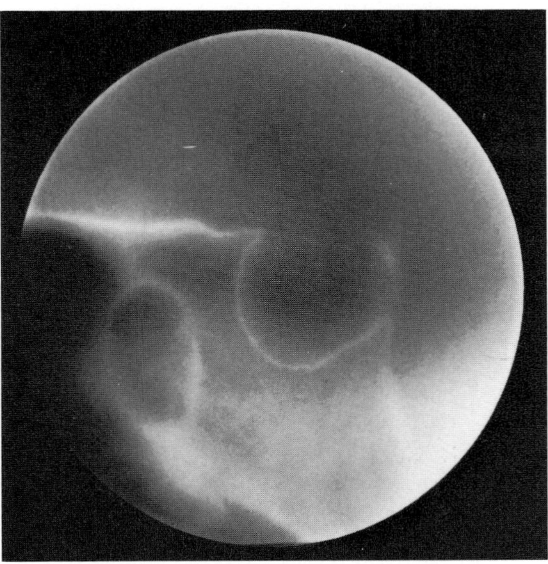

FIG. 5. Poorly pneumatized sphenoid. Exposure of the sella is difficult.

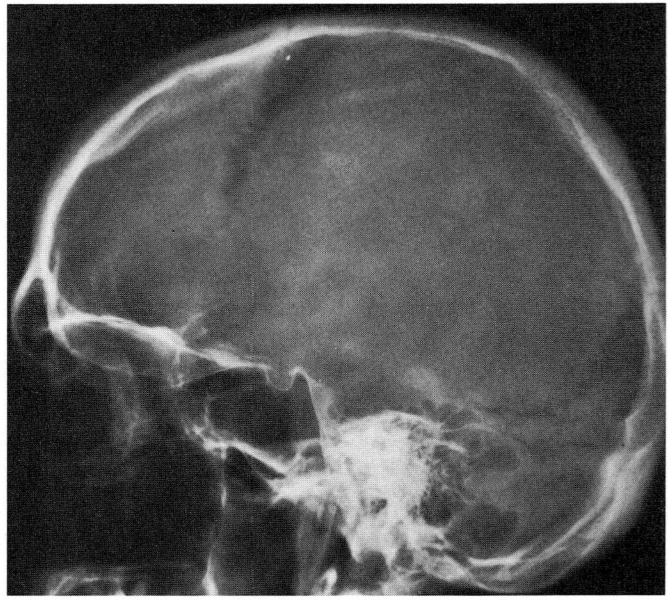

FIG. 6. Highly pneumatized, delicate sphenoid fracture may occur.

or erosion of the sella from large intrasellar lesions has been recognized as a predisposing factor to complications, usually hemorrhage (2,4,5,15).

Sphenoid Complications

Inaccurate insertion and overzealous spreading of the transsphenoidal speculum may result in significant problems. If inserted at an incorrect angle, the speculum may guide the surgeon through the floor of the anterior fossa rather than the sphenoid and sella, leading to potential intracranial damage or CSF rhinorrhea. Use of the speculum spreader may produce diastasis of the hard palate as well as fracture of facial bones and/or the cribriform plate. The mucosa of the sphenoid sinus may be responsible for postoperative complications of sinusitis and/or mucocele (14).

Nasal Complications

Postoperative nasal problems may be grouped into two categories: functional and cosmetic. Functional disturbances include olfactory dysfunction and/or nasal respiratory obstruction. Technical difficulties with the dissection of the nasal mucosa may lead to symptomatic nasal septal perforation, with crusting, epistaxis, nasal airway obstruction, chronic superficial infection, loss of cartilage, and the inevitable saddle nose deformity. Inadequate hemostasis during surgery may lead to extensive facial swelling, ecchymosis, and postoperative epistaxis. Cosmetic complications are usually related to excessive resection of the anterior nasal spine and septal cartilage. Despite experience and care, the vagaries of scar formation may produce nasal tip deformities (Fig. 7), sagging, or saddle nose deformity with widening of the base of the nose. Usually the cosmetic imperfections are preventable and the functional dysfunctions treatable. Nasal airway obstruction can usually be corrected by reoperation with restructuring of septal components. Olfactory dysfunction is rare, occurring in only one patient; however, it is annoying and "impossible" to repair. Symptomatic septal perforations (six patients) can be repaired by flap techniques using neighboring tissues, although we favor a nonsurgical closure using a Silastic septal button, which is frequently successful.

Endocrinologic Complications

Acute symptomatic hypopituitarism may occur in patients not properly prepared for the stress of pituitary surgery. Diabetes insipidus may develop after

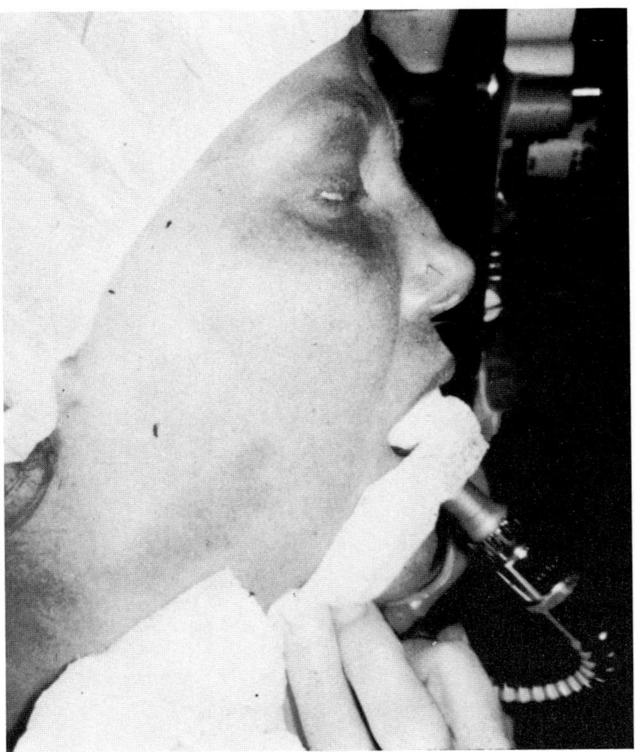

FIG. 7. Nelson–Salassa syndrome. Nasal deformity followed transsphenoidal surgery elsewhere.

manipulation of the posterior pituitary gland and/or the infundibulum and, if inadequately managed, may lead to serious electrolyte imbalance. Diabetes insipidus usually is transient. Patients with Cushing's disease and acromegaly have a tendency to bleed more vigorously than others, rarely forcing abandonment of the surgical procedure. One should always be alert for patients with one of the multiple endocrine neoplasia (MEN) syndromes as, postoperatively, associated endocrinologic problems (i.e., hyperparathyroidism, diabetes mellitus) may occur and complicate management of the patient.

MAYO CLINIC EXPERIENCE

Between November 1, 1972 and August 31, 1978, 505 transsphenoidal procedures were performed on 489 patients (Table 1). The majority of the patients were treated for pituitary adenoma, and only a small number had undergone hypophysectomy as an ablative procedure.

The seven fatalities are listed in Table 2. These were related to technical errors in three cases and to less-avoidable factors in the others. There were four instances of vascular occlusion, producing one immediate and one late fatality (Table 3). The two patients with fatal intracerebral hemorrhage and

TABLE 1. *Transsphenoidal surgery: Mayo Clinic 1972–1978*

Indication	No. of patients	No. of operative procedures
Pituitary adenoma		
"Nonfunctioning" adenomas	135	138
Acromegaly	99	101
Prolactin adenomas	108	109
Cushing's disease	35	35
Nelson–Salassa syndrome	21	23
FSH adenoma	1	1
TSH adenoma	1	1
Total	400	408
Craniopharyngioma	23	26
Chordoma	8	9
Hypophysectomy—cancer	14 (15)[a]	15
Hypophysectomy—diabetic retinopathy	3 (4)	3 (4)
Empty sella	13 (15)	14
CSF rhinorrhea (primary)	3	3
CSF rhinorrhea (secondary)	(7)	(7)
Other (miscellaneous)	25	27
Total no.	489	505
Mortality	7 (1.43%)	

[a]Numbers in parentheses represent number of procedures.
FSH = follicle-stimulating hormone. TSH = thyroid-stimulating hormone.

TABLE 2. *Postoperative fatalities with transsphenoidal surgery: Mayo Clinic 1972–1978*[a]

Cause of death	Pituitary adenomas	All cases
Hypothalamic injury	1	1
Meningitis		1
CSF leak, meningitis		1
Carotid artery injury	1	1
Intracranial hematoma	2	2
Vascular occlusion, circle of Willis		1
Total	4	7

[a]Total of 489 patients, 505 procedures.

the two who lost vision following intracerebral hemorrhage had very large tumors, and complications might have been avoided had they been managed by the transcranial route. Three of these four patients had previously undergone craniotomy as treatment for the tumor.

CSF rhinorrhea and meningitis are now rare complications and are seldom fatal. Table 4 lists the common complications seen with transsphenoidal surgery. Subarachnoid hemorrhage may occur regardless of whether the diaphragm is violated. There were five instances of visual loss, four permanent and one transient. This unfortunate complication is more than offset by the results of transsphenoidal microsurgery in patients with visual impairment due to pituitary tumors; in these cases vision improved in 81% of our patients.

TABLE 3. *Major postoperative complications with transsphenoidal surgery: Mayo Clinic 1972–1978*[a]

Complication	With pituitary adenomas	With all cases
Vascular occlusion		
Basilar thrombosis, late death		1
Left carotid artery occlusion, stroke	1	1
Left carotid artery, transient ischemic attack	1	1
Circle of Willis, fatal		1
Intracranial hematoma		
Fatal	2	2
Producing visual loss	2	2
CSF rhinorrhea		
Reoperated	2	7
Transient		1
Meningitis		
Fatal		2
Successfully treated		1

[a]Total 489 patients, 505 procedures.

TABLE 4. *Postoperative complications with transsphenoidal surgery: Mayo Clinic 1972–1978*[a]

Complication	In patients with pituitary adenomas	In all patients
Major complications		
Subarachnoid hemorrhage	2	2
Permanent visual loss	3	4
Subarachnoid hemorrhage		
Optic nerve infarct		
Surgical trauma		
Intracranial hematoma		
Transient visual loss	1	1
Hemorrhage from intercavernous sinus	1	1
Lesser complications		
Transient third nerve palsy	1	2
Transient sixth nerve palsy		1
Diabetes insipidus, "permanent"	5	9
Nasal septal perforation	4	6
Palatal diastasis		2
Late complications		
Death, malignant pituitary tumor	2	2
Death, basilar artery thrombosis		1
Visual loss, late subdural hematoma (11 months)	1	1
Transient third nerve palsy, during radiotherapy (3 months)	1	1

[a]Total 489 patients, 505 procedures.

The less-devastating complications, which left the patients with no significant persisting disability, are also listed in Table 4. Late complications are cited in Table 4 as well.

The complications reported here are similar to those in other large series using transsphenoidal surgery. If this report is compared with the earlier analysis of our first 185 patients (11), it is evident that the mortality and complication rates decrease as our experience with this highly effective operative technique continues.

REFERENCES

1. Bergland, R. M., Ray, B. S., and Torack, R. M. (1968): Anatomical variations in the pituitary gland and adjacent structures in 225 human autopsy cases. *J. Neurosurg.*, 28:93–99.
2. Deborsu, F. L. (1959): Difficultés de la vöie transphènöidale de l'operation de l'adènom de l'hypophyse. *Neurochirurgia (Stuttg)*, 1:209–215.
3. Guiot, G. (1973): Transsphenoidal approach in surgical treatment of pituitary adenomas: General principles and indications in non-functioning adenomas. In: *Excerpta Medica International Congress Series No. 303*, pp. 159–178. Excerpta Medica, Amsterdam.
4. Guiot, G., and Cheibani, G. (1972): Risques et problémes de l'exérèse transsphenoidale des adènomes hypophysaires. *Nouv. Presse Med.*, 1:2117–2119.
5. Guiot, G., Derome, P., Demailly, P., and Hertzog, E. (1968): Complication inattendue de l'exérèse complete de volumineux adènomes hypophysaires. *Rev. Neurol. (Paris)*, 118:164–167.

6. Halstead, A. E. (1910): Remarks on the operative treatment of tumors of the hypophysis. *Surg. Gynecol. Obstet.*, 10:494–502.
7. Hardy, J. (1973): Transsphenoidal surgery of hypersecreting pituitary tumors. In: *Excerpta Medica International Congress Series No. 303*, pp. 179–193. Excerpta Medica, Amsterdam.
8. Henderson, W. R. (1939): Pituitary adenomata: A follow-up study of surgical results in 338 cases (Dr. Harvey Cushing's series). *Br. J. Surg.*, 26:811–921.
9. Hirsch, O. (1959): Life-long cures and improvements after transsphenoidal operation of pituitary tumors. *Acta Ophthalmol. [Suppl.] (Kbh)*, 56:1–60.
10. Jordan, R. M., and Kerber, C. W. (1978): Rupture of a parasellar aneurysm with a coexisting pituitary tumor. *South. Med. J.*, 71:741–742.
11. Laws, E. R., Jr., and Kern, E. B. (1976): Complications of transsphenoidal surgery. *Clin. Neurosurg.*, 23:401–416.
12. Lippman, H. H., Onofrio, B. M., and Baker, H. L. (1971): Intrasellar aneurysm and pituitary adenoma: Report of a case. *Mayo Clin. Proc.*, 46:532–535.
13. Newfield, P., Ablin, M. S., Chestnut, J. S., and Maroon, J. (1978): Air embolism during transsphenoidal pituitary operations. *Neurosurgery*, 2:39–42.
14. Schoen, D. (1970): Mukozele des keilbeines nach hypophysektomie. *Fortschr. Geb. Roentgenstr. Nuklearmed.*, 112:114–116.
15. Svien, H. J., Kennedy, W. C., and Kearns, T. P. (1963): Results of surgical treatment of pituitary adenoma: The factor of the excessively enlarged sella. *J. Neurosurg.*, 20:669–674.
16. White, J. C., and Ballantine, H. T., Jr. (1961): Intrasellar aneurysms simulating hypophyseal tumors. *J. Neurosurg.*, 18:34–50.

Subject Index

W